PAIN
SOURCEBOOK

Health Reference Series

AIDS Sourcebook
Allergies Sourcebook
Alternative Medicine Sourcebook
Alzheimer's, Stroke & 29 Other Neurological Disorders Sourcebook
Arthritis Sourcebook
Back & Neck Disorders Sourcebook
Blood & Circulatory Disorders Sourcebook
Burns Sourcebook
Cancer Sourcebook
Cancer Sourcebook for Women
Cardiovascular Diseases & Disorders Sourcebook
Communication Disorders Sourcebook
Congenital Disorders Sourcebook
Consumer Issues in Health Care Sourcebook
Contagious & Non-Contagious Infectious Diseases Sourcebook
Diabetes Sourcebook
Diet & Nutrition Sourcebook
Ear, Nose & Throat Disorders Sourcebook
Endocrine & Metabolic Diseases & Disorders Sourcebook
Environmentally Induced Disorders Sourcebook
Fitness & Exercise Sourcebook
Food & Animal Borne Diseases Sourcebook
Gastrointestinal Diseases & Disorders Sourcebook
Genetic Disorders Sourcebook
Head Trauma Sourcebook
Health Insurance Sourcebook
Immune System Disorders Sourcebook
Kidney & Urinary Tract Diseases & Disorders Sourcebook
Learning Disabilities Sourcebook
Men's Health Concerns Sourcebook
Mental Health Disorders Sourcebook
New Cancer Sourcebook
Ophthalmic Disorders Sourcebook
Oral Health Sourcebook
Pain Sourcebook
Pregnancy & Birth Sourcebook
Public Health Issues Sourcebook
Respiratory Diseases & Disorders Sourcebook
Sexually Transmitted Diseases Sourcebook
Skin Disorders Sourcebook
Sports Injuries Sourcebook
Substance Abuse Sourcebook
Women's Health Concerns Sourcebook

SOUTH COLLEGE
709 Mall Blvd.
Savannah, GA 31406

Blood & Circulatory Disorders Sourcebook

Basic Information about Disorders Such As Anemia, Hemorrhage, Shock, Embolism, and Thrombosis, along with Facts Concerning Rh Factor, Blood Banks, Blood Donation Programs, and Transfusions

Edited by Linda M. Ross. 600 pages. 1998. 0-7808-0203-9. $75.

Burns Sourcebook

Basic Information about Heat, Chemical, Electrical, and Sun Burns, along with Facts about Burn Treatment and Recovery, and Reports on Current Research Initiatives

Edited by Allan R. Cook. 600 pages. 1998. 0-7808-0204-7. $75.

Cancer Sourcebook

Basic Information on Cancer Types, Symptoms, Diagnostic Methods, and Treatments, Including Statistics on Cancer Occurrences Worldwide and the Risks Associated with Known Carcinogens and Activities

Edited by Frank E. Bair. 932 pages. 1990. 1-55888-888-8. $75.

"This publication's nontechnical nature and very comprehensive format make it useful for both the general public and undergraduate students."
— *Choice*, Oct '90

"This compact collection of reliable information, written in a positive, hopeful tone, is an invaluable tool for helping patients and patients' families and friends to take the first steps in coping with the many difficulties of cancer." — *Medical Reference Services Quarterly*, Winter '91

"An important resource for the general reader trying to understand the complexities of cancer."
— *American Reference Books Annual*, '91

Cancer Sourcebook for Women

Basic Information about Specific Forms of Cancer That Affect Women, Featuring Facts about Breast Cancer, Cervical Cancer, Ovarian Cancer, Cancer of the Uterus and Uterine Sarcoma, Cancer of the Vagina, and Cancer of the Vulva; Statistical and Demographic Data; Treatments, Self-Help Management Suggestions, and Current Research Initiatives

Edited by Allan R. Cook and Peter D. Dresser. 524 pages. 1996. 0-7808-0076-1. $75.

"This timely book is highly recommended for consumer health and patient education collections in all libraries." — *Library Journal*, Apr '96

REFERENCE

"The availability under one cover of all these pertinent publications, grouped under cohesive headings, makes this certainly a most useful sourcebook."
— *Choice*, Jun '96

"Laudably, the book portrays the feelings of the cancer victim, as well as her mate . . . .both benefit from the gold mine of information nestled between the two covers of this book. It is hard to conceive of any library that would not want it as part of its collection. Recommended."
— *Academic Library Book Review*, Summer '96

". . . written in easily understandable, non-technical language. Recommended for public libraries or hospital and academic libraries that collect patient education or consumer health materials."
— *Medical Reference Services Quarterly*, Spring '97

New Cancer Sourcebook

Basic Information about Major Forms and Stages of Cancer, Featuring Facts about Primary and Secondary Tumors of the Respiratory, Nervous, Lymphatic, Circulatory, Skeletal, and Gastrointestinal Systems, and Specific Organs; Statistical and Demographic Data, Treatment Options, and Strategies for Coping

Edited by Allan R. Cook. 1,313 pages. 1996. 0-7808-0041-9. $75.

"This book is an excellent resource. The dialogue is simple, direct, and comprehensive."
— *Doody's Health Sciences Book Review*, Nov '96

"The amount of factual and useful information is extensive. The writing is very clear, geared to general readers. Recommended for all levels."
— *Choice*, Jan '97

Cardiovascular Diseases & Disorders Sourcebook

Basic Information about Cardiovascular Diseases and Disorders, Featuring Facts about the Cardiovascular System, Demographic and Statistical Data, Descriptions of Pharmacological and Surgical Interventions, Lifestyle Modifications, and a Special Section Focusing on Heart Disorders in Children

Edited by Karen Bellenir and Peter D. Dresser. 683 pages. 1995. 0-7808-0032-X. $75.

". . . comprehensive format provides an extensive overview on this subject." — *Choice*, Jun '96

"Easily understood, complete, up-to-date resource. This well executed public health tool will make valuable information available to those that need it most, patients and their families. The typeface, sturdy non-reflective paper, and library binding add a feel of quality found wanting in other publications. Highly recommended for academic and general libraries."
— *Academic Library Book Review*, Summer '96

Continues next page

Communication Disorders Sourcebook

Basic Information about Deafness and Hearing Loss, Speech and Language Disorders, Voice Disorders, Balance and Vestibular Disorders, and Disorders of Smell, Taste, and Touch

Edited by Linda M. Ross. 533 pages. 1996. 0-7808-0077-X. $75.

"This is skillfully edited and is a welcome resource for the layperson. It should be found in every public and medical library."
— Doody's Health Sciences Book Review, May '96

Congenital Disorders Sourcebook

Basic Information about Disorders Acquired during Gestation, Including Spina Bifida, Hydrocephalus, Cerebral Palsy, Heart Defects, Craniofacial Abnormalities, Fetal Alcohol Syndrome, and More, along with Current Treatment Options and Statistical Data

Edited by Karen Bellenir. 607 pages. 1997. 0-7808-0205-5. $75.

Consumer Issues in Health Care Sourcebook

Basic Information about Consumer Health Concerns, Including an Explanation of Physician Specialties, How to Choose a Doctor, How to Prepare for a Hospital Visit, Ways to Avoid Fraudulent "Miracle" Cures, How to Use Medications Safely, What to Look for when Choosing a Nursing Home, and End-of-Life Planning

Edited by Wendy Wilcox. 600 pages. 1998. 0-7808-0221-7. $75.

Contagious & Non-Contagious Infectious Diseases Sourcebook

Basic Information about Contagious Diseases like Measles, Polio, Hepatitis B, and Infectious Mononucleosis, and Non-Contagious Infectious Diseases like Tetanus and Toxic Shock Syndrome, and Diseases Occurring as Secondary Infections Such As Shingles and Reye Syndrome, along with Vaccination, Prevention, and Treatment Information, and a Section Describing Emerging Infectious Disease Threats

Edited by Karen Bellenir and Peter D. Dresser. 566 pages. 1996. 0-7808-0075-3. $75.

Diabetes Sourcebook

Basic Information about Insulin-Dependent and Noninsulin-Dependent Diabetes Mellitus, Gestational Diabetes, and Diabetic Complications, Symptoms, Treatment, and Research Results, Including Statistics on Prevalence, Morbidity, and Mortality, along with Source Listings for Further Help and Information

Edited by Karen Bellenir and Peter D. Dresser. 827 pages. 1994. 1-55888-751-2. $75.

"Very informative and understandable for the layperson without being simplistic. It provides a comprehensive overview for laypersons who want a general understanding of the disease or who want to focus on various aspects of the disease."
— Bulletin of the MLA, Jan '96

Diet & Nutrition Sourcebook

Basic Information about Nutrition, Including the Dietary Guidelines for Americans, the Food Guide Pyramid, and Their Applications in Daily Diet, Nutritional Advice for Specific Age Groups, Current Nutritional Issues and Controversies, the New Food Label and How to Use It to Promote Healthy Eating, and Recent Developments in Nutritional Research

Edited by Dan R. Harris. 662 pages. 1996. 0-7808-0084-2. $75.

"It is so refreshing to find a reliable and factual reference book. Recommended to aspiring professionals, librarians, and others seeking and giving reliable dietary advice. An excellent compilation."
— Choice, Feb '97

"Recommended for public and medical libraries that receive general information requests on nutrition. It is readable and will appeal to those interested in learning more about healthy dietary practices."
— Medical Reference Services Quarterly, Fall '97

Ear, Nose & Throat Disorders Sourcebook

Basic Information about Disorders of the Ears, Nose, Sinus Cavities, Tonsils, Adenoids, Pharynx, and Larynx, along with Statistical and Demographic Data and Reports on Current Research Initiatives

Edited by Linda M. Ross. 600 pages. 1998. 0-7808-0206-3. $75.

Endocrine & Metabolic Diseases & Disorders Sourcebook

Basic Information for the Layperson about Disorders Such As Graves' Disease, Goiter, Cushing's Syndrome, and Hormonal Imbalances, along with Reports on Current Research Initiatives

Edited by Linda M. Ross. 600 pages. 1998. 0-7808-0207-1. $75.

Continues on back end sheets

Health Reference Series

Volume Thirty-two

PAIN SOURCEBOOK

Basic Information about Specific Forms of Acute and Chronic Pain Including Headaches, Back Pain, Muscular Pain, Neuralgia, Surgical Pain, and Cancer Pain Along with Pain Relief Options such as Analgesics, Narcotics, Nerve Blocks, Transcutaneous Nerve Stimulation, and Alternative Forms of Pain Control Including Biofeedback, Imaging, Behavior Modification, and Relaxation Techniques.

Edited by
Allan R. Cook

Omnigraphics, Inc.
Penobscot Building / Detroit, MI 48226

BIBLIOGRAPHIC NOTE

This volume contains individual documents and excerpts from periodic publications issued by the following government agencies: Agency for Health Care Policy and Research (AHCPR); National Institute of Arthritis and Musculoskeletal and Skin Diseases (NIAMS); National Institutes of Health (NIH); Food and Drug Administration (FDA); U.S. Department of Health and Human Services (DHHS); and National Center for Research Resorces (NCRR).

This volume also includes copyrighted materials reprinted with permission from the following sources: American Chiropractic Association; Department of Orthotics and Prosthetics, Duke University; American Chronic Pain Association; American Council for Headache Education; HDI Publishers; St. Joseph Mercy—Oakland, *SmartHealth*; *Journal of Obstetric, Gynecologic, & Neonatal Nursing*, Lippincott-Raven; Susan Lang; Mayo Foundation for Medical Education and Research; Medical Economics, *Patient Care*; Medtronic, Inc.; National Headache Foundation; New York Times; Scientific American; and the Trigeminal Neuralgia Association.

All copyrighted material is reprinted with permission. Document numbers where applicable and specific source citations are provided on the first page of each chapter. Every effort has been made to secure all necessary rights to reprint the copyrighted material. If any omissions have been made, please contact Omnigraphics to make corrections for future editions.

Edited by Allan R. Cook

Peter D. Dresser, Managing Editor, Health Reference Series
Karen Bellenir, Series Editor, Health Reference Series

Omnigraphics, Inc.

Matthew P. Barbour, Production Manager
Laurie Lanzen Harris, Vice President, Editorial
Peter E. Ruffner, Vice President, Administration
James A. Sellgren, Vice President, Operations and Finance
Jane J. Steele, Marketing Consultant

Frederick G. Ruffner, Jr., Publisher

Copyright 1998, Omnigraphics, Inc.

Library of Congress Cataloging-in-Publication Data

Pain sourcebook ; basic information about specific forms of acute and chronic pain including headaches, back pain, muscular pain, neuralgia, surgical pain and cancer pain along with pain relief options such as analgesics, narcotics, nerve blocks, transcutaneous nerve stimulation, and alternative forms of pain control including biofeedback, imaging, behavior modification, and relaxation techniques / edited by Allan R. Cook.
    p. cm. — (Health reference series ; 32)
  Includes bibliographical references and index.
  ISBN 0-7808-0213-6 (lib. bdg. : alk. paper)
  1. Pain. I. Cook, Allan R. II. Series.
RB127.P346 1997   97-37833
616'.0472—dc21   CIP

This book is printed on acid-free paper meeting the ANSI Z39.48 Standard. The infinity symbol that appears above indicates that the paper in this book meets that standard.

Printed in the United States of America

Table of Contents

Preface ix

Part I: Understanding Pain

Chapter 1—Getting to Know Pain 3
Chapter 2—Suffer No More: Why Pain Is Bad for You
 and How to Get Relief... 19
Chapter 3—Chronic Pain: Hope through Research 31
Chapter 4—Assessment and Measurement of Acute
 Pain 55
Chapter 5—Probing the Underpinnings of Pain 69

Part II: Headaches

Chapter 6—The Ache and the Head 75
Chapter 7—Headache Misery May Yield to Proper
 Treatment.. 79
Chapter 8—Tension-Type Headache 89
Chapter 9—The Migraine Aura 93
Chapter 10—Headache: Myth, Misunderstanding, and
 Mistreatment... 95
Chapter 11—The Eye and Headache 97
Chapter 12—Results of a National Poll of Migraine
 Sufferers 101

Chapter 13—Sleep: Searching a New Frontier for
  Answers 111
Chapter 14—What Can Be Done About Headache? 115
Chapter 15—How to Find a Headache Doctor 131

Part III: Backaches

Chapter 16—Back Talk: Advice for Suffering Spines 135
Chapter 17—The New Thinking on Low-back Pain 149
Chapter 18—Understanding Acute Low-back Problems 173
Chapter 19—Chiropractic Manipulation and Federal
  Guidelines on Low Back Pain Treatment 183
Chapter 20—Neck Pain and Disorders of the Cervical
  Spine 187

Part IV: Some Other Common Forms of Nerve and Muscle Pain

Chapter 21—Trigeminal Neuralgia (Tic Douloureaux) 193
Chapter 22—Bell's Palsy: A Painful, Disfiguring Ailment 205
Chapter 23—Fibromyalgia 209
Chapter 24—Thoracic Outlet Syndrome 213
Chapter 25—Carpal Tunnel Syndrome and Other
  Repetitive Strain Injuries (RSIs) 217
Chapter 26—Making a Stand Against Leg Cramps 227
Chapter 27—Spinal Stenosis: A Subtle Source of Leg Pain 235
Chapter 28—Knee Pain: Strong Enough to Stop the Pain 239
Chapter 29—Heel Pain: It's Usually a Symptom of Plantar
  Fasciitis 241
Chapter 30—No Strain, No Pain: The Bottom Line in
  Treating Hemorrhoids 245
Chapter 31—Painful Menstruation and Menstrual
  Cramps 251

Part V: Surgical Pain

Chapter 32—Acute Pain Management: Operative or
  Medical Procedures and Trauma 263
Chapter 33—Pains Following an Amputation 383
Chapter 34—Anesthesia: Safer and More Choices 385

Chapter 35—Calming Fears, Easing Pain: Children's
       Anesthesia Is Tricky 389

Part VI: Cancer Pain

Chapter 36—Cancer Pain: What Is It? How Do I Talk
       About It? 397
Chapter 37—Relieving Cancer Pain with Medicines 407
Chapter 38—Relieving Cancer Pain without Medicines 425

Part VII: Managing Pain

Chapter 39—Multidisciplinary Teams: The Integrated
       Approach to the Management of Pain 447
Chapter 40—Guidelines to Help Select a Pain Unit 461
Chapter 41—The Challenge of Relieving Pain 465
Chapter 42—Pain, Pain Go Away: An FDA Guide to
       Nonprescription Pain Relievers (OTC) 477
Chapter 43—Taking Nonsteroidal Anti-Inflammatory
       Drugs (NSAIDs) 483
Chapter 44—Aspirin: Potent Pain Relief, but Misuse Can
       Be Dangerous 487
Chapter 45—A Burning Question: When Do You Need
       an Antacid? 499
Chapter 46—Taking Beta Blocker Drugs 507
Chapter 47—Patches, Pumps, and Timed Release: New
       Ways to Deliver Drugs 511
Chapter 48—Treating Chronic Pain with Implantable
       Therapies 517
Chapter 49—Integration of Behavioral and Relaxation
       Techniques for the Treatment of Chronic
       Pain and Insomnia 527
Chapter 50—What Can Be Done When the Pain Won't
       Go Away? 543
Chapter 51—Living With Chronic Pain: A How-to-
       Manage Manual for Families of Chronic
       Pain Patients 549
Chapter 52—Aggressive Pain Management as an
       Alternative to Euthanasia for the Terminally
       Ill Patient 605

Part VII: Pain Resources

Chapter 53—Finding Help 617

Index **631**

Preface

About this Book

Pain is the brain's way of telling the body that something is wrong. It serves as a stimulus to protect against serious harm. Some pain, however, continues long after its message has been received. Pain that never leaves completely or returns periodically can be debilitating. Such chronic pain needs to be managed effectively and constantly because, by definition, it cannot be cured.

Every year, approximately half of all Americans seek some form of relief from persisting pain. In fact, pain is the most common complaint doctors receive. Despite its frequency, an estimated 50 to 100 million Americans remain under-treated for their pain, and half of the more than 23 million who undergo surgery each year do not receive adequate pain control. Under-treatment can also be problematic in children because some doctors believe that children's undeveloped nervous systems make them immune to most pain.

This book contains basic information for the layperson on the nature and mechanism of pain, and gives attention to common complaints associated with pain. It also considers advances in the treatment methods used to combat the affliction and in the attitudes of the medical profession toward the need to treat pain as a real illness.

How to Use this Book

This book is divided into parts and chapters. Parts focus on broad areas of interest and chapters on specific topics within those areas.

Part I: Understanding Pain describes pain. It identifies different types of pain, offers information about pain assessment, and describes some trends in current research as well as changes in the ways the medical establishment approaches the treatment of pain.

Part II: Headaches looks specifically at pains in the region of the head and differentiates between some important types of headaches and their appropriate treatments.

Part III: Backaches focuses on the spinal region, one of the most common sites of pain, and considers a variety of strategies for coping with these frequent complaints.

Part IV: Some Other Common Forms of Nerve and Muscle Pain broadens the examination of pain to include other common problems such as neuralgia, fibromyalgia, repetitive strain injuries, muscle cramps, and menstrual pain, along with information about their causes and treatments.

Part V: Surgical Pain looks into the operating room to reveal how surgeons and anesthesiologists assist their patients to cope with the physical and mental trauma of invasive procedures.

Part VI: Cancer Pain focuses entirely on cancer pain and offers strategies for dealing with this common source of chronic pain.

Part VII: Managing Pain explores a wide variety of treatment options currently being used to provide patients with relief from pain. Information about the choices that remain when that pain relief efforts fail is also included.

Part VIII: Pain Resources brings together a listing of organizations and materials that can offer more help.

Acknowledgements

Many people and organizations have contributed the material in this volume. The editor gratefully acknowledges the assistance and cooperation of the American Council for Headache Education; American Chiropractic Association; Department of Orthotics and Prosthetics, Duke University; American Chronic Pain Association; American Council for Headache Education; IIDI Publishers; St. Joseph Mercy—

Oakland *SmartHealth*; *Journal of Obstetric, Gynecologic, & Neonatal Nursing*, Lippincott-Raven; Susan Lang; Mayo Foundation for Medical Education and Research; Medical Economics, *Patient Care*; Medtronic, Inc.; National Headache Foundation; New York Times; Scientific American; and the Trigeminal Neuralgia Association.

Special thanks to Margaret Mary Missar for her patient search for the documents that make up this volume, Karen Bellenir for her technical assistance and advice, Bruce the Scanman and special assistant Mike for their optical translations, David Cook for his text-cleaning assistance and Valerie Cook for her sharp-eyed verification.

Note from the Editor

This book is part of Omnigraphics' Health Reference Series. The series provides basic information about a broad range of medical concerns. It is not intended to serve as a tool for diagnosing illness, in prescribing treatments, or as a substitute for the physician/patient relationship. All persons concerned about medical symptoms or the possibility of disease are encouraged to seek professional care from an appropriate health care provider.

Part One

Understanding Pain

Chapter 1

Getting to Know Pain

Attitude, Medication and Therapy Are Keys to Control

Pain is universal. You can trace its trail through time—from a toothache evident in fossil remains of a human jawbone to today's drugstore shelves packed with pain relievers. Almost half of all Americans seek treatment for pain each year, 7 million from newly diagnosed back pain alone.

Pain is complex. Sometimes it's beneficial. A sharp stab alerts you to injury when you burn your finger, hurt your back or break a bone. But other pain—the day-after-day ache of arthritis or the anguish of cancer—serves no useful purpose, and its relentlessness can become overwhelming.

Above all, pain is unique. The varieties of misery are as many as its sufferers. Your pain is an interplay of your own particular biological, psychological and cultural makeup.

New insight into these components is changing the concept of pain management. Pain is no longer seen as just a companion of disease or injury. It can become a damaging process in its own right that requires early and aggressive treatment.

In addition, effective management increasingly focuses on your attitude as well as medication and other therapies. You must understand the reasons for your pain and how to control it.

©1996. Reprinted from a June 1996 supplement to *Mayo Clinic Health Letter* with permission of the Mayo Foundation for Medical Education and Research, Rochester, Minnesota 55905. For subscription information, please call 1-800-333-9038. Reprinted with Permission.

By working closely with your doctor and health-care team, you can learn to manage your pain and enjoy a more fulfilling family, work and leisure life.

Exercise, relaxation techniques, and physical, occupational and psychological therapies play important treatment and prevention roles. And new drug delivery systems can keep some types of pain under continuous control. But despite these advances, some painful conditions are still inadequately treated.

Physical Sensation

Most pain originates when special nerve endings, called nociceptors (no-si-SEP-turs), detect an unpleasant stimulus. You have millions of nociceptors in your skin, bones, joints, muscles and internal organs. There may be as many as 1,300 in just one square inch of skin.

Some nociceptors sense sharp blows, others heat. One type senses pressure, temperature and chemical changes. Nociceptors can also detect inflammation due to injury, disease or infection. Nociceptors use nerve impulses to relay pain messages to networks of nearby nerve cells (your peripheral nervous system). Messages then travel along nerve pathways to your spinal cord and brain (your central nervous system). Each cell-to-cell relay is almost instantaneous, thanks to chemical facilitators called neurotransmitters. These chemicals flow from one nerve cell to the next in less than a thousandth of a second.

Some nerve pathways are faster than others. One type makes connections with many surrounding nerve cells en route. They transmit more slowly. You feel this type of pain as dull, aching and generalized. Another type relays impulses almost instantaneously and signals sharp pain focused in one spot.

Scientists believe that pain signals must reach a threshold before they're relayed. This "gate control" theory holds that specialized nerve cells in your spinal cord act as gates that open to allow pain messages to pass, depending on the strength and nature of the pain signal.

A Message-routing Section in Your Brain

Pain signals travel from your peripheral nerves to your spinal cord to your thalamus, a message sorting and switching station in your brain. The thalamus sends two types of messages. One goes to your cerebral cortex, the thinking part of your brain, which assesses the location and severity of damage. The second is a "stop-pain" message back to the injury site to tell local nociceptors to stop

Getting to Know Pain

sending any more pain messages. Once alerted, your brain doesn't need additional warning. But sometimes, this mechanism fails and pain persists.

Meanwhile, your cerebral cortex relays the pain message it received to your brain's limbic center. Your limbic center produces emotions, such as sadness or anger, in response to pain messages. Your limbic center can affect the way your cerebral cortex perceives pain messages, and can lessen or intensify your pain.

Your cerebral cortex also sends messages to your autonomic nervous system, which controls vital body functions such as breathing, blood flow and pulse rate.

Several types of neurotransmitters (proteins and hormones produced in your brain or nervous system) can increase or decrease pain signals. A hormone—one of the prostaglandins—speeds transmission of pain messages and makes nerve endings more sensitive to pain. And a protein called substance P continuously stimulates nerve endings at the injury site and within your spinal cord, increasing pain messages.

Serotonin and norepinephrine (nor-ep-i-NEF-rin) seem to decrease pain by causing nociceptors to release natural pain-relievers called endorphins (see "Stimulating your body's natural painkillers").

Stimulating Your Body's Natural Painkillers

As early as 6,000 years ago, Sumerian Healers used opium, a drug derived from the poppy plant, to relieve pain. Today, researchers know that your brain has special receptors for morphine-like substances.

Morphine, a potent narcotic painkiller used to treat acute pain and pain associated with terminal illness, is derived from opium.

Researchers also know that your brain and spinal cord make their own morphine-like pain relievers, called endorphins (en-DOR-fins) and enkephalins (en-KEF-uh-lins). When they attach to morphine receptors, these natural pain relievers help relay "stop-pain" messages back to the site of tissue damage.

You can stimulate the release of endorphins through aerobic exercise. Duration of exercise appears to be more important than intensity. Doing low-intensity aerobic exercises for 30 to 45 minutes at a time, five or six days a week, may produce an effect. Be sure to build up slowly. Even exercising three or four days a week may produce some effect.

You should have a complete medical evaluation before beginning any exercise program that is more vigorous than walking if:

- You are age 40 or older.
- You have been sedentary.
- You have risk factors for coronary artery disease.
- You have chronic health problems.

The Emotional Component

Pain is not simply a matter of passing messages up and down your spinal cord. When a pain signal reaches your brain, it passes through a filter of your personal experience. Your emotional and psychological state at the moment, memory of past pain experiences, outlook and stress level all affect how you interpret a pain message and your ability to tolerate it. Your upbringing and cultural attitude toward pain also play a role. And your age, level of information about your pain, and even lack of sleep may have an impact.

The emotional responses of shock, fear and anxiety can increase your perception of pain. For example, a minor pain sensation, such a dentist's probe, combined with anxiety can cause undue pain.

But your emotional state can also diminish major pain messages. One pain study compared survivors of a major battle in World War II with men in the general population of a major U.S. city, matched injury for injury. The combat veterans required less pain relief than those in the general population.

People who learn from upbringing and cultural background that the normal response to pain is great suffering and distress actually experience more pain than people who grow up in an environment where pain is often ignored. The common expressions "suffer in silence," "bite the bullet," "grin and bear it," and "no pain, no gain" point to American cultural patterns that discourage acknowledgment of pain.

Types and Characteristics of Pain

In general, doctors divide pain into two general categories—acute and chronic.

- **Acute**. Acute pain is temporary, related to the physical sensation of tissue damage. It can last from a few seconds to several months, but generally subsides as normal healing occurs. Examples include a burn, a fracture, an overused muscle, or pain after surgery. Cancer pain may be long-lasting but acute due to ongoing tissue damage.

- **Chronic**. Chronic pain lingers long beyond the time of normal healing. Some chronic pain is due to damage or injury to nerve fibers themselves (neuropathic pain). Although it may begin as acute pain, neuropathic pain often develops gradually and becomes chronic pain that's difficult to treat.

Chronic pain can result from diseases, such as shingles and diabetes, or from trauma, surgery or amputation (phantom pain). It can also occur without a known injury or disease. Like a gate that's blocked open, nerves continue to send pain messages even though there is no continuing tissue damage.

Chronic pain ranges from mild to disabling and can last from a few months to many years. Significant emotional and psychological components may develop. The essential ingredient is that the chronic pain changes your behavior. For example:

You experience the actual physical sensation of acute pain—the immediate, sharp stab in arthritic finger joints as you try to open a lid. Next is the emotional response—your anger and frustration with fumbling fingers. Eventually, behavior changes may occur. You may avoid using aching fingers and hands. Your hands become weak from inactivity, and you depend on others for assistance.

Chronic pain can result in lowered self-esteem, sadness, anger and depression. Over the long term, a sense of helplessness to control chronic pain can lead you to develop characteristic "pain behavior." Behavioral changes can become habitual—crutches that can undermine your ability to effectively manage your pain (see "Caution: Pain behavior can become addicting").

Caution: Pain Behavior Can Become Addicting

If you have chronic pain, you may fall into a "sick Role"

Endless rounds of tests, diagnostic procedures and doctor visits searching for a cause and cure may promote the feeling of being a victim of pain. Feelings of uselessness, helplessness and worthlessness can follow.

Initially, you may even enjoy some benefits from this sickness role—extra attention or relief from responsibilities. But eventually, you become mired in a cycle of inactivity, isolation and pain.

There's rarely a single cause or simple cure for chronic pain. How you cope is more important than the pain relief you get. Here are tips:

- **Stay active**. Focus on the things you can do. Try new hobbies and activities. If possible, get plenty of exercise. An activity that intially causes some pain doesn't necessarily cause damage or worsen chronic pain.

- **Focus on others**. By volunteering in your community, you pay more attention to other's problems and less to your own.

- **Accept your pain**. Don't deny or exaggerate how you feel, but be clear and honest about your current capabilities. And be practical about what you can accomplish.

- **Stay healthy**. Eat and sleep on a regular schedule. Reduce stimulants such as caffeine and nicotine. They may intensify some pain.

Evaluating Pain

Pain is subjective, but there are ways to measure it. Doctors may use questionnaires, have you fill out a pain-rating scale, or have you select words that best describe your pain (see "The language of pain").

When repeated attempts to find a cause fail, and treatments aren't effective, you may benefit from a team approach offered by a pain clinic. A thorough evaluation may involve specialists in anesthesiology, neurology, psychology and psychiatry, rheumatology, physiatry and physical therapy. The goal is to treat all facets of your pain.

Specialized tests can evaluate how your body senses nerve impulses and how the impulses travel through your nervous system. Imaging techniques, such as X-rays, computed tomography (CT), magnetic resonance imaging (MRI), bone scans and ultrasound, may help detect problems in bones, muscles, joints and soft tissue.

Treat Pain Early and Aggressively

For many years, standard practice called for treating moderate to severe acute pain with injections of narcotic medication "as needed." This method often resulted in delays and widely varying levels of pain relief. Your pain rose and fell based on the dose timing. For most people, pain relief was effective only part of the time. Even today, pain is often undertreated.

Inadequate pain control can occur for many reasons. The choice, dose and timing of medication are critical in obtaining effective relief. Also, patients and their doctors may be unduly concerned about the use of narcotics in treating acute pain. But addiction is rare when narcotics are used for short-term relief of acute pain. It may become a problem when narcotics are inappropriately used for chronic pain relief. Addiction is not an issue in treatment of pain from a terminal illness.

Adequate acute pain control following surgery is important because it can allow you to recover your strength faster and start walking earlier. This can help you avoid problems, such as pneumonia and blood clots, due to inactivity.

Inadequately treated acute pain can prolong recovery and make you more susceptible to chronic pain. Continued pain messages enhance subsequent pain responses. Peripheral pain receptors become more sensitive. And continued pain may cause long-lasting modifications in nerve cells along spinal cord pain pathways. These changes make established pain harder to suppress.

As pain persists, feelings of anxiety, stress, anger, helplessness and depression can worsen. Tension and pain may initiate a downward pain spiral that's difficult to break. Early, aggressive treatment, and working with your doctor to prepare a pain plan, can help prevent this (see "Make a pain plan").

Make a Pain Plan

Whether you have short-lived or long-standing pain, or whether you're facing a simple diagnostic procedure or complicated surgery, discuss a pain plan with your doctor.

Find out how much pain you might have, how long it might last, and how it will be treated. Ask about alternatives if initial treatment doesn't adequately relieve your pain.

Clear communication allows you and your health-care team to monitor and modify your pain plan to maximize control.

Pain-relieving Medications

Pain treatment often includes medications and nondrug therapies (see "Achieving pain relief without medication"). Over-the-counter pain-relieving (analgesic) drugs include:

- **NSAIDs**. Nonsteroidal anti-inflammatory drugs, or NSAIDs (enSAYDS), are used to treat acute pain from inflammation, such as from arthritis. They relieve pain by inhibiting production of pain-intensifying neurotransmitters activated by tissue damage. NSAIDs include aspirin (Anacin, Bayer, Bufferin), ibuprofen (Motrin, Advil, Nuprin), naproxen sodium (Aleve) and ketoprofen (Orudis KT). All can cause gastrointestinal bleeding. All are also available in prescription form.

- **Acetaminophen**. Acetaminophen (Tylenol) is used to treat pain and control fever, but has only a limited effect on inflammation. It doesn't cause gastrointestinal bleeding like NSAIDs. Prolonged, high-dose use will cause kidney and liver damage.

Drugs available only by prescription include:

- **Narcotics**. These drugs are the most effective medication for moderate to severe pain. They're used for cancer pain and acute pain when the cause is known and other medications are ineffective. Narcotics also have an important role in the treatment of pain associated with terminal illness. They're not approved for chronic pain.

Narcotics include drugs derived from opium (opiates), such as morphine and codeine, and synthetic narcotics (opioids), such as oxycodone, methadone and meperidine (Demerol).

Side effects can include drowsiness, nausea, constipation, mood changes, and with prolonged use, addiction.

- **Antidepressants**. These medications may offer some relief for people with chronic pain, whether or not they also have depression. Amitriptyline (Elavil), trazodone (Desyrel) and imipramine (Tofranil) may be used with other analgesics. These drugs aren't addicting. They're especially useful for neuropathic, head and cancer pain. Side effects can include drowsiness, constipation and mouth dryness.

- **Anticonvulsants**. Developed for epilepsy, these drugs, such as phenytoin (Dilantin) and carbamazepine (Tegretol), can also help control chronic nerve pain. Side effects include drowsiness and confusion.

Other drugs may be used for specific types of pain.

Corticosteroid medications may help relieve pain due to inflammation and swelling. Prolonged use can result in widespread problems, such as bone thinning, cataracts and increased blood pressure.

Tramadol (Ultram) is a synthetic analgesic used primarily for chronic pain, but is also prescribed for acute pain. Side effects may include dizziness, (drowsiness, nausea, constipation and sweating.

Sumatriptan (Imitrex), now available in tablet form, may reduce pain from migraine headache by constricting blood vessels in your brain. Because the drug may increase blood pressure and constrict arteries to your heart, it's not used for people with uncontrolled high blood pressure or heart disease.

Capsaicin (Zostrix), a topical cream made from an extract of red peppers, can help relieve skin sensitivity resulting from shingles. It's also used to treat pain from arthritis, cluster headaches, diabetic neuropathy and pain after mastectomy. You may have an initial burning sensation where the cream is applied. Benefits are temporary so you'll need repeated application. Capsaicin probably relieves pain by interrupting transmission of pain messages from nociceptors.

Achieving Pain Relief Without Medication

Drug-free methods of pain relief may work by "sensory overload." They send a barrage of nerve messages to your brain and crowd out the pain messages that would otherwise be transmitted.

They may also stimulate the production of endorphins, your body's natural painkillers.

Methods include:

- **Electrical stimulation**. Transcutaneous electrical nerve stimulation (TENS) delivers a tiny electrical current to key points on a nerve pathway.

  The current, delivered through electrodes taped to your skin, isn't painful. TENS is thought to work by stimulating the release of endorphins.

  Electrical stimulation can also be delivered to areas under your skin, in your spinal cord or in your brain.

- **Acupuncture**. Acupuncture reduces the perception of pain by using tiny needles painlessly inserted along nerve pathways. Acupuncture is thought to work by stimulating the release of endorphins.

- **Heat, cold, massage, whirlpool.** Vigorous rubbing and heat from a heating pad or whirlpool bath can overload your sensory nerves.

  Physical therapists can apply deep heat to painful areas with an electronic heating technique called diathermy.

- **Surgery.** Surgery is rarely recommended for long-term pain control, and does not always provide relief unless it cures the underlying problem.

Managing Pain

Short-lived acute pain generally responds to medication and goes away with healing (see "Handling acute pain,"). But persistent pain can lead to depression, inactivity, deconditioning and increased dependence on others.

Chronic pain can interfere with sleep and eating habits, exercise, social activity and work. Breaking this cycle usually requires a coordinated approach offered in a pain rehabilitation program. Physical, occupational and behavioral therapies, and assistance with the psychological components of chronic pain, are the cornerstones of successful treatment. Here are some strategies for coping with chronic pain:

- **Relaxation techniques.** Stress increases muscle tension and worsens pain. Relaxation techniques—such as meditation and yoga—involve activities in which you focus on something other than your pain. You can do many at home. Listening to music, visualizing a relaxing scene, trying a new hobby or visiting a friend may also help. These techniques can alter peripheral and central pain processes and are especially effective for chronic headache and muscle tension.

  Biofeedback may also help by teaching you to be aware of autonomic pain responses such as skin temperature, muscle tension, blood pressure and heart rate, and how to modify these.

  Ask your doctor about where to find help in learning relaxation and biofeedback techniques.

- **Occupational therapy.** This helps you return to ordinary tasks around your home and work. Focusing on home responsibilities, work or volunteer activities—perhaps for limited hours at first—is a first step in pain rehabilitation.

Getting to Know Pain

- **Physical therapy and exercise**. You may fear exercise will increase pain, but if you start gently and increase gradually, exercise usually doesn't cause injury or additional pain. A regular program should include stretching, strengthening activities and aerobic exercise, such as walking, swimming or cycling. Slow stretching can relax muscles and release tension. If you have chronic back pain, you may get enough relief from muscle-strengthening exercises alone, thereby avoiding surgery.

- **Family therapy**. Chronic pain can change personalities and unravel relationships. The person with pain feels guilt and family members become stressed taking over additional responsibilities and new roles. The key is to maintain your normal responsibilities and roles as much as possible.

A Part of Life

Pain may be universal—perhaps even unavoidable. But it doesn't have to control your life. The keys to successful pain control are early treatment, ongoing assessment, and clear communication between you and your doctor.

The Language of Pain

Finding the right words to describe your pain will help your doctor find the right diagnosis and treatment.

Begin with the basics and describe the location, intensity, frequency, and what makes the pain better or worse. Then convey the quality of your pain. Use words such as stinging, penetrating, dull, throbbing, achy, nagging or gnawing. These words may give your doctor a clearer understanding of your pain. Once pain passes, it's difficult to reconstruct your precise sensation in words. By keeping a pain diary, you can write a detailed description of your pain while you have it.

When Pain Signals an Emergency

Pain is your body's warning system. If you have sudden, severe pain of no known cause and you haven't had this pain before, see your physician. The following types of pain may signal medical emergencies and require urgent care:

- **Head pain**. An unusual, sudden or severe headache, sometimes together with changes in vision, speech or sensation, may signal a brain hemorrhage or stroke. Head pain accompanied by a fever, vomiting, confusion or drowsiness may indicate a sepious brain infection (meningitis).

- **Eye pain**. Any sudden, severe pain in your eye or eyes may indicate a possible vision-damaging problem.

- **Chest pain**. Seek emergency care for any sudden chest pain of unknown cause. Intense pain or heavy pressure in your chest lasting more than 15 minutes may signal a heart attack. Pain may radiate to your left shoulder, arm(s), back, teeth, jaw or neck. Heart attack symptoms may also resemble severe indigestion and be accompanied by nausea, vomiting, shortness of breath, sweating and restlessness.

  Sudden, sharp chest pain that worsens with a deep breath or cough may signal a blockage of the pulmonary artery (pulmonary embolism). A rupture in your aorta (aortic aneurysm), the main artery that carries blood from your heart, is a life-threatening emergency. This condition may produce severe chest pain, but pain may also be subtle.

- **Abdominal pain**. Any sudden, severe, unfamiliar stomach or abdominal pain lasting longer than 30 minutes requires immediate attention. Intense pain in your upper abdomen may indicate a perforated stomach ulcer or ruptured spleen. Sharp pain extending up under your right shoulder may signal gallstones.

  Appendicitis often produces a dull pain around your navel with tenderness on the lower right side of your abdomen.

- **Pelvic pain**. Pain with urination or a severe, intense pain that moves downward from your side toward your groin may point to a kidney stone. If you could be pregnant, abdominal pain and cramping, often accompanied by dizziness and vaginal bleeding, may indicate a ruptured ectopic pregnancy. Both conditions require immediate treatment.

- **Pain in your arms or legs**. Sudden and severe pain accompanied by paleness and coldness in an arm or leg may mean an artery has become blocked by a blood clot. When a blood clot

Getting to Know Pain

occurs in a deep vein, usually in your leg, you may have tenderness, pain, swelling and even a fever. Because the clot could break loose and lodge in a lung, seek immediate treatment.

Medication Delivery Systems

A Variety of Drug Delivery Systems Can Help Provide Effective Pain Relief

Medications can be delivered by a variety of techniques to provide pain control (analgesia):

- **Self-controlled analgesia**. You control administration of a predetermined dose of medication. Self-controlled analgesia is usually used postoperatively in the hospital. You push a button and a controlled amount of drug is automatically delivered through an intravenous (IV) tube. Benefits include eliminating delays in dispensing medication and decreasing anxiety about adequate relief.

- **Implantable epidural and spinal infusion**. Pioneered at Mayo Clinic in the 1970s for unrelenting cancer pain, these techniques use a catheter implanted into your spinal canal to give a steady infusion of pain medication. Implantable drug delivery systems, which can provide adequate control for most cancer pain, are used only when other measures are ineffective.

- **Skin patch**. The opioid medication fentanyl (Duragesic) is available as a skin (transdermal) patch. It's used primarily for people who can't take medication by mouth. Wearing the patch gradually increases blood levels of fentanyl over 12 to 18 hours. This method is used for relatively constant pain, such as cancer pain, rather than for rapid pain relief. The patch can reduce variability—the peaks and troughs—in pain relief that may occur with oral or injected medications. Side effects include nausea and skin irritation.

- **Pain-relief lollipop**. Fentanyl, sweetened with sucrose, is also used in hospital settings in a lollipop form. Drugs are readily absorbed by mucous membranes lining your mouth because these membranes contain many blood vessels.

The lollipop form, called oral transmucosal fentanyl citrate (OTFC), provides reliable analgesia within 20 to 40 minutes when used as a premedication before painful medical procedures. It's also used for pain relief in the emergency room, following surgery, and for episodes of severe cancer pain.

Adults who use it often require less potent anesthesia during surgery and less pain medication afterwards. In children, the OTFC lollipop decreases anxiety and provides analgesia within 30 minutes.

New research shows that buprenorphine (Buprenex), a potent synthetic morphine, can be delivered via a lozenge placed under your tongue. It's been successfully used in clinical trials for premedication and for postoperative and cancer pain. Buprenorphine is available as an injection, but is not yet approved for use in lozenge form.

Handling Acute Pain

Here are some techniques for handling acute pain:

- **Know what to expect.** Ask about pain you'll have after surgery and how to control it. Studies show people report less pain, need less medication and have shorter hospital stays when they understand how much discomfort to expect, how long it will last, and how to cope with it.

- **Take medications on schedule**. To keep pain under control continuously, take medications when pain first begins, and on a schedule. It's more difficult to control pain once it's taken hold. And take medication before any activity that might worsen pain.

- **Report pain that won't go away**. Tell your nurse or doctor about pain that's not relieved as expected. Pain can be a sign of other problems.

- **Learn relaxation techniques**. Relaxing muscles reduces pain. Techniques such as deep breathing and jaw relaxation are easy to learn and you can use them anywhere.

Getting to Know Pain

- **Change strategies**. Inadequately treated acute pain may slip toward chronic pain any time, but most often between three and six months after the onset of pain. The transition is often imperceptible and marked by frustration because a cause hasn't been found and treatment hasn't worked.

  Refocusing on your pain as chronic rather than acute helps put it in perspective.

Chapter 2

Suffer No More: Why Pain Is Bad for You and How to Get Relief

In the dark ages of pain management 20 years ago, the nurses waited for my repeated cries of suffering before giving me a painkiller after abdominal surgery. In 1980, when my father-in-law lay dying in agony with cancer, the medical staff said he couldn't have more morphine to quell his suffering "for fear of addiction," and our entire family cried with him as we sweated out the intervals between shots. And even as recently as 10 years ago, many chronic pain sufferers were told their condition was "all in their mind" and little could be done.

Today, pain experts agree that these approaches to pain are outdated, unhealthy, inhumane, and yet still all too common.

Tragically, some 50 to 100 million Americans suffer from pain when most could experience significant relief. Pain is the most common complaint to doctors and costs the country millions of dollars in medical bills and lost workdays. "Pain destroys relationships, is disabling, feeds depression, and makes the future impossible to contemplate for millions of citizens," says Norman J. Marcus, M.D., director of the New York Pain Treatment Program at Lenox Hill Hospital. Yet it is "one of the most serious, most treatable, and most under-treated conditions in American medicine," adds University of Florida College of Medicine neurologist Stephen Nadeau.

One reason millions suffer needlessly is that many doctors overlook pain as a side effect of illness when, in fact, "pain is as serious and as legitimate a medical condition as diabetes or heart disease,"

©1997 Susan S. Lang. This article first appeared in the November 1994 issue of *Good Housekeeping*. Reprinted with permission.

Table 2.1. Guide to Over-the-Counter (OTC) Pain Relievers

Pain Reliever	Acetaminophen	Aspirin	Ibuprofen	Naproxen
Brands	Tylenol, Panadol Pamprin, store brands	Anacin, Bayer, Bufferin, store brands	Advil, Motrin, Nuprin, store brands	Aleve
Uses	In adults, all are equivalent at helping to reduce fevers, relieve temporary headaches, and relieve minor aches and pains.			
		At full doses, taken regularly, these three anti-inflammatory drugs are equally effective for inflammatory conditions such as muscle sprains, joint aches, and pains, back pain, headaches, and the minor aches and pains of arthritis. Individuals, however, may find that they respond better, or have fewer side effects, with one than another.		
How long a dose lasts	4 hours	4 hours	6 to 8 hours	8 to 12 hours
Advantages / Benefits	Most gentle on the stomach	Tends to be cheapest. Regular low doses may reduce the risk of colon cancer, and high blood pressure in pregnant women.	Very similar medications. Best choice for alleviating menstrual cramps. Both very effective for migraine headaches and dental pain. At OTC doses, less irritating to the stomach than aspirin.	
Disadvantages / Precautions	Has very weak anti-inflammatory properties, so not so good for muscular or back pains.	Avoid giving to children for fevers; ringing in the ears is a symptom of taking too much.	Both fairly expensive. If stronger doses are needed, it may be cheaper to purchase prescription-strength pills than to take numerous OTC pills.	
		May cause upset stomach, mild heartburn, or stomach pain. Take with milk or food if such discomfort occurs. All anti-inflammatories carry the risk of gastrointestinal bleeding or ulceration and impaired kidney function, and should be used with caution by people with histories of ulcers of kidney problems.		
			If you are allergic or sensitive to asprin, you will be allergic or sensitive to these drugs.	
**Read the label carefully. Do not exceed recommended doses without a doctor's approval.**				

says Richard Patt, M.D., deputy chief of the pain and symptom section at the M.D. Anderson Cancer Center in Houston, Texas. Many doctors and patients also believe that enduring pain is a sign of strong character and erroneously fear that using painkillers for pain will cause addiction. While it is true that narcotics (opioids) such as morphine can cause a physical dependence, that can be dealt with by gradually reducing the doses to withdraw from the medication. Addiction, on the other hand, involves a psychological craving to use the drug for nonmedical purposes that overwhelms the addict's life.

"Although the situation is improving both here and abroad, pain is commonly under-recognized and mismanaged," says Dr. Patt. A virtual revolution has occurred in the past 20 years in how specialists view and treat pain, but all too many patients and doctors still hold outdated notions about "toughing pain out."

Surgical Pain

In the "old" days, post-surgical patients had to ask for a shot each time they needed relief. Now many physicians know that patients will be far more comfortable and need less medication if the pain is *prevented* from peaking with scheduled doses of medication given around the clock, regardless of the pain intensity. That's why many surgical patients wake up in the recovery room with an electronically controlled pump automatically delivering preset intravenous doses of an opioid such as morphine at regular intervals. Tom Schneider, 45, a psychotherapist in upstate New York, woke up from his shoulder surgery last year with the pump attached. Whenever the pain intensified, he simply pressed a button for an extra dose without having to ask.

"We let patients regulate their own doses within boundaries," explains Judith Paice, R.N., Ph.D., a clinical nurse specialist in pain management at Rush-Presbyterian-St. Luke's Medical Center in Chicago. Schneider could push for an extra dose only after a preset interval. If he had needed numerous "escape" doses to relieve the pain, the medical staff would have re-evaluated Schneider and likely increased the pump's preset doses, understanding that each patient's response to pain is different.

Gone too are the days when doctors and nurses determined whether a patient's complaints of pain were justified. "We always use the patient's self-report of pain," says Paice. Many doctors now ask patients to rank their pain on a scale from zero (no pain) to 10 (excruciating) and accept the patient's assessment as valid.

Yet, despite all the advances in pain control, about half the surgical cases in this country are still needlessly under-medicated. That's why, in 1992, the government issued guidelines for surgical pain (see "For More Information" later in this chapter and the chapter "Acute Pain Management" later in this volume).

Cancer Pain

Surgical patients are not the only ones under-treated; cancer patients too often do not get adequate pain relief. By the time Mary Stevenson was diagnosed with lung cancer late last year, the pain in her hip and shoulder was excruciating. She could barely walk, couldn't hold or feed her new baby or play with her two-year-old daughter. "Before I went to the pain clinic, my days were hell," recalls Stevenson, of Pittsburgh. "I just lay in bed and wanted to die." Doctors at the Pain Management Center at the Fox Chase Cancer Center in Philadelphia had her try several forms of morphine. Today, she uses a skin patch that releases a morphine-like drug (fentanyl) through the skin; she can walk, lift the baby, and sit on the floor and play with her daughter.

Yet far too many cancer patients—some 40 to 60 percent—still needlessly suffer, despite a powerful arsenal of modern medications and alternative therapies, says Charles S. Cleeland, Ph.D., who heads the University of Wisconsin, Madison Pain Research Group. The reasons:

- Many doctors inadequately assess pain and are intimidated by state and federal regulations that discourage large or frequent doses of opioids;

- patients hesitate to report their pain; and

- both patients and medical staff fear the side effects of these strong medications when, with proper use, they can be minimized or managed.

Although recent federal guidelines for cancer pain management (see "For More Information" and the chapter on Managing Cancer Pain) may go a long way in enlightening physicians that unrelieved cancer pain is tragic and totally unnecessary, cancer pain specialists stress that patients and their families play an important role, too. "Consumers need to be active participants in the prevention of cancer pain," says Michael Levy, M.D., Ph.D., director of the Pain Management Center at Fox Chase Cancer Center. "Patients need to know that cancer pain can be controlled, but they must also help by knowing how to accurately assess their pain and report it to their nurses and physicians."

Far too many cancer patients are reluctant to complain or use the valuable time with their doctors to discuss pain. Others deny their pain has intensified for fear it would mean the disease has progressed. "Complaining about pain is not a sign of weakness, and patients who are reluctant to discuss it are doing themselves an enormous disservice," says Dr. Patt.

Chronic Pain

Chronic pain remains an even greater challenge because the pain may persist for months or years after recovery with no end in sight. Also, many of the 50 million chronic pain sufferers in this country become increasingly inactive, which can make their situation even worse. Chronic pain costs the nation anywhere from $100 million to $50 billion a year in medical costs, lost income, lost productivity, and compensation costs.

"Although we've been making a lot of headway in convincing practitioners that cancer pain should be adequately treated, it's been much more difficult to convince folks that chronic pain should be adequately treated too," says Carol Warfield, M.D., director of the Pain Management Center at Beth Israel Hospital in Boston. "Many people still feel there's a lot of malingering going on."

Guadalupe Delacruz, a 36-year old mother of five, was paralyzed from the waist down in an accident 23 years ago. Eleven years ago, she started having such intense pain in her partially paralyzed shoulder that she had to stuff a washcloth in her mouth to muffle her cries whenever the pain escalated. "It was so intense, stabbing deep into my rib cage, that I couldn't help but scream," says the Chicago housewife. During that time, she was unable to care for her five children.

Her doctor had her try 10 nerve blocks, a half-dozen medications, TENS (a painless electrical stimulation of nerves that can provide dramatic relief for some), chiropractic, and physical therapy before she consulted the pain management team at Rush-Presbyterian-St. Luke's Medical Center in Chicago five years ago. After some trial and error, the team finally brought her pain down to a tolerable level with low doses of morphine taken on schedule every three hours. Delacruz can now function normally; she can wash and dress her little ones, cook, and drive the kids to school. She is physically dependent on the morphine, which is a normal response, but her doctors are confident that this will not lead to an addiction.

Although the use of daily morphine is becoming more common for some chronic pain conditions, most patients don't need it and can obtain significant relief, when all else fails, from a comprehensive chronic pain program that addresses the complex nature of pain. These programs often focus on rehabilitation by building strength and endurance and increasing mobility; psychotherapy to enhance coping skills; medication regimens (often including an anti-depressant not only to treat depression but to relieve nerve pain and improve sleep); exercises; stress management such as relaxation training, hypnosis, and biofeedback; and physical and occupational therapy to relearn how to perform daily activities without causing further pain.

"Chronic pain is incurable by definition, so we need to manage it like we manage diabetes or epilepsy—as a problem that we need to live with but one that remains in the background," says Jennifer Kriegler, M.D., director of the Pain Center at Mt. Sinai Medical Center in Cleveland.

Many chronic pain patients need to get out of bed, strengthen muscles that have atrophied, and return to work or remain active and productive despite the pain. "Physical therapy plays a vital role in helping those in chronic pain, by improving motor skills, range of motion, strength, mobility, posture, body movements, and endurance," says Marilyn Moffat, P.T., Ph.D., president of the American Physical Therapy Association. "Physical therapists also teach patients the proper ways to sit, stand, lift, carry, and perform other activities of daily living."

Molly Nadel (not her real name), 45, for example, suffered intense and chronic pain in her neck and upper back months after a car rammed into the rear of her car in 1989. "I was completely flat on my back for months. I could hardly sit, couldn't even lift a carton of milk, and my husband had to cut my food," says Nadel. Although Nadel eventually went back to work as a business manager in a large office in Cleveland, she was always in pain. Out of desperation, she enrolled in Dr. Kriegler's program.

"It really saved my life. I became a productive person again." Nadel learned how to drink out of a cup with a straw instead of bending her head back and how to work at her computer without straining herself. She also took ibuprofen, which helped with the musculoskeletal pain, and fluoxetine (Prozac), an anti-depressant, which reduced the nerve pain.

Suffer No More: Why Pain Is Bad for You and How to Get Relief

"Patients cannot take for granted that they will receive state-of-the-art pain relief, because changes in medicine can be slow," says Dr. Patt. "Doctors and patients need to disregard old-fashioned notions about toughing out pain and understand that pain can undermine our body's best defenses against illness and disease, not to mention the suffering and toll on the quality of life that pain exacts."

So, don't hurt. Relieve the pain. It's good for your health.

Common Misconceptions about Chronic Pain

A lot of head and back pain is "all in your head"; in other words, it's often just a psychological problem.

False. Pain may be exacerbated by stress as are a number of other medical conditions, but the vast majority of pain cases are not caused by stress or other psychological conditions.

For many chronic pain conditions, nothing can be done and you just need to accept your disability.

False. Although chronic pain can't be "cured," more than one-third of the sufferers will experience significant relief with help and another third will admit their life was significantly improved from a comprehensive program. The remainder will learn how to cope better with their pain, although they may not be significantly helped.

No one with chronic pain should be put on opioid medications.

False. Although these drugs are not the first course of action, some patients require regularly scheduled doses of an opioid to control their pain. They are still able to drive, work, and function normally.

Bed rest and inactivity can help relieve chronic pain; you should try to be only as active as your pain allows.

False. Immobility results in a loss of muscle tone and strength that can cause more pain when you do try to move. A goal for chronic pain patients is to maintain the same activity level every day, regardless of pain or the lack of it. This avoids "good" and "bad" days and the urge to overdo it when pain is low. "Patients learn that: by restraining themselves on days when their pain is low, they experience fewer days of severe pain as well as far more productive days," says Jennifer Kriegler, M.D., director of the Pain Center at Mt. Sinai Medical Center in Cleveland.

Chronic pain is harmless.

False. Chronic pain can actually damage nerve cells in the spinal cord, causing hyper-sensitivity to the same stimuli. As a result, it is important to reduce pain as soon as possible so it does not become a permanent pain syndrome.

Common Myths about Pain

Pain is to be expected with surgery, cancer, and other illnesses. Although uncomfortable, pain, itself is harmless.

False. Pain stresses the body by sapping valuable energy that's critically needed at times of surgery and illness. Pain also interferes with the ability to eat and sleep. The resulting fatigue can reduce the availability of nutrients to your organs and thus impede recovery. Pain may also interfere with your pursuit of treatments and activities keep you in bed when it's best to be mobile, and release hormones that boost blood pressure and increase water retention. Unrelieved pain may also take a serious toll on your immune system. It's even been shown to promote tumor growth in animals.

Furthermore, people whose pain is well controlled after surgery heal faster, walk sooner, breathe better and more deeply, go home sooner (thereby reducing health costs), and get back to work earlier than those whose pain is not well controlled. They are also much less likely to develop complications such as pneumonia, lung collapse, and blood clots.

Doctors tend to over-prescribe narcotic (opioid) medications such as morphine, and I should avoid them as much as possible because they can be addictive.

False on both counts. In fact, doctors tend to under-prescribe pain relievers, and even when they do appropriately prescribe them, more than half of all patients do not take the medications correctly, thereby undermining even the best medical management. Furthermore, studies show that patients who take opioids for pain almost never become addicted. The risk of addition is only about 1 in 10,000 patients.

When it comes to painkillers, it's best to wait as long as possible before taking the medication.

False. Doctors have learned that much less medication will be needed if it is taken preventatively or as soon as pain starts. By taking the medication at regular intervals to prevent the pain from surging, you'll have fewer side effects and less discomfort.

Suffer No More: Why Pain Is Bad for You and How to Get Relief

If I use strong painkillers now, they will gradually lose their effectiveness, and then I won't have anything to take if the pain gets worse.

False. Although some people will need larger doses of strong painkillers (such as morphine) over time as their bodies grow tolerant of the medication or their pain increases, there is no upper limit of doses for opioids and their pain relieving effect does not wear out. However, patients may not be able to tolerate the side effects associated with very high doses.

New Trends in Pain Relief

1. Using "old medications" in new ways.

As fears of addiction wane, morphine and other opioids are being more commonly used for severe pain. But instead of injections, doctors are increasingly using oral medications, pumps that automatically give doses at predetermined intervals, medicated skin patches, and nasal sprays. By combining an opioid with a non-steroidal anti-inflammatory medication, much lower doses of opioids may be used, thereby reducing the risk of side effects.

In some cases, delivering morphine or similar opioids directly to the spine with pumps, catheters, or implants can provide dramatic relief. Epidural spinal injections of steroids can provide several months of relief for back pain.

2. Using non-pain relievers to treat pain.

Many medications not normally prescribed for pain have analgesic effects, including anti-depressants (which also improve sleep) and anti-convulsants. Calcium channel blockers that are used to treat irregular heartbeats can reduce nerve pain; anti-spasmodic medications can relieve muscle spasms; tranquilizers may reduce painful muscle tension and spasms; and high blood pressure medications may reduce chronic pain.

3. Taking pain medication at regular intervals, rather than "as needed."

Doctors have learned that around-the-clock (atc) dosing—continuously taking medications at set intervals—is far more effective than "as needed." It requires more medication to relieve a wave of pain that has begun than to prevent it from occurring in the first place. By providing medications around the clock, patients don't have to wait for medication, feel more in control, and receive fewer injections.

4. Letting patients control their own medication.

Doctors now know that letting patients regulate when and how much pain medication to take results in more pain relief and less medication use and abuse. With no objective measure of pain, more doctors and nurses are acknowledging that a person's pain level is what he or she says it is.

5. Treating pain before surgery.

By numbing the area of a surgical incision with an anesthetic (even when the patient is under general anesthesia) or injecting morphine, doctors may be able to reduce the amount of pain and pain medication needed *after* surgery.

6. Using other opioids instead of Demerol after surgery.

The use of Demerol is falling out of favor because it may be toxic and accumulate in the body. This side effect does not occur with non-steroidal anti-inflammatory drugs, which are used for mild to moderate post-operative pain, or other opioids, which are used for moderate to severe pain.

7. Increasing use of non-traditional methods such as relaxation, breathing and visualization exercises, biofeedback, hypnosis, and acupuncture.

These alternative methods are becoming increasingly accepted by both patients and doctors, and are becoming part of mainstream pain therapy. Biofeedback—the use of painless electrodes to monitor muscle tension, heart rate, brain activity, and other body functions—is particularly useful in learning how to master relaxation techniques.

For More Information

For the free booklet *Pain Control after Surgery: Patient's Guide*, call 800 358-9295.

For the free booklet *Management of Cancer Pain: Adult Patient's Guide;* call 800-4-CANCER.

Suffer No More: Why Pain Is Bad for You and How to Get Relief

To find an accredited pain treatment center nearby, you may write:

The Commission on Accreditation of Rehabilitation Facilities,
101 N. Wilmot Rd., Suite 500,
Tucson, AZ
85711

For more information, write:

National Chronic Pain Outreach Association
7979 Old Georgetown Rd., Suite 100,
Bethesda, MD
20814-4948

American Pain Society,
5700 Old Orchard Rd.,
Skokie, IL 60077

— by Susan S. Lang

Susan S. Lang is a senior science writer at Cornell University, is co-author (with Richard Patt, M.D.) of the cancer pain book *You Don't Have to Suffer* (Oxford University Press, 1994).

Chapter 3

Chronic Pain: Hope through Research

What was the worst pain you can remember? Was it the time you scratched the cornea of your eye? Was it a kidney stone? Childbirth? Rare is the person who has not experienced some beyond-belief episode of pain and misery. Mercifully, relief finally came. Your eye healed, the stone was passed, the baby born. In each of those cases, pain flared up in response to a known cause. With treatment, or with the body's healing powers alone, you got better and the pain went away. Doctors call that kind of pain, **acute pain**. It is a normal sensation triggered in the nervous system to alert you to possible injury and the need to take care of yourself.

Chronic pain is different. Chronic pain persists. Fiendishly, uselessly, pain signals keep firing in the nervous system for weeks, months, even years. There may have been an initial mishap—a sprained back, a serious infection—from which you've long since recovered. There may be an ongoing cause of pain— arthritis, cancer, ear infection. But some people suffer chronic pain in the absence of any past injury or evidence of body damage. Whatever the matter may be, chronic pain is real, unremitting, and demoralizing—the kind of pain New England poet Emily Dickinson had in mind when she wrote:

> *Pain—has an Element of Blank—*
> *It cannot recollect*
> *When it begun—or if there were*
> *A time when it was not.*

NIH Publication No. 90-2406. November 1989.

The Terrible Triad

Pain of such proportions overwhelms all other symptoms and becomes the problem. People so afflicted often cannot work. Their appetite falls off. Physical activity of any kind is exhausting and may aggravate the pain. Soon the person becomes the victim of a vicious circle in which total preoccupation with pain leads to irritability and depression. The sufferer can't sleep at night and the next day's weariness compounds the problem—leading to more irritability, depression, and pain. Specialists call that unhappy state the "terrible triad" of suffering, sleeplessness, and sadness, a calamity that is as hard on the family as it is on the victim. The urge to do something—anything—to stop the pain makes some patients drug dependent, drives others to undergo repeated operations or worse, resort to questionable practitioners who promise quick and permanent "cures."

"Chronic pain is the most costly health problem in America," says one of the world's authorities on pain. He and others estimate annual costs, including direct medical expenses, lost income, lost productivity, compensation payments and legal charges, at close to $50 billion. Here's how that adds up:

- **Headache**. At least 40 million Americans suffer chronic recurrent headaches and spend $4 billion a year on medications. Migraine sufferers alone account for 65 million workdays lost annually.

- **Low back pain**. Fifteen percent of the adult U.S. population has had persistent low back pain at some time in their lives. Five million Americans are partially disabled by back problems, and another two million are so severely disabled they cannot work. Low back pain accounts for 93 million workdays lost every year and costs over $5 billion in health care.

- **Cancer pain**. The majority of patients in intermediate or advanced stages of cancer suffer moderate to severe pain. More than 800,000 new cases of cancer are diagnosed each year in the U.S., and some 430,000 people die.

- **Arthritis pain**. The great crippler affects 20 million Americans and costs over $4 billion in lost income, productivity and health care.

Other pain disorders like the neuralgias and neuropathies that affect nerves throughout the body, pain due to damage to the central nervous system (the brain and spinal cord), as well as pain where no physical cause can be found—psychogenic pain—swell the total to that $50 billion figure.

Many chronic pain conditions affect older adults. Arthritis, cancer, angina—the chest-binding, breath-catching spasms of pain associated with coronary artery disease—commonly take their greatest toll among the middle-aged and elderly. *Tic douloureux* (**trigeminal neuralgia**) is a recurrent, stabbing facial pain that is rare among young adults. But ask any resident of housing for retired persons if there are any tic sufferers around and you are sure to hear of cases. So the fact that Americans are living longer contributes to a widespread and growing concern about pain.

Neuroscientists share that concern. At a time when people are living longer and painful conditions abound the scientists who study the brain have made landmark discoveries that are leading to a better understanding of pain and more effective treatments.

In the forefront of pain research are scientists supported by the National Institute of Neurological Disorders and Stroke (NINDS), the leading Federal agency supporting research on pain. Other Federal agencies important in pain research include the National Institute of Mental Health (NIMH), the National Institute of Dental Research (NIDR) and the National Cancer Institute (NCI). Within the last decade both the International Association for the Study of Pain and the American Pain Society have been established and grown into flourishing professional organizations attracting young as well as established research investigators and practicing physicians.

Sounding the Pain Alarm

Part of the inspiration for the new groups has come from a deeper understanding of pain made possible by advances in research techniques. Not long ago neuroscientists debated whether pain was a separate sense at all, supplied with its own nerve cells and brain centers like the senses of hearing or taste or touch. Maybe you hurt, the scientists reasoned, because nerve endings sensitive to touch are pressed very hard. To some extent, that is true: Some nerve fibers in your skin will be stimulated by a painful pinch as well as a gentle touch. But neuroscientists now know that there are many small nerve cells with extremely fine nerve fibers that are excited exclusively by intense, potentially harmful stimulation. Scientists call the nerve cells **nociceptors**, from the word noxious, meaning physically harmful or destructive.

Some nociceptors sound off to several kinds of painful stimulation—a hammer blow that hits your thumb instead of a nail; a drop of acid; a flaming match. Other nociceptors are more selective. They are excited by a pinprick but ignore painful heat or chemical stimulation. It's as though nature had sprinkled your skin and your insides with a variety of pain-sensitive cells, not only to report what kind of damage you're experiencing, but to make sure the message gets through on at least one channel.

Broadcasting the News

That same dispersion of forces continues once pain messages reach the central nervous system. Suppose you touch a hot stove. Some incoming pain signals are immediately routed to nerve cells that signal muscles to contract, so you pull your hand back. That streamlined pathway is a reflex, one of many protective circuits wired into your nervous system at birth.

Meanwhile the message informing you that you've touched the stove travels along other pathways to higher centers in the brain. One path is an express route that reports the facts: where it hurts, how bad it is, and whether the pain is sharp or burning. Other pain pathways plod along more slowly, the nerve fibers branching to make connections with many nerve cells (neurons) *en route*. Scientists think that these more meandering pathways act as warning systems alerting you of impending damage and in other ways filling out the pain picture. All the pathways combined contribute to the emotional impact of pain—whether you feel frightened, anxious, angry, annoyed. Experts called those feelings the "suffering" component of pain.

Still other branches of the pain news network are alerting another major division of the nervous system, the **autonomic nervous system**. That division handles the body's vital functions like breathing, blood flow, pulse rate, digestion, elimination. Pain can sound a general alarm in that system, causing you to sweat or stop digesting your food, increasing your pulse rate and blood pressure, dilating the pupils of your eye, and signaling the release of hormones like epinephrine (adrenaline). Epinephrine aids and abets all those responses as well as triggering the release of sugar stored in the liver to provide an extra boost of energy in an emergency.

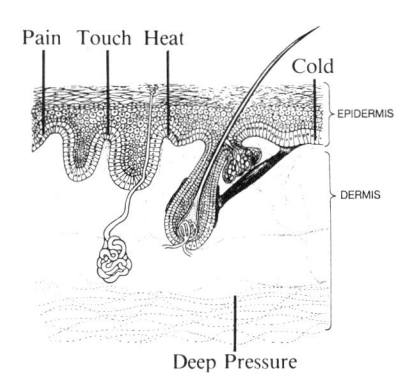

Figure 3.1 *Your skin is supplied with a variety of nerve endings sensitive to touch, pressure, heat, cold—and pain. The pain fibers are extremely fine in diameter, branching to form bare nerve endings.*

Censoring the News

Obviously not every source of pain creates a full-blown emergency with adrenaline-surging, sweat-pouring, pulse-racing responses. Moreover, observers are well aware of times and places when excruciating pain is ignored. Think of the quarterback's ability to finish a game oblivious of a torn ligament, or a fakir sitting on a bed of spikes. One of the foremost pioneers in pain research adds his personal tale, too, of the time he landed a salmon after a long and hearty struggle, only then to discover the deep blood-dripping gash on his leg.

Acknowledging such events, neuroscientists have long suspected that there are built-in nervous system mechanisms that can block pain messages.

Now it seems that just as there is more than one way to spread the news of pain, there is more than one way to censor the news. These control systems involve pathways that come down from the brain to prevent pain signals from getting through.

The Gate Theory of Pain

Interestingly, a pair of Canadian and English investigators speculated that such pain-suppressing pathways must exist when they devised a new "gate theory of pain" in the mid-sixties. Their idea was that when pain signals first reach the nervous system they excite

Pain Sourcebook

activity in a group of small neurons that form a kind of pain "pool." When the total activity of these neurons reaches a certain minimal level, a hypothetical "gate" opens up that allows the pain signals to be sent to higher brain centers. But nearby neurons in contact with the pain cells can suppress activity in the pain pool so that the gate stays closed. The gate-closing cells include large neurons that are stimulated by non-painful touching or pressing of your skin. The gate could also be closed from above, by brain cells activating a descending pathway to block pain.

The theory explained such everyday behavior as scratching a scab, or rubbing a sprained ankle: the scratching and rubbing excite just those nerve cells sensitive to touch and pressure that can suppress the pain pool cells. The scientists conjectured that brain-based pain control systems were activated when people behaved heroically—ignoring pain to finish a football game, or to help a more severely wounded soldier on the battlefield.

The gate theory aroused both interest and controversy when it was first announced. Most importantly, it stimulated research to find the conjectured pathways and mechanisms. Pain studies got an added boost when investigators made the surprising discovery that the brain itself produces chemicals that can control pain.

The landmark discovery of the pain-suppressing chemicals came about because scientists in Aberdeen, Scotland, and at the Johns Hopkins University Hospital in Baltimore were curious about how morphine and other opium-derived painkillers, or analgesics, work.

For some time neuroscientists had known that chemicals were important in conducting nerve signals (small bursts of electric current) from cell to cell. In order for the signal from one cell to reach the next in line, the first cell secretes a chemical "neurotransmitter" from the tip of a long fiber that extends from the cell body. The transmitter molecules cross the gap separating the two cells and attach to special receptor sites on the neighboring cell surface. Some neurotransmitters *excite* the second cell—allowing it to generate an electrical signal. Others *inhibit* the second cell—preventing it from generating a signal.

When investigators in Scotland and at Johns Hopkins injected morphine into experimental animals, they found that the morphine molecules fitted snugly into receptors on certain brain and spinal cord neurons. Why, the scientists wondered, should the human brain—the product of millions of years of evolution—come equipped with receptors for a man-made drug? Perhaps there were naturally occurring brain chemicals that behaved exactly like morphine.

The Brain's Own Opiates

Both groups of scientists found not just one pain-suppressing chemical in the brain, but a whole family of such proteins. The Aberdeen investigators called the smaller members of the family **enkephalins** (meaning "in the head"). In time, the larger proteins were isolated and called **endorphins**, meaning the "morphine within." The term endorphins is now often used to describe the group as a whole.

The discovery of the endorphins lent weight to the general concept of the gate theory. Endorphins released from brain nerve cells might inhibit spinal cord pain cells through pathways descending from the brain to the spinal cord. Endorphins might also be activated when you rub or scratch your itching skin or aching joints. Laboratory experiments subsequently confirmed that painful stimulation led to the release of endorphins from nerve cells. Some of these chemicals then turned up in cerebrospinal fluid, the liquid that circulates in the spinal cord and brain. Laced with endorphins, the fluid could bring a soothing balm to quiet nerve cells.

A New Look at Pain Treatments

Further evidence that endorphins figure importantly in pain control comes from a new look at some of the oldest and newest pain treatments. The new look frequently involves the use of a drug that prevents endorphins and morphine from working. Injections of this drug, naloxone, can result in a return of pain which had been relieved by morphine and certain other treatments. But, interestingly, some pain treatments are not affected by naloxone: Their success in controlling pain apparently does not depend on endorphins. Thus nature has provided us with more than one means of achieving pain relief.

- **Acupuncture**. Probably no therapy for pain has stirred more controversy in recent years than acupuncture, the 2,000-year-old Chinese technique of inserting fine needles under the skin at selected points in the body. The needles are agitated by the practitioner to produce pain relief which some individuals report lasts for hours, or even days. Does acupuncture really work? Opinion is divided. Many specialists agree that patients report benefit when the needles are placed near where it hurts, not at the body points indicated on traditional Chinese acupuncture charts. The case for acupuncture has been made by investigators who argue that local needling of the skin excites endorphin systems of pain control. Wiring the needles to stimulate nerve endings electrically (electro-acupuncture) also activates endorphin systems, they believe. Further, some experiments have shown that there are higher levels of endorphins in cerebrospinal fluid following acupuncture.

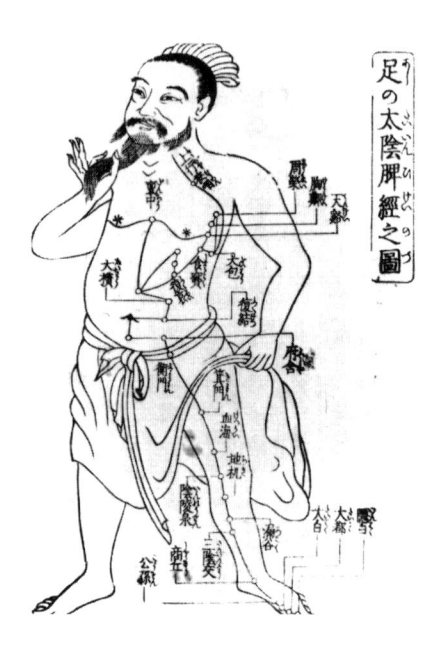

Figure 3.2. Acupuncture points are indicated in this Japanese version of the traditional Chinese teaching.

Those same investigators note that naloxone injections can block pain relief produced by acupuncture. Others have not been able to repeat those findings. Skeptics also cite long-term studies of chronic pain patients that showed no lasting benefit from acupuncture treatments. Current opinion is that more controlled trials are needed to define which pain conditions might be helped by acupuncture and which patients are most likely to benefit.

- **Local electrical stimulation**. Applying brief pulses of electricity to nerve endings under the skin, a procedure called transcutaneous electrical nerve stimulation (TENS), yields excellent pain relief in some chronic pain patients. The stimulation works

Chronic Pain: Hope through Research

best when applied to the skin near where the pain is felt and where other sensibilities like touch or pressure have not been damaged. Both the frequency and voltage of the electrical stimulation are important in obtaining pain relief.

- **Brain stimulation**. Another electrical method for controlling pain, especially the widespread and severe pain of advanced cancer, is through surgically implanted electrodes in the brain. The patient determines when and how much stimulation is needed by operating an external transmitter that beams electronic signals to a receiver under the skin that is connected to the electrodes. The brain sites where the electrodes are placed are areas known to be rich in opiate receptors and in endorphin-containing cells or fibers. Stimulation-produced analgesia (SPA) is a costly procedure that involves the risk of brain surgery. However, patients who have used this technique report that their pain "seems to melt away." The pain relief is also remarkably specific: The other senses remain intact, and there is no mental confusion or cloudiness as with opiate drugs. NINDS is currently supporting research on how SPA works and is also investigating problems of tolerance: Pain may return after repeated stimulation.

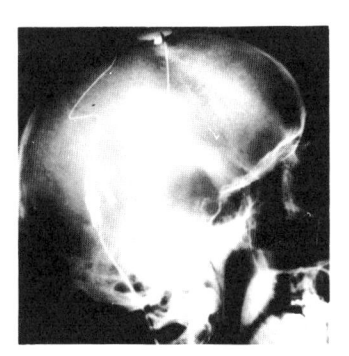

Figure 3.3. X-Ray showing implanted electrodes for stimulating the cells that produce pain relievers. The patient controls the stimulation by operating an external transmitter.

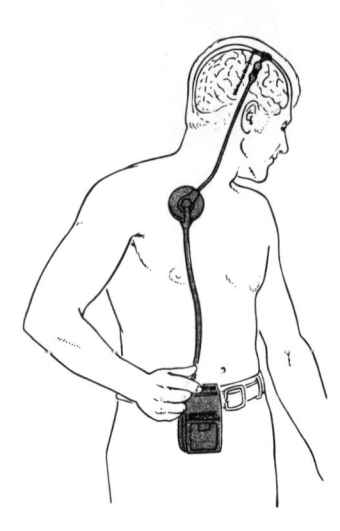

Figure 3.4. *Electrostimulator used by patient with chronic pain. The small electrical impulses stimulate the brain to produce naturally-occurring pain-relieving substances.*

- **Placebo effects**. For years doctors have known that a harmless sugar pill or an injection of salt water can make many a patient feel better—even after major surgery. The placebo effect, as it has been called, has been thought to be due to suggestion, distraction, the patient's optimism that something is being done, or the desire to please the doctor (*placebo* means "I will please" in Latin).

Now experiments suggest that the placebo effect may be neurochemical, and that people who respond to a placebo for pain relief—a remarkably consistent 35 percent in any experiment using placebos—are able to tap into their brains' endorphin systems. To evaluate it, two NINDS- and NIDR-supported investigators at the University of California at San Francisco designed an ingenious experiment. They asked adults scheduled for wisdom teeth removal to volunteer in a pain experiment. Following surgery, some patients were given morphine, some naloxone, and some a placebo. As expected, about a third of those given the placebo reported pain relief. The investigators then gave these people naloxone. All reported a return of pain.

How people who benefit from placebos gain access to pain control systems in the brain is not known. Scientists cannot even predict

Chronic Pain: Hope through Research

whether someone who responds to a placebo in one situation will respond in another. The San Francisco investigators suspect that stress may be a factor. Patients who are very anxious or under stress are more likely to react to a placebo for pain than those who are more calm, cool, and collected. But dental surgery itself may be sufficiently stressful to trigger the release of endorphins—with or without the effects of placebo. For that reason, many specialists believe further studies are indicated to analyze the placebo effect.

As research continues to reveal the role of endorphins in the brain, neuroscientists have been able to draw more detailed brain maps of the areas and pathways important in pain perception and control. They have even found new members of the endorphin family: Dynorphin, the newest endorphin, is reported to be 10 times more potent a painkiller than morphine.

At the same time, clinical investigators have tested chronic pain patients and found that they often have lower-than-normal levels of endorphins in their spinal fluid. If you could just boost their stores with manmade endorphins, perhaps the problems of chronic pain patients could be solved.

Not so easy. Some endorphins are quickly broken down after release from nerve cells. Other endorphins are longer lasting, but there are problems in manufacturing the compounds in quantity and getting them into the right places in the brain or spinal cord. In a few promising studies, clinical investigators have injected an endorphin called beta-endorphin under the membranes surrounding the spinal cord. Patients reported excellent pain relief lasting for many hours. Morphine compounds injected in the same area are similarly effective in producing long-lasting pain relief.

But spinal cord injections or other techniques designed to raise the level of endorphins circulating in the brain require surgery and hospitalization. And even if less drastic means of getting endorphins into the nervous system could be found, they are probably not the ideal answer to chronic pain. Endorphins are also involved in other nervous system activities such as controlling blood flow. Increasing the amount of endorphins might have undesirable effects on these other body activities. Endorphins also appear to share with morphine a potential for addiction or tolerance.

Meanwhile, chemists are synthesizing new analgesics and discovering painkilling virtues in drugs not normally prescribed for pain. Much of the drug research is aimed at developing non-narcotic painkillers. The motivation for the research is not only to avoid introducing potentially addictive drugs on the market, but is based on the observation that narcotic drugs are simply not effective in treating a variety of chronic pain conditions. Developments in nondrug treatments are also progressing, ranging from new surgical techniques to physical and psychological therapies like exercise, hypnosis, and biofeedback.

New and Old Drugs for Pain

When you complain of headache or low back pain and the doctor says take two aspirins every four hours and stay in bed, you may think your pain is being dismissed lightly... not at all. Aspirin, one of the most universally used medications is an excellent painkiller. Scientists still cannot explain all the ways aspirin works, but they do know that it interferes with pain signals where they usually originate, at the nociceptive nerve endings outside the brain and spinal cord: peripheral nerves. Aspirin also inhibits the production of chemicals manufactured in the blood to promote blood clotting and wound healing: prostaglandins. Unfortunately, prostaglandins, released from cells

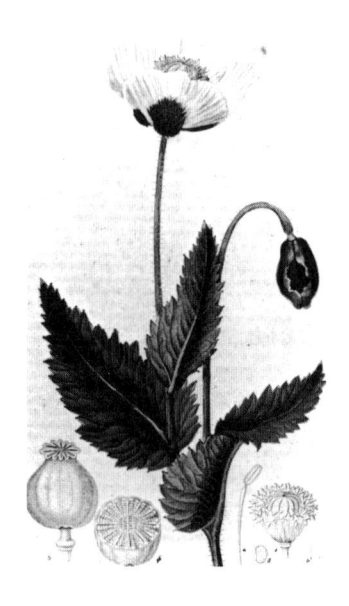

Figure 3.5. The natural source of opiates is the opium poppy. While opiate drugs are potent painkillers, they are ineffective in treating chronic pain disorders.

at the site of injury, are pain-*causing* substances. They actually sensitize nerve endings, making them—and you—feel more pain. Along with increasing the blood supply to the area, the chemicals contribute to inflammation—the pain, heat, redness and swelling of tissue damage.

Some investigators now think that the continued release of pain-causing substances in chronic pain conditions may lead to long-term nervous system changes in some patients that make them hypersensitive to pain. People suffering such *hyperalgesia* can cry out in pain at the gentlest touch, or even when a soft breeze blows over the affected area. In addition to the prostaglandins, blister fluid and certain insect and snake venoms also contain pain-causing substances. Presumably these chemicals alert you to the need for care—a fine reaction in an emergency, but not in chronic pain.

There are several prescription drugs that usually can provide stronger pain relief than aspirin. These include the opiate-related compounds codeine, propoxyphene (Darvon®), morphine, and meperidine (Demerol®). All these drugs have some potential for abuse, and may have unpleasant and even harmful side effects. In combination with other medications or alcohol, some can be dangerous. Used wisely, however, they are important recruits in the chemical fight against pain.

In the search for effective analgesics physicians have discovered pain-relieving benefits from drugs not normally prescribed for pain. Certain anti-depressants as well as anti-epileptic drugs are used to treat several particularly severe pain conditions, notably the pain of shingles and of facial neuralgias like *tic douloureux*.

Interestingly, pain patients who benefit from anti-depressants report pain relief before any uplift in mood. Pain specialists think that the anti-depressant works because it increases the supply of a naturally produced neurotransmitter, serotonin. (Doctors have long associated decreased amounts of serotonin with severe depression.) But now scientists have evidence that cells using serotonin are also an integral part of a pain-controlling pathway that starts with endorphin-rich nerve cells high up in the brain and ends with inhibition of pain-conducting nerve cells lower in the brain or spinal cord. Anti-depressant drugs have been used successfully in treating the excruciating pain that can follow an attack of shingles.

Anti-epileptic drugs have been used successfully in treating tic douloureux, the riveting attacks of facial pain that affect older adults. The rationale for the use of the anti-epileptic drugs (principally carbamazepine—Tegretol®) does not involve the endorphin system.

It is based on the theory that a healthy nervous system depends on a proper balance of incoming and outgoing nerve signals. Tic and other facial pains or neuralgias are thought to result from damage to facial nerves. That means that the normal flow of messages to and from the brain is disturbed. The nervous system may react by becoming hypersensitive: It may create its own powerful discharge of nerve signals, as though screaming to the outside world "Why aren't you contacting me?" Anti-epileptic drugs—used to quiet the excessive brain discharges associated with epileptic seizures—quiet the distress signals associated with tic and may relieve pain that way.

Psychological Methods

Psychological treatment for pain can range from psychoanalysis and other forms of psychotherapy to relaxation training, meditation, hypnosis, biofeedback, or behavior modification. The philosophy common to all these varied approaches is the belief that patients can do something on their own to control their pain. That something may mean changing attitudes, feelings, or behaviors associated with pain, or understanding how unconscious forces and past events have contributed to the present painful predicament.

- **Psychotherapy**. Freud was celebrated for demonstrating that for some individuals physical pain symbolizes real or imagined emotional hurts. He also noted that some individuals develop pain or paralysis as a form of self-punishment for what they consider to be past sins or bad behavior. Sometimes, too, pain may be a way of punishing others. This doesn't mean that the pain is any less real; it does mean that some pain patients may benefit from psychoanalysis or individual or group psychotherapy to gain insights into the meaning of their pain.

- **Relaxation and meditation therapies**. These forms of training enable people to relax tense muscles, reduce anxiety, and alter mental state. Both physical and mental tension can make any pain worse, and in conditions such as headache or back pain, tension may be at the root of the problem. Meditation, which aims at producing a state of relaxed but alert awareness, is sometimes combined with therapies that encourage people to think of pain as something remote and apart from them. The methods promote a sense of detachment so that the patient thinks of the pain as confined to a particular body part over which he or she has marvelous control. The approach may be particularly helpful when pain is associated with fear and dread, as in cancer.

- **Hypnosis**. No longer considered magic, hypnosis is a technique in which an individual's susceptibility to suggestion is heightened. Normal volunteers who prove to be excellent subjects for hypnosis often report a marked reduction or obliteration of experimentally induced pain, such as that produced by a mild electric shock. The hypnotic state does not lower the volunteer's heart rate, respiration, or other autonomic responses. These physical reactions show the expected increases normally associated with painful stimulation.

  The role of hypnosis in treating chronic pain patients is uncertain. Some studies have shown that 15 to 20 percent of hypnotizable patients with moderate to severe pain can achieve total relief with hypnosis. Other studies report that hypnosis reduces anxiety and depression. By lowering the burden of emotional suffering, pain may become more bearable.

- **Biofeedback**. Some individuals can learn voluntary control over certain body activities if they are provided with information about how the system is working—how fast their heart is beating, how tense are their head or neck muscles, how cold are their hands. The information is usually supplied through visual or auditory cues that code the body activity in some obvious way—a louder sound meaning an increase in muscle tension, for example. How people use this "biofeedback" to learn control is not understood, but some masters of the art report that imagery helps: They may think of a warm tropical beach, for example, when they want to raise the temperature of their hands. Biofeedback may be a logical approach in pain conditions that involve tense muscles, like tension headache or low back pain. But results are mixed.

- **Behavior modification**. This psychological technique (sometimes called operant conditioning) is aimed at changing habits, behaviors, and attitudes that can develop in chronic pain patients. Some patients become dependent, anxious, and homebound—if not bedridden. For some, too, chronic pain may be a welcome friend, relieving them of the boredom of a dull job or the burden of family responsibilities. These psychological rewards—sometimes combined with financial gains from compensation payments or insurance—work against improvements in the patient's condition, and can encourage increased drug dependency, repeated surgery, and multiple doctor and clinic visits.

There is no question that the patient feels pain. The hope of behavior modification is that pain relief can be obtained from a program aimed at changing the individual's lifestyle. The program begins with a complete assessment of the painful condition and a thorough explanation of how the program works. It is essential to enlist the full cooperation of both the patient and family members. The treatment is aimed at reducing pain medication and increasing mobility and independence through a graduated program of exercise, diet, and other activities. The patient is rewarded for positive efforts with praise and attention. Rewards are withheld when the patient retreats into negative attitudes or demanding and dependent behavior.

How effective are any of these psychological treatments? Are some superior to others? Who is most likely to benefit? Do the benefits last? The answers are not yet in hand. Patient selection and patient cooperation are all-important. Analysis of individuals who have improved dramatically with one or another of these approaches is helping to pinpoint what factors are likely to lead to successful treatment.

Surgery to Relieve Pain

Surgery is often considered the court of last resort for pain: When all else fails, cut the nerve endings. Surgery can bring about instant, almost magical release from pain. But surgery may also destroy other sensations as well, or, inadvertently, become the source of new pain. Further, relief is not necessarily permanent. After six months or a year, pain may return.

For all those reasons, the decision for surgery must always involve a careful weighing of the patient's condition and the outlook for the future. If surgery can mean the difference between a pain-racked existence ending in death, versus a pain-free time in which to compose one's life and see friends and family, then surgery is clearly a humane and compassionate choice.

There are a variety of operations to relieve pain. The most common is cordotomy: severing the nerve fibers on one or both sides of

Chronic Pain: Hope through Research

the spinal cord that travel the express routes to the brain. Cordotomy affects the sense of temperature as well as pain, since the fibers travel together in the express route.

Besides cordotomy, surgery within the brain or spinal cord to relieve pain includes severing connections at major junctions in pain pathways, such as at the places where pain fibers cross from one side of the cord to the other, or destroying parts of important relay stations in the brain like the thalamus, an egg-shaped cluster of nerve cells near the center of the brain.

In addition, surgeons sometimes can relieve pain by destroying nerve fibers or their parent cell bodies outside the brain or spinal cord. A case in point is the destruction of sympathetic nerves (a part of the autonomic nervous system) to relieve the severe pain that sometimes follows a penetrating wound from a sharp instrument or bullet.

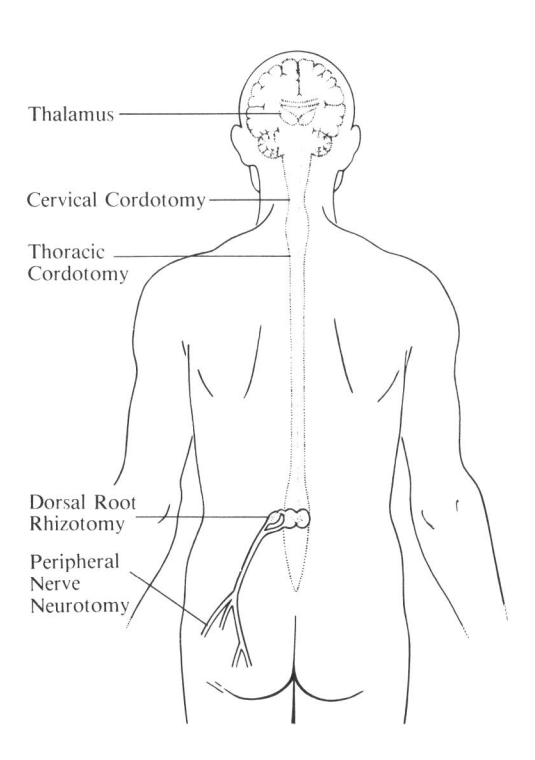

Figure 3.6 This diagram shows sites along the spinal cord where nerve fibers can be severed to relieve pain.

When pain affects the upper extremities, or is widespread, the surgeon has fewer options and surgery may not be as effective. Still, skilled neurosurgeons have achieved excellent results with upper spinal cord or brain surgery to treat severe intractable pain. These procedures may employ chemicals or use heat or freezing treatments to destroy tissue, as well as the more traditional use of the scalpel.

Recently, Harvard Medical School surgeons reported success with a new brain operation called cingulotomy to relieve intractable pain in patients with severe psychiatric problems. The nerve fibers destroyed are part of a pathway important in emotions and motivation. The surgery appears to eliminate the discomfort and suffering the patient feels, but does not interfere with other mental faculties such as thinking and memory.

Prior to operating, physicians can often test the effectiveness of surgery by using anesthetic drugs to block nerves temporarily. In some chronic pain conditions—like the pain from a penetrating wound—these temporary blocks can in themselves be beneficial, promoting repair of nerve damage.

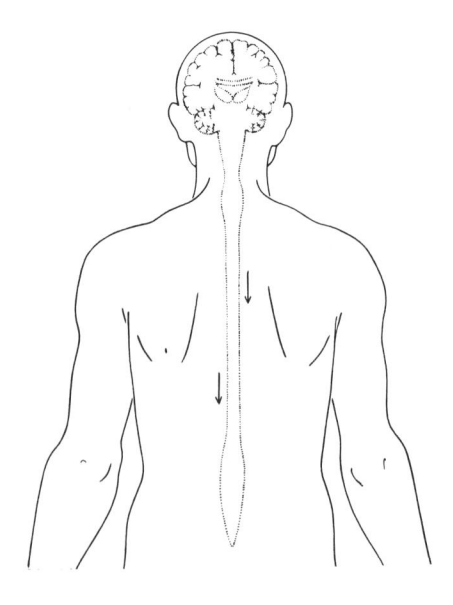

Figure 3.7 This diagram shows nerve fibers descending from the brain to the spinal cord where they can inhibit pain in various areas.

Chronic Pain: Hope through Research

How do these current treatments apply to the more common chronic pain conditions? What follows is a brief survey of major pain disorders and the treatments most in use today.

The Major Pains

- **Headache**. Tension headache, involving continued contractions of head and neck muscles, is one of the most common forms of headache. The other common variety is the vascular headache involving changes in the pressure of blood vessels serving the head. Migraine headaches are of the vascular type, associated with throbbing pain on one side of the head. Genetic factors play a role in determining who will be a victim of migraine, but many other factors are important as well. A major difficulty in treating migraine headache is that changes occur throughout the course of the headache. Blood vessels may first constrict and then dilate. Changing levels of neurotransmitters have also been noted. While a number of drugs can relieve migraine pain, their usefulness often depends on when they are taken. Some are only effective if taken at the onset.

  Drugs are also the most common treatment for tension headache, although attempts to use biofeedback to control muscle tension have had some success. Physical methods such as heat or cold applications often provide additional if only temporary relief.

- **Low back pain**. The combination of aspirin, bed rest, and modest amounts of a muscle relaxant are usually prescribed for the first-time low back pain patient. At the initial examination, the physician will also note if the patient is overweight or works at an occupation such as truck-driving or a desk job that offers little opportunity for exercise. Some authorities believe that low back pain is particularly prevalent in Western society because of the combination of overweight, bad posture (made worse if there is added weight up front), and infrequent exercise. Not surprisingly, then, when the patient begins to feel better, the suggestion is made to take off pounds and take on physical exercise. In some cases, a full neurological examination may be necessary, including an x-ray of the spinal cord called a myelogram, to see if there may be a ruptured disc or other source of pressure on the cord or nerve roots.

Sometimes x-rays will show a disc problem which can be helped by surgery. But neither the myelogram nor disc surgery is foolproof. Milder analgesics (aspirin or stronger non-narcotic medications) and electrical stimulation—using TENS or implanted brain electrodes—can be very effective. What is *not* effective is long-term use of the muscle-relaxant tranquilizers. Many specialists are convinced that chronic use of these drugs is detrimental to the back patient, adding to depression and increasing pain. Massage or manipulative therapy are used by some clinicians but other than individual patient reports their usefulness is still undocumented.

- **Cancer pain.** The pain of cancer can result from the pressure of a growing tumor or the infiltration of tumor cells into other organs. Or the pain can come about as the result of radiation or chemotherapy. These treatments can cause fluid accumulation and swelling (edema), irritate or destroy healthy tissue causing pain and inflammation, and possibly sensitize nerve endings. Ideally, the treatment for cancer pain is to remove the cancerous tissue. When that is not possible, pain can be treated by any or all of the currently available therapies: electrical stimulation, psychological methods, surgery, and strong painkillers.

- **Arthritis pain.** Arthritis is a general descriptive term meaning an affliction of the joints. The two most common forms are *osteoarthritis* that typically affects the fingers and may spread to important weight-bearing joints in the spine or hips, and *rheumatoid arthritis*, an inflammatory joint disease associated with swelling, congestion, and thickening of the soft tissue around joints. Recently, a distinguished panel of pain experts commenting on arthritis reported that "in all probability aspirin remains the most widely used ... and important drug ... although it may cause serious side effects." In the 1950's, the steroid drugs were introduced and hailed as lifesavers—important anti-inflammatory agents modeled after the body's own chemicals produced in the adrenal glands. But the long-term use of steroids has serious consequences, among them the lowering of resistance to infection, hemorrhaging, and facial puffiness—producing the so-called "moonface."

Besides aspirin, current treatments for arthritis include several nonsteroid anti-inflammatory drugs like indomethacin and ibuprofen. But these drugs, too, may have serious side effects.

Chronic Pain: Hope through Research

TENS and acupuncture have been tried with mixed results. In cases where tissue has been destroyed, surgery to replace a diseased joint with an artificial part has been very successful. The "total hip replacement" operation is an example.

Arthritis is best treated early, say the experts. A modest program of drugs combined with exercise can do much to restore full function and forestall long-term degenerative changes. Exercise in warm water is especially good since the water is both relaxing and provides buoyancy that makes exercises easier to perform. Physical treatments with warm or cold compresses are helpful sources of temporary pain relief.

- **Neurogenic pain**. The most difficult pains to treat are those that result from damage to the peripheral nerves or to the central nervous system itself. We have mentioned *tic douloureux* and shingles as examples of extraordinarily searing pain, along with several drugs that can help. In addition, tic sufferers can benefit from surgery to destroy the nerve cells that supply pain-sensation fibers to the face. "Thermocoagulation"—which uses heat supplied by an electrical current to destroy nerve cells—has the advantage that pain fibers are more sensitive to the treatment resulting in less destruction of other sensations (touch and temperature).

  Sometimes specialists treating tic find that certain blood vessels in the brain lie near the group of nerve cells supplying sensory fibers to the face, exerting pressure that causes pain. The surgical insertion of a small sponge between the blood vessels and the nerve cells can relieve the pressure and eliminate pain.

  Among other notoriously painful neurogenic disorders is pain from an amputated or paralyzed limb—so called "phantom" pain—that affects up to 10 percent of amputees and paraplegia patients. Various combinations of anti-depressants and weak narcotics like Darvon® are sometimes effective. Surgery, too, is occasionally successful. Many experts now think that the electrical stimulating techniques hold the greatest promise for relieving these pains.

- **Psychogenic pain**. Some cases of pain are not due to past disease or injury, nor is there any detectable sign of damage inside or outside the nervous system. Such pain may benefit from any of the psychological pain therapies listed earlier. It is also possible that some new methods used to diagnose pain may be useful. One method gaining in popularity is thermography, which measures the temperature of surface tissue as a reflection of blood flow. A color-coded "thermogram" of a person with a headache or other painful condition often shows an altered blood supply to the painful area, appearing as a darker or lighter shade than the surrounding areas or the corresponding part on the other side of the body. Thus an abnormal thermogram in a patient who complains of pain in the absence of any other evidence may provide a valuable clue that can lead to a diagnosis and treatment.

Where to Go for Help

People with chronic pain have usually seen a family doctor and several other specialists as well. Eventually they are referred to neurologists, orthopedists, or neurosurgeons. The patient/doctor relationship is extremely important in dealing with chronic pain. Both patients and family members should seek out knowledgeable specialists who neither dismiss nor indulge the patient; physicians who understand full well how pain has come to dominate the patient's life and the lives of everyone else in the family.

Many specialists today refer chronic pain patients to pain clinics for treatment. Over 800 such clinics have opened their doors in the United States since a world leader in pain therapy established a pain clinic at the University of Washington in Seattle in 1960.

Pain clinics differ in their approaches. Generally speaking, clinics employ a group of specialists who review each patient's medical history and conduct further tests when necessary. If the applicant is admitted, the clinic staff designs a personal treatment program that may include individual and group psychotherapy, exercise, diet, ice massage for pain (especially before bedtime), electrical stimulation techniques, and the use of a variety of analgesic but non-narcotic drugs. The aim is to reduce pain medication and so improve the patient's pain problem that when he or she leaves the hospital it is with the prospect of resuming more normal activities with a minimal requirement for analgesics and a positive self-image.

Contrary to what many people think, pain clinic patients are not malingerers or hypochondriacs. They are men and women of all ages, education, and social back ground, suffering a wide variety of painful conditions. Patients with low back pain are frequent, and so are people with the complications of diabetes, stroke, brain trauma, headache, arthritis, or any of the rarer pain conditions. The majority of patients participate for two or three weeks and usually report substantial improvement at discharge. One young man who had suffered painful chest injury as a result of a factory accident said he literally "felt taller" after his pain clinic experience. Followup at three- and six-month intervals, and at lengthier intervals thereafter, is an essential part of the program, both to evaluate the long-term effectiveness of treatment and to initiate a further course of treatment or counseling if necessary.

Pain clinics have the virtue that they bring together people with pain problems that have left them feeling isolated, helpless, and hopeless. But not everyone with a pain problem may need the support of a group or residence in a hospital. The important factors are that the pain patient—and the family—understand all the ramifications of pain, and the many and varied steps that can now be taken to undo what chronic pain has done. As a result of the strides neuroscience has made in tracking down pain in the brain—and in the mind—we can expect more and better treatments in the years to come. The days when patients were told "I'm sorry, but you'll have to learn to live with the pain" will be gone forever.

Voluntary Health Organizations

Several lay organizations are directly concerned with pain problems. They are excellent sources of additional information, research updates, and specific help and referrals:

American Chronic Pain Association, Inc.
257 Old Haymaker Road
Monroeville, PA 15146
(412) 856-9676

National Chronic Pain Outreach Association, Inc.
4922 Hampden Lane, Dept. "P"
Bethesda, MD 20814
(301) 652-4948

National Headache Foundation
5252 N. Western Avenue
Chicago, IL 60625
(312) 878-7715
(800) 843-2256 (toll-free)
(800) 523-8858 (toll-free in Illinois)

In addition, many organizations concerned with specific diseases, such as arthritis or heart disease, provide information and advice about attendant pain problems.

Pain Clinics

While there is no official certifying agency accrediting pain clinics throughout the country, there are many excellent clinics, often affiliated with university-associated medical centers. Your family doctor or university medical center may be able to refer you to reputable clinics nearby. If not, physicians can request a worldwide pain clinic directory published by:

American Society of Anesthesiologists
515 Busse Highway
Park Ridge, IL 60068

NINDS Information

For additional information concerning NINDS research on pain write:

Office of Scientific and Health Reports
National Institute of Neurological Disorders and Stroke
Building 31, Room 8A06
National Institutes of Health
9000 Rockville Pike
Bethesda, MD 20892
(301) 496-5751

Chapter 4

Assessment and Measurement of Acute Pain

Pain is a personal and individual experience. Pain assessment is a multi-dimensional process. A process is outlined that begins at admission and is systematically performed throughout the period of care. This process involves the patient in goal setting and selection of the instruments that will be used to assess the level of pain. Objective and subjective indicators of pain are described, but emphasis is on the patient's self-report as the major indicator of pain. Several instruments are described that help the patient and nurse to communicate more effectively. Using a variety of instruments allows the patient to select one that is most meaningful. Visual analog and verbal descriptor scales are described, as are how to use them in assessment of pain and evaluation of interventions. The emphasis is on assessment of the adult patient.

Pain is a physiologic process, modified by the human experience. Pain is unique to the individual and unique to each experience. No two persons experience pain in the same way, and no two pain experiences are the same for one individual. This automatically creates problems for assessment of the experience. Pain frequently serves the purpose of notifying the individual of actual or potential tissue damage. However, untreated pain is detrimental. Untreated or inadequately treated pain interferes with healing in adults, young children, and infants (Acute Pain Management Guideline Panel,

©1995 Lippincott-Raven. *Journal of Obstetric, Gynecologic and Neonatal Nursing*. Reprinted with permission.

1992). As nurses, and as sentient beings, we make the basic assumption that pain is not a desirable experience and that nurses play a major role in the recognition and treatment of pain. However, no other manifestation of illness or injury creates as much difficulty for health care professionals and their clients as does pain.

Pain is classified as acute, malignant, or chronic. Acute pain occurs in response to the sudden onset of injury, disease, surgery, or medical procedures. Acute pain has an identifiable source. Malignant pain occurs with progressive disorders, such as cancer. The source of malignant pain is organic. Chronic pain is pain of long duration without organic lesions or pain that persists after the precipitating damage has healed (Watt-Watson & Donovan, 1992). This chapter deals with the assessment of acute pain. Information about the assessment and management of malignant pain is presented in the Cancer Pain Management Guideline Panel (1994).

It has been documented that acute pain frequently goes unrecognized and is inadequately treated in children and adults (Altimier, Norwood, Dick, Holditch-Davis, & Lawless, 1994). Much of the failure to effectively treat pain may lie in mistaken beliefs about pain and its management that make it difficult to assess. Watt-Watson and Donovan (1992) identify many of the "misbeliefs" held by nurses and patients that are problematic for effective pain therapy. Two of these misbeliefs are especially pertinent to pain assessment: nurses believe that patients in pain will have behavioral or physiologic signs, and they believe that patients will tell a nurse they are in "pain." The nurse who holds these misbeliefs may inadequately assess and treat acute pain in a patient who reports that she aches but is lying quietly in bed and occasionally sleeping. Education to correct these misbeliefs is necessary as part of a thorough approach to the management of pain. This is important for each nurse, for each member of the health care team, and for the institution.

Current Standards of Care

Current pain assessment protocols often indicate that the patient should be asked about pain or level of comfort at the beginning of each shift. Nurses expect patients will request pain medication if it is needed at other times. Patients may or may not be asked how well the medication worked. This approach frequently leads to undertreatment (Watt-Watson & Donovan, 1992).

In 1990, the Agency for Health Care Policy and Research (AHCPR) established an interdisciplinary panel with representation from medicine, nursing, pharmacy, physical therapy, ethics, and consumers. This panel reviewed research, practices, technologies, and any existing guidelines for the management of acute pain in adults, infants and children. The *Clinical Practice Guideline* (Acute Pain Management Guideline Panel, 1992) forms the standard against which patient care may be judged in the United States. The underlying assumption of this standard is that, although it is not possible to eliminate all acute pain, it is expected that each patient will be appropriately assessed, and a variety of interventions will be applied to prevent or relieve pain.

In these guidelines, emphasis is placed on an interdisciplinary approach, with active involvement of the patient, and clear lines of responsibility for assuring that pain management becomes a major emphasis for all persons dealing with the individual. This belief is consistent with that of other authors in medicine (Melzack, 1983) and nursing (McCaffery & Beebe, 1989). The basis for effective pain management is accurate assessment, intervention and reassessment of the patient.

Definitions of Pain

The definition of pain we use will guide our assessment strategies. In 1979, the International Association for the Study of Pain (IASP) published a definition of pain that is used in research and to guide clinical practice. The IASP defined pain as "an unpleasant sensory and emotional experience associated with actual or potential tissue damage, or described in terms of such damage" (IASP, 1979, p. 250). This definition emphasizes the subjective nature of pain. The accompanying discussion indicates that this subjective experience of pain may occur in the absence of objectively detectable biologic stimuli. If we use this definition of pain, our assessments focus on and value most highly the subjective reports of the experience. We look for what patients say they are experiencing, with attention to identifying the source of the pain as a means of effective treatment.

Watt-Watson and Donovan carry the definition further by including factors that may influence how the individual perceives pain as a "complex perceptual and affective experience determined by the unique history of the individual, by the meaning of the stimulus to him, by his 'state of mind' at the moment, and by the sensory nerve patterns evoked by physical stimulation" (Watt-Watson & Donovan, 1992, p. 19). Using this definition will guide us to expand our assessment to look at the individual's past experiences with pain and its treatment to more completely understand the patient's perceptions. This broader definition indicates the multiple components of pain. With each of these definitions, assessment of pain relies on our valuing the patient's experience; our interaction with the patient is the key factor. In no instance are patients required to "prove" that they are experiencing pain. However, it often is difficult for the patient to effectively communicate the experience. For this reason, a comprehensive approach to the prevention and treatment of pain is needed.

Pain Measurement or Pain Assessment

There are similarities between assessment and measurement of pain, but the goals are distinct, so the process and instruments used may be different. Pain measurement is an attempt to quantify the individual experience of pain and to convert the experience into terms that can be compared for all individuals. Pain measurement looks at the commonalties of the pain experience: intensity, nature of sensation, and effects of pain. Pain measurement attempts to decrease the idiosyncratic components of pain. Pain measurement is needed in quantitative research to compare groups of individuals when testing the overall effectiveness of various nursing or medical interventions. Pain measurement denotes control, consistency, and normative values. Pain measurement is an important concept for identifying and testing new approaches to the prevention and treatment of pain. Without testing, each interaction with a patient would be a process of trial and error.

There are other terms and definitions used in pain research and measurement, including sensation, threshold, and tolerance. These terms are not useful in clinical practice, and our concerns are with the nature of the pain experience to the patient, including the questions: where is the pain, how intense is it, and how bothersome is it to the patient. Once interventions have been implemented, we are concerned with the extent to which the pain is reduced or the relief that the patient reports.

Pain assessment is a broader process than is measurement. For the nurse in clinical practice, pain assessment is the process of identifying the occurrence, location, intensity, and meaning of pain to *individual* patients. Although the same instrument may be used to obtain information about pain in the individual and in groups of people, the uses of the resulting information differ. For example, normative data about pain ratings for women in labor or women who have had certain types of gynecologic surgery are helpful in research but

Assessment and Measurement of Acute Pain

are inappropriate when dealing with a specific patient. Each occurrence is individual, and comparisons, if any, are from one time of assessment to the next within the individual patient. Pain assessment is part of the overall nursing process. It is a continuous process. No attempt is or should be made to evaluate one person's pain with another's or to compare this individual to a standard of intensity before intervening to relieve the pain.

Pain Assessment Process

Pain assessment is a process of interaction between the nurse and client to guide goal setting and interventions and to evaluate the effectiveness of the intervention in light of these mutually established goals. This process begins at the first contact between the patient and the health care team. Assessment of pain is the foundation for overall treatment and is based on the nursing process. As assessment is an ongoing process within the nursing process; pain assessment is an ongoing one.

A comprehensive approach to pain assessment involves determining the probable sources of pain, multiple factors that influence its occurrence, the nature of the pain (location, intensity, quality, effect), its meaning to the patient, and a history of how the patient has dealt with prior pain. This comprehensive approach begins in the earliest contacts between the patient and the nurse. If possible, assessment of pain should begin before the pain occurs.

If the patient is admitted for surgery, the assessment should begin as part of the preoperative teaching. A candid discussion of what may be expected in terms of pain and the measures to be taken to manage pain should begin at this time. The best time to discuss what is likely to occur, to discover expectations of pain and its treatment, and to begin to set goals for treatment is when the patient is not in pain. Because patients often are admitted directly to the preoperative area on the day of surgery, nurses with the opportunity to do this assessment are not the ones who will be using the information.

Thus, each institution should use a standard format that encourages communication among nurses. This format should include preferred terminology, assessment instrument to be used, desired level of pain control, and measures used in the past to decrease pain. These data should provide the heading for the pain assessment flow sheet and the basis for the ongoing assessment.

This process places pain management in the open and helps to dispel myths that patients and health professionals may hold. The first part of assessment is to identify the preferred terminology: what words does the patient use to describe pain. Exploring this terminology will not increase the pain the person experiences, but it will clarify the experience and help the nurse to ask the right questions. Asking the patient, "Are you having discomfort?" may be appropriate *if* one has first determined that "discomfort" is a word used by the patient to describe some level of pain. It may result in erroneous answers if the patient does not think of pain in the same terms.

In addition to determining the patient's preferred pain vocabulary, it is important to choose an assessment instrument. The assessment instrument allows the patient and the nurse to gauge the level of pain the patient is experiencing with consistency from one assessment to another. Several instruments should be available for the patient to make a choice that is easy to use and meaningful. This gives the patient and nurse an indicator of changes in pain and the need for modifications in management.

A good time to discuss the expectations of treatment and frequently used interventions is during the choosing of an instrument. It is important to discuss a variety of interventions and medications that may be used and combined. If this is not done, the patient who fears overmedication or believes that narcotics are to be avoided until the last resort may hesitate to report moderate levels of pain. This patient may be under-medicated. It also is important for the patient who fears medication will not be administered until the pain level is great and thus tends to report higher levels of pain.

These interactions between the patient, the physician, and the nurse are the basis of the plan for pain management: how does the patient communicate pain, what are the goals for pain management, and what interventions will be used to achieve these goals. For the plan to be effectively implemented, continuous assessment needs to be performed by the nurse. This assessment should be done frequently, which may be as often as every two hours during the first post-operative day. Later, routine assessments may be done less frequently. However, an assessment should be made with each report of increased or sudden pain and again after interventions. A patient who is assessed frequently the first day, will learn to recognize pain early and to request assistance appropriately. Assessment should be done when the patient is active. If assessment is done with the patient lying quietly in bed, the patient may be lying in the only comfortable position possible. An artificially low rating will be obtained at that moment, but the patient may resist activities that facilitate recovery and healing.

Assessment and Measurement of Acute Pain

Physiologic and Behavioral Indicators

Routine assessment calls for determining the presence of pain, its location and intensity, and the patient's response to therapy. The assessment phase of the nursing process calls for the use of objective and subjective data. The nurse can look for objective signs that may trigger additional assessment; however, these signs often are inaccurate representations of what the patient is experiencing or may be transient in nature. Objective data include physiologic responses, such as sweating, pallor, or elevated pulse, respirations, or blood pressure. However, these physiologic manifestations of pain may last for only a few minutes because the body seeks to adapt (Carrieri, Lindsey, West, 1986). Changes in vital signs may be an early sign that pain is present and should stimulate additional assessment; however, absence of changes should not support the conclusion that pain is not present.

The second form of objective data is patient behavior. These are the most commonly used indicators of the existence of pain. Behavior includes facial expressions, such as frowning, looking worried, grimacing, or clenched teeth. Behavioral cues also include soft sounds (such as moaning, gasping, or sighing) and the louder sounds of crying, grunting, and screaming. Additional behaviors that nurses assess relate to body movement. There may be rocking, rubbing the area involved (such as the child with otitis media), or rubbing another area in an attempt to distract oneself (such as the person with abdominal pain who rocks back and forth while rubbing the tops of her legs). Other behaviors noted are attempts to not move the affected part, to hold the abdomen, or to curl as tightly as possible into one position in the bed.

These are gross indicators of pain in some individuals. These behavioral manifestations of pain are influenced by cultural patterns and individual coping patterns. The patient using coping mechanisms such as sleeping, reading, or talking with visitors may show no outward signs of pain but would report the pain as moderate to severe. The presence of physiologic and behavioral signs may indicate that pain is present, the absence of such signs may not indicate that pain is absent. The presence of these signs calls for immediate assessment of the subjective aspects of pain: what is the patient experiencing. The patient's self-report is the most compelling indicator of pain. It is inappropriate to rely solely on vital signs and behaviors to assess pain (Beyer, McGrath, & Berde, 1990; Teske, Daut, & Cleeland, 1983) or to wait for these signs to perform additional assessment.

Self-Report of Pain

The subjective assessment of the amount of pain and the distress caused by the pain is the basis for intervention. Pain is a subjective experience and can be effectively assessed only from the patient's point of view. The patient's self-report of the occurrence and intensity of pain and the distress experienced is the most useful measure of pain; it forms the basis for the rest of the assessment and thus for the nursing process. To effectively use this self-report, the patient and nurse need to communicate effectively. A common terminology is important; do the words mean the same to nurse and patient. What words or descriptors does the person use when describing pain? When asked if she is having pain, she may say no and mean that she aches, but not use the word "pain" until the pain is so severe that she cannot cope with it, by which time pain management must play catch-up. Thus, it is important to discuss the words the patient usually uses to describe pain, as well as a brief hierarchy of how the words are used. With this basis, it is possible to discuss assessment instruments that can be used with this patient.

Assessment Instruments

The instruments chosen to assess pain should be appropriate for the individual's cognitive ability and acceptable to the patient. There are several basic types of instruments in several formats that can be used in the clinical setting. One of the more extensive is the McGill Pain Questionnaire. In the shortened, one-page version, there are

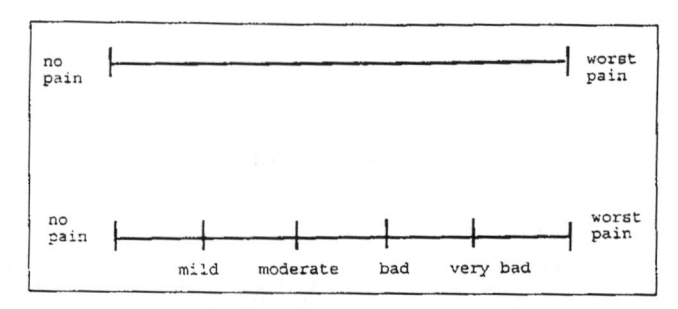

Figure 4.1. Sample pain assessment scale formats (Upper) Visual analog scale. (Lower) Combined visual analog and verbal descriptors. (Note that the lines are not shown full size here).

Assessment and Measurement of Acute Pain

three parts front and back body outline for indicating location of the pain; a pain intensity scale measured from 0 for "no pain" to 5 for "excruciating"; and the pain rating index (Melzack, 1983, 1987). The pain rating index consists of 78 words that describe the sensory, affective, and evaluative aspects of pain. The patient is to select the words that describe the pain being experienced. Numerical scores can be calculated from these selections. Even the shortened version takes 10 to 20 minutes to complete (Lowe, 1989). This instrument is useful in the research of acute pain (Wells, 1991) and in the assessment of chronic pain (Wilkie, Savedra, Holzemer, Tesler, & Paul, 1990) but takes too long to administer and is awkward to interpret when used in the routine assessment of acute pain.

Several assessment instruments should be available for the patient and nurse to determine the most meaningful and useful for each patient. There are two types of instruments commonly used with adults: visual analog scales (VAS) and verbal descriptor scales (VDS). The VAS is simple to use but requires that the patient be able to conceptualize pain in this manner. The VAS consists of a blank line anchored at each end of the line by adjectives that describe the extremes of pain. For ease of measurement, a 10-centimeter line usually is used. The VAS may be vertical or horizontal, according to the patient's preference. The anchoring adjectives commonly used are "no pain" and "worst possible pain." See Figure 4.1 for an example of a VAS. The anchors may be changed to agree with the terminology used by the patient.

If the patient uses "hurt," instead of "pain," this could be substituted. The patient is asked to place a mark on the line that best indicates the pain being experienced. Measuring from the "no pain" end of the line to the mark made by the patient gives a numeric rating of the intensity of the pain. Lee and Kieckhefer (1989) and Wewers and Lowe (1990) provide in-depth evaluations of the VAS as a measurement instrument.

To use the VAS, a clear and concise explanation of the scale and how to complete it must be given. Practice with the scale should be done at this point to identify and correct any problems with using the scale. If the patient has difficulty reading or understanding English, the VAS can be translated into the patient's language. Initial instructions in use of the scale must be given by someone fluent in the language. This is important because instructions will include a discussion of what will happen after the patient completes the scale. It also is important to evaluate the patient's physical ability to use the scale. Can the patient see the scale clearly, and does the patient have the fine motor ability to mark it? If not, another approach should be used.

Another approach to self-report of pain is the VDS. This often is easier for a patient to comprehend. The VDS involves a list of adjectives that describe increasing levels of pain, such as "no pain, mild, moderate, severe, very severe, worst possible" (Acute Pain Management Guideline Panel, 1992). The list may be presented in writing or read to the patient. The patient selects the adjective that best describes the pain. Numbers can be attached to the adjectives if a numeric score is desired or useful in documenting the patient's response. The possible responses to the list cited here would range from 0 to 6. The format for presenting these descriptors depends upon the patient's ability to read and to communicate verbally.

There are variations on these types of approaches. One such variation is to use the line and anchors from the VAS and to present the intermediate descriptors at equal intervals along the line. See Figure 4.1 for an example. This may create problems for the researcher because responses tend to clump around the descriptors (Wewers & Lowe, 1990), but it may help the patient to communicate the nature of pain with these intervening descriptors. Another variation is to use a numeric rating scale that asks the patient to rate the pain being experienced on a scale of 0 to 5 or 0 to 10, with 0 being no pain and the top number being the worst possible pain. These variations may be easier for patients with limited fine motor skills because the patient may point to a rating without having to write or speak. Patients should be given options when selecting the instrument to use. The VAS may be too abstract for some. Kremer, Atkinson, and Ignelzi (1981) found that more adults preferred the VDS to the VAS. Eleven percent of adults had difficulty completing the VAS, whereas all were able to use the VDS. A choice between two formats should be offered. This contributes to the individual's sense of control, participation in care planning, and management of pain.

Planning Interventions

Pain assessment scales help the patient and nurse to understand the patient's experience. They provide a basis for intervention. Knowing the site, the nature of the pain, and its intensity are part of the information needed to select appropriate interventions. The other necessary component is goal identification: what level of relief does the patient desire, and what interventions are acceptable to reach this level? For example, pain from an episiotomy may respond to a combination of therapies such as analgesics, sitz baths, and instruction in how to sit properly. The analgesic may deal with the pain centrally, but the other interventions may decrease the original stimulus and thus reduce the amount of analgesic needed or the length of time it is required. Interventions depend upon the cause, location, and intensity of pain.

Evaluation of Pain Management

This brings us to the final step in the assessment process. Evaluation of the effectiveness of pain management should be as routine as the initial assessment. The effectiveness or relief of pain is evaluated in relation to the original pain and the patient's goals for pain management. A simple way to evaluate effectiveness is to use the same pain scale. Remind the patient of the rating originally given to the pain and ask the patient to rate the pain currently being experienced. The difference between the two ratings is an indicator of the relief obtained. If the second pain rating is higher than the patient's goal for pain management, additional interventions or a change in the pain management plan may be needed.

Conclusion

Management of acute pain is an involved process that requires the full participation of the patient, physician, nurse, and other health care professionals. In addition, family members often are participants in this process. The nurse is responsible for continuing assessment and intervening to control pain. Support from the institution in the form of education in pain theories, pain assessment and multiple approaches to treatment of many kinds of pain is needed. The nurse also needs access to a variety of assessment instruments and a documentation system that facilitates communication of information to all members of the health team. To effectively perform this responsibility, a systematic approach is needed by the individual nurse. However, success with pain management depends on the standards, expectations, and support provided by the institution.

References

Acute Pain Management Guideline Panel. (1992). *Acute Pain Management: Operative or Medical Procedures and Trauma. Clinical Practice Guideline.* AHCPR Publication No. 92-0032. Rockville, MD: Agency for Health Care Policy and Research, Public Health Service, US Department of Health and Human Services.

Altimier, L., Norwood, S., Dick, M.J., Holditch-Davis, D., & Lawless, S. (1994). Postoperative pain management in preverbal children: The prescription and administration of analgesics with and without caudal analgesia. *Journal of Pediatric Nursing*, 9, 226-232.

Beyer, J. E., McGrath, P. J., & Berde, C. B. (1990). Discordance between self-report and behavioral measures in 3-7 year old children following surgery. *Journal of Pain and Symptom Management*, 5, 350-356.

Cancer Pain Management Guideline Panel. (1994). *Cancer Pain Management: Clinical Practice Guideline.* AHCPR Publication No. 94-0592. Rockville, MD: Agency for Health Care Policy and Research, Public Health Service, US Department of Health and Human Services.

Carrieri, V. K., Lindsey, A. M., & West, C. M. (1986). *Pathophysiological Phenomena in Nursing: Human Responses to Illness.* Philadelphia: WB Saunders.

International Association for the Study of Pain. (1979). Pain terms: A list with definitions and notes on usage. *Pain*, 6, 249-252.

Kremer, E., Atkinson, J. H., & Ignelzi, R.J. (1981). Measurement of pain: Patient preference does not confound pain measurement. *Pain*, 10, 241-248.

Lee, K. A., & Kieckhefer, G. M. (1989). Measuring human responses using visual analogue scales. *Western Journal of Nursing Research*, 11, 128-132.

Lowe, N. R. (1989). Explaining the pain of active labor: The importance of maternal confidence. *Research in Nursing and Health*, 12, 237-238.

McCaffery, M., & Beebe, A. (1989). *Pain: Clinical Manual for Nursing Practice.* St. Louis: Mosby.

Melzack, R. (1983). *Pain Measurement and Assessment.* New York: Raven Press.

Melzack, R. (1987). The short-form McGill Pain Questionnaire. *Pain*, 30, 191-197.

Teske, K., Daut, R. L., & Cleeland, C. S. (1983). Relationships between nurses' observations and patients' self-reports of pain. *Pain*, 16, 289-296.

Watt-Watson, J. H., & Donovan, M. I. (Eds.). (1992). *Pain Management: Nursing Perspective*. St. Louis: Mosby Yearbook.

Wells, N. (1991). Pain and distress during abortion. *Health Care for Women International*, 12, 293-302.

Wewers, M. E., & Lowe, N. K. (1990). A critical review of visual analogue scales in the measurement of clinical phenomena. *Research in Nursing & Health*, 13, 227-236.

Wilkie, D. S., Savedra, M. C., Holzemer, W. L., Tesler, M. D., & Paul, S. M. (1990). Use of the McGill Pain Questionnaire to measure pain: A meta-analysis. Nursing Research, 39, 36-41.

—by Margaret Jorgensen Dick, RN, Ph.D.

Margaret Jorgensen Dick is an associate professor in the School of Nursing of the University of North Carolina at Greensboro.

Address for correspondence:
Margaret Jorgensen Dick, RN, Ph.D,
2523 Cottage Place
Greensboro, NC 27455

Chapter 5

Probing the Underpinnings of Pain

When a stranger with somewhat irrational behavior suddenly appears and claims to be a member of the family, an investigation is in order. Maybe the newcomer is an impostor and not a member of the family after all, or perhaps his quirks must be understood and explained before he can be accepted. Such was the situation when researchers in Europe discovered a peptide—a chain of amino acids—in the mouse brain that apparently belonged to a family of natural pain killers, known as opioids. But their research showed that the new peptide intensified the sense of pain. Intrigued by the possibility that there might be a subfamily of opioid molecules with effects diametrically opposite those of other members, NCRR grantee Dr. Sukhbir S. Mokha decided to investigate.

"Neurons communicate with each other through a complex and tightly regulated system of chemicals and receptors, many of which we still don't know about," says Dr. Mokha, associate professor of physiology at Meharry Medical College in Nashville, Tennessee, where an NCRR Research Centers in Minority Institutions grant has helped to strengthen neuroscience studies. Within moments of receiving a painful stimulus, an intricate network of signals springs into action inside the body, relaying the message from the source to the spinal cord and brain. In addition to an obvious response to remove the source of pain; such as jerking a singed hand away from heat and other, long-term processes are set into motion. "If we want to be able

---

NCRR Reporter, January/February 1997.

to control pain, we need to know the intricacies of various chemical modulators in the nervous system," Dr. Mokha says.

Using a special technique called microiontophoresis, the scientists applied small amounts of the new peptide named nociceptin or orphanin FQ for its apparent pain-enhancing effects and orphan status directly on trigeminal neurons and examined how it modified their responses. Trigeminal neurons sense stimuli to the face such as a pinch on the cheek. "We observed that nociceptin inhibited responses not just to pain but also to various non-painful stimuli," he says. In contrast, scientists in the two independent research groups that first studied nociceptin reported in 1995 that the peptide enhanced the response to pain when injected into the brains of mice.

The Meharry researchers also found that nociceptin reduced the responses evoked by stimulation of another type of receptor called the NMDA-receptor, which plays a key role in mediating pain signals and in generating the chronic pain that follows nerve injuries or inflammation. The responses evoked by certain non-NMDA receptors were also similarly dampened. The NMDA and non-NMDA receptors are pore-containing proteins situated in the membranes of neurons; they serve as channels for the passage of ions and hence generation of electrical current. The pores open and close when neurotransmitters that are released in response to pain or other stimuli bind to receptors. According to Dr. Mokha, researchers in Sweden and Britain have also shown that nociceptin inhibits spinal cord reflexes and responses of spinal cord neurons to painful stimuli.

"All these results indicate that nociceptin may be an analgesic [pain dampener] rather than a pain enhancer as originally thought," says Dr. Mokha. "The next step would be to look into the mechanisms of action in more detail to determine how nociceptin modulates pain."

But the paradox remains unresolved. Why does nociceptin evoke opposite responses in the laboratories of different researchers? One possible answer, suggests Dr. Mokha, is that nociceptin acts differently in different species: the molecule's effects were first observed in a mouse, though all subsequent tests showing the pain-dampening effects were conducted in the rat model. Nevertheless, researchers agree that it does seem odd that the same compound would act so differently in animals that are quite closely related in evolution, given that molecules often have the same effect in very unrelated species.

There is also a second, more probable albeit more complicated explanation for nociceptin's apparent different effects in mice and rats. "It is possible that the injection of any substance directly into the brains of mice might induce a stress response, accompanied by the

Probing the Underpinnings of Pain

release of hormones and other chemicals that in turn trigger a host of reactions by the nervous system, including mechanisms to dampen pain," Dr. Mokha suggests. Perhaps nociceptin blocks this stress-induced analgesia. Recent evidence from researchers at Oregon Health Sciences University in Portland suggests that this explanation might be correct. "When administered into the brain, nociceptin did, in fact, act like an anti-opioid agent in rats and mice and reduced the stress-induced analgesia in mice," Dr. Mohka says. In contrast, at the spinal cord level it consistently acts like an analgesic and enhances the pain-dampening effects of opioids in rats.

Regardless of its end effects, nociceptin and its nerve receptor continue to excite Dr. Mokha and other researchers. "The actions of nociceptin appear to be as complicated as those of dynorphin, a well-known opioid molecule that binds to the kappa-opioid receptor," he notes. Dr. Mokha's immediate goal is to clarify the role of nociceptin in modulating both acute and chronic pain mechanisms, but he predicts that future research in the field will take off in many directions. He suggests that the peptide might affect a number of nervous system functions, including diverse sensory perceptions, motor functions, learning, and memory.

It appears that the newcomer, after all, will be accepted as a valued member of the opioid family, rather than being rejected as the oddball.

—*by Neeraja Sankaran*

These studies were supported by the Research Infrastructure area of the National Center for Research Resources, the National Institute of Dental Research, and the National Science Foundation.

Additional Reading

Wang X.-M., Zhang, K. M., and Mokha, S. S., Nociceptin (Orphanin FQ), an endogenous ligand for the ORL-1 (opioid-receptor-like-1) receptor, modulates responses of trigeminal neurons evoked by excitatory amino acid and somatosensory stimuli. *Journal of Neurophysiology* 76: 3568-3572, 1996.

Zhang, K. M., Wang X.-M., and Mokha, S. S., Opioids modulate N-methyl-D-aspartic acid (NMDA)-evoked responses of neurons in the superficial and deeper dorsal horn of the medulla (trigeminal nucleus caudalis). *Brain Research* 719: 229-233, 1996.

Meunier, J. C., Mollereau, C., Toll, L., et al., Isolation and structure of the endogenous agonist of opioid receptor-like ORL1 receptor. *Nature* 377: 532-535, 1995.

Reinscheid, R. K., Nothacker, H. P., Bourson, A., et al., Orphanin FQ: A neuropeptide that activates an opioid-like G protein-coupled receptor. *Science* 270: 792--794, 1995.

Part Two

Headaches

Chapter 6

The Ache and the Head

When we burn a finger or bang a knee, we know what causes the pain. We also understand that the pain, however unpleasant, serves a purpose. It shouts the message, "Stop what you're doing—it's dangerous! And take care of this problem." With a headache, the mechanisms causing the pain, and the reason for the pain, are much less clear.

The brain itself has no sense of pain. The pain-sensitive parts of the head are the scalp and its blood supply, the head and neck muscles, the nasal sinuses, some of the arteries of the brain, the membrane surrounding the brain (the dura mater), and some of the neck and brain nerves. Although the pain is not in the brain, we would not feel pain in the head or any other part of the body without the brain's involvement.

The brain and the nerves communicate by means of a special group of chemicals called neurotransmitters. The neurotransmitters are essential for all nervous system functioning, including muscle contraction, sensory perception, thought, mood, and awareness of pain. Changes in the availability of the neurotransmitter serotonin are believed to have a primary role in the genesis of a migraine, and perhaps of other forms of headache as well. A number of migraine medications, including the antidepressants and sumatriptan, act to stabilize the brain's supply of serotonin.

©1995 *Headache*. American Council for Headache Education Newsletter Volume 6, Issue 4. Reprinted with permission. For more information, please call 1-800-255-ACHE.

Pain Sourcebook

Nerve signals, moving at speeds up to 100 feet per second, warn of danger, and we yank our finger off the hot stove before we are aware of what we are doing. The reflex of withdrawing the injured finger doesn't need the brain's involvement. It occurs at the level of the spinal cord. The pain signal is first processed by the brain stem at the base of the brain (see illustration). The brain stem regulates many body processes, such as breathing and heart rate, that are involuntary and unconscious.

From the brain stem the pain signals pass upward to the thalamus, which lies at the very center of the brain. It partially interprets and relays sensory nerve signals to other parts of the brain. The thalamus is closely connected to the hypothalamus, a major regulator of sleep, appetite and other cycles. The hypothalamus is thought to have a role in cluster headaches and migraine. We become "aware" of pain, perceive it, and other sensations when the nerve signals reach the cortex, the wrinkled outer "gray matter" of the brain.

Neurotransmitters and other chemicals in the nervous system modulate perception of pain, magnifying or minimizing the pain in response to environmental factors or emotions. The endorphins, the body's natural opium-like chemicals, can reduce perception of pain.

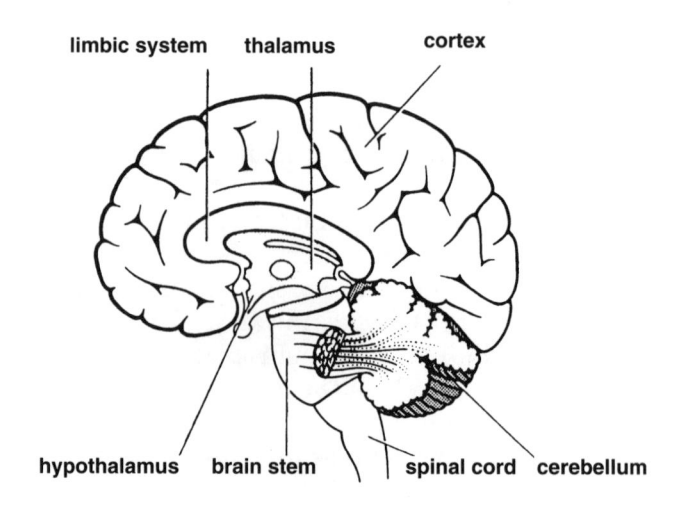

Figure 6.1. The Main Regions of the Brain

The Ache and the Head

Narcotic drugs mimic these natural pain-relieving chemicals. Athletes who suffer serious injuries during competition or persons injured while undergoing extreme stress sometimes report feeling very little pain. (At other times or for other people, stress may increase pain or be experienced as pain.)

Other chemicals, including one known as "substance P," increase pain awareness. Serotonin has a role in controlling the release of substance P. Substance P, histamine, bradykinin, prostaglandins and other irritating chemicals are released by injured tissues. Nerves supplying the irritated tissue relay the "bad news" to the brain, and a pain is experienced in the tissue itself, or elsewhere along the path of the nerve. Aspirin and other NSAID (nonsteroidal anti-inflammatory drugs) relieve pain by suppressing some of these irritating substances.

The pain-sensing and -responding pathways of the brain and body work in a complex feedback system. The brain stem, which first receives the pain message, also has an important role in regulating pain perception—in effect determining how bad the pain should be. As we learn more about the role of the brain stem and other pain centers in the brain, we hope to develop better nonaddictive drugs that will act at this level to "influence" the brain's "decisions" about the painfulness of the injury, trigger or irritant that launches the pain response.

The pain of occasional headache, like the pain of a hurt finger, can be educational. It can tell us that too much alcohol, too little sleep, or excessive eye strain should be avoided, or that we need to find better ways of coping with daily stress. Most chronic headache sufferers, in contrast, are believed to have abnormalities in the complex chemistry of the brain and nerves. They may be more sensitive to the effects of some of the pain-triggering chemicals of the body, or have an imbalance in some of the key neurotransmitters involved in pain response, such as serotonin.

Glossary

brain stem: essential to many life processes; contains the pathways connecting the brain and spinal cord; now known to have an important role in migraine.

cerebellum: responsible for coordination of movements; not known to have a role in headache or pain perception.

cortex: responsible for sensory perception, decision-making, many aspects of behavior and the integration of these functions.

hypothalamus: an internal "clock" and regulator that coordinates many body functions and cycles; believed to have a role in migraine and cluster headache.

limbic system: governs instinct and emotional reactions; believed to have a role in the emotional response to pain; the cingulate cortex is usually considered part of the limbic system.

thalamus: a central relay station for processing and forwarding sensory impulses, including pain.

spinal cord: carries pain and other sensory information from the trunk and limbs to the brain; communicates the brain's commands to the nerves controlling the body's muscles.

Chapter 7

Headache Misery May Yield to Proper Treatment

"My headaches started when I was taking birth control pills. The pain was intense, first right above my eyes, then spreading below the eyes. It might start on one side and the next day switch to the other side. Nearly every week I'd be sick two or three days like I had the flu—vomiting, aching, and yawning all the time. All I wanted to do was sleep."

"After I went off the pill, the headaches were sporadic. I'd go for years with very little trouble. Surprisingly, during my pregnancies, they disappeared. But they returned with a vengeance at menopause, and I was sick more than I wasn't sick. I could hardly stand it."

Janice Bailey, of Tucson, Ariz., describes her decades-long battle with "sick headaches," the most common symptom of a disabling condition called migraine. Attacks often follow exposure to a trigger—such as birth control pills.

Migraine is only one of the 12 headache types (with more than 60 sub-types) classified in 1988 by the International Headache Society for use in diagnosis. Migraine, cluster, and tension-type headaches are the main varieties. Numerous physical disorders underlie the nine other types.

Chronic headaches plague more than 45 million Americans, reports the National Headache Foundation, of Chicago.

Still, the vast majority of headaches are temporary, "requiring no more than an over-the-counter analgesic," says Russell Katz, M.D.,

---

FDA Consumer, September 1992.

deputy director of the Food and Drug Administration's division of neuro-pharmacological drugs, which reviews anti-migraine drugs. "Headaches from life-threatening conditions such as tumors are uncommon," he says.

An important tool in diagnosing headache is the patient's medical history, says Stuart Stark, M.D., director of the Headache Program for The Neurology Center in Alexandria, Va

"The history usually is sufficient to determine the specific type of headache," he says. "But when headaches are debilitating, a diagnostic workup is warranted."

Workups often include taking pictures of the brain with a radiological procedure such as computed tomography or magnetic resonance imaging. To rule out certain causes, further procedures may be needed—blood tests, for instance. "We particularly look at the blood count," Stark says, "to see whether the blood is too thick or too thin. Blood that clots abnormally can be caused by disease, such as lupus (a rheumatic disease)."

Most Common Headache Types

- **Migraine headaches** usually throb and affect one or both sides of the head. Physical activity tends to worsen the pain. Patients also may have nausea, vomiting, light and noise sensitivity, or other symptoms. Some sufferers have warnings, such as visual disturbances. Attacks last from a few hours to days, recurring from several times a week to once every few years. Women get migraines more frequently than men.

- **Cluster headaches** occur as a series of one-sided headaches that are sudden and excruciating and continue for 15 minutes to four hours. Cluster attacks last 4 to 12 weeks, and are followed by remission as long as months or years. Other symptoms on the painful side include nasal congestion, drooping eyelid, and irritated, teary eye. Most cluster patients are men.

- **Tension-type headaches** may last a few hours, a few days, or be chronic. The pain is described as a tight band around the head, but it can affect any scalp, face, neck, and shoulder muscles. Some patients, especially those with chronic tension headaches, also suffer from stress, anxiety or depression.

Headache Misery May Yield to Proper Treatment

Migraine

Migraine headaches affect 16 million to 18 million Americans, of whom nearly two-thirds are women, the National Headache Foundation says. Since migraine is believed to be mostly an inherited condition, children, even babies, may be "migraineurs," as victims of this headache are called.

"Abdominal colic could be a form of migraine," Stark says. "If the mother or father has had migraines, it's worth considering the colic as a possible prelude to a migraine condition. About all you can treat a baby with is liquid Tylenol, but the colic could alert you to watch for symptoms as the child grows."

The two main migraine sub-types are "migraine with aura" (formerly called "classic migraine") and "migraine without aura" (formerly called "common migraine"). Attacks can last from several hours to several days.

About 10 percent of migraine patients have auras—certain neurological (nerve-related) symptoms that precede the headache by 5 to 30 minutes but sometimes persist into the headache phase. Aura symptoms include visual disturbances such as flashing lights or zigzag lines or even temporary vision loss. Others are a pins-and-needles feeling on one side of the face or body followed by numbness, or numbness without the tingling. Less frequent signs are speech problems, confusion, and weakness on one side.

Migraines without auras may be accompanied by vague warning signs, including mood swings, mental fuzziness, and fluid retention.

Bailey says she often was very tired before an attack. "I'd yawn and yawn," she says. "But mainly it was just an overall feeling. I'd know I'd better not eat much if I had that feeling."

Patients describe their pain with words such as intense, throbbing, pounding. They feel it in the forehead, temple, ear, jaw, or, like Bailey, around the eye. Most migraines are one-sided. Some start on one side but spread to the other.

Besides headache, symptoms include nausea, vomiting, appetite loss, diarrhea, sensitivity to light and noise, fever, chills, flu-like achiness, and sweats. Attacks range in frequency from several times a week to once every few years.

About 5 percent of migraineurs don't have headaches. "They may have vomiting, dizziness, or ringing in the ears," Stark says. "Since migraine is a condition of the brain, literally any neurologic symptom can occur."

But Where Does a Migraine Come from?

A longstanding theory holds that blood vessels in the scalp and on the brain's surface constrict. This reduces the brain's oxygen supply to produce the aura some patients have. The same vessels, reacting to the brain's need for oxygen, open up, or dilate, releasing pain-causing chemicals called prostaglandins, other chemicals that increase sensitivity to pain, and still others that induce painful inflammation and swelling.

Stark is among the neurologists who subscribe to a newer theory that migraine stems from a chemical change deep within the brain, where the body uses the neuro-transmitter serotonin abnormally. (Neuro-transmitters are chemical messengers that nerve cells use to tell each other what to do.)

Working with other chemicals, serotonin regulates blood vessel constriction and dilation. It can both sharpen and deaden pain. While serotonin's role in migraine isn't completely understood, areas of the brain responsive to serotonin are often involved in migraine. The hypothalamus, for instance—which regulates involuntary bodily functions such as menstruation, sleep and hunger—has cells sensitive to serotonin. Such cells also appear in large amounts in the stomach and intestinal walls. Certain serotonin cells stop "firing" during sleep, which often ends a migraine attack.

"Serotonin acts on the electrical impulses sent out by nerve cells in and around the blood vessels in the brain," Stark explains. "We believe that in a migraine attack, the serotonin isn't properly used for some reason, so that the electrical wave of impulses becomes diminished, or depressed. The wave, called 'spreading depression,' reduces blood flow through the vessels leading to the back of the brain.

"This is when the aura occurs. The symptoms depend on which areas of the brain are included in the wave. Spreading depression is believed present in all migraine attacks, even in people who don't have auras."

"After the spreading depression subsides, the blood vessels start leaking fluid, inflaming the outside of the vessels. The inflammation causes the pain, which can extend to all the nerve cells supplying the blood vessels, not just those in the area of the spreading depression."

The spreading depression correlates with the aura, but not the headache, Stark says. In other words, a depressed wave limited to one side of the head can lead to pain on both sides.

Also, some scientists believe a disturbance in the brain's trigeminal nerve contributes to migraine headache by causing the release of "substance P," which causes inflammation.

Headache Misery May Yield to Proper Treatment

If these theories are correct, changes in the head's blood vessels, impulses deep within the brain, and the pain pathway in the trigeminal nerve may all play a part in migraine pain.

Given the theory that most migraineurs are predisposed to their condition, migraine has been described as a cocked gun waiting to go off—except that this gun has many triggers.

A trigger for Bailey was cigarette smoke. "At a party where lots of people were smoking and there wasn't good air flow, I'd nearly always get sick," she says. "Once I was sick, smells such as glue, pesticides or perfume egged it on."

Reaction to stress is a common trigger. Others include fatigue, lack of sleep, glaring lights, excessive noise, weather, certain drugs that cause blood vessels to swell, and hormonal fluctuation—as happens around menstruation, at menopause, and during use of birth control pills.

Foods trigger migraines, too. Keeping a food diary can help identify sensitivities.

As for headache prevention and treatment, FDA has approved a number of anti-migraine drugs. Their benefits vary from person to person and must be weighed against the risks, some of which are serious.

"One preventive drug is Inderal [propranolol]," says FDA's Katz. "It was initially approved to treat high blood pressure and heart problems, and only accidentally found to prevent migraine. It's not useful after the headache begins." FDA approved Inderal, a beta blocker, for preventing migraine in 1979. It's the only beta blocker with this indication. Inderal's effect in migraine is not well-understood.

The other drug approved for preventing migraine is Sansert (methysergide), one of several ergot drugs, which constrict blood vessels. Sansert can't be given continuously for more than six months, so its use is limited.

"Effective drugs to stop a particular attack of migraine once it has started," Katz says, "include analgesics and ergotamines. Whichever is used, it must be taken early in the attack to be most effective." For occasional mild migraines, he says, over-the-counter (OTC) pain relievers or prescription drugs with a low dose of codeine are usually adequate.

"Isometheptene combined with dichloralphenazone and acetaminophen—Midrin or Isocom—may also be helpful early in an attack," Katz says. "Antiemetics can relieve the associated nausea and vomiting in migraine."

OTC analgesics for headache include aspirin, Tylenol (and other brands of acetaminophen), and Advil, Motrin IB, and Nuprin (and other brands of ibuprofen). Ergot drugs include Ergomar, Ergostat, Cafergot, Wigraine, and D.H.E. 45.

Cluster Headache

"This piercing pain," the man cries to his wife. His hand goes to his right eye, which is teary and red with irritation.

Tingling on one side of the face or body and visual sensation, such as flashing lights and zig-zag lines are the most common symptoms of the migraine aura, a pre-headache phenomenon in about 10 percent of migraine sufferers. Many scientists believe the aura correlates with a brain wave of depressed electrical impulses called spreading depression. According to this theory, spreading depression occurs in all migraine attacks, even those without auras. For a half hour, the man has been pacing, unable to keep still. Pausing to stub out his cigarette, he clenches and unclenches his fists, then wipes sweat from his right brow with a tissue. He blows his nose.

Finally, the pain is over. He collapses in a chair to wait, fearing the pain will return yet a fourth time today.

The patient is a fictitious composite of symptoms and behavior typical of cluster headache sufferers.

Cluster headache is so-named because it recurs in clusters, several times a day, for several weeks or months. A cluster may start at a certain time of year, perhaps with a change of season. Each headache lasts from 15 minutes up to four hours, but the cluster attack—repeated headaches—can go on for weeks or months. When the cluster series is over, in 90 percent of patients, it won't recur for months or years. The cause is unknown.

Nearly a million Americans have cluster headaches, the National Headache Foundation reports. Most cluster patients are men, usually smokers. Cluster has been called the "suicide headache," "demon of headaches," and, because it often wakens the person, "alarm clock headache."

Nearly always, only the blood vessels of one carotid artery are affected, making the intense, steady pain one-sided—usually centered behind the eye and in the temple.

Also, the pupil on the pain side may constrict, the eyelid may droop, and the brow may sweat. Nasal congestion may lead the person to suspect a sinus infection, but sinus headaches don't start and stop several times a day. Unlike migraineurs, who want to curl up in bed, cluster victims can't sit still.

Why these symptoms accompany cluster headache has not been established. One theory suggests involvement of the nerves supplying that area according to Seymour Diamond, M.D., executive director of the National Headache Foundation and head of the Diamond Headache Clinic in Chicago.

Headache Misery May Yield to Proper Treatment

One hundred percent oxygen inhaled through a mask for 8 to 15 minutes often stops an attack, Stark says. Painkillers tend not to work, he says. Drugs such as Cafergot lessen some acute attacks. Sansert is sometimes prescribed for prevention.

"We aren't certain how drugs work in cluster" Stark says.

Tension-type Headache

The tension-type headache usually involves increased tension in the scalp and neck muscles. It has also been called "muscle contraction headache," "psychogenic headache," "stress headache," "ordinary headache," and "tension headache."

As some of those names suggest, tension-type headaches are the most common, accounting for 90 percent of headaches not due to disease, and are most often caused by anxiety and stress—for instance, a mile-long traffic tie-up, work deadlines, standing sixth in a grocery check-out line, money worries.

Others susceptible to tension-type headache, Katz says, are people with poor posture, beauticians and others who move their neck and shoulders a lot, and people who work at stationary, repetitive tasks, as on an assembly line.

The pain often involves most of the head, from the forehead to the nape of the neck, and feels like a dull ache, as though the head were being pressed in a vise. Neck and shoulder muscles may be tense. The pain may go away after an hour. It may last several days.

"Usually, OTC pain relievers, hot packs, and relaxation will relieve occasional tension headaches," Katz says.

Patients with chronic tension-type headaches often are depressed. The depression may result from the pain itself, wrote Stephen Silberstein, M.D., and Marsha Silberstein, M.D., in recent articles in *Pain Management*. For these patients, some doctors prescribe antidepressants.

Other headaches are associated with physical problems, including dysfunction of the temporomandibular joint (which connects the jaw to the skull), brain disease, a blow to the head, arthritis, whiplash, metabolic disorders such as an overactive thyroid gland, and dental, sinus or ear infection. Treatment is based on the underlying cause.

Thanks to increasing knowledge about headaches, most headaches can be prevented or treated, if not cured. Bailey, for instance, has been treated with Inderal since 1983. Does she still have sick headaches?

"I don't know," she says. "I haven't quit taking my medicine long enough to find out."

Help for Headache Sufferers

In addition to over-the-counter products, a number of prescription drugs are available to treat headaches. Some migraine preparations also are approved to treat cluster headaches. One labeled as only "possibly" effective for migraine is approved for tension headache.

Anti-migraine drugs should be taken under medical supervision. Though they provide benefits, they can cause side effects, some of which are serious. Scientists don't know exactly how they work. The drugs' names, approved formulations and uses, and probable ways they achieve their effects are:

- **Ergotamine tartrate** (Ergomar, Ergostat) tablets, dissolved under the tongue, are used short-term to prevent cluster headaches in some patients and to treat migraine and cluster. This drug constricts blood vessels and inhibits pain-causing fluid leakage from vessels in the brain's outer membrane. It interacts with brain "receptors" for serotonin (a chemical messenger that nerve cells use to tell each other what to do).

- **Ergotamine tartrate/caffeine** (Cafergot, Cafermine, Ercaf, Ercatab, Ergo-Caff, Gotamine, Lanatrate, Migergot, Wigraine) tablets and/or suppositories are used to treat the same headaches as ergotamine alone. Caffeine increases ergotamine's effect, reducing the amount of ergotamine needed.

- **Dihydroergotamine mesylate injection** (D.H.E. 45), an ergotamine derivative, is used like ergotamine. However, it can be injected in a muscle or given intravenously and may be more effective for a given attack.

- **Methysergide maleate** (Sansert) tablets are used to prevent vascular headaches that occur once or more a week or are uncontrollable by other treatments. Thus, it is not used once an attack begins. It should not be taken continuously longer than six months. Sansert blocks serotonin transmission.

- **Isometheptene mucate/dichloralphenazone/acetaminophen** (Amidrin, I.D.A., Iso-Acetazone, Isocom, Midrin, Migratine, Migrazone, Migrex, Mitride) capsules are used to treat tension headache and, the labeling says, "possibly" migraine. (FDA recognizes a potential benefit in migraine but requires more research to prove it is fully effective.) Isometheptene constricts vessels, dichloralphenazone mildly sedates, and acetaminophen relieves pain.

- **Propranolol hydrochloride** (Inderal) tablets are used to prevent migraine. This drug may block communication between certain nerve cells.

FDA is reviewing data to support marketing of a migraine preparation called Imitrex (sumatriptan succinate), formulated as an injection patients can administer. The drug acts on serotonin receptors.

Last fall, an advisory panel to FDA on nervous system drugs recommended unanimously that Imitrex be considered approvable for treating migraine headaches. The panel concluded that more evidence was needed to prove safety and efficacy for use in cluster headaches.

Danger Signals

Sometimes a headache can signal a serious condition requiring prompt medical attention. According to the National Institute of Neurological Disorders and Stroke in Bethesda, Md., a doctor should be consulted if a headache:

- is accompanied by confusion, unconsciousness or convulsions
- involves pain in the eye or ear
- is accompanied by fever
- is accompanied by nausea
- occurs after a blow to the head
- is persistent in someone previously free of headaches
- is recurrent, especially in children
- interferes with normal life.

For more information, contact:

The Neurology Institute
P.O. Box 5801
Bethesda, MD 20824
Telephone (1-800) 352-9424 or,

The National Headache Foundation
5252 N. Western Ave.
Chicago, IL 60625
Telephone (1-800) 843-2256

NHF offers a list of headache clinics and a state list of National Headache Foundation physician members interested in treating headache.

—by Dixie Farley

Dixie Farley is a staff writer for *FDA Consumer*.

Chapter 8

Tension-Type Headache

Tension-type headache has undergone many name changes in the past 30 years. It has been referred to as tension headache, stress headache, muscle-contraction headache, and since 1988, tension-type headache. It refers to the most common of all headaches; it is more common than migraine and all its variants and subtypes. This form of headache affects almost all individuals at one time or another, occurring most often with anxiety or stress and at times increasing in frequency in headache-prone individuals with depression. This is the type of headache refered to in newspapers, magazines, and television advertisements when promoting a particular brand of analgesic or pain killer. Sometimes these over-the-counter remedies will alleviate headache distress in migraine sufferers as well. Individuals with tension-type headache may also suffer from migraine or cluster headache. They may have migraine one day and a tension-type headache another day, or one type may lead to another.

One of the reasons this form of headache has had numerous titles is that the exact mechanism is not completely understood. Its characteristics sometimes suggest a blend into migraine. Medications, at times effective for one type, may similarly alleviate the other. Scientific investigations dating back to the 1950s suggest there are vascular mechanisms involved that are also found in migraine without aura

---

©1995 the National Headache Foundation. Reprinted with permission. Permission to reprint granted by the National Headache Foundation, Chicago, IL. For more information on headache causes and treatments, call the NHF at (800) 843-2256.

(common migraine without the visual symptoms). During the early 1960s, Dr. Arnold Friedman and his co-investigators at Montefiore Hospital demonstrated and confirmed the earlier work of Dr. Harold Wolff and his research investigators showing that blood vessel and circulatory changes occurred in what was then known as tension or muscle-contraction headache. I was fortunate to have worked at Montefiore Hospital with patients suffering from tension and migraine headache and studied their circulatory changes. This early work, plus studies in some patients with tension-type headache, revealed increased muscle spasm or tension in the muscles of the scalp, particularly the rear of the head as well as the upper neck muscles overlying the spine and shoulders.

Many studies have been conducted since. The impression today is that in some patients heightened muscle contraction may be present, as well as changes in the smaller blood vessels of the muscles overlying the skull and muscles of the neck (usually those near the cervical spine). However, not all patients with tension-type headache exhibit these muscular changes. Furthermore, not every tension-type headache is associated with anxiety or stress. A similar type of head pain follows head injury with or without concussion, temporomandibular (jaw) joint and jaw muscle problems, and infections of structures of the head and neck. Arthritis of the cervical spine and other abnormalities of the spine may be associated with similar headache symptoms. The International Headache Society met in 1988 to classify all

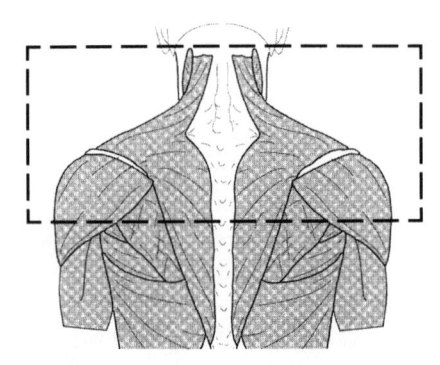

Figure 8.1. Muscles of the neck and upper shoulder areas that may be involved during tension-type headache.

Tension-Type Headache

types of headache and affix this new title to distinguish patients with physical problems from this group of acute and chronic tension-type headache sufferers.

Even more important than the name is what can be done to help individuals with tension-type headache. Since many people suffer from stressful events resulting in head pain, relaxation exercises and biofeedback may be extremely helpful. It is also important to use common sense, if possible avoiding circumstances that may induce moderate or severe anxiety and headache. The unrestricted use of over-the-counter pain relievers, as well as the excessive use of certain prescription medications, may produce rebound headache. Medications containing caffeine, if used in excess of the manufacturers' recommendations, can also produce rebound headache. Frequent headache sufferers may benefit by avoiding food and beverages containing caffeine. Some patients may require treatment for depression if it is associated with tension-type headache.

Numerous medications exist for the acute relief of tension-type headache. Acetaminophen, aspirin, ibuprofen, and naproxen are effective and the addition of caffeine appears to enhance the effect of aspirin and acetaminophen. However, it should be emphasized this is effective therapy for an occasional acute headache. When headache becomes chronic and occurs several times a week or more, alternate therapy is recommended. Preventive medication may include various anti-depressant compounds from one of many categories.

Co-existing migraine and tension-type headache may warrant a combination of medications with migraine-preventive properties. Certain muscle-relaxing compounds provide short-term relief. Patients with chronic tension-type headache should seek competent medical help or consultation to be sure no serious co-existing medical or neurological problem is present before embarking on therapy.

In summary, tension-type headache comes in two forms: acute and chronic. One step in diagnosis is to preclude serious or co-existing medical-neurological causes of the headache symptoms. Tension-type headache is extremely common and affects all age groups but is most often seen in the teens through fifties. It does not appear to be inherited and it occurs more frequently in females. Symptoms are often described as a tight hatband sensation, although only one side of the head may be affected, and often the neck and upper shoulders as well. The pain is described as steady and tightening but may throb in some patients, particularly if migraine co-exists. Analgesics with caffeine are often effective in acute occasional attacks. Prescription compounds containing butal-bital are highly effective in more painful attacks.

Chronic or frequent headache can benefit from relaxation exercises, biofeedback, and at times preventive drugs. Sometimes it may be necessary to avoid analgesics, prescription pain relievers, and excessive caffeine intake for a satisfactory outcome and to reduce headache frequency. If the chronic form is resistant to treatment, highly specialized care, including hospitalization, is sometimes required in the most difficult-to-treat circumstances. Many questions remain unanswered about this very common and at times disabling disorder. Treatment, however, has advanced in the past decade, and many physicians and health professionals are presently engaged in the study and treatment of this type of headache.

—by Arthur H. Elkind, M.D., Director,
Elkind Headache Center,
Mt. Vernon, New York.

Chapter 9

The Migraine Aura

About 15 percent of migraine sufferers have a warning that the headache is coming on. They experience a change in brain function called an **aura.** It is usually a visual symptom, such as an arc of sparkling (scintillating) zigzag lines or a blotting out of vision or both. But any other brain-related symptom may occur, such as numbness of one side of the face and hand, weakness, unsteadiness, or altered consciousness. In past years these symptoms were thought to be caused by spasm of blood vessels supplying parts of the brain, and the headache was thought to be due to subsequent expansion (dilation) of blood vessels in the head. We now know that it is not that simple.

Headache follows certain changes that take place in the nerves to the major blood vessels in the head. The aura is due to changes that take place in the **cortex**, the outer layer of the brain.

The nerve cells of the brain are always active. This can be seen by the electrical activity they generate on the electroencephalogram (EEG). In experiments with animals, the EEG shows a depression (lowering) of nerve cell activity below a spot on the cortex of the brain that has been stimulated. Surrounding the area of depressed activity is a zone in which nerve cells have become **hyperactive**. It's thought that a similar pattern of decreased and increased nerve cell activity occurs in the brain of a person with migraine, following the stimulus of a migraine "trigger."

©1995 American Council for Headache Education. Reprinted with Permission. For more information, please call 1-800-255-ACHE.

When the activity of nerve cells is depressed, there is impairment of function in the part of the body controlled by these cells. For example, there may be a loss of vision or of strength. Increased activity of brain nerve cells may result in flashing lights or tingling in the face and hand. In the experiments with animals, the depression of nerve cell activity slowly spreads beyond the initial spot of stimulation. This phenomenon is called **spreading depression**. It is preceded by a wave of increased nerve cell activity.

This slowly spreading depression of nerve cell activity is believed to account for the pattern of development of the typical aura. In the migraine aura, symptoms build up gradually and move slowly from one visual region or one part of the body to another. For example, the migraine aura sufferer may first notice a black spot in the field of vision. This black spot is often surrounded by flashing lights or bright zigzag lines. The size of the black spot gradually enlarges over a period of minutes. The combination of loss of vision (negative symptoms) with flashing lights or zigzag lines (positive symptoms) is a typical and distinctive feature of migraine aura. The negative symptom is due to depressed nerve activity; the positive visual symptoms are due to the zone of hyperactive nerve cells. In contrast, a sudden shutting off of blood supply to the brain (as might occur with a blood clot) causes a sudden loss of function. In this case, there is no gradual "march" of visual symptoms or numbness, and positive visual symptoms do not occur.

What starts this sequence of events that leads to the aura and headache?

The answers to that question are not fully understood. We do know that migraine sufferers have an inborn susceptibility to factors that normally do not trigger headaches. In people with migraine, changes in body chemistry, such as menstruation, certain foods, and dozens of environmental influences, such as a change in weather, may trigger an attack.

These internal or external events stimulate different nerves of the brain, and these nerves relay the stimuli to one or more nerve centers in the **brain stem**, the lower portion of the brain that connects with the spinal cord. From these brain stem centers, another set of nerve impulses is sent to the cortex of the brain, causing the aura. The sequence of biochemical events that results in the headache may also begin in these brain stem centers.

—by Seymour Solomon, M.D., Headache Unit,
Montefiore Medical Center, New York, NY

Chapter 10

Headache: Myth, Misunderstanding, and Mistreatment

A Symptom or an Illness?

For most people, headache is an annoying temporary symptom, or a signal of a more basic, underlying condition. Headache as a symptom may be caused by the flu, a hangover, or more rarely by serious conditions such as brain tumors. Three hundred other disorders may cause headache as well. With resolution or treatment of the underlying problem, headache, the symptom, usually disappears.

But for many others, recurring and perhaps daily head pain is an illness that can bring with it years or even a lifetime of pain, isolation, rejection, and self-doubt. This is the plight of headache illness victims, like those with other poorly understood or poorly recognized illnesses. But, like no other condition of such magnitude, headache is uniquely subject to myth, misunderstanding and mistreatment.

The Myths

There are countless myths about headache—too many in fact to address here. But among the most troubling is the belief that headache is due to disturbed emotions or an inability to deal with the stress of daily living. To a large measure, this misunderstanding may reflect a hidden prejudice against women, who are more likely than men to

---

©1995 *Headache*, American Council for Headache Education Newsletter. April 1995 Issue. Reprinted with permission. For more information, please call 1-800-255-ACHE.

suffer from headache. In fact, the greater vulnerability of women to headache is due to biological triggers—primarily fluctuations in estrogen levels—not emotional or psychological factors.

The Misunderstandings

Recurring headache can be a chronic medical condition, comparable to diabetes, epilepsy, or hypertension. Many types of headaches are known to be inherited. For example, over 80 percent of migraine sufferers have a family history of headache. Contrary to widespread belief, the illness of headache arises from a biological vulnerability. Scientific data indicate that chronic head pain patients suffer disturbances related to changes in brain chemistry. Sufferers require and deserve the same attention and concern accorded other significant, and at times, less disabling conditions.

The Mistreatments

Patients with headache have been given pain killers to the point of toxicity and addiction, then stereotyped and rejected for seeking additional pain killers. In short, the headache patient has been denied the professional commitment and standards of care that the illness of headache deserves and desperately requires.

Things are now changing. New research that identifies the basic mechanisms of headache is challenging many of these myths, misunderstandings and mistreatments.

—by Joel R. Saper, M.D.,
Past Chairman, ACHE

Chapter 11

The Eye and Headache

The eye, and much of the head and face, share sensory innervation (the distribution or supply of nerves to a part) from the first and second branches of the trigeminal nerve. Thus, it is not surprising that causes of headache that are not related to the eye often refer pain to the eye and eye socket and that many eye and eye-related problems refer pain to other parts of the head.

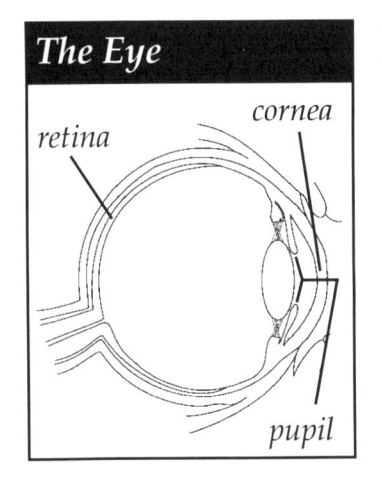

Figure 11.1.

Headache from Ocular or Orbital Causes

Head pain from eye or eye socket disease could be the result of eyestrain, corneal and conjunctival disease (such as infections or dry eyes), glaucoma, uveitis (intraocular inflammation), ocular ischemic syndrome (poor blood flow to the eye), and eye socket problems (infections, inflammation, or cancer). A good general rule of thumb is that if the eye

---

©1995 National Headache Foundation. Reprinted with permission. Permission to reprint granted by the National Headache Foundation, Chicago, IL. For more information on headache causes and treatments, call the NHF at (800) 843-2256.

Parts of the Trigeminal Nerve

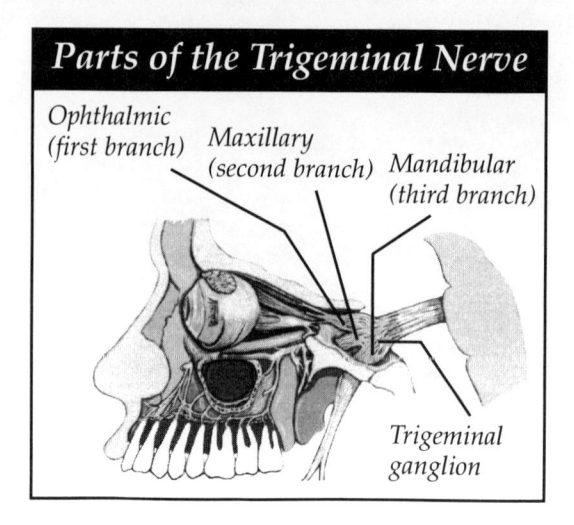

Ophthalmic (first branch)
Maxillary (second branch)
Mandibular (third branch)
Trigeminal ganglion

Figure 11.2.

is white (that is, uninflamed) it is not the primary cause of eye ache or headache. Any eye pain or headache associated with loss of vision or double vision needs prompt evaluation by a physician.

By and large, the need for glasses is overrated as a cause of true headache. However, uncorrected vision problems or mild eye misalignment problems can cause a mild, dull nonspecific pain around the eyes (asthenopia) that is described variously as an aching sensation or a strained feeling. "Tired eyes" is a common lay term for asthenopia. This problem is always made better by resting the eyes or getting new glasses, if indicated.

In patients over the age of 40, dry eyes can cause a significant amount of ocular discomfort, and artificial tears are the treatment of choice.

A sudden, sharp stabbing pain in the eye upon awakening, associated with tearing, is usually due to poor adherence of the cellular covering of the cornea, leading to a small corneal abrasion or recurrent erosion syndrome. This problem is rare and is treated with ocular lubricants at bedtime.

Acute angle closure glaucoma is a condition in which the pressure within the eye rises rapidly due to obstruction of normal outflow pathways. The pain is severe and throbbing, intensifies over a period of hours, and is associated with blurred vision and ocular redness. Nausea, vomiting, and lethargy are often present. Because the pupil often becomes unresponsive to light, this condition is sometimes

The Eye and Headache

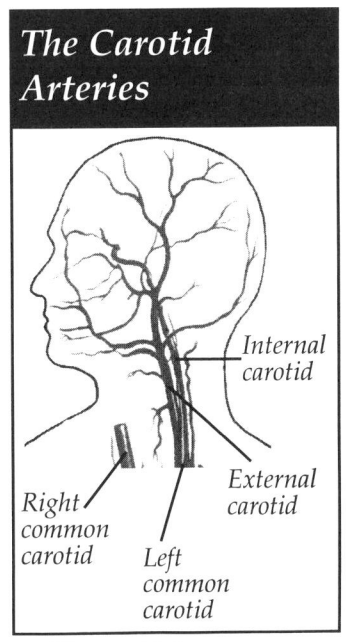

The Carotid Arteries

Figure 11.3.
(Labels: Internal carotid; External carotid; Right common carotid; Left common carotid)

misdiagnosed as a cerebral aneurysm in emergency room settings. Permanent blindness can result unless the condition is treated immediately by laser.

Some patients with diabetes, carotid artery occlusion, or prior blood flow problems to the retina of the eye develop neovascular glaucoma. Here, eye pressure elevates because blood vessels grow in and obstruct the outflow channels for aqueous fluid. Laser treatment is often used in this condition as well.

Uveitis, or intraocular inflammation, is associated with a number of systemic diseases, especially of the rheumatologic (arthritis-like) variety. The pain is usually throbbing and is made worse by exposure to bright light.

The ocular ischemic syndrome (poor blood flow to the eye) usually results from obstruction of the carotid artery in the neck due to atherosclerotic disease. The pain is constant, aching, and is localized to the face, brow, and temple. It is most often worse when standing. Visual loss in the affected eye when exposed to bright light is a common symptom.

A number of orbital (eye socket) problems are associated with pain. These conditions include orbital inflammations, infections, and primary or metastatic tumors. Double vision and protrusion of the eye are common in orbital diseases.

Nonocular Causes of Eye Pain

Nonocular problems that are associated with eye pain include migraine; third, fourth, or sixth cranial nerve palsy; trigeminal neuralgia; cavernous sinus syndromes; giant cell (temporal) arteritis, and *herpes zoster ophthalmicus*.

If you suffer from eye pain or discomfort, ask your physician for a careful evaluation of your symptoms.

—by Robert L. Tomsak, M.D., Ph.D.,
Section of Neuro-Ophthalmology,
The Mt. Sinai Medical Center, Cleveland, Ohio.

Chapter 12

Results of a National Poll of Migraine Sufferers

The AASH-Gallup Poll

This chapter presents the results of a national telephone survey of migraine sufferers conducted by the Gallup Organization on behalf of the American Association for the Study of Headache (AASH) and the American Council for Headache Education (ACHE). The survey was written and the data were reviewed and analyzed by Drs. Fred Sheftell (ACHE President), Seymour Solomon (ACHE Chairman), Lawrence Newman, Walter Stewart and Richard Lipton.

Why the AASH-Gallup Poll?

This survey was conducted as part of AASH's ongoing effort to improve patient care through medical education and headache research. AASH recognized that migraine sufferers who see their doctor and particularly those who seek treatment from headache specialists represent only a small minority of all migraine sufferers. The survey was intended to provide a snapshot of migraine sufferers all over the United States, whether or not they were actively seeking care. Through this survey AASH learned more about the symptoms and the consequences of migraine in the community.

©1995 *Headache*. American Council for Headache Education Newsletter. November 1995 issue. Reprinted with permission. For more information, please call 1-800-255-ACHE.

Pain Sourcebook

AASH also hoped to develop a report card on medical care, to help us identify both strengths and weaknesses in health care delivery for migraine sufferers. AASH hoped to determine which migraine sufferers consult doctors, why they consult, what treatment people receive and whether or not they are satisfied with it. For the people who do not seek care AASH wanted to determine the severity of their illness, their reasons for not seeking care and their satisfaction with the self-treatment options they utilize.

The answers to some of these questions were presented at the AASH Annual Scientific Meeting, held in Boston in June 1995. AASH is using this information to improve our educational programs for health care providers, while ACHE will use the results to identify and better address the needs of headache sufferers in the community. AASH felt that the survey results were of interest not only for doctors but for headache sufferers as well.

How Was the Survey Conducted?

The Gallup Organization selected a random sample of households in the United States and contacted them by telephone. Phone calls were completed to over 10,000 U.S. households. In each household, one individual, age 18 or older, was selected to participate in the interview. The initial part of the interview was designed to identify

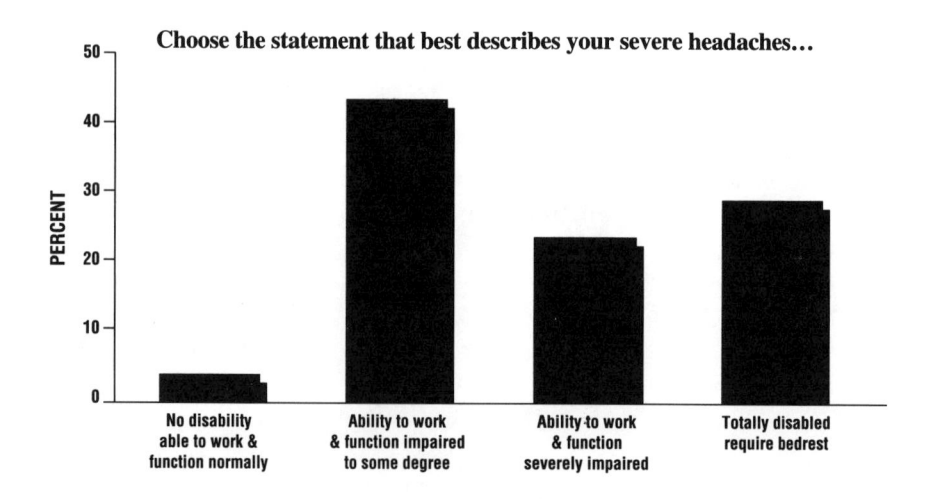

Choose the statement that best describes your severe headaches...

Figure 12.1.

Results of a National Poll of Migraine Sufferers

people whose symptoms met the diagnostic criteria for migraine developed by the International Headache Society (IHS). These criteria are based on the type and pattern of headache pain as well as the symptoms which come with the pain (such as nausea or sensitivity to light). Using the IHS criteria, the study identified 1,014 migraine sufferers.

With this approach, AASH was able to identify a nationally representative sample of over 1,000 migraine sufferers including those who had never seen a doctor about their headaches or been diagnosed as having migraine. Of course, a telephone interview is no substitute for an evaluation by a doctor. However, AASH is aware from prior research that this approach accurately identifies most people with migraine. Each migraine sufferer was then asked a series of follow-up questions about symptoms, severity, medical treatment, and the impact of the migraines on social and work life.

How Bad Is it? Pain and Disability

Among the 1,014 migraineurs interviewed, over half (54 percent) said that their severe headaches occurred less than once a month, but 29 percent reported severe headaches that occurred several times a month. About one in seven migraineurs said they had an attack once a week or more often.

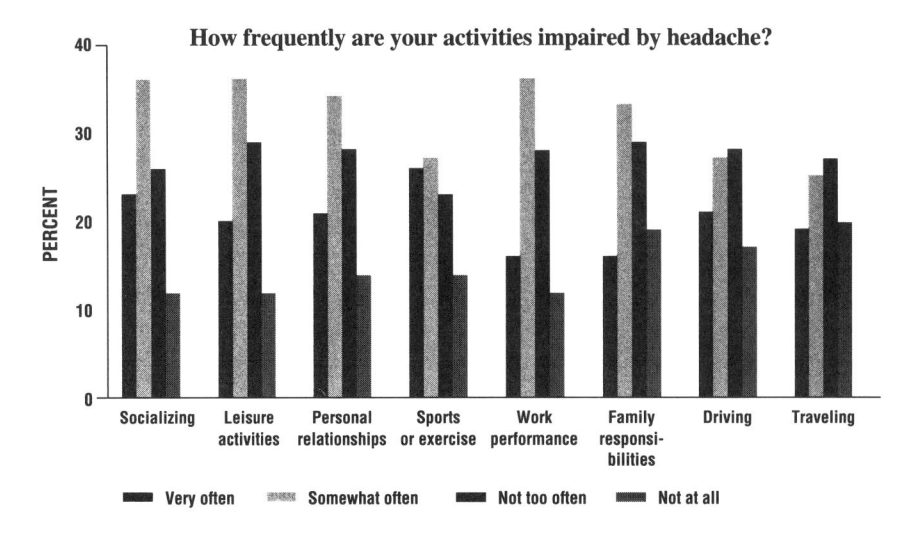

Figure 12.2.

Pain Sourcebook

The migraineurs were then asked to rate the severity of the migraine on a scale of one to ten, where "0" equals no pain at all and "10" equals pain "as bad as it can be." Most rated their pain an "8" or higher, and just over one-third gave their pain a "10." Asked about how their worst headaches affected their level of functioning, using a similar one-to-ten scale, most migraineurs rated their level of impairment at "7" or greater.

The migraineurs interviewed reported missing an average of three days of work, school or homemaker work because of headache in the past three months. In that same period, they reported going to work with a severe headache an average of five days. They estimated their level of functioning at an average of 60 percent on these days.

Asked about the impact of their condition on a variety of normal activities, most migraineurs said that their headaches interfered with most activities. Six in ten (59 percent) report their migraine limits their socializing very often or somewhat often. Similarly, 58 percent say that their headaches limit their leisure activities very often or somewhat often; and 55 percent say that their personal relationships are impaired by their headaches. Roughly half report similar levels of impairment in exercise and sports participation (53 percent), work performance (52 percent), performance of family responsibilities (49 percent), driving (48 percent) and traveling (44 percent).

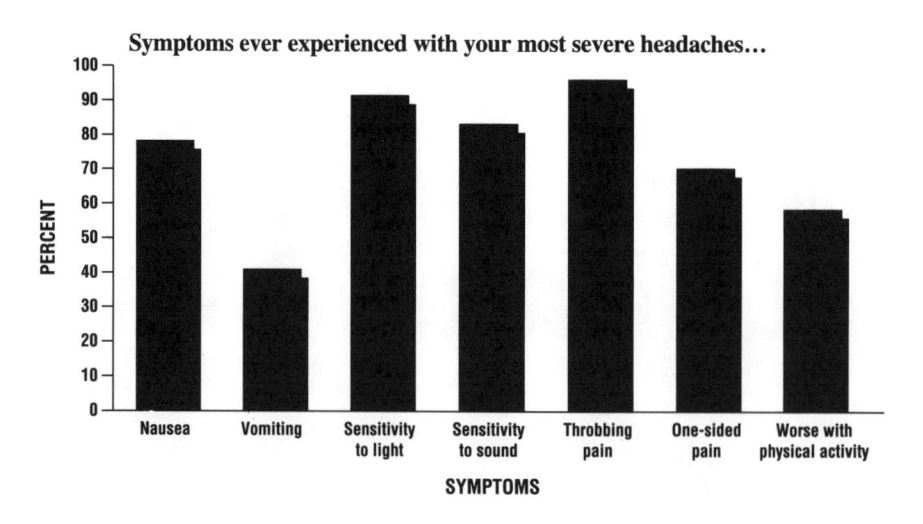

Figure 12.3.

Results of a National Poll of Migraine Sufferers

What Are the Symptoms?

Among those surveyed, 17 percent experience aura with their migraine and 84 percent have migraine without aura. Nine in ten migraineurs (91 percent) describe sensitivity to light and 84 percent experience sensitivity to sound during their attacks. Most describe the level of sensitivity as moderate. However, four in ten report that their sensitivity to light is severe (29 percent) or very severe (10 percent). Similarly, 31 percent say that the sensitivity to sound is severe, and 8 percent describe it as very severe.

More than three-quarters of the migraineurs in the survey said that they sometimes experienced nausea during some of their attacks—a little under half (46 percent) of these have nausea at least half the time during their severe attacks. About 42 percent of all migraineurs interviewed said they experience vomiting during their attacks—of these, 38 percent vomit during at least half of their attacks. Only about 12 percent said they took something to treat their nausea.

Nausea is an important symptom because it is used to help diagnose migraine. It is also important because gastrointestinal (GI) symptoms can interfere with the effectiveness of migraine treatments taken by mouth. Even when people can swallow a pill and keep it down, absorption through the GI tract may be slower, so that they get little benefit from the medicine.

What Do You Take for it?

A little more than half (54 percent) of migraineurs said they have taken at least one type of prescription medication for their headaches at one time, and virtually all have used at least one kind of over-the-counter (OTC) pain reliever. Of those who have tried OTCs, 20 percent said that these medicines were very successful, and 45 percent said they were somewhat successful in relieving their headache. Another 14 percent said the OTC pain relievers were not at all successful in relieving their headache pain.

More than one-third (36 percent) report using a prescription medication taken by mouth. Only 8 percent use nasal sprays, 6 percent use injections, and 4 percent use suppositories. This is an important finding, since non-oral medications are often recommended for migraineurs with nausea. However, of the migraineurs with nausea, an overwhelming majority (84 percent) of those surveyed said they preferred a pill to a nasal spray if a new, effective medication were offered to them. If a pill does not work, a nasal spray is the preferred second choice.

Have You Seen a Doctor? Did You Get Help?

On average, the adult migraineurs interviewed have suffered from migraines for about sixteen years. Over half (56 percent) said that they had seen a doctor at least once for their headaches. Of these, only half (51 percent) said that their doctor had diagnosed their condition as migraine.

Among those who have ever seen a physician about their headaches, a little over a third (36 percent) are currently being treated. A little over half (56 percent) of those say that they are very satisfied with the care and treatment they are receiving, and another 30 percent described themselves as fairly satisfied with their treatment.

On average, those migraineurs currently seeing a doctor say they have consulted three different doctors about their headaches. Those who have not seen a doctor for more than a year were asked about their reasons. Close to half (47 percent) said their doctor gave them a treatment that works. Another 37 percent said that their headaches were not a serious problem. Some said that treatment was expensive (32 percent) and/or that the doctor did not help (30 percent).

Those migraineurs (44 percent) who have never seen a doctor about their headaches were also asked about their reasons. Over three-quarters (78 percent) said that OTC medicines helped. Three in five (59 percent) said that their headache problem was not serious. Forty percent

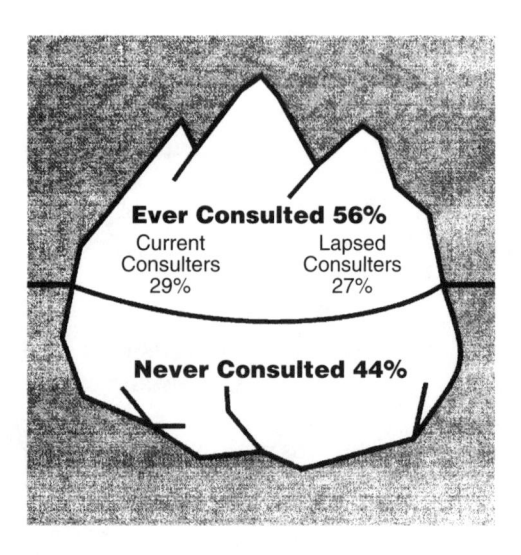

Figure 12.4. The Consultation Iceberg

Results of a National Poll of Migraine Sufferers

said they found a treatment elsewhere and 38 percent said treatment was expensive. One in five (20 percent) believes a doctor cannot help their severe headaches.

Migraine Awareness: The Need for Patient and Physician Education

Surprisingly, less than half of the respondents (49 percent) with the symptom profile of migraine realized that their condition was migraine. Of these less than half (46 percent—about 21 percent of all the migraineurs) had been diagnosed by a doctor. Those who did not believe they had migraines tended to identify their condition as stress, sinus or tension headache.

Only half of those who saw a doctor reported being given a diagnosis of migraine, suggesting physician error or miscommunication/lack of communication between the physician and the patient. Knowing that the headaches are migraine has important implications for treatment and prevention, including identifying and avoiding the individual's migraine triggers. Since most of those interviewed sought help from their primary care physician, there is a need to offer educational programs to this group of providers to ensure that headache sufferers receive a proper diagnosis to guide treatment.

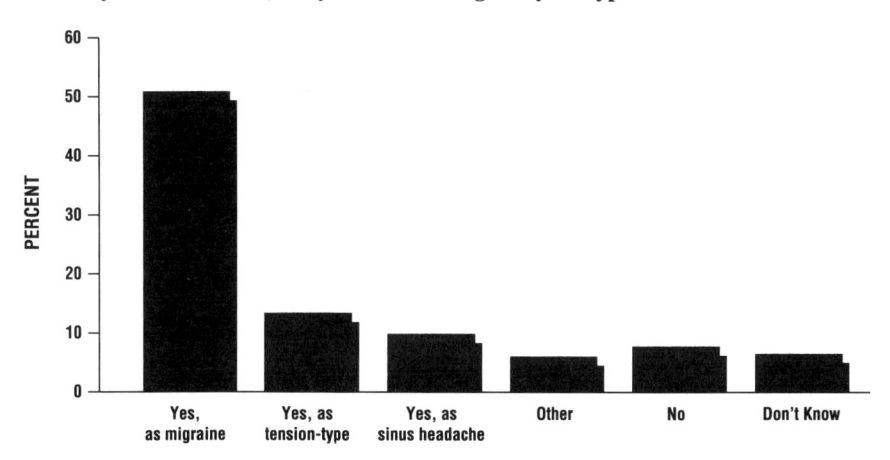

Figure 12.5.

Pain Sourcebook

Migraine is a highly variable condition—a minor nuisance for some, severely disabling for others. Self-care is appropriate when:

- the headache pattern is stable,
- medication use is relatively infrequent (less than two or three days per week),
- the medication provides a satisfactory level of pain relief, and
- there is little or no disability.

However, many of those who don't seek care would benefit from seeing a physician and trying suggested lifestyle changes and prescription medication.

Clearly, many people with migraine don't know they have it and treat themselves with OTC pain relievers. While this self-treatment can be satisfactory for those with mild to moderate headaches, many self-treaters reported significant pain and impairment. Those with nausea may be getting little benefit from their oral pain relievers, and the lack of a proper diagnosis limits the effectiveness of self-care and prevention measures.

To improve recognition and understanding of migraine, more educational efforts are needed at both the health care provider and consumer levels. AASH and ACHE have parallel missions to provide

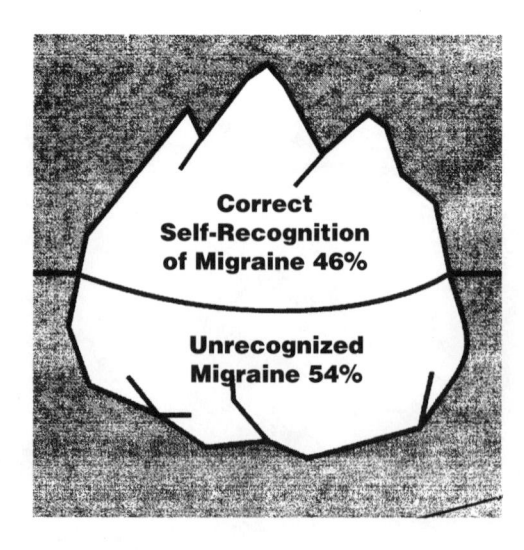

Figure 12.6. Migraine Recognition Iceberg

educational interventions that will improve awareness of migraine and its prevention and treatment. Since most of the migraineurs interviewed are not seeing a doctor, educational programs that operate outside the traditional health care system are required to reach and inform these headache sufferers.

Major Findings and Their Implications

Problem:

- A majority of migraineurs have not been diagnosed as having migraine.

- The treatments they are using are not providing optimal symptom control.

Response:

- AASH: Educate doctors in diagnosing and treating migraine.

- ACHE: Increase community outreach to help migraineurs educate themselves and "network" to achieve better care.

—by Richard B. Lipton, M.D.

Chapter 13

Sleep: Searching a New Frontier for Answers

Seeking knowledge in the field of pain and headache disorders is like the mission of the Starship Enterprise. Re-worded it could say: "To explore strange new symptoms, seek out new knowledge and understanding, and to boldly learn what no man or woman has learned before."

One frontier worth exploration is the relationship between sleep and headaches. After reviewing the numerous facts collected in patient histories, the emergence of a common thread in sleep disturbances reported by some patients went beyond simple insomnia. Some patients couldn't fall asleep and would lie awake for hours.

Others would have difficulty staying asleep and would awaken multiple times throughout the night. Some could even relate the exact times of arousal. Migraine sufferers noted that if they were sleep deprived even one night (insomnia) or had their sleep disturbed (such as noise from a dog or cat), a migraine could be triggered. Many of my migraine patients do not realize that sleep problems are one of their triggers. Patients with tension-type headaches almost always experience difficulty in their sleep patterns. Some go without a normal night's sleep for so long they don't even consider a poor night's sleep as abnormal or part of the problem.

Careful assessment can help determine if the sleep disturbance causes the headache or is caused by the headache.

©1995 National Headache Foundation. Reprinted with permission. Permission to reprint granted by the National Headache Foundation, Chicago, IL. For more information on headache causes and treatments, call the NHF at (800) 843-2256.

Unraveling the puzzle is complex and requires a thorough examination of the patient. Co-existing or other medical problems must be explored. Anxiety and adjustment disorders, many types of depression, sleep apnea, previous head trauma, medical and psychiatric causes, and medication abuse must be considered. Almost weekly I discover patients chronically using sedative benzodiazepines (Xanax, Valium, Ativan, and so on) or hypnotics at bedtime. Although they help patients fall asleep, they rob patients of the most important stage of sleep if used repetitively—that stage of sleep when the body relaxes and its neurological systems shut down—stage IV sleep. Referred to as "super sleep," it is the restoration part of the sleep cycle and we suffer when it is disrupted. Using sedatives on a short-term basis in the way they are intended is acceptable, but many patients with sleep problems are unable to limit their use because they either have an undiagnosed sleep disorder or they become hooked and can't fall asleep without using them. Hypnotics such as Ambien, chloral hydrate, Doriden, Dalmane, Restoril, and Doral are known as "knock out drops" and rarely provide restorative sleep. These should only be used on a short-term basis for simple insomnia.

The use of hypnotics and sedatives is a double-edged sword. Their long-term abuse or misuse may cause interruption of sleep (sleep rebound) that can create or aggravate tension-type headaches or be a trigger for migraines. For the migraine sufferer who has occasional sleep deprivation such as jet lag or a bad day at work, the short-term use of an hypnotic may avoid triggering a migraine.

The most commonly known diagnosed sleep disorder is sleep apnea. It has been known to cause or trigger migraines, tension headaches, and many other symptoms associated with non-restorative sleep. One of my patients developed migraines without aura and did not respond to normal treatment. A sleep study uncovered true sleep apnea. Now he sleeps with oxygen but is free of headaches. This exemplifies a case where diagnosing and treating a sleep disorder rather than using drugs controlled the migraine.

Another young male patient did not respond well to migraine prophylactics (Inderal and Elavil) or sleep repairing medication. The headaches were reduced from one to two per week to two or three per month, which was helpful but not impressive control. A sleep diary gave us no further clues. One day I overheard a discussion by his family about their dog. Man's best friend was awakening the patient around 2:00 A.M. He would mechanically perform the required duties in a groggy state, return to bed, and forget the incident. It never occurred to him that this was disturbing his sleep and robbing him of stage IV sleep! When canine duties were shifted to another member of his family, the prophylactic drugs finally worked.

A nurse I treat for migraines was discussing a recent headache. It had kept her awake until 3:00 A.M. at which time she self-injected Imitrex. She could not recall any trigger factors, yet two nights before she suffered a loss in her family and had not slept well either night. More questioning yielded more evidence that when her sleep was disturbed due to a stressful event, she would suffer a migraine. In this case of insomnia with an identifiable cause, prescribing a simple, short-term hypnotic like Ambien helped. Her sleep diary confirmed that identifying the sleep disturbance and using Ambien for no more than one or two nights avoided night migraines.

In 1993, I was fortunate to attend lectures by four prominent neurologists on the topic of headache. They described the effects of disturbing the sleep of normal subjects causing them to miss stage IV sleep. Subjects became irritable and experienced short-term memory loss, a depressed state, loss of energy, and most importantly, they all developed tension-type headaches. When allowed to return to normal sleep patterns, the headaches persisted. A neurologist from The University of Colorado, stated that their treatment for headache relief was medication to repair sleep architecture. The drugs that did this best were certain tricyclic anti-depressants, specifically Elavil or Pamelor and a few others.

In conclusion, sleep is the essence for a fruitful, happy life. Without it there is anger, fatigue, frustration, memory problems, and despondency, not to mention headaches. Working together, the patient and physician can explore the sleep frontier to examine its relevance for each patient. After a careful medical interview resulting in a thorough patient history, your doctor may suggest you keep a sleep diary. A close look at your nighttime sleeping habits may offer some insight into potential daytime (or nighttime) relief.

—by Jay D. Bayer, D.O.

Pain Management and Evaluation
Greencastle, Pennsylvania

Chapter 14

What Can Be Done About Headache?

Today, thanks to medical research, doctors have a much better understanding about what causes headache and what can be done about it. They know, for example, that headache is a real biological disorder, caused by chemical changes in the brain which are frequently inherited. Chronic headache is not just due to "nerves" although stress can be an important aggravating factor. Rather than simply taking painkillers advertised on television, headache sufferers now can choose from a variety of surprisingly effective treatment programs. If you or someone you're close to has chronic headache, read this chapter about the various specific headache treatments available today, including stress reduction, biofeedback, exercise, and medications for both relief and prevention of headache. Then read the companion chapters describing the different types of headaches.

For best results managing headache, it's important to understand what happens during a headache and to take a look at how lifestyle—diet, sleep habits, stress, and exercise—can affect headaches. It helps to get in touch with the body through biofeedback and relaxation techniques. Headache sufferers may need to examine emotional factors in their lives, and may wish to explore how counseling, physical therapy, and massage can be helpful. Finally, each headache sufferer must be willing to work with his or her doctor to find the most effective medications for relief of his or her

© ACHE American Council for Headache Education, 875 Kings Highway, Suite 200, Woodbury, NJ 08096-3172. Reprinted with permission. For more information, please call 1-800-255-ACHE.

particular headache problem, since response to medication can vary from one person to another.

Diet and Headache

Can food allergies cause headache? Should certain foods be avoided?

There is very little evidence that food allergies have anything to do with headaches. Certain foods do contain substances called amines that may affect the brain and trigger migraines in susceptible or headache-prone individuals, but not through an allergic mechanism. Cheese, chocolate, and citrus, the "three Cs," are the most common offending foods, but only a minority of headache sufferers are affected. Some headache patients can eat these potential troublemakers when their lives are running smoothly, but during times of stress or fatigue, or at certain times of the menstrual cycle, these same substances may trigger attacks.

It's generally thought that a hereditary chemical imbalance in the brain causes susceptibility or proneness to headaches. This chemical imbalance involves serotonin, one of the neurotransmitters, or chemicals that transmit messages from one cell to another. Factors such as fatigue, irregular sleep patterns, stress, or hormone changes associated with the menstrual cycle may change the level or threshold of headache susceptibility or proneness, so that certain food "triggers" can set an attack in motion. Alcohol, especially red wine, is often mentioned by migraine sufferers as a trigger, especially when other factors have "set the stage."

What about food additives?

Nitrites, which are found in cured or processed meats such as turkey, ham, hot dogs, and sausage, can cause problems for some people, and so can monosodium glutamate, or MSG, which is found in Accent, meat tenderizers, canned meats and fish, and some Chinese restaurant food. This common food additive sometimes masquerades under a variety of other names, such as "textured protein" or "natural flavoring." New food labeling requirements will make it harder to conceal MSG.

Eating salty snack food has been linked to headache attacks by some studies. Use of aspartame (Nutrasweet®, Equal®) has been associated with a high frequency of headache in some studies, but not

What Can Be Done About Headache?

in others. Until this issue is settled, headache sufferers, especially those with migraine, should avoid this artificial sweetener.

Even though the foods and beverages mentioned don't cause problems for all headache sufferers, avoiding them for a while to see if this helps is worth trying. If you think diet may be an important factor in your attacks, a dietitian who has a special interest in this subject can be helpful. Keeping a headache diary can also help you spot troublesome foods or beverages, but remember that there may be a "lag period," commonly 3-12 hours but occasionally as long as a day, between the time a particular food or beverage is used and onset of the headache. It's also good to remember that some headaches may be triggered by a combination of foods. For example, you may be able to eat cheese by itself, but not in a pizza with pepperoni, which has cured meat containing nitrites and may also be a headache trigger.

I've heard that caffeine can sometimes cause headache, but caffeine is also used in some painkillers. How can you explain this?

Sometimes it's easy to forget that caffeine is a drug. It's found not only in coffee but also in tea and many soft drinks. Caffeine is a stimulant that can speed up the heart, raise blood pressure, and interfere with relaxation. A good rule is to drink no more than two caffeinated beverages per day, or less if headaches are frequent. Strangely, once a headache has begun, caffeine can be helpful. This is because caffeine is an "adjuvant"—it enhances the effects of pain medicine. That's why caffeine is added to many over-the-counter medications used to treat headache.

Like some other drugs, caffeine can cause headache if over used by a rebound mechanism once the body comes to depend on it. This is the reason why it's probably not a good idea to avoid caffeine altogether on the weekend if you are accustomed to having one or more cups per day. If you decide to cut down on caffeine, it's best to do so very gradually.

What other diet factors are important?

Skipping meals, which can allow blood sugar levels to drop, seems to be one of the most common triggers mentioned by migraine patients. Anyone prone to frequent headaches should avoid skipping meals. A better idea is to have meals at regular intervals during the day, and to eat some protein at least three times during each day.

Stress Reduction, Rest, and Emotions

Can emotional upset cause headache attacks?

Feelings of worry, anxiety, or anger don't usually cause headache by themselves, but they may aggravate headache. Many people are not fully in touch with the emotions that may be affecting their health. Headache sufferers may benefit from exploring their feelings with their physician, or with a clinical psychologist or counselor. Learning stress reduction and stress management techniques can also be helpful.

How can friends and family help?

Friends and family members need to be informed about what's happening. Headache sufferers should tell their family and friends when pain is developing and the level of that pain (mild, moderate, or severe); share their plan for responding to the pain, for example with relaxation, medication, etc.; and at the same time make any requests of their family or friends.

Some headache sufferers may pretend that nothing is wrong or be ashamed to admit they are having a headache attack, heroically trying to carry on even when they are in significant pain. This is unfortunate, since such behavior denies family members and friends the opportunity to understand their headaches or to be helpful.

How about sleep habits?

While it's important to get enough rest, avoid oversleeping as well. It's best to go to bed and get up at about the same time each day, since this helps to regulate and stabilize the brain's important biological clocks. To make up for loss of sleep after a late night, set the alarm clock no more than one hour later than usual and then try taking a rest or nap later in the day if necessary.

Some people with frequent headaches either have difficulty falling asleep or wake up too early in the morning and are then unable to get back to sleep. If this is a problem, it should be discussed with a physician. Luckily, some of the treatments used to prevent headaches—medications, exercise, avoiding too much caffeine, and relaxation or biofeedback training—can help relieve sleep disturbances as well.

What Can Be Done About Headache?

Gaining Control with Biofeedback

What is biofeedback?

Many people can learn to control, at least to some degree, the internal reactions of their bodies through biofeedback training. The basic principle is simple: The more aware we are of a bodily process, the more control we can learn to exercise over it. With the help of a biofeedback therapist using a computer to monitor what is going on in the body, people can learn to become aware of bodily functions that normally aren't noticed, and then can learn to gain some control over those functions.

How can this kind of control be learned?

The signals from the computer and monitoring devices used in biofeedback training put you in more direct touch with your body. Biofeedback can be compared in some respects to a mirror, but a mirror of your inner responses instead of your outer appearance. Using the electronic "mirror" of the biofeedback computer helps you to change these inner responses.

How does biofeedback training work?

Biofeedback training can be thought of as another way to stabilize the erratic brain centers responsible for chronic headaches. The benefits appear to be long-lasting, and there are no problems with side effects. Biofeedback training is usually conducted by a biofeedback therapist or psychologist. People who choose this form of treatment are connected to monitoring devices and a computer that shows skin temperature and the level of muscular tension. This is a completely painless process.

Prescribed relaxation exercises affect the centers in the brain that control circulation, blood vessels, and the level of tension in the muscles. Measurable changes then begin to take place in the body as the patient learns to relax muscles around the head and neck reduce blood pressure, slow the pulse, and even relax the tiny muscles in the walls of blood vessels. The instruments can be thought of as aids to help get started. It's like using training wheels on a bicycle. Pretty soon they are no longer needed.

Does biofeedback training always work?

Numerous studies over the years show that most headache sufferers are able to reduce the intensity or duration of their attacks by at least half using this approach. As a bonus, most people feel more relaxed in general and more able to cope with the stresses and strains of everyday life. Since biofeedback training takes several months to be effective, physicians often take a combined approach by treating the headache problem with medication while biofeedback is learned.

Exercise, Physical Therapy, and Massage

How can exercise help ward off headaches?

Regular and vigorous physical exercise such as brisk walking, jogging, swimming, riding a bicycle, rowing, or aerobic dancing can be very relaxing and calming. Some headache specialists believe that such exercise may release substances in the brain called endorphins, which are powerful natural painkillers. The improved physical condition and the generally healthier, more attractive appearance that results from regular physical exercise gives a feeling of increased energy and well-being and can also build self-confidence. If you enjoy competitive games such as tennis or golf, taking a more playful approach may be helpful rather than viewing each game as a grim struggle.

If you're over 30 and not accustomed to regular exercise, you should be sure that no medical conditions are present that could cause problems before starting any of the more vigorous activities such as jogging. This means you may need to check with your physician. The simplest exercise program of all, and one of the safest, consists of regular brisk walking. One program is to walk 4 or 5 days each week, starting with about 15 to 20 minutes at a time and gradually working up to between 30 minutes and an hour as your schedule permits. Don't forget to wear comfortable shoes such as the special walking, aerobic, or jogging shoes now widely available. Never walk so fast that you flunk the "breath test"—that is, become so breathless that you can't carry on a conversation in a normal voice. Exercise can be an important part of any headache prevention program.

Can physical therapy and massage help? What's the difference?

Along with headache, there are often tightness and pain in neck muscles and upper back muscles, or less often, in the muscles involved in chewing. Physical therapists use heat, ultrasound, ice, and other measures to reduce this muscular tightness and the associated pain. Physical therapists also may use hands-on treatment to loosen and "mobilize" soft tissues, including muscles, tendons, and ligaments.

What Can Be Done About Headache?

Massage is generally provided by a massage therapist. The goal here is not only to reduce muscle tightness and pain, but also to help bring about a generally relaxed state. Usually a massage therapist works with major muscle groups all over the body, but he or she may focus on those that are particularly tight and uncomfortable.

Relief Medicines

What are some of the over-the-counter drugs that work for headache?

Some people with mild head pain can get relief with common painkillers such as aspirin, acetaminophen, or ibuprofen tablets. But, even these drugs should not be used more than two or, at most, three days per week to avoid rebound headache, which will be explained later. People with more severe headaches usually require more potent medications. An example would be the drug naproxen sodium, an anti-inflammatory drug and pain killer that is now available over the counter. Although stronger than aspirin, this drug isn't habit forming and is usually well tolerated with few side effects, although it can sometimes cause stomach burning or irritation. Often these over-the-counter painkillers are combined with caffeine, evidence suggests that the addition of caffeine can increase pain relief.

If over-the-counter medicines don't relieve headache, what other medications can doctors prescribe? Are there medicines specifically designed for headache?

Luckily, specific relief medicines are available that can stop or reduce the intensity of most chronic or recurrent headaches. These medicines are not painkillers in the usual sense, but they are thought to act directly on centers in the brain and blood vessels over the surface of the brain to restore stability and proper function. If your doctor prescribes such a medication, you should keep it handy or carry it with you. Since the medication may affect other parts of the body, it's important not to take a larger dose than is prescribed.

What kinds of specific medicines are available?

There are several different kinds of specific relief medications. Some are pills, and some are rectal suppositories. Suppositories are absorbed more quickly than pills and may be more effective although less convenient. Some people with especially violent attacks may even need to inject themselves with relief medications, just as diabetics give themselves insulin. Other medications may be given by use of an inhaler.

Specific Relief Medicines for Headache

How often can a person with headache take relief medication?

It's important to understand that if some relief medications are taken too frequently, they may lose their effectiveness and may even aggravate the headaches through a rebound mechanism. For example, if your doctor prescribes an ergot medication for you, then you should not take it more often than two days in a given week, and should not take it two days in a row. This is called the "rule of two." Your doctor may also restrict the use of other relief drugs and is your best source of advice about how frequently each medication can be used safely.

Does specific relief medication always work to stop the attack?

In medicine, very few treatments work all the time for everybody. For headaches having a clear-cut migraine or "vascular" pattern, relief medications are usually effective if the dose is properly adjusted. If an attack is already underway upon awakening, it's impossible to know how long ago it started, but in this situation it's probably best to try the relief medicine anyway.

Are there any medications that can be taken for relief of headache attacks that won't cause drowsiness so that I can continue working or other activities?

People with headache often ask this question. Most of the specific relief medications either don't cause drowsiness at all or don't cause drowsiness to the extent that bed rest is necessary. However, after taking relief medication, a person suffering from headache may need to rest in a quiet place without bright lights for about one-half hour in order to give the drug a chance to work. An ice pack, such as the reusable gel packs that can be kept in the freezer, may give some additional relief at this time.

If the specific relief drugs plus an ice pack don't give complete relief in the case of a stubborn attack, then rest or a short nap may be necessary for the nervous system to stabilize itself. In this situation, many physicians prescribe a mildly sedating "backup" medication or

What Can Be Done About Headache?

Table 14.1. Specific Relief Medicines for Headache

CATEGORY	EXAMPLES	ROUTE	MAJOR SIDE EFFECTS
serotonin agonist	DHE-45	injection	less nausea than with ergots
sumatriptan receptor subtype agonist	Imitrex®	injection	flushing, chest or neck tightness, tingling
ergots	Cafergot® Wigraine®	tablets, or suppositories	nausea, cramps, sometimes agitation
sympathomimetic agents	Midrin®	tablets	drowsiness, dizziness

Table 14.2. Nonspecific Relief Medicine for Headache

CATEGORY	EXAMPLES	ROUTE	MAJOR SIDE EFFECTS
narcotics	Codeine	tablets	nausea, drowsiness
	Demerol®	tablets, injection	dizziness, addiction, constipation
	Stadol®	nasal spray; injection	sedation
barbiturate-containing compounds	Fiorinal® Fioricet®, Esgic® Phrenilin®	tablets, capsules	drowsiness, dizziness, can be habit-forming
antinauseants	Phenergan® Thorazine® Compazine®	tablets, suppositories	drowsiness, dizziness
nonsteroidal anti-inflammatory drugs (NSAIDs)	Anaprox® Ansaid®	tablets	stomach irritation or bleeding, fluid retention
steroids	Decadron®	tablets, injection	stomach irritation, fluid retention

"rescue" medication that also has nausea-relieving properties. Sometimes this is given as a rectal suppository, a helpful form for patients with vomiting as a prominent part of their headache attacks. It may be necessary to take several doses of this medication to get the desired effects: taking the sharp edge off the pain, relieving any nausea, and allowing rest and preferably sleep.

How about narcotics? Won't they get rid of pain?

We live in a world where people often want quick answers, especially where pain is concerned. Unfortunately, real life isn't as simple as television ads suggest. Narcotics can be prescribed by a physician when pain is severe, but these drugs can also be habit-forming or addicting. Also, the more frequently they are used, the less effective they become. In addition, they may have other unpleasant side effects such as nausea, constipation, and a general "drugged" or groggy feeling.

Since there are other ways to relieve primary headaches and some very specific medications are now available, it's usually best to avoid or minimize the use of narcotics and other potentially habit-forming medications, especially when headaches are frequent.

Nonspecific Relief Medicine for Headache

What can be done for headache that strikes frequently or daily?

People with a proneness to headache may get into a pattern of having daily or almost daily headache. For some, migraine-type headache attacks may become so frequent that they finally blend together with no clear-cut beginning or ending of individual episodes. Taking some relief medications too frequently for headache may even make debilitating headaches more likely to strike on a daily basis. Daily or almost daily use of even such over-the-counter medications as aspirin, acetaminophen, and ibuprofen—or more commonly, combination sedative/painkillers—appears to interfere with the brain centers that regulate the flow of pain messages into the nervous system, thus worsening the headache disorder.

Each of us has a system in the brain to block pain. If you've ever burned your finger, you know that the pain may be very intense. After a short while, however, the pain starts to lessen. The body's natural pain-blocking system, which involves chemicals known as endorphins, acts to relieve the pain. Daily use of painkillers seems to

What Can Be Done About Headache?

interfere with this process and can lead to rebound headaches. Stopping daily use of painkillers and sedatives—without doing anything else—will almost always result in a considerable improvement in daily headaches as the body's own pain-fighting mechanisms gradually start to function properly again. This means that even if a person is only taking over-the-counter painkillers—but on a daily or almost daily basis—they will have to be given up until the body's own pain-fighting mechanisms recover. Daily use of painkillers and sedatives may also interfere with the action of the medications used to prevent headaches. Overuse of such common over-the-counter drugs as aspirin, ibuprofen, and acetaminophen can also cause other problems such as peptic ulcer, intestinal bleeding, ringing in the ears, dizziness, and kidney damage.

Do you mean that headache patients who give up daily painkillers may actually feel better rather than worse?

Yes, that's correct. Some people have little difficulty giving up painkillers, although they may experience temporary worsening of their headaches for a week or so. Those who have been depending on them for a long time to "get through the day," or who have been taking some of the stronger prescription painkillers, may have more difficulty. They may need to enter the hospital briefly when stopping medications to avoid a severe "rebound" headache. Specific anti-migraine medications (DHE-45) can be given by intravenous drip in the hospital to break the "pain cycle." In any case, physicians who specialize in treating headache can help patients through this transition period. As an added bonus, when people are no longer taking the daily painkillers, then preventive medications will work much better.

Preventive Medications

What do you mean by preventive medications?

Several medications that are taken daily to prevent headaches have come into widespread use over the last several years. Some of them are drugs used for other medical conditions that were accidentally discovered to help headache. They have truly brought about a revolution in treatment for people with frequent or especially severe attacks! While none of them actually cures the often inborn tendency toward chronic headache, all have the ability to stabilize and regulate the brain centers and brain chemicals thought to be responsible for the problem. By doing so, they reduce both the frequency and severity of headache attacks. These medications include certain anticonvulsants, some of the antidepressants, beta blockers, calcium channel blockers, ergot derivatives, and nonsteroidal anti-inflammatory drugs (NSAIDs). Researchers around the world are continuing to investigate new preventive drug therapies for headache.

Can these preventive drugs be habit forming or cause side effects?

These drugs are not habit-forming, but any medication can cause unwanted side effects. Doctors who prescribe these medications must work with their patients to carefully regulate the dosage so that side effects are minimized—starting with a small dosage and building up gradually. Side effects of these drugs are usually not serious but may cause some minor inconvenience, generally much more acceptable than the headaches. Depakote, Sansert, and Nardil are generally considered among the most effective of the preventive drugs but occasionally cause more serious side effects. So, careful monitoring is required if these drugs are used. To be effective, all of these preventive medications must be taken one or more times each day. It may

Table 14.3. Preventive Medications

CATEGORY	EXAMPLES	MAJOR SIDE EFFECTS
anticonvulsants	Depakote®	nausea, drowsiness, weight gain, tremor, rare liver inflammation
antidepressants	Elavil®, Pamelor®, Sinequan®	weight gain, dry mouth, constipation, fatigue
	Nardil®	weight gain, fluid retention, dietary precautions
	Prozac®, Zoloft®, Paxil®	insomnia, restlessness
beta blockers	Inderal®, Corgard® Tenormin®, Lopressor®	fatigue, depression, weight gain, memory disturbance, faintness, diarrhea, impotence
calcium channel blockers	Calan®, Isoptin® Cardizem®	constipation, dizziness
ergot derivatives	Sansert®, Methergine®	weight gain, leg cramps, rare scar tissue formation
NSAIDs	Naprosyn®, Anaprox®, Ansaid®	stomach irritation or bleeding, fluid retention

What Can Be Done About Headache?

be necessary to experiment to discover which preventive drug or combination of drugs works best to reduce the attacks, since none of them is effective in all cases.

How long does it take for these drugs to work? How long do you have to take them?

Careful daily records of headache frequency and severity while these medications are being used will permit the treating physician to judge how they are working. Since most of them require some time to stabilize the brain centers, headache sufferers must have the courage and commitment to give them time to act over a month or more, even if quick results aren't obtained. These drugs definitely don't give the "20-second relief" promised by television ads. Once good headache control has been achieved and maintained for six months or a year, it may be possible to taper down and stop preventive medications without having the headaches come back as frequently as before. In other cases, it's necessary to take the medications for several years.

It sounds like there are many things I can do myself to relieve my headaches. Is this correct?

Yes, a doctor can be helpful, but there are many things people can and must do themselves. The best results are achieved when the doctor and the patient form a committed team to tackle the problem together. Usually, the more treatment approaches that are taken, the better the chances of managing the headache problem successfully. Remember that headache, like diabetes, arthritis, high blood pressure, and many other common disorders that doctors treat, generally can't be cured, but usually can be controlled.

There's one more thing that can be very helpful. At the end of this chapter is a daily headache record form, or what's called a "headache diary." Many headache sufferers find keeping a headache diary an extremely helpful way to identify triggers and to track their progress. If headaches only occur occasionally (less than once a week), it's only necessary to fill out the form on headache days. Rate the severity of the attacks on a one-to-three scale as explained in the instructions.

Since people with headache react to many different triggers, and since these triggers vary from one person to another, it's helpful to note the circumstances surrounding each attack, including life events, foods, feelings, stress levels or anything else that could contribute both to attacks of headache or—equally important—to days free of pain.

Severity Scale:

0. Headache-free
1. Mild headache, allowing normal activity
2. Moderate headache, disturbing but not preventing normal activity
3. Severe headache, normal activity is impossible. Bed rest may be necessary.

Relief Measures

1. Ice Pack
2. Bed rest
3. Dark room
4. Medication (list name and dosage)
5. Relaxation techniques
6. Other (please specify)

Headache Triggers

1. Alcohol
2. Chocolate
3. Aged cheese
4. Citrus fruits
5. Cured meats
6. MSG
7. NutraSweet®
8. Skipped meals
9. Nuts
10. Onions
11. Salty foods
12. Excess caffeine
13. Stress
14. Fatigue
15. Missed medication
16. Eyestrain or other visual triggers

What Can Be Done About Headache?

HEADACHE DIARY (Circle dates of menstrual flow)

Date	Severity 0 1 2 3	Relief Measures	Headache Triggers
1			
2			
3			
4			
5			
6			
7			
8			
9			
10			
11			
12			
13			
14			
15			
16			
17			
18			
19			
20			
21			
22			
23			
24			
25			
26			
27			
28			
29			
30			
31			

Chapter 15

How to Find a Headache Doctor

Having a chronic pain condition means you are likely to spend much time and money in physicians' offices, and perhaps in emergency rooms as well. Achieving pain control requires a strong working partnership with a physician who is caring, knowledgeable, and compatible. He or she may be a headache expert, a neurologist or other specialist, or your family doctor. The key element is not necessarily the doctor's area of practice. What matters most is the doctor's respect for the reality of your pain and your mutual willingness to trust each other and to keep trying.

Think of your first appointment as an interview. You will need to be able to answer the doctor's questions about the history and pattern of your headaches. You should also be asking questions to evaluate the doctor's ability and willingness to help you.

Questions to Ask the Doctor

- Have you treated many patients with migraine or other headache conditions?
- What do you think causes headaches like mine?
- Do you think headache conditions like mine are treatable?

©1995 *Headache*. American Council for Headache Education Newsletter. April 1995 issue. Adapted from *Migraine: The Complete Guide*, by the American Council on Headache Education, with Lynne M. Constantine and Suzanne Scott. A 1994 Dell Trade Paperback, Reprinted with permission. For more information, please call 1-800-255-ACHE.

- If the drug prescribed doesn't work for me or has too many side effects, are there other alternatives we can try?
- Will you give me a written treatment plan to follow?

In listening to the doctor's responses, you want to know that he or she has experience with headache, knows the most recent biochemical theories of headache and believes it to be treatable, but is aware that multiple strategies may be necessary. A doctor who has either too little or too much confidence that a medical treatment will resolve chronic headaches is not likely to be the best choice. Continuing the relationship may only frustrate both of you.

The partnership concept implies that both parties have a role to play in keeping the patient healthy. Here are some equally important questions to ask yourself.

- Am I willing to follow the doctor's treatment plan, even if it means making lifestyle changes that are hard for me?
- Am I going to be honest with this doctor about what I did or didn't do that might have had an impact on treatment success?
- Will I stick with this relationship even if the treatment prescribed doesn't bring me pain relief right away?

Just as with any other type of relationship, good communication, openness and realistic expectations are essential prerequisites for a successful doctor-patient relationship.

Part Three

Backaches

Chapter 16

Back Talk: Advice for Suffering Spines

"Some days," says Linda, "my back hurts so much that I can't stand to have clothes touching me."

If misery loves company, Linda's got plenty of it. At least once in their lives, about 80 percent of Americans will experience a bout of low back pain that can range from a dull, annoying ache to absolute agony. According to *American Family Physician*, on any given day 6.5 million Americans are under some sort of treatment for low back pain.

After headaches, low back pain is the second most common ailment in the United States and is topped only by colds and flu in time lost from work. Low back pain has been described as a 20th century epidemic, the nemesis of medicine, and an albatross of industry. When all the costs connected with it are added up—job absenteeism, medical and legal fees, social security disability payments, workmen's compensation, long-term disability insurance—the bill to business, industry and the government has been estimated to total at least $16 billion each year. Those most often affected are young adults in their most productive years, from ages 17 to 45.

There's no mystery in why Linda's back hurts. Her spine will never be the same because an automobile accident left her with four fractured vertebrae and a destroyed disc. Though accidents are responsible for a fair share of back pain, most backaches are not caused by anything so dramatic.

FDA Consumer, April 1989.

Sedentary Lifestyles

It is believed that many cases of low back pain are due to stresses on the muscles and ligaments that support the spine. Our sedentary jobs and lifestyle make us vulnerable to this type of damage. Too much time in front of the TV, not enough exercise, poor posture, and poor sleeping habits (including sleeping on the stomach) weaken muscles. Weak muscles, especially abdominal muscles, cannot support the spine properly. Obesity, which afflicts 34 million Americans, is another factor—it increases both the weight on the spine and the pressure on the discs.

When the body is in poor shape, it doesn't take much to overstretch (strain) a muscle or put a small tear in (sprain) a ligament. The medical word for backaches arising from either of these conditions is lumbosacral strain (or sprain). Sometimes, a sudden twist or fall can bring on muscle spasm—sudden, involuntary contractions that can be excruciatingly painful. A spasm immobilizes the muscles over the injured area, possibly acting as a kind of splint to protect muscles or joints from further damage.

Jobs that involve bending and twisting, or lifting heavy objects repeatedly—especially when the loads are beyond a worker's strength—are no better for the back than are sedentary jobs. Certain occupations, such as truck driving or nursing, are particularly hard on the back. The truck driver must contend with sitting for long periods (actually worse for the back than standing), the vibration of the vehicle, and lifting and straining at the end of the day when muscles are fatigued and more susceptible to damage. (Truck driving ranks first in workmen's compensation cases for low back pain.) Football, gymnastics, and other strenuous sports can also damage the lower back.

Slipped Discs

Because many people are familiar with the term "slipped" disc, this problem is mistakenly believed to be the chief cause of most low back pain. But in fact, slipped discs are responsible for only 5 percent to 10 percent of the cases. Actually, the term itself is inaccurate because the disc doesn't slip at all; it bulges out between two vertebrae. In some cases, the tough tissues that contain the disc are weakened by injuries that allow the soft gel-like center to protrude. If the protrusion presses on a nerve root, pinching it against the bone, the result is pain in the area of the body served by that nerve. Doctors can tell which disc in the lower back is causing the problem by the part of the body affected, usually the legs.

The protruded part of the disc does not slip back into place. Scar tissue forms around the protrusion and walls it in. If the outer tissues continue to be stressed, they will weaken further and, in time, the slightest activity—a sneeze or cough—may cause the disc to burst through its capsule, or rupture.

As might be expected, pain from disc disease can rank pretty high on the pain index. To make matters worse, if a nerve root is irritated in any one place, it tends to become irritable along its whole length. A ruptured disc that presses on nerve roots in the low back (lower lumbar or high sacral areas) causes sciatica, a condition in which sharp, shooting pains begin in the buttock and run down the back of the thigh and the inside of the leg to the foot. Tingling, numbness and weakness may follow. If the pressure on the nerve root is not relieved, the leg muscles will eventually waste away, or atrophy.

"When sciatica occurs," explains Todd L. Samuels, M.D., Department of Neurology, Georgetown University Hospital, Washington, D.C., "we can pinpoint the specific nerve root or roots that are compressed in most cases by carefully examining the strength of individual muscles and deep tendon reflexes, and by noting where there's loss of sensation."

Samuels says that conservative treatment such as strict bed rest, anti-inflammatory medication, and muscle relaxants often relieve the acute symptoms. In intractable cases, surgery may be necessary to relieve pressure on the nerve root.

A large protrusion may also press on the nerves that branch off the end of the spinal cord (cauda equina), causing back pain, loss of sensation in the buttocks, thighs or genital organs, and bowel and bladder disturbances. When this, or any other symptoms of nerve root pressure, occur, help should be sought immediately.

Anatomy of a Backache

Knowing a little about the spine and its parts makes it easier to understand why things can go wrong with the back. Though humans are born with 33 separate vertebrae (the bones that form the spine), by adulthood most have only 24. The nine vertebrae at the base of the spine grow together. Five form a triangular bone called the sacrum—those two dimples in most everyone's back are where the sacrum joins the hipbones (the sacroiliac joint). The lowest four form the tailbone, or coccyx, often united with the sacrum above.

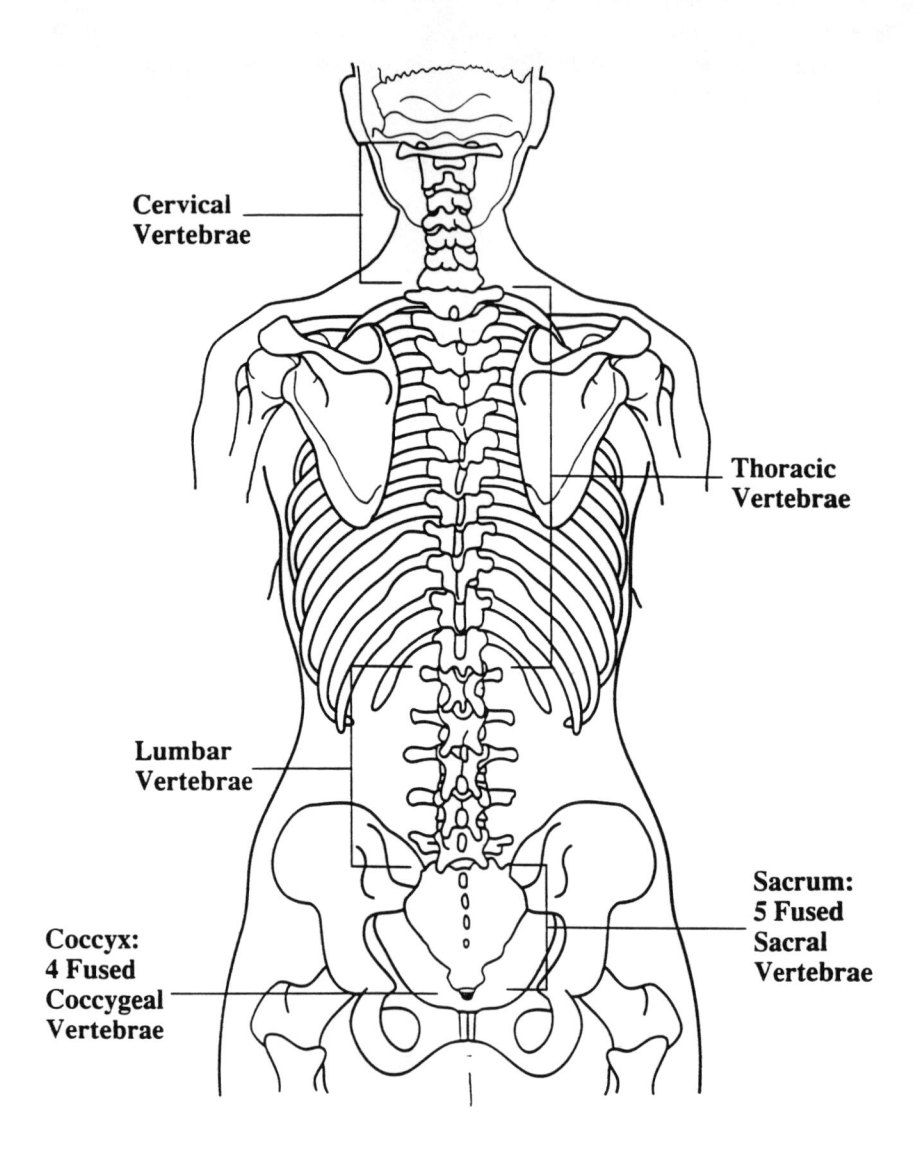

Figure 16.1. The Human Spine

Back Talk: Advice for Suffering Spines

Physicians use a code to identify the vertebrae. The seven in the neck, the cervical vertebrae that support and provide movement for the head, are called C1 to C7. The thoracic vertebrae, numbered Tl to T12, join with and are supported by the ribs, which protect the heart and lungs. Because they're fairly rigid, thoracic vertebrae don't permit much movement, and, consequently, aren't injured as often as the other vertebrae. The lumbar vertebrae below the thoracic vertebrae and above the sacrum, are most frequently involved in back pain, because they carry most of the body's stress. They are known as Ll to L5.

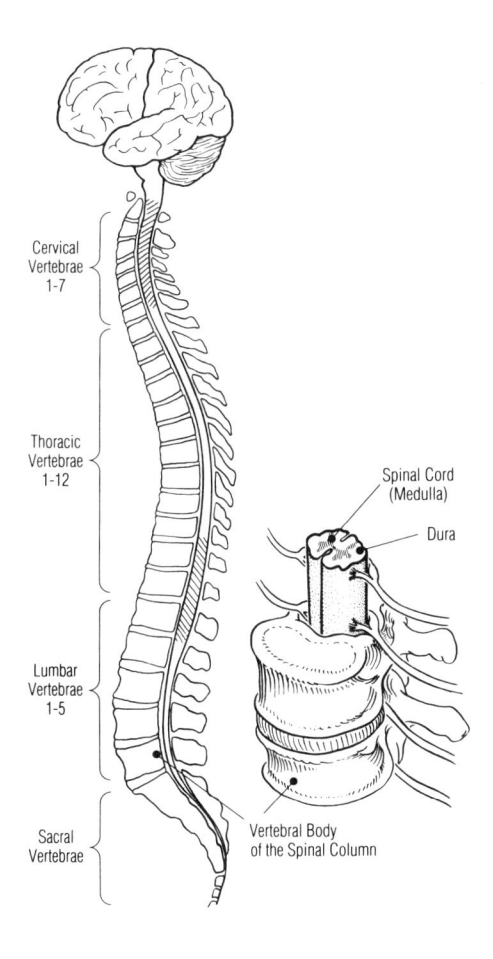

Figure 16.2. The cervical vertabrae are numbered C1 to C7. The thoracic vertebrae are numbered T1 to T12. The lumbar vertebrae are numbered L1 to L5.

Pain Sourcebook

The vertebrae are not stacked one on top of the other in a straight line; each rests on the one below at an angle, forming an S-curve when viewed from the side. The vertebrae would collapse like a house of cards without tough ligaments that secure one to another, and strong muscles and tendons that keep the spinal column upright.

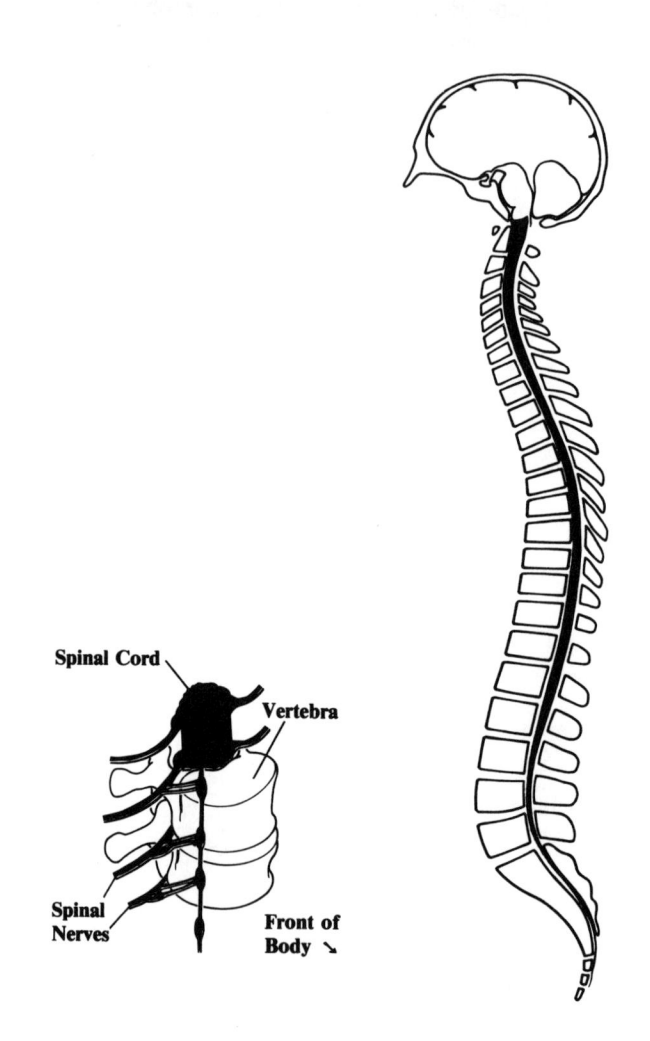

Figure 16.3. *The spinal cord extends from the brain to the lower back. The detail shows the snug fit of the cord inside the spinal column. Both incoming and outgoing nerve signals are carried in the spinal nerves which exit from the sides of the cord through the spaces in the certebrae.*

Back Talk: Advice for Suffering Spines

Sandwiched between each pair of adjacent vertebrae is a spinal disc, 23 discs in all. Discs are flat, round structures—about one-quarter to three-quarters of an inch thick—of tough outer rings of tissue that contain a soft, white jelly-like center. Each disc is connected to the vertebrae above and below it by flat, circular plates of cartilage. The discs not only keep the vertebrae apart, but act as shock absorbers. They compress when weight is put on them, and spring back when the weight is removed.

While we need the strong, solid parts of the lumbar vertebrae (vertebral bodies) to bear the body's weight, only joints will allow us to bend backward and forward, twist and turn. These joints are found in a ring-like structure of bone, known as the arch, at the rear of each vertebra. The arch has a hollow center and little bones that go off in several directions, serving as anchors for muscles and ligaments. A pair of vertical bones projecting upward and another pair projecting downward—the facet joints—glide on similar smooth surfaced bones in the vertebrae above and below them, creating an interlocking column of bones. The hollow areas of the arches form a channel (spinal canal) that encloses and protects the spinal cord. The only parts of the spine that we can feel with our fingers are projections from the bony rings called spinous (thorn-like) processes. Each spinous process bends down slightly over the one below to form an extra shield for the spinal cord.

The spinal cord, an extension of the brain, extends as far as L1, where it ends in a sheaf of nerves (*cauda equina*) resembling a horse's tail. Throughout the length of the spine, 31 pairs of nerves branch off from the spinal cord and serve all parts of the body, transmitting sensory messages to the brain (the pot is hot), and messages from the brain to the muscles (withdraw your hand). Where the nerves exit from the spinal cord through spaces (foramina) between adjacent vertebrae, they are called nerve roots. Few people are aware that when the neck is bent forward as far as it will go, the whole spinal cord moves upwards in the spinal canal. Anything that prevents the cord and nerves from moving freely, such as abnormal bone growth within the spinal canal, will cause tingling or pain.

Thirty-three vertebrae, 23 discs, 31 pairs of spinal nerves, 140 muscles that hook on to the vertebrae, plus ligaments, tendons, cartilage—all very complicated and all potential sources of back trouble. Small wonder that in 80 percent of the cases doctors can't pinpoint exactly what is causing, the ailing back.

Pain That Comes with Aging

Degenerative conditions that go along with aging can also cause low back pain. The bloom may still be on the cheek, but things are slowly falling apart within. Muscles reach their peak capacity by age 20, then decline without proper exercise. Disc degeneration begins in the early 20s. Though discs in babies are about 90 percent water, by age 70 fluid loss reduces the water content to 70 percent, flattening the discs. (Because discs constitute 25 percent of the spine's length, as the discs become flatter and less elastic, people lose height: Most of us can expect to be about a half inch to two inches shorter in old age.) When discs shrink, they lose their ability to act as shock absorbers, putting greater stress on supporting ligaments, causing back pain.

Back pain can also result from osteoporosis, a disorder that robs bones of calcium and makes them porous, so that vertebrae crush or fracture easily. Though both men and women lose bone density after age 35, the disease appears most often in women past menopause. It is thought that failure to develop adequate bone mass during youth, lack of exercise, and a diet low in calcium and other nutrients may be contributing factors. Smoking and over-consumption of alcohol may also be involved.

Spinal joints are also affected by various types of arthritis. One type that most of us will experience, if we live long enough, is degenerative joint disease, or osteo-arthritis. The cartilage that cushions joints gradually breaks down, resulting in back pain and stiffness, especially in the morning. Osteo-arthritis may appear as early as the 20s and 30s, though without symptoms, and nearly everybody has it by age 70.

A particularly distressing type of arthritis is ankylosing spondylitis. The lower back and sacroiliac joints become stiff and swollen. Muscle spasm and back pain may be so severe that bending over is the only way to relieve it. If untreated, in some cases the inflamed spinal joints may fuse, preventing the individual from straightening up. The disease affects more men than women, usually starting between the ages of 20 and 40, though it can begin as early as 10. The cause is unknown, but it is believed that some people may be genetically susceptible to this disorder. Posture-maintaining exercises, hot baths, painkillers, and non-steroidal anti-inflammatory drugs may help relieve symptoms.

Referred Pain

To add insult to injury, pain can be "referred" to the back from other parts of the body. Prostate problems in men, a retroverted or "tipped" uterus in women, peptic ulcers, colitis, gallbladder disease, heart disease, cancer that has spread to the spine from other organs (most often the breast, lung, prostate and kidney), and many other conditions can all be felt as back pain. People can also be born with abnormalities or develop conditions, such as scoliosis that predispose them to back pain when they grow older. Infections of the spine, although rare, can also cause back pain. And it is possible to have severe back pain of a psychological, rather than physiological, nature.

The good news is that acute low back pain, especially when caused by lumbosacral strain, often goes away by itself in a few days to a few weeks. Sometimes it's not even necessary to see the doctor. Rest is the basic treatment. A day or two in bed to take the weight off the spine, some aspirin or other pain reliever, an ice bag or a hot water bottle on the back—whichever feels more comfortable—are usually all that's needed. Even disc problems respond to rest; the protruding tissue shrinks, and pressure on the nerve lessens.

But rest can be overdone. Dr. Alf Nachemson, the eminent Swedish orthopedist who designed the Volvo automobile seat for good back support, noted at a National Institutes of Health conference on low back pain in 1988 that recovery is quicker when people are moderately active, even if they feel some pain. He warned that prolonged bed rest is not beneficial because it weakens muscles.

Manipulation by chiropractors or osteopaths appears to afford short-term relief in some cases. (But when the problem is disc herniation or osteoporosis, manipulation may make matters worse.)

It is reassuring to know that with or without treatment some 60 percent of back pain sufferers go back to work within a week, and nearly 90 percent return within six weeks.

When to See a Doctor

But, if there's no relief from pain after a few days in bed, or if pain is severe or recurs, it's time to see the family doctor. There's no time to waste if radiating pain, numbness, tingling or weakness occurs in the arms or legs, or if the bowel or bladder doesn't function properly. It also makes sense to consult the doctor if a child or elderly person has back pain. Fever or vomiting with the pain may indicate infection.

Because so many conditions can contribute to back pain, it's not always easy to pinpoint the cause, even using the best technology available. Nevertheless, if the pain won't let up and the cause can't be determined after the doctor has taken a complete medical history and conducted a comprehensive physical examination, referral to a specialist may be needed.

Specialists—orthopedists, neurologists, neurosurgeons, rheumatologists, internists—have an array of diagnostic tests at their disposal:

- **X-rays** can show bone deformities or fractures of the spine. Although the discs themselves cannot be seen, vertebrae that appear too close together may indicate that the disc has ruptured or degenerated. Though helpful in diagnosing certain diseases, such as ankylosing spondylitis and osteoporosis, X-rays are more valuable for what they rule out—for example, cancer or tuberculosis—than for what they reveal.

- **CAT-scans (computerized axial tomography)** are special X-rays used with a computer to produce images of a "slice" of anatomic tissue. They're good for looking at the spinal cord, spinal bones, fractures, osteoarthritis damage, narrowed spinal canal (spinal stenosis), tumors, and spinal cord infections.

- **Magnetic resonance imaging (MRI)** uses a strong magnetic field and a computer to create highly detailed images of soft tissues, such as muscles, cartilage, ligaments, tendons, blood vessels, and, to a lesser extent, bone. MRI can also show disc degeneration, protrusion and rupture, infection, and other spinal disorders.

- A **myelogram** is another type of X-ray examination. Before taking X-rays, the radiologist injects a contrast medium (dye) into the spinal canal. This dye blocks X-rays and outlines the spinal cord and spinal nerves. Myelograms can show a ruptured disc.

- An **electromyogram (EMG)** is a graphic record of muscle contraction that can show nerve and muscle damage.

When Surgery Is Called for

Although physicians prefer to treat even severe cases of low back pain conservatively with bed rest and painkillers, surgery is clearly called for if pressure on a nerve root causes severe pain lasting for weeks, or if progressive damage to the nerves results in leg weakness or paralysis. Every year, about 200,000 Americans undergo surgery for persistent back pain.

Back Talk: Advice for Suffering Spines

"There are several operations that we do to relieve back pain . . . The most common one is the removal of the slipped disc or herniated disc," says Edward R. Laws Jr., M. D., professor and chairman of neurosurgery at George Washington University, Washington, D.C. "We get at the slipped disc by removing only a very small part of the bone—the arch of the vertebra. [This procedure is called a laminectomy.] Then we remove the part of the disc that's out of place and any other loose fragments that are accessible."

Another condition that requires laminectomy is spinal stenosis, an unusual narrowing of the space inside the spinal canal. A narrow spinal canal may cause pressure on the nerve roots and, in rare cases, on the cord itself. "That's the second most common operation that we do" says Laws. "Some people are born with a narrow spinal canal . . . [others have] buildup of ligaments and bone spurs that narrow the spinal canal. They occur as a result of wear and tear, of having the spine work against gravity over time."

"In some cases, we do spinal fusion," continues Laws. "The spine is made up of a number of joints, and if a joint is unstable and slips, [causing] nerve root pinching, we can stop the slipping by fusing two vertebrae together." To do this, surgeons insert fragments of the patient's own bone, usually taken from the hip, to bridge the space between two adjacent vertebrae. In time, the bones grow together. Fusion relieves pain but reduces mobility.

A 1987 NIH report to Congress estimated that fewer than 1 in 10 people with low back pain requires surgery. Of these, about one-fifth have unsuccessful outcomes—a rather unsettling statistic. "I can see where some analyses would turn out that way, because if you take all comers and look at how the patients do three, four, five years after surgery, only about 75 percent have really great results," comments Laws. "Sometimes, the wrong operation is done, or an operation is done on a patient who could have gotten by without one. There's no doubt that there are a lot of mighty sore backs out there." To avoid unnecessary surgery, it is wise to get a second opinion.

A Drug Instead of the Knife

In a small percentage of cases, sciatic pain caused by a herniated disc that would normally require surgery is treated by some physicians with chymopapain. This drug, approved by FDA in 1982, is an enzyme found in papaya that is used to tenderize meat, make beer, and clear cloudy contact lenses. Injected into the disc's jelly-like center, chymopapain dissolves the disc, thus lessening pressure on the nerve root. The drug has had its champions and detractors ever since it was introduced, but when used in patients in whom conservative treatment has failed and who are candidates for surgery, it can be very successful. Its advantages over surgery are a shorter hospital stay, less expense, less scarring, and less trauma. Since some people are highly allergic to the drug, skin tests must be done first to detect chymopapain sensitivity in candidates for treatment.

A relatively new technique called aspiration percutaneous lumbar diskectomy (APLD) may be useful for people allergic to chymopapain and those for whom general anesthesia is risky. Using X-ray pictures as a guide, the neurosurgeon or orthopedist inserts a long, thin needle called a nucleotome probe into the center of the protruding disc. The physician loosens the disc material by moving the probe back and forth. A pump attached to the probe suctions up the material and carries it away.

APLD takes about 40 minutes, requires about 10 days recuperation, and costs a great deal less than laminectomy. However, not everybody is a suitable candidate for this procedure. It cannot be used on those who have severely ruptured discs or spinal stenosis.

To Prevent Recurrences

People who've had one backache are not anxious to have another. There are some things they can do to help prevent recurrences:

- Exercise regularly to strengthen back and abdominal muscles. Walking, swimming, bike riding, and walking in chest-deep water are particularly helpful in building up trunk and thigh muscles.

- Before participating in sports that are recommended by the doctor, warm up by gently stretching for a few minutes to reduce tension and strain.

- Stop smoking. (Some researchers believe that a cigarette smoker's cough may contribute to low back pain by putting pressure on the discs.)

- Lose weight, if necessary, to lessen strain on the back.

- Maintain correct posture. Sit with shoulders back and feet flat on the floor, or on a footstool or chair rung. Stand with head and chest high, neck straight, stomach and buttocks held in, and pelvis forward.

Back Talk: Advice for Suffering Spines

- Use comfortable, supportive seats while driving.
- Use a firm mattress, and sleep on the side with knees drawn up or on the back with a pillow under bent knees.
- Lift by bending at the knees, rather than the waist, using leg muscles to do most of the work.
- Avoid standing or working in any one position for too long. Shift weight from one leg to another.
- Try to reduce emotional stress that causes muscle tension.

—by Evelyn Zamula

Evelyn Zamula is a free-lance writer in Potomac Md.

Chapter 17

The New Thinking on Low-back Pain

Bed rest is out, exercise is in. Routine use of medications and invasive modalities is discouraged. And the best way to return to daily activities, the experts say, is never to abandon them in the first place.

A paradigm shift is occurring in the diagnosis and treatment of low-back problems, one that seems almost tailor-made for the era of managed care:

- It's a common problem. Back-related complaints are second only to the common cold as a reason for office visits to primary care physicians in the United States.

- It's an expensive problem—the leading cause of disability in patients younger than 45 and one that costs the health system upwards of $20 billion a year.

- It's an overtested and often overtreated problem (imaging, surgery, medication), due in part to the fact that many research studies have not been well-defined.

The new thinking, though not universally embraced, emphasizes not only treating the pain but also keeping the patient up and about

---

©1995 Medical Economics from July 15, 1995 *Patient Care*. Reprinted with permission of *Patient Care*.

as much as possible to avoid the debilitation that results from inactivity. The salient features are incorporated in the Clinical Practice Guidelines on acute (less than three months' duration) low-back problems in adults, released in December 1994 by the Agency for Health Care Policy and Research (AHCPR)[1]:

- Bed rest is not the cornerstone of therapy it was once thought to be. True, it may provide brief symptomatic relief for some patients with severe pain, but increasing evidence indicates that it slows healing and contributes to debilitation.

- The new mantra is to emphasize the likelihood of spontaneous recovery of reasonable activity tolerance within four weeks for about 90 percent of patients with low-back complaints and to encourage either continued activity or a return to activity, including work, as soon as it is feasible.

- If bed rest is out, exercise is in—general fitness exercises as well as specific strengthening exercises for the back and, in some cases the trunk. These can help build tolerance until normal activities can be resumed.

- Imaging studies are often not needed and, unless there are "red flags" of possibly serious conditions, should be considered later rather than sooner, for those who are slowest to recover with time and modest intervention. Apart from their cost and radiation dose, imaging tests have great potential to mislead by showing age-related or other changes that may bear no relation to current symptoms.

- Back pain in and of itself is not a surgical condition, and only a minority of patients with related leg symptoms even need a surgical evaluation. In most cases, primary care physicians can successfully manage these complaints themselves, calling on physical therapists, physiatrists, and other professionals to address specific needs of patients who are slow to recover.

- Because of the generally good prognosis, most patients can be reassured that today's problem need not turn into tomorrow's disability. The severity will most likely lessen within a few days, unless patients avoid normal activity long enough to get out of shape.

The New Thinking on Low-back Pain

The conservative tide is balanced by the use of red flags to recognize the serious and potentially life-threatening undertow of back problems that need prompt attention and, in some instances, aggressive intervention. Your challenge is to avoid unnecessary, sometimes confusing, and expensive tests and unnecessary referrals for the majority of patients while not missing the rare patients whose back pain masks a tumor, infection, fracture, or serious neurologic impairment.

Regardless of the findings, a strong therapeutic alliance with your back patients is essential. Cementing the relationship with empathy and education is the best kind of "spinal fusion" you can provide.

Making a Diagnosis—When You Can

Keep in mind that 80-85 percent of low-back pain does not carry a specific diagnosis; the often-used term "lumbar strain" is a diagnosis by default. Many low-back symptoms have been blamed on sprains, strains, soft-tissue injuries, fibromyalgia, disk syndrome, facet syndrome, and arthritis—even though no diagnostic tests are available to document such causes.

Your initial evaluation should seek red flags that identify patients with a serious cause for their symptoms, especially those with neurologic deficits who may be candidates for a surgical evaluation. However, even in patients with herniated disks and nerve root compression, conservative treatment that helps keep the patient as active as possible—acetaminophen, nonsteroidal anti-inflammatory drugs (NSAIDs), and manipulation—may avoid the need for surgery.

It's also important to identify psychosocial factors that may influence management, amplify the patient's experience of pain, or increase the likelihood that an acute problem will turn into a chronic one. These factors may include substance abuse, depression, other psychiatric conditions, or involvement in disability-related litigation or compensation claims.

The History

Don't let a wait-and-see attitude lull you into a false sense of security when a patient presents with nonspecific back problems. A thorough history and physical examination, including neurologic screening and the straight-leg raising test, are needed the first time a patient comes to you in pain.

In taking the history, focus on function: What does the pain prevent you from doing (at home and at work)? Do you feel unsafe performing those activities? Or just uncomfortable? How long have your activities been limited? Within that framework, helpful questions to ask include:

- Where is the pain? Primarily in the back? In the leg? Both? Pain drawings and visual analog scales can be helpful in determining the pain's location. Pain intensity is best noted in terms of what the symptoms keep the patient from doing.

- Is the pain constant or intermittent?

- Is it worse at night?

- Is it just as bad or worse when you're resting as it is when you're active? Is there anything you do that makes the symptoms better or worse?

- Do you have other symptoms besides pain—numbness, weakness, stiffness?

- Have you had similar episodes of back problems before? (This may be the first time the patient has sought medical attention for back pain, but a careful history may reveal repeated traumas over a number of years that were self-treated with OTC medications, heating pads, etc.)

- Does lifting bother your back? The answer to this question can set the stage for educational efforts later on.

The AHCPR guidelines call on physicians to search for signs of serious underlying causes of back problems, such as tumor, infection, *cauda equina* syndrome, and fracture. Red flags for tumor or infection include:

- Age older than 50 or younger than 20; older age is a particular risk factor for malignancy or vertebral compression fracture
- Personal history of cancer
- Unexplained weight loss, recent fever or chills, lymphadenopathy, or other constitutional symptoms
- Pain that is worse when supine; pain at rest that is as bad as pain during periods of activity
- Severe pain at night, significantly worse than daytime pain.

The New Thinking on Low-back Pain

For spinal infection, additional risk factors include recent urinary tract infection or other bacterial infection, IV drug use, or immune suppression resulting from HIV infection, a transplant, or corticosteroid use. Severe guarding of lumbar motion in all planes is also a clue to tumor, infection, fracture, or inflammatory arthropathies.

Compression of the *cauda equina*, whether from a fracture, dislocation, spinal stenosis, or a massively herniated disk, is a medical emergency that calls for immediate consultation. Red flags include:

- Recent onset of bladder dysfunction (urinary retention, increased frequency, overflow incontinence)
- Saddle anesthesia; sensory loss in the perianal or perineal area
- Severe or progressive neurologic deficits in the lower extremities
- Unexpected laxity of the anal sphincter
- Major motor weakness in the quadriceps (knee extension weakness) and in the ankle plantar flexors, evertors, and dorsiflexors (footdrop).

Advise patients to contact you promptly if they experience increasing numbness or weakness in the back or extremities or any bowel or bladder problems.

Red flags for fracture include:

- A history of major trauma (fall from a height, motor vehicle accident)
- A history of minor trauma (including minor falls) or strenuous lifting, especially in older patients or those at risk for osteoporosis.

The Physical Examination

Two key considerations in the physical examination are (1) the presence or absence of pain radiating to the leg (sciatica), especially if it extends below the knee and (2) the presence or absence of neurologic deficits, based on assessment of muscle strength, reflexes, and sensation. This initial neurologic examination provides a baseline for future reference; it is the progression of neurologic deficits that typically signals the need for a surgical evaluation.

That's why follow-up is essential: The pain may remain the same, but the patient's neurologic status may change. Consider a return visit within 3 to 7 days in patients with severe pain, progressive symptoms by history, mild neurologic compromise on initial examination, or inconsistent findings due to guarding or pain on motion. A follow-up visit

Pain Sourcebook

(Decision points in heavy outline)

```
Your adult patient has acute onset of low-back pain or back-related leg symptoms that limit daily activities.
    │
    ▼
Perform a thorough history and physical examination, including neurologic screening and straight-leg raising.
    │
    ▼
Are there any red flags for serious conditions?
    ├── YES ──► The red flags indicate possible...
    │             ├── spinal fracture.
    │             │     └── Order plain X-ray film of lumbosacral spine. If after 10 days you still suspect a fracture, consider a bone scan or consultation.
    │             ├── cancer or infection.
    │             │     └── Order a CBC, ESR, and urinalysis. If still suspicious, consider a consult or order an X-ray film or bone scan.
    │             └── cauda equina syndrome.
    │                   └── Obtain immediate consultation for emergency studies and definitive care.
    └── NO ──► Return to full normal activities. Continue exercise program, now including muscle conditioning. Reevaluate if symptoms recur.
```

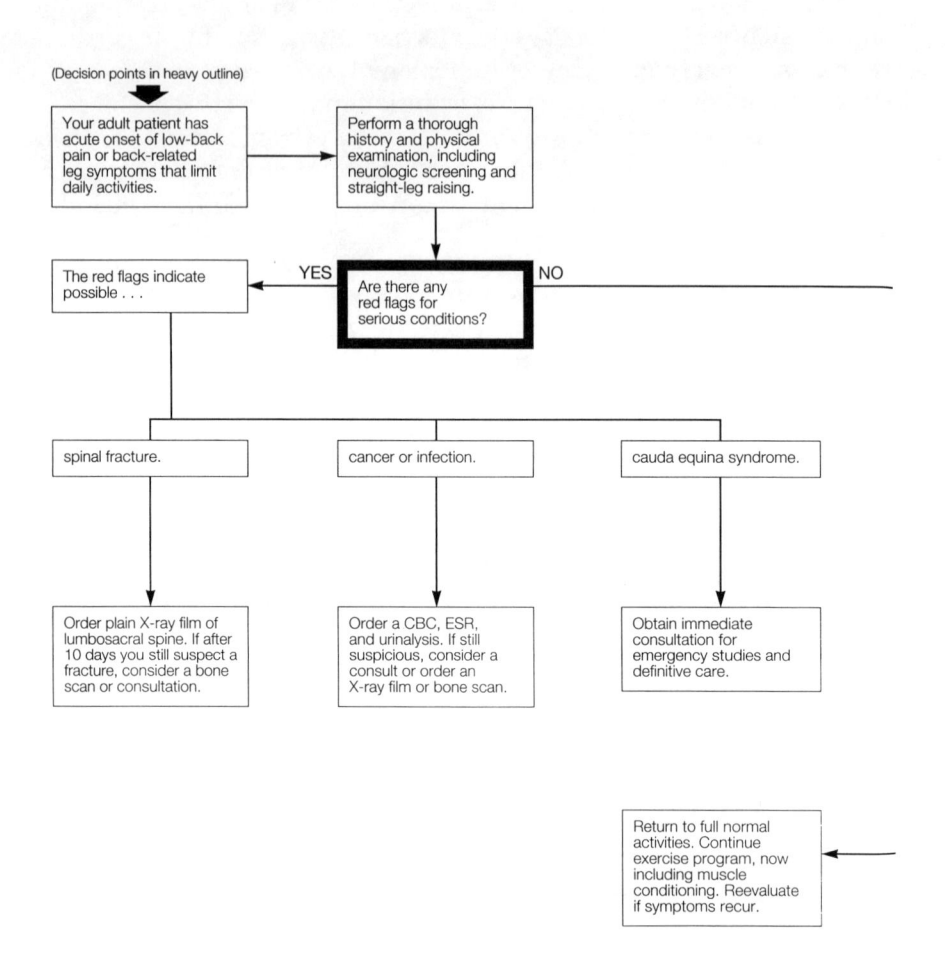

Note: For detailed algorithms on the various phases of managing low-back problems, see Bigos S, Bowyer O, Braen G, et al: *Acute Low Back Problems in Adults*. Clinical Practice Guideline Number 14. Agency for Health Care Policy and Research publication No. 95-0643. Rockville, Md, Public Health Service, US Dept of Health and Human Services, 1994.

Copyright © 1995 by Medical Economics, Montvale, N.J. No part of this FlowChart may be reproduced or extracted in any form without written permission.

Figure 17.1a. Evaluating acute low back pain

The New Thinking on Low-back Pain

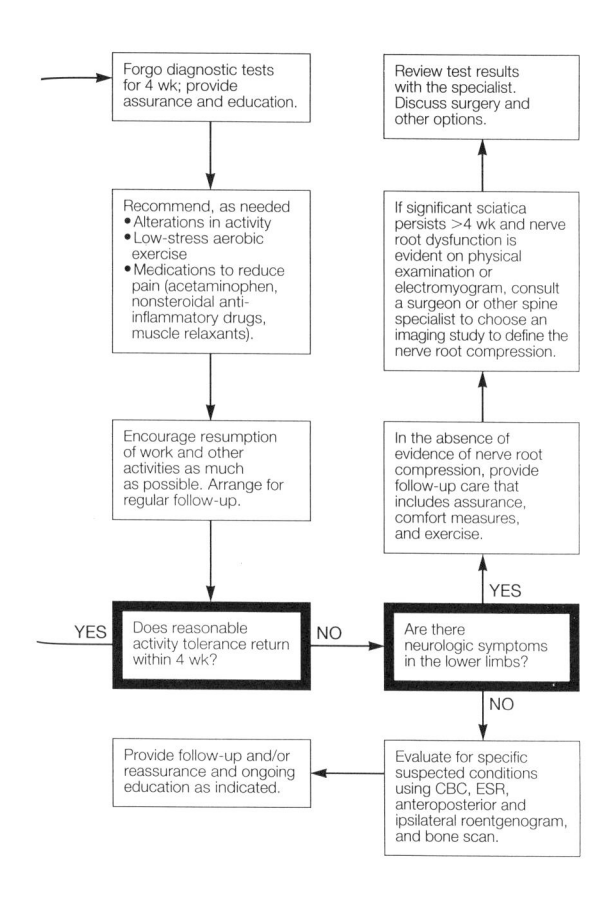

Figure 17.1b. Evaluating acute low back pain

in 10 to 14 days is probably sufficient for the patient with low-back pain and no evidence of neurologic compromise.

Observe the patient for a limp, other efforts to compensate for pain or discomfort, and any problems with coordination. Though some patients may magnify their symptoms, the true malingerer is rare. Clues to a psychological component include a patient's report that back or leg pain is unrelenting, that pain and numbness involve the entire leg, or that the leg "gives way." Also consider psychosocial factors if the reported pain level seems out of sync with the physical findings, or if the patient says that nothing helps and everything seems to make the pain worse. Most embellishments, however, should be interpreted as an attempt to convince you to take the patient's plea for help more seriously.

How Not to Miss a Herniated Disk

Herniation of disks is part of the aging process. Most herniations seem to be silent, but occasionally they can cause back-related leg pain and even radiculopathy. This occurs in only about 5 percent of patients who present with acute low-back symptoms. Neural compression from a herniated disk can cause a patient with mild back pain to have abrupt onset of unilateral numbness, tingling, or lancinating pain in the leg. A non-elderly patient with a herniated disk is generally more comfortable standing than sitting. The pain is exacerbated by forward flexion, and a Valsalva's maneuver may cause more leg pain than back pain.

More than 90 percent of radiculopathy due to herniated disks involves the L5 or S1 nerve root at the L4-L5 or L5-S1 disk level. The same sites are involved in virtually any type of neurologic loss that fits a nerve root distribution. Thus, most of these problems can be detected by testing ankle reflex (S1 dysfunction), foot and great toe dorsiflexion (L5), and light touch or pinprick sensation over the medial (L4), dorsal (L5), and lateral (S1) aspects of the foot. Also look for signs of muscle weakness, including inability to toe walk (S1), perform repetitive toe rises (S1), heel walk (L5), or do a single squat and rise (L4).

The straight-leg raising test suggests disk herniation, especially if the patient experiences pain below the knee at less than 70 degrees of raising. The raised-leg pain is aggravated by dorsiflexion of the ankle and internal limb rotation and relieved by ankle plantar flexion or external limb rotation. An even stronger indication of nerve root compression is crossover pain—when straight raising of the well leg elicits pain in the leg with sciatica.

The New Thinking on Low-back Pain

Other Considerations

- *Spinal Stenosis* is rare in patients younger than 60. Consider this diagnosis in patients older than 60 who have pseudoclaudication—leg pain that limits walking, causing the patient to sit or squat to rest, but characterized by normal peripheral pulses. In contrast to patients with herniated disks, patients with spinal stenosis have less pain when sitting and when the spine is flexed. Straight-leg raising may be normal. Studies indicate that conservative management is often successful; in any event, surgery is rarely considered in the first three months of symptoms.

Table 17.1. Possible causes of low back pain

Systemic causes
Malignancy (metastatic breast, lung, or prostate cancer; multiple myeloma, lymphoma, leukemia, primary spinal cord or extradural tumors)

Infection (endocarditis, vertebral osteomyelitis, diskitis, epidural abscess)

Abdominal aortic aneurysm

Renal, GI, or pelvic disease

Rheumatologic and structural conditions
Ankylosing spondylitis

Psoriatic arthritis

Reiter's syndrome

Arthritis associated with inflammatory bowel disease

Osteoporosis

Spondylosis (narrowing of disk space and arthritic changes of facet joint)

Spondylolisthesis (forward displacement of one or more lumbar vertebrae)

Disk problems
Vertebral disk herniation

Cauda equina syndrome

Spinal stenosis

Source: Wipf JE, Deyo RA: Low back pain. *Med Clin North Am* 1995; 79(2):231-246.

- *Abdominal aortic aneurysm* may be signaled by a severe, sharp tearing pain that comes and goes and is not necessarily related to activity. Check for a pulsatile mass in the abdomen, especially in patients 60 and older. Order an ultrasound study if you suspect an expanding aortic abdominal aneurysm.

- *Spondylolysis* stress fracture is uncommon in adults but is increasingly seen in adolescents involved in sports activities.

- A variety of other conditions may cause back pain (see Table 17.1).

Back Pain in Young Athletes: a Different Story.

The causes of low-back pain in adolescents, especially those involved in organized sports, may be significantly different from the causes in adults. And, in contrast to the decidedly conservative drift in the management of adult back pain, youngsters with low-back pain may need prompt and more aggressive intervention.

A recent study at Children's Hospital, Boston, compared the diagnoses of low-back complaints in 100 adults (aged 21 to 77, mean age of 31.9) and 100 athletically active adolescents (aged 12 to 18).[5] The adolescents had been treated at a sports medicine clinic and the adults at a back pain clinic. The pertinent findings:

- Nearly half of the adolescents (47 of 100) had a spondylolysis stress fracture of the *pars interarticularis*, compared with just five of the adults. Overall, 73 of 100 adolescents had an injury to the posterior elements of the spine.

- The most common diagnosis among adults was discogenic back pain (48 of 100), which includes herniation and/or degeneration of the lumbar disk. Discogenic back pain was diagnosed in just 11 of the 100 adolescents.

- 27 adults had muscle tendon strain, compared with six adolescents, suggesting that the muscles and tendons of the back are more resilient in younger people when exposed to stress.

- 26 adolescents had hyperlordotic mechanical back pain; no adults did.

Early intervention with bracing or activity modification can lead to complete healing and avoid the need for surgery, the authors say,

The New Thinking on Low-back Pain

but delays may result in nonunion of the *pars interarticularis* fracture, causing persistent pain and, in some cases, disability. They recommend that every child presenting with low-back pain of recent onset, a history of repetitive hyperextension training, and an examination showing pain on provocative hyperextension testing should receive X-rays of the lumbar spine (anteroposterior, lateral, and oblique views).

Imaging Studies

In the absence of any red flag conditions, the AHCPR guidelines suggest delaying all imaging studies, including X-rays, for one month. The algorithm you want to avoid is the one that leads from unnecessary imaging to inappropriate surgical referral, based on coincidental or irrelevant findings. Imaging studies of patients who have no back symptoms may still show items that could be labeled as "spinal pathology," including bulging or herniated disks, degenerative disk disease, spurring, and spinal stenosis.

The crucial point is to correlate the history and any measures of physiologic change before considering imaging tests. The management of back pain is plagued by a lack of physiologic-to-imaging correlation. As Stanley J. Bigos, M.D., chairman of the AHCPR panel and a consultant for this chapter, describes it, an MRI may show you a "telephone" but doesn't tell you whether the phone is ringing (i.e., producing symptoms). It's unusual to discover anything on plain x-ray films that actually affects treatment. As for CT and MRI, they are useful

Table 17.2 Acute low back pain

Test	Order when
Needle electromyography (EMG), H-reflex tests of lower limb*	Assessing questionable nerve-root dysfunction in patients with leg symptoms lasting >4 wk (regardless of whether back pain is present)
Sensory evoked potentials	Assessing suspected spinal stenosis and spinal cord myelopathy
Bone scan	Evaluating suspected spinal tumor, infection, or occult fracture; bone scan is contraindicated in pregnancy

*Electrophysiologic testing is not recommended if radiculopathy is obvious and specific on physical examination.
Tests not recommended: Thermography, surface EMG and F-wave response tests, diskography, CT-diskography

Source: Bigos S, Bowyer O, Braen G, et al: *Acute Low Back Problems in Adults*. Clinical Practice Guideline Number 14. Agency for Health Care Policy and Research publication No. 95-0643. Rockville, Md, Public Health Service, US Dept of Health and Human Services, 1994.

in delineating possible causes of back pain but are regarded by the AHCPR guidelines as primarily helpful in confirming a physiologically based diagnosis and planning any surgery needed.

Order a bone scan if you suspect an occult fracture, tumor, or infection, on the basis of red flag findings, lab tests, or films. Bone scans are contraindicated in pregnant patients. For recommendations on these and other special tests see Table 17.2.

Treatment—What Works?

In the treatment of low-back problems, the paradigm shift is away from passive therapies and toward greater self-reliance and a return to activity as soon as feasible. A "wait and see" interval could turn into a period of deconditioning: The more patients can do on their own and the sooner they can do it, the greater the physical as well as psychological benefits.

Instead of focusing on the pain, encourage patients to think in terms of what they can realistically continue to do: The goal is to avoid the back injury that results from resting too much; staying active will help the patient to avoid deconditioning and ensuing debilitation. If tolerance for certain daily tasks is not feasible, exercise is an alternative.

You can also explore ways to minimize time lost from work, suggesting to a supervisor that the patient be allowed to do less strenuous forms of labor for a specified period. The patient can usually document specific tasks that are too difficult to perform, on the job or at home.

It's important to know the patient's expectations and to show empathy. Listen carefully to all complaints; other diagnoses may need attention as well. You can reassure most patients that you suspect no serious problem and that a full recovery can be expected. Those with back symptoms and physically demanding jobs will need to develop realistic expectations and understand that a quick cure is not possible.

Bed Rest and Home Therapy

Not so long ago, a heart attack was followed by 30 days of bed rest. Today in an uncomplicated myocardial infarction, patients are up and moving about within 24 to 48 hours. The same thinking is now applied to acute low-back problems: Bed rest for 2-4 days may help the patient with both back and leg pain but is not considered helpful for

The New Thinking on Low-back Pain

others. More than four days of bed rest has a debilitating effect. During a period of rest, the patient should still get up and around from time to time.

A practical alternative to bed rest is to counsel the patient to avoid or limit activities that can irritate the spine—not just heavy lifting but also prolonged unsupported sitting. Some clinicians prescribe a program of home therapy, such as placing a bag of ice and water (or a bag of frozen vegetables) on the affected area for 15 to 20 minutes at a time a few times each day. A damp, warm washcloth underneath the bag will keep the skin from getting too cold. Cooling the area may help to lower muscle tone that is contributing to the pain. Alternating the cold treatment with 5 to 10 minutes of heat (hot pack, heating pad, or warm shower) may also provide some relief.

Exercise

Exercise is the central component in the management of back pain. Its basic purpose and value are to encourage the patient to be active.

Start by maintaining or building general endurance with stationary bicycling, walking, and swimming. Aerobic exercises like these can usually be started within the first two weeks of symptoms and the regimen gradually increased, from 5 to 10 minutes a day to up to 20 to 30 minutes of continuous activity per day. Brisk walking is a more viable option than jogging. Keep the exercise prescription realistic and provide regular encouragement, otherwise the patient may abandon the effort and lose endurance by resting too much. Any activity—even 2 to 3 minutes a day to start—is better than no activity.

There is less agreement on which strengthening exercises are most helpful. These exercises may aggravate pain in the early stages and are probably best delayed until after 2 to 4 weeks of aerobic fitness exercises. Some recent trials prove the benefit of active extension exercises to condition paraspinous muscles, though elderly patients with facet degeneration and posterior spurring may not be able to tolerate them. Some physical therapists theorize that passive extension exercises benefit those who were injured in a flexed position, and vice versa. Simple stretching exercises and back exercise machines have not been proved to be effective according to the AHCPR guidelines.

General endurance exercises and specific back muscle conditioning may also help to avoid the recurrence of symptoms in patients with a previous history of back pain who are currently asymptomatic.

Manipulation

The AHCPR guidelines conclude that spinal manipulation is a reasonable alternative to medication in the short term for patients with uncomplicated low-back pain, especially if the manipulation keeps patients active. Not advocated are the "maintenance" treatments of spinal manipulation that continue for months or years. Manipulation has not been proven to be of benefit in patients with sciatica or chronic back pain, though some practitioners say they have found it helpful in patients with nondiscogenic sciatica.

Practitioners of manipulation are many and include osteopathic physicians, physical therapists, chiropractors, and allopathic physicians who are willing to take the requisite training in manual medicine. If manipulation does not allow the patient to maintain activity or exercise enough to build activity tolerance within the first month of care, therapy should be discontinued and the patient reevaluated.

Medication

Consider prescribing pain medication on a fixed daily dosage rather than saying "Take the medicine when it hurts." The same concept applies for the duration of the therapy: Prescribe for a fixed time period rather than saying "Take the medicine until the pain goes away."

Many patients will do well on simple pain medication such as acetaminophen and NSAIDs, including aspirin. Muscle relaxants are an option, but they have not been shown to be more effective than NSAIDs, not have combinations of muscle relaxants and NSAIDs proved more effective than NSAIDs alone. Opioids offer another option, though they are no more effective than safer analgesics. Consider narcotic analgesics for patients with acute, severe pain and sciatica; many clinicians advise limiting the prescription to one week at a time, while others feel confident prescribing them pro re nata (as needed) for a short period of time.

Injections

The AHCPR guidelines provide a mild vote of confidence in epidural corticosteroid injections "for short-term relief of radicular pain after failure of conservative treatment and as a means of avoiding surgery." The panel turned thumbs-down on most other types of injection, including trigger-point, ligamentous, and facet joint injections, as well as epidural corticosteroids, anesthetics, or opioids in patients without radiculopathy.

Injections of chymopapain (Chymodiactin) into a small- or medium-sized herniated disk are suggested as an alternative (albeit a less effective one) to laminotomy for direct nerve-root compression. However, the International Intradiscal Therapy Society, an organization of orthopedic surgeons and neurologists, says the AHCPR guidelines underestimate the value of chymopapain as an alternative to surgery, especially with respect to its relative safety.

Chymopapain injections are meant to break down the herniated material from inside the disk that is indirectly putting pressure on the nerve root; some studies, however, indicate that the body naturally degrades this material over time. Chymopapain injections are not likely to be successful in patients with sequestered disk material or stenosis of the spinal canal or lateral recess.

Some physician groups maintain that injections are clinically much more useful than described in the AHCPR document. They say, for example, that facet injections and sacroiliac joint injections help relieve back pain originating below the lumbosacral junction. Studies documenting such effectiveness are lacking, however.

Referral and Follow-up

Before making any referrals, be sure to conduct a thorough diagnostic evaluation of your own. Think about referring the patient who is still greatly limited and not improving after 1 to 2 months of conservative therapy. Referral is also appropriate when neurologic signs are conflicting or confusing. Your first call need not be to a surgeon; consider the value of someone who specializes in the evaluation and care of patients with back problems, occupational illness, or pain problems in general. If you are not prepared to offer manipulation yourself, for example, you can usually make a local referral and continue to monitor and offer encouragement. Some patients entrenched in chronic pain or difficult pain syndromes may need to be cared for by a multidisciplinary team.

Physical Therapy

A good working relationship with a physical therapist can be established in most primary care settings. The most helpful benefits a physical therapy program can offer to a patient with back pain are a structured, supervised exercise program and further education about its importance. This approach is favored over the use of modalities such as heat, cold, ultrasound, and transcutaneous electrical nerve stimulation (TENS). There is no strong evidence at present that those interventions make a difference in the course of acute low-back pain.

In addition to patients with persistent pain, patients whose jobs are at risk when limited by back pain and others in need of further education may benefit from a referral to a physical therapist, physiatrist, or occupational medicine specialist. Rather than issue a blanket prescription for physical therapy, convey your expectations and establish regular communications. Review the endurance program and any exercises to condition the back muscles or trunk, and ask for regular progress reports.

Typically, a patient limited by back pain may continue a therapy program for 10 to 12 sessions (about one month). The treatment approach should also include an ongoing home-exercise program of 10 to 15 minutes a day.

Surgery

Rates of back surgery in this country vary widely by geographic region and even within the same state, suggesting a lack of uniform criteria. For properly selected patients (about 1 percent of all patients with back pain), surgery speeds pain relief, although it will not strengthen the spine. Surgery benefits less than 40 percent of those who do not have obvious surgical indications. Even among those who have such indications, more than 80 percent recover, with or without surgery.

The most compelling reason to call a surgeon is the combination of:

- Severe and disabling sciatica
- Progression of signs and symptoms or persistence without notable improvement
- Documented progressive neurologic loss, matched by
- Evidence of disk herniation with nerve root impingement, not responding to treatment.

Thus, consider a surgical referral if the patient has radicular findings in a dermatomal distribution, measurable nerve-root compression on the straight-leg raising test, numbness in the foot, and failure to regain reasonable activity tolerance after 4 to 6 weeks of conservative treatment. Surgical consultation is not necessary if a patient has a possible herniated disk but no evidence of nerve root compromise or no significant limitations in daily activity. One of the criteria for surgery is that nerve root compression and other imaging findings correspond to radicular signs on physical examination.

The New Thinking on Low-back Pain

Education

The first step in educating patients is to let them know that back pain is ubiquitous in our society but not usually disabling. Most patients don't fully appreciate the importance of the back until they experience pain. It may be helpful to remind them that anyone can wrench the back by reaching the wrong way for a glass of juice or bending over to pick up a paper clip, especially after being deconditioned by inactivity.

A wealth of educational materials on back pain is available from a variety of organizations (see "Helpful sources of information on back pain,"). Although formal back school is probably not necessary outside the workplace, some "back basics" courses given by hospitals and other health organizations may assist patients in gaining helpful tips about daily activities that stress the back.

Other risk factors that slow recovery from back symptoms include obesity and cigarette smoking—factors that need to be addressed in their own right. Younger patients who perceive themselves to be in good shape may be the most difficult to teach about back pain. But proper care of the back is an appropriate subject for patient education throughout life.

Why Less Is More

Why are experts today advocating a conservative approach to the management of acute low-back problems? Recent studies offer some insights:

Fit in Finland. A study in Finland focused on municipal employees who came to an occupational health care center in Helsinki with acute, nonspecific low-back pain or exacerbations of chronic pain.[2]

The average age was 40, and 60 percent of the patients were women. Subjects were randomly assigned to one of three groups:

- Two days of complete bed rest, with only essential walking allowed.

- Light back-mobilizing exercises (back extension and lateral bending movements, 10 repetitions every other hour).

- Avoidance of bed rest and continuation of routine activities as much as possible within the limits of pain (the control group).

More than 90 percent of patients in each of the three groups received prescriptions for anti-inflammatory drugs or analgesics. At the three-week follow-up, patients in the bed rest group had spent an average of 22 hours at rest, versus five hours for those in the exercise group and two hours for those in the control group. The control group fared significantly better with respect to time lost from work—4.1 days versus 5.7 days for the exercise group and 7.5 days for the bed rest group. This benefit continued at the 12-week follow-up. Controls also scored higher in the self-assessed ability to perform one's job.

Not sleepless in Seattle. Another study, conducted in a Seattle HMO, suggests that a conservative approach produces comparable outcomes and patient satisfaction at a significantly lower cost. Investigators categorized primary care physicians as high-, low-, or moderate frequency prescribers in the treatment of acute or chronic back pain.[3] Doctors in the high-frequency group prescribed bed rest and medications such as opioids and sedative-hypnotics twice as often as did those in the low-prescribing group. Low prescribers put more emphasis on self-care and early return to activity.

After one month, the percentage of patients who reported moderate or severe limitation of activity was highest in the high-prescribing group (46 percent of patients) and lowest in the low-prescribing group (30 percent). Activity limitation was comparable in all three groups at one and two years of follow-up, but after one year the costs of care were 79 percent higher in patients treated by high-prescribing physicians.

Satisfaction with medical care was comparable in all three groups, but patients of low-frequency prescribers were more satisfied with the education they received about back pain.

A choice in China. In China, a study at a primary care clinic focused on a functional approach to the treatment of back pain-emphasizing exercise and health education and eschewing medication as much as possible.[4]

The results:

- Two patients with acute back pain recovered within two weeks with no use of medication or formal treatment modalities.
- Of 30 patients with chronic back pain, 23 had 50 to 100 percent relief within eight weeks.
- No patients reported loss of work time due to back pain.

The New Thinking on Low-back Pain

Treatment Recommendations for Acute Low-back Problems

The Clinical Practice Guidelines on acute low-back problems, issued December 1994 by the Agency for Health Care Policy and Research, make the following recommendations for therapeutic intervention:

Bed Rest

- Bed rest for 2 to 4 days may be an option for patients with symptoms of leg pain but is generally not helpful to others with uncomplicated low-back pain.
- For any patient, bed rest for more than four days may lead to debilitation.

Exercise

- Low-stress aerobic exercise in the first month of symptoms can prevent the deconditioning that results from inactivity. Most patients can start aerobic exercises (walking, stationary bicycling, swimming, etc.) in the first two weeks.
- Exercise for trunk muscles, especially back extension exercises, gradually increased, are helpful, especially if symptoms persist. They may aggravate symptoms in the first two weeks, however.
- Gradually increased exercise quotas seem to work better than telling patients to stop exercising if pain occurs.
- Back stretching exercises and back exercise machines are not usually helpful.

Medications

- **Acceptable**: Acetaminophen and nonsteroidal anti-inflammatory drugs (NSAIDs), including aspirin.
- **Optional**: Muscle relaxants, though they have not been shown to be more effective than NSAIDs. Combinations of muscle relaxants and NSAIDs are not more effective than NSAIDs alone.
- **Another Option**: Opioids, though no more effective than safer analgesics.

- **Not Recommended**: Oral corticosteroids, colchicine (unlabeled use for colchicine) Some clinicians, however, find oral steroids helpful in cases of lower back and leg pain due to nerve root impingement by acute disk herniation.

Manipulation

- Can be helpful in patients without radiculopathy in the first month of symptoms.
- Should be discontinued and the patient reevaluated if no improvement occurs within one month.
- Not recommended for the long term.

Physical Modalities

- Patients can be instructed on the use of heat and cold at home.
- Not recommended are spinal traction, biofeedback, trigger-point injections, facet joint injections, needle acupuncture, and epidural injections of anesthetics or opioids. (Some clinicians feel, however, that translumbar or caudal epidural injections, as well as selective nerve-root blocks, may have a role in back pain associated with radiculopathy or sizeable disk herniations that do not respond to conservative management.)
- Epidural corticosteroid injections are not recommended for patients who experience low-back pain without radiculopathy. Epidural corticosteroids may provide short-term relief in patients with persistent radiculopathy and thus help avoid the need for surgery.
- Lumbar corsets may be helpful as a preventive measure for people whose work or other activity poses a risk of back strain, but their benefits have not been carefully documented.

Referral to a Spine Specialist

- Consider Surgical Evaluation if after one month of conservative treatment sciatica remains severe and disabling, its symptoms either progress or persist without improvement, and there is evidence of nerve-root compromise. (An alternative is to consult a nonsurgical spine specialist such as a physiatrist, occupational medicine specialist, or pain management specialist.)

The New Thinking on Low-back Pain

- Chymopapain (Chymodiactin) injection is an acceptable, though less efficacious, alternative to surgery for patients with a herniated disk and nerve-root compromise.

- Standard diskectomy and microdiskectomy are appropriate surgical procedures for herniated disks with nerve-root dysfunction; percutaneous diskectomy and other new methods cannot be recommended at present.

- Conservative management of spinal stenosis can often avoid the need for surgery in elderly patients who function well in activities of daily living. No surgical referral is required in the first three months of symptoms; any surgical decision should take into account the persistence and neurogenic claudication, associated limitations, and evidence of nerve-root compromise.

- Spinal fusion is not recommended in the first three months of symptoms unless there is spinal fracture or dislocation or complications of tumor or infection. Spinal fusion may be considered in patients with the combination of degenerative spondylolisthesis, spinal stenosis, and radiculopathy, following decompressive laminectomy for stenosis.

Helpful Sources of Information on Back Pain

Publications

Acute Low Back Problems in Adults: Assessment and Treatment

Department of Health and Human Services AHCPR Publications Clearinghouse Box 8547
Silver Spring, MD 20907-8547
(800) 358-9295 (voice mail, 24 hours a day)

This and all other AHCPR Clinical Practice Guidelines are also available online through the National Library of Medicine (Health Services/Technology Assessment Text).

Back in Action: A Guide to Understanding Your Low-Back Pain and Learning What You Can Do About It

A brochure published by the Group Health Cooperative of Puget Sound, University of Washington Schools of Medicine and Public Health, and Seattle Veterans Affairs Medical Center. It can be ordered through the AHCPR Clearinghouse listed above.

American Medical Association Pocket Guide to Back Pain

This 80-page minibook discusses the anatomy of the back, offers tips on preventing injury, and describes back problems ranging from muscle aches and pains to trauma, infections, and other disorders. $4.99. For information on bulk discounts, write to Special Markets, Random House, Inc., 201 E 50th St.. New York. NY 10022.

Good News for Bad Backs

Robert L. Swezey, MD, and Annette M. Swezey. Published in 1993 by Cequal Publishing Co., 1328 Sixteenth St., Santa Monica, CA 90404. A video by Dr. Swezey titled "No More Back Pain" is also available.

Organizations

American Academy of Orthopaedic Surgeons
6300 N. River Rd.
Rosemont, IL 60018-4262
(708) 823-7186

American Academy of Physical Medicine and Rehabilitation (AAPMR)
IBM Plaza
Suite 2500
Chicago, IL 60611-3604
(312) 464-9700

Within the AAPMR is a group of physiatrists with a special interest in musculoskeletal medicine and the spine, known as the **Physiatric Association of Spine, Sports and Occupational Rehabilitation (PASSOR)**. They can be reached at the address and phone number above.

American College of Occupational and Environmental Medicine
55 W. Seegers Rd.
Arlington Heights, IL 60005-3919
(708) 228-6850

American Congress of Rehabilitation Medicine
5700 Old Orchard Rd.
1st fl.
Skokie, IL 60077-1057
(708)966-0095

The New Thinking on Low-back Pain

American Osteopathic Association
142 E Ontario St.
Chicago, IL 60611
(800) 621-1773

In addition, hospitals and local chapters of organizations such as the American Red Cross often sponsor courses for patients on proper back care.

References

1. Bigos S, Bowyer 0, Braen G, et al: *Acute Low Back Problems in Adults. Clinical Practice Guideline* Number 14. Agency for Health Care Policy and Research publication No. 95-0643. Rockville, Md, Public Health Service, US Dept of Health and Human) Services, 1994.

2. Malrnivaara A, Hakkinen U, Aro X, et al: The treatment of acute low back pain--bed rest, exercises, or ordinary activity? *N Engl J Med* 1995;332:351

3. Von Korff M, Barlow W, Cherkin D, et al Effects of practice style in managing back pain. *Ann Intern Med* 1994;121:187-195.

4. Chang WD, Wang YS, Chou CS, et al: Functional approach to treatment of back pain in primary care; A preliminary report. Chung Hua I *Hsueh Tsa Chih* (Taipei) 1994;53;338-345.

5. Micheli LJ, Wood R: Back pain in young athletes: Significant differences from adults in causes and patterns. *Arch Pediatr Adolesc Med* 1995;149;15-18.

—Prepared by Jeff Forster, editor

Chapter 18

Understanding Acute Low-back Problems

About the Back and Back Problems

The human spine (or backbone) is made up of small bones called vertebrae. The vertebrae are stacked on top of each other to form a column. Between each vertebra is a cushion known as a disc. The vertebrae are held together by ligaments, and muscles are attached to the vertebrae by bands of tissue called tendons.

Openings in each vertebra line up to form a long hollow canal. The spinal cord runs through this canal from the base of the brain. Nerves from the spinal cord branch out and leave the spine through the spaces between the vertebrae.

The lower part of the back holds most of the body's weight. Even a minor problem with the bones, muscles, ligaments, or tendons in this area can cause pain when a person stands, bends, or moves around. Less often, a problem with a disc can pinch or irritate a nerve from the spinal cord, causing pain that runs down the leg, below the knee called sciatica.

Purpose

This chapter is about acute low back problems in adults. If you have a low back problem, you may have symptoms that include:

- Pain or discomfort in the lower part of the back.
- Pain or numbness that moves down the leg (sciatica).

AHCPR Publication No. 94-0644. December 1994. Clinical Practice Guideline No. 14, Consumer Version.

Pain Sourcebook

Low back symptoms can keep you from doing your normal daily activities or doing things that you enjoy.

A low back problem may come on suddenly or gradually. It is acute if it lasts a short while, usually a few days to several weeks. An episode that lasts longer than three months is not acute.

If you have been bothered by your lower back, you are not alone. Eight out of ten adults will have a low back problem at some time in their life. And most will have more than one episode of acute low back problems. In between episodes, most people return to their normal activities with little or no symptoms.

This chapter will tell you more about acute low back problems, what to do, and what to expect when you see a health care provider.

Causes of Low Back Problems

Even with today's technology, the exact reason or cause of low back problems can be found in very few people. Most times, the symptoms are blamed on poor muscle tone in the back, muscle tension or spasm, back sprains, ligament or muscle tears, or joint problems. Sometimes

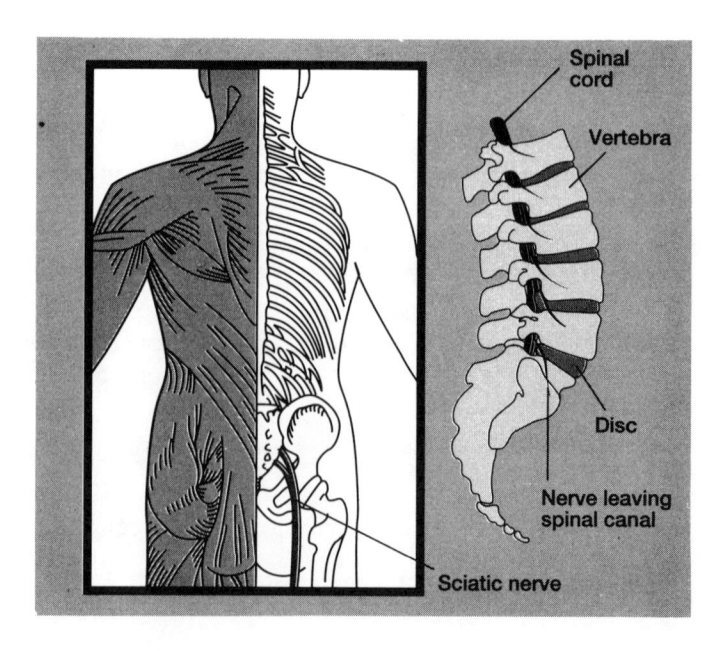

Figure 18.1.Muscles of the back and the spine

Understanding Acute Low-back Problems

nerves from the spinal cord (see Figure 18.1) can be irritated by slipped discs causing buttock or leg pain. This may also cause numbness, tingling, or weakness in the legs.

People who are in poor physical condition or do work that includes heavy labor or long periods of sitting or standing are at greater risk for low back problems. These people also get better more slowly. Emotional stress or long periods of inactivity may make back symptoms seem worse.

Low back problems are often painful. But the good news is that very few people turn out to have a major problem with the bones or joints of the back or a dangerous medical condition.

Things to Do about Low Back Problems

Seeing a Health Care Provider

Many people who develop mild low back discomfort may not need to see a health care provider right away. Often, within a few days, the symptoms go away without any treatment.

A visit to your health care provider is a good idea if:

- Your symptoms are severe.
- The pain is keeping you from doing things that you do every day.
- The problem does not go away within a few days.

If you also have problems controlling your bowel or bladder, if you feel numb in the groin or rectal area, or if there is extreme leg weakness, call your health care provider right away.

Your health care provider will check to see if you have a medical illness causing your back problem (chances are you will not). Your health care provider can also help you get some relief from your symptoms.

Your health care provider will:

- Ask about your symptoms and what they keep you from doing.
- Ask about your medical history.
- Give you a physical exam.

Talking about Your Symptoms

Your health-care provider will want to know about your back problem. Here are some examples of the kinds of questions he or she may ask you:

- When did your back symptoms start?
- Which of your daily activities are you not able to do because of your back symptoms?
- Is there anything you do that makes the symptoms better or worse?
- Have you noticed any problem with your legs?
- Around the time your symptoms began, did you have a fever or symptoms of pain or burning when urinating?

Talking about Your Medical History

Be sure to tell your health care provider about your general health and about illnesses you have had in the past. Here are some questions your health care provider may ask you about your medical history:

- Have you had a problem with your back in the past? If so, when?
- What medical illnesses have you had (for example, cancer, arthritis, or diseases of the immune system)?
- Which medicines do you take regularly?
- Have you ever used intravenous (IV) drugs?
- Have you recently lost weight without trying?

You should also tell your health-care provider about anything you may be doing for your symptoms: medicines you are taking, creams or ointments you are using, and other home remedies.

Having a Physical Exam

Your health-care provider will examine your back. Even after a careful physical examination, it may not be possible for your health care provider to tell you the exact cause of your low back problem. But you most likely will find out that your symptoms are not being caused by a dangerous medical condition. Very few people (about 1 in 200) have low back symptoms caused by such conditions. You probably won't need special tests if you have had low back symptoms for only a few weeks.

Getting Relief

Your health care provider will help you get relief from your pain, discomfort, or other symptoms. A number of medicines and other treatments help with low back symptoms. The good news is that most people start feeling better soon.

Proven Treatments

Medicine often helps relieve low back symptoms. The type of medicine that your health care provider recommends depends on your symptoms and how uncomfortable you are:

- If your symptoms are mild to moderate, you may get the relief you need from an over-the-counter (nonprescription) medicine such as acetaminophen, aspirin, or ibuprofen. These medicines usually have fewer side effects than prescription medicines and are less expensive.

- If your symptoms are severe, your health care provider may recommend a prescription medicine.

For most people, medicine works well to control pain and discomfort. But any medicine can have side effects. For example, some people cannot take aspirin or ibuprofen because it can cause stomach irritation and even ulcers. Many medicines prescribed for low back pain can make people feel drowsy. These medicines should not be taken if you need to drive or use heavy equipment. Talk to your health care provider about the benefits and risks of any medicine recommended. If you develop side effects (such as nausea, vomiting, rash, dizziness), stop taking the medicine, and tell your health-care provider right away.

In addition, your health care provider may recommend one or more of the following to be used alone or along with medicine to help relieve your symptoms:

- **Heat or cold applied to the back.** Within the first 48 hours after your back symptoms start, you may want to apply a cold pack (or a bag of ice) to the painful area for 5 to 10 minutes at a time. If your symptoms last longer than 48 hours, you may find that a heating pad or hot shower or bath helps relieve your symptoms.

- **Spinal manipulation.** This treatment (using the hands to apply force to the back to adjust the spine) can be helpful for some people in the first month of low back symptoms. It should only be done by a professional with experience in manipulation. You should go back to your health care provider if your symptoms have not responded to spinal manipulation within four weeks.

Keep in mind that everyone is different. You will have to find what works best to relieve your own back symptoms.

Other Treatments

A number of other treatments are sometimes used for low back symptoms. While these treatments may give relief for a short time, none have been found to speed recovery or keep acute back problems from returning. They may also be expensive. Such treatments include:

- Traction.
- TENS (transcutaneous electrical nerve stimulation).
- Massage.
- Biofeedback.
- Acupuncture.
- Injections into the back.
- Back corsets.
- Ultrasound.

Physical Activity

Your health-care provider will want to know about the physical demands of your life (your job or daily activities). Until you feel better, your health care provider may need to recommend some changes in your activities. You will want to talk to your health care provider about your own personal situation. In general, when pain is severe, you should avoid:

- Heavy lifting.
- Lifting when twisting, bending forward, and reaching.
- Sitting for long periods of time.

The most important goal is for you to return to your normal activities as soon as it is safe. Your health care provider and (if you work) your employer can help you decide how much you are able to do safely at work. Your schedule can be gradually increased as your back improves.

Understanding Acute Low-back Problems

Bed Rest

If your symptoms are severe, your health care provider may recommend a short period of bed rest. However, bed rest should be limited to two or three days. Lying down for longer periods may weaken muscles and bones and actually slow your recovery. If you feel that you must lie down, be sure to get up every few hours and walk around—even if it hurts. Feeling a little discomfort as you return to normal activity is common and does not mean that you are hurting yourself.

About Work and Family

Back problems take time to get better. If your job or your normal daily activities make your back pain worse, it is important to communicate this to your family, supervisor, and coworkers. Put your energy into doing those things at work and at home that you are able to do comfortably. Be productive, but be clear about those tasks that you are not able to do.

Things You Can Do Now

While waiting for your back to improve, you may be able to make yourself more comfortable if you:

- Wear comfortable, low-heeled shoes.

- Make sure your work surface is at a comfortable height for you.

- Use a chair with a good lower back support that may recline slightly.

- If you must sit for long periods of time, try resting your feet on the floor or on a low stool, whichever is more comfortable.

- If you must stand for long periods of time, try resting one foot on a low stool.

- If you must drive long distances, try using a pillow or rolled-up towel behind the small of your back. Also, be sure to stop often and walk around for a few minutes.

- If you have trouble sleeping, try sleeping on your back with a pillow under your knees, or sleep on your side with your knees bent and a pillow between your knees.

Exercise

A gradual return to normal activities, including exercise, is recommended. Exercise is important to your overall health and can help you to lose body fat (if needed). Even if you have mild to moderate low back symptoms, the following things can be done without putting much stress on your back:

- Walking short distances.
- Using a stationary bicycle.
- Swimming.

It is important to start any exercise program slowly and to gradually build up the speed and length of time that you do the exercise. At first, you may find that your symptoms get a little worse when you exercise or become more active. Usually, this is nothing to worry about. However, if your pain becomes severe, contact your health care provider. Once you are able to return to normal activities comfortably, your health care provider may recommend further aerobic and back exercises.

If You Are Not Getting Better

Most low back problems get better quickly, and usually within four weeks. If your symptoms are not getting better within this time period, you should contact your health care provider.

Special Tests

Your health care provider will examine your back again and may talk to you about getting some special tests. These may include x-rays, blood tests, or other special studies such as an MRI (magnetic resonance imaging) or CT (computerized tomography) scan of your back. These tests may help your health-care provider understand why you are not getting better. Your health care provider may also want to refer you to a specialist.

Certain things, such as stress (extra pressure at home or work), personal or emotional problems, depression, or a problem with drug

Understanding Acute Low-back Problems

or alcohol use can slow recovery or make back symptoms seem worse. If you have any of these problems, tell your health care provider.

About Surgery

Even having a lot of back pain does not by itself mean you need surgery. Surgery has been found to be helpful in only 1 in 100 cases of low back problems. In some people, surgery can even cause more problems. This is especially true if your only symptom is back pain.

People with certain nerve problems or conditions such as fractures or dislocations have the best chance of being helped by surgery. In most cases, however, decisions about surgery do not have to be made right away. Most back surgery can wait for several weeks without making the condition worse.

If your health-care provider recommends surgery, be sure to ask about the reason for the surgery and about the risks and benefits you might expect. You may also want to get a second opinion.

Prevention of Low Back Problems

The best way to prevent low back problems is to stay fit. If you must lift something, even after your back seems better, be sure to:

- Keep all lifted objects close to your body.
- Avoid lifting while twisting, bending forward, and reaching.
- You should continue to exercise even after your back symptoms have gone away. There are many exercises that can be done to condition muscles of your body and back. You should talk to your health care provider about the exercises that would be best for you.

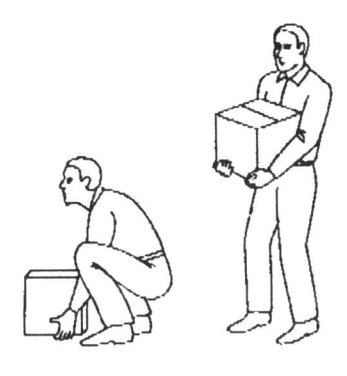

Figure 18.2. Safe lifting and carrying positions

When Low Back Symptoms Return

More than half of the people who recover from a first episode of acute low back symptoms will have another episode within a few years. Unless your back symptoms are very different from the first episode, or you have a new medical condition, you can expect to recover quickly and fully from each episode.

While Your Back Is Getting Better

It is important to remember that even though you are having a problem with your back now, most likely it will begin to feel better soon. It is important to keep in mind that you are the most important person in taking care of your back and in helping to get back to your regular activities. It may also help you to remember that:

- Most low back problems last for a short amount of time and the symptoms usually get better with little or no medical treatment.

- Low back problems can be painful. But pain rarely means that there is serious damage to your back.

- Exercise can help you to feel better faster and prevent more back problems. A regular exercise program adds to your general health and may help you get back to the things you enjoy doing.

For Further Information

The information in this chapter was based on the *Clinical Practice Guideline, Acute Low Back Problems in Adults*. The Guideline was developed by a non-Federal panel of experts sponsored by the Agency for Health Care Policy and Research. Other guidelines on common health problems are available, and more are being developed.

For more information about guidelines or to receive a free copy of *Understanding Acute Low Back Problems*, call toll-free 800-358-9295, or write to:

Agency for Health Care Policy and Research
Publications Clearinghouse
P.O. Box 8547
Silver Spring, MD 20907

Note: The picture of the muscles of the back in Figure 18.1 was taken from another AHCPR-sponsored publication, *Back in Action*.

Chapter 19

Chiropractic Manipulation and Federal Guidelines on Low Back Pain Treatment

Background

On December 8, 1994, The Agency for Health Care Policy and Research (AHCPR) of the U.S. Department of Health and Human Services, released an extensive study of diagnostic and treatment methods for acute low back pain. This condition is the most common health complaint experienced by working Americans today, and a condition which costs the economy at least $50 billion a year in lost wages and productivity.

The AHCPR panel—a 23-member committee of medical doctors, nurses, chiropractic doctors, experts in spine research, physical therapists, a psychologist, an occupational therapist and a consumer representative—concluded, among other things, that:

- spinal manipulation is a recommended treatment for acute low back problems in adults;

- conservative treatment such as manipulation should be pursued—in most cases—before surgical interventions are considered;

- prescription drugs such as oral steroids, antidepressant medications and colchicine are not recommended for acute low back problems.

©1995 American Chiropractic OnLine (ACA OnLine). Source: http://www.cais.net/aca/. Reprinted with permission.

The Facts about Chiropractic Care for Low Back Pain

- If the AHCPR Guideline is followed by medical gatekeepers, HMOs and other managed care groups, the end result will be significant savings to the overall health care system, because patients will have direct access to chiropractic care.

- The RAND Corporation reported from its analysis of literature on manipulation that 94 percent of all manipulation services are performed by doctors of chiropractic.

- According to the latest Gallup Poll conducted for the ACA, over 18 million Americans have sought chiropractic care. Ninety percent of those chiropractic users considered their treatment effective, 80 percent were satisfied with the services received, and 73 percent felt that most or all of their care expectations were met

- Patients are more satisfied with chiropractic treatment for back problems than with any other form of care, according to a recent Harris Poll.

- In a 1993 study, the Ontario Ministry of Health determined there should be a "shift in policy to encourage and prefer chiropractic services for most patients with low-back pain," and chiropractic should be "fully insured (and) fully integrated" into the Ontario health care system. It went on to state that chiropractors should be added to all hospital staffs and that low back pain patients currently under the care of medical physicians should be transferred to chiropractic physicians for evaluation and/or treatment.

- The mean compensation costs paid out by the Utah Workers' Compensation Board for patients treated by doctors of chiropractic was only 10 percent of that paid out for patients treat by other physicians. (*Journal of Occupational Medicine*, 1991.)

- As many as 80 percent of Americans will suffer from back pain at some point in their lives.

- Back symptoms are the leading cause of disability for Americans under age 45.

- Twenty percent of all American military medical discharges are due to low back pain.

Chiropractic Manipulation and Federal Guidelines

Further Resources about the AHCPR Guidelines and How They Impact the Chiropractic Profession:

These materials are available online at http://www.cais.net/aca/ or contact the American Chiropractic Association by calling its Department of Marketing at 1-800-986-INFO.

Summary: A Detailed Summary and Discussion of the AHCPR Guidelines by Howard Balduc, DC, Former ACA Vice President of Professional Information Development.

Legal Implications: An article by Tom Daly, ACA Legal Council, about the potential legal effect of the recent AHCPR Guideline for Doctors of Chiropractic.

News Releases: ACA Press Releases about the AHCPR Guidelines, highlighting why the guidelines should clear the way for direct access to chiropractors in managed care health plans.

Media Coverage: A summary of some of the positive media coverage the AHCPR Guidelines have generated for the chiropractic profession.

How to obtain the AHCPR Guidelines: Ordering instructions for the full set of AHCPR Guidelines, and other related materials published by ACA. The Guideline on Acute back pain is extracted as the previous chapter of this Sourcebook. To receive more information about guidelines or to receive a free copy of *Understanding Acute Low Back Problems*, call toll-free 800-358-9295, or write to:

Agency for Health Care Policy and Research
Publications Clearinghouse
P.O. Box 8547
Silver Spring, MD 20907

Online, go to http://text.nlm.nih.gov/ftrs/pick?dbName=lbpp&ftrsK= 33341&cp=1&t=868227432&collect=ahcpr

Manipulation for My Back Problem?: An Informative Guide for Patients outlining the benefits of manipulation for back problems, adapted from a brochure available from ACA Press

Questions and Answers About Manipulation: Adapted from ACA's booklet, What is Manipulation & How Can it Help Me? Available from

ACA Press. This article is also reprinted in Omnigraphics' *Back and Neck Disorders Sourcebook*.

AMA Publication on Back Pain Ignores AHCPR Findings: In its review of the new publication by the American Medical Association (AMA) titled AMA Pocket Guide to Back Pain, the Foundation for Chiropractic Education and Research (FCER) asks, "Why did the AMA ignore the results of the AHCPR clinical practice guideline in preparing this new publication?"

Results of a Nationwide Survey: Results of a survey of Americans regarding attitudes on practitioners and treatments for back pain. See also Omnigraphics' *Back and Neck Disorders Sourcebook*.

Chapter 20

Neck Pain and Disorders of the Cervical Spine

What is the cervical spine?

The spine consists of small bones, called vertebrae, that are linked in a column extending down the center of the back from the base of the head to the buttocks area. The cervical spine consists of the top seven vertebrae of the vertebral column. The top vertebra next to the base of the skull is called the atlas. The second vertebra is called the axis. These two vertebrae are different in shape and function from the other vertebrae of the spine. Discs which act as cushions rest between vertebrae and facilitate movement of the vertebral column. The spinal cord runs through a hollow channel in each vertebra, and nerves carrying impulses to all areas of the body branch off from the spinal cord between the vertebrae.

What are some causes of neck pain?

Neck pain may be caused by injury, postural strain on the neck, a variety of diseases, or pain radiating from another site, such as the jaw. In acute cervical sprains where the head is thrust forward and then backward on impact (whiplash), pain or spasm in the neck may begin up to 48 hours after the accident. Neck symptoms which are worse in the morning and improve during the day suggest an inflammatory disease, but may be simply due to a sleeping position that puts

---

A fact sheet prepared by the National Institute of Arthritis and Musculoskeletal and Skin Diseases, April, 1992.

the neck in an awkward position (bending backwards or sideways). Occupations that require repetitive or prolonged flexion, extension, or rotation of the neck may cause problems. Pain that is accentuated by coughing, sneezing, or jolting suggests a disc problem, such as a herniation (slipped disc). In the case of a disease, like arthritis, degenerative (deteriorating or eroding) changes and partial dislocation may result from destruction of bone, disc, cartilage, ligaments, and other soft tissue. This condition is known as spondylosis. Although uncommon, tumors and infections may also cause cervical problems.

What are some symptoms of cervical spine disorders?

The signs of a problem involving the cervical spine depend on the location, extent, and cause of the problem. Symptoms may be due to pressure on the spinal cord (myelopathy) or on the nerve roots as they extend from the cord (radiculopathy). The first signs are stiffness and/or pain in the neck. There may also be tingling or, in more severe cases, numbness of the hands, arms, and shoulders or tingling that radiates upward to the base of the head or down the back. Rarely, weakness or numbness may extend into the legs or feet, and there may be a loss of bowel or bladder function.

Eye, ear, nose, and throat symptoms are sometimes associated with cervical disease. Irritation of nerves that branch upward from the cervical spine may cause blurred vision that is altered by moving the neck, increased tearing, and pain at the back of the eye. A need to repeatedly clear the throat or difficulty speaking and the feeling of being unable to get enough breath may also be symptoms of nerve irritation in the neck. Heart palpitations and a rapid heart beat may result from hyperextension of the neck.

How are cervical problems diagnosed?

Physical examination is sometimes all that is needed to diagnose a cervical problem. Often, however, additional diagnostic techniques are used. An x-ray may be all that is needed to see an obvious problem in the cervical spine. Various diagnostic techniques may be used to determine the nature and extent of a cervical problem. These include myelography, CT scan, and/or MRI. Cervical discography may play a role in the management of patients with degenerative conditions when the diagnosis cannot be determined by the other tests. An injection for pain (analgesic) is sometimes used to determine the pain pattern (where the pain is most acute and where it radiates).

Neck Pain and Disorders of the Cervical Spine

What are conservative treatments for neck pain?

The goal of therapy for cervical spine problems is to relieve pain and reverse any neurological problems. For minor neck stiffness, exercises that stretch the muscles in the neck, massage, and heat may be all that is necessary to relieve pain. When the cause of pain is more than a temporary stiffness, resolution of pain by these conservative measures may take weeks or months. Rigid or soft cervical collars may be suggested. Soft collars, unlike rigid ones, only partially constrain neck motion, but they do support the head and remind the person to limit motion. However, these collars rarely reverse neurologic symptoms associated with more severe conditions, such as a partial dislocation of a cervical vertebra. People whose pain or stiffness is due to inflammation, rather than structural damage, often respond to treatment with nonsteroidal anti-inflammatory drugs. Physical therapy treatments may include range of motion and strengthening exercises, heat, cold, ultrasound, cervical traction, and the use of cervical support pillows. Narrowing of the spinal canal or intervertebral foramina with pain spreading along nerve pathways may respond to corticosteroid (anti-inflammatory steroid) injection. Pain treatment centers play an important role in helping patients cope with chronic neck pain. In addition to the traditional treatments mentioned, many centers offer behavioral modification, biofeedback, acupuncture, and acupressure.

What surgery might be necessary to treat cervical problems?

Most people with neck problems can be effectively treated non-operatively. Except in cases of injury, surgical intervention should not be considered until the patient has undergone an adequate trial of non-operative management. People with progressive neurological deterioration (e.g., persistent numbness, weakness, and interference with movement) may be candidates for cervical surgery, as may those with severe and persistent neck pain, even in the absence of neurological symptoms. There are two basic surgical approaches to the cervical spine: anterior and posterior. Anterior procedures, in which an incision is made in the front of the neck, primarily include removal of the disc with or without fusion. (Fusion creates a bony bridge between two or more vertebrae.) When a fusion is performed, bone is usually taken from the patient's hip, but bone from a donor or other source outside the body might also be considered. Patients with disc herniations and central cord compression are most often candidates for the anterior approach. Posterior procedures include surgical removal of all or part of one or more of the bony arches of the vertebrae that surround the spinal cord to relieve pressure on the cord or nerve extending from it (called a laminectomy). Disc material may be removed at the same time.

What can be expected after surgery?

Following surgery a hard collar is usually placed around the neck, and this may be worn day and night for a few weeks. When the doctor feels the neck has healed sufficiently, the hard collar may be replaced by a soft one, and eventually, no collar will be needed. Because the muscles of the neck may become weakened with prolonged wear of a collar, these devices are worn no longer than necessary. After removal of the collar, exercises to strengthen the neck muscles may be prescribed to help restore a full range of motion to the neck.

What can be done to protect the neck from future problems?

Following are some of the steps a person can take to guard against neck problems:

- When at a desk, sit straight, rather than bending forward or leaning over work—place work material so that it is unnecessary to bend or turn your head to see it;

- Sit in a chair with arm rests;

- Hold a phone receiver in your hand, not handless supported on the shoulder by the head;

- Use a foot stool if you must reach into a high cupboard or shelf;

- Don't read or watch TV with the head propped forward on a pillow or arm of a sofa;

- When lying down, place a pillow under the head and neck in a position that keeps the neck straight.

Part Four

Some Other Common Forms of Nerve and Muscle Pain

Chapter 21

Trigeminal Neuralgia (Tic Douloureux)

Chapter Contents

Section 21.1—Background 192
Section 21.2—TN's Jolting Symptoms and the
              Drugs That Help 193
Section 21.3—Glycerol Can Be Shot of Relief for
              Persistent Pain.. 198
Section 21.4—When Pain Returns after Surgery 201

Section 21.1

Background

©1995 Trigeminal Neuralgia Association. PO Box 340, Baranegat Light, NJ 08006. Phone (609) 361-1014, fax (609) 361-0982.
Reprinted with permission.

Trigeminal neuralgia (tic douloureux) is a disorder of the fifth cranial (trigeminal) nerve that causes episodes of intense, stabbing, electric shock-like pain in the areas of the face where the branches of the nerve are distributed—lips, eyes, nose, scalp, forehead, upper jaw, and lower jaw. Something as simple and routine as brushing the teeth, putting on makeup or even a slight breeze can trigger an attack resulting in sheer agony for the individual. Trigeminal neuralgia [TN] is not a fatal disease, but it is universally considered to be the most painful affliction known to adult men and women. Initial treatment of TN is through the use of anticonvulsant drugs, such as tegretol or baclofen. Should the medication be ineffective or if it produces undesirable side effects neurosurgical procedures are available to relieve pressure on the nerve or to reduce nerve sensitivity.

Trigeminal Neuralgia (Tic Douloureux)

Section 21.2

TN's Jolting Symptoms and the Drugs That Help

©1995 Trigeminal Neuralgia Association. Reprinted with permission.

There should be little difficulty in diagnosing trigeminal neuralgia if doctors take a careful patient history and watch for clues that are very specific to this jolting pain.

TN rarely occurs in patients under age 30. The pain is of high intensity, typically lasting 20 to 30 seconds and then disappearing, only to be followed by another sudden jab later.

The pain also usually is triggered by a light touch to a particular area or two of the face, especially around the nose and mouth. Often patients say they seem to feel a sense of numbness or deadness in the face, although an exam usually doesn't bear that out.

One of the biggest clues, though, is not what TN patients say but what they do. In almost every other facial pain syndrome, patients will be found massaging the painful area or rubbing it or applying heat or cold.

With TN, exactly the opposite occurs. The patient goes to great lengths to avoid any stimulation of the face or mouth whatsoever. Thus it's characteristic of TN patients to avoid touching the face, washing the face, shaving, biting, chewing or anything else that stimulates the trigger zones and produces the pain.

Many factors may produce TN. These include aging, a persistent viral infection of the trigeminal ganglion (the cluster of nerve cells just before the nerve splits out into its three branches in the face) or an abnormality that is compressing the trigeminal nerve, such as a blood vessel, tumor, cyst or aneurysm (a blood vessel bulging at a weak area).

In about 3 percent of the cases, multiple sclerosis is at the root of the pain. MS plaques can form on the trigeminal nerve and destroy the nerve's protective coating.

Besides giving doctors descriptions of pain that are as accurate as possible, TN patients also should have a magnetic resonance imaging (MRI) scan of the brain to search for tumors and aneurysms.

If those disorders are ruled out, most doctors agree that medical treatment is the best first step. How a patient responds to medications also can help nail down a definite diagnosis of TN. If, for example, a patient presumed to have TN does not rapidly respond to carbamazepine (e.g., Tegretol) in 24 to 48 hours, the diagnosis is then seriously in doubt.

If the patient does respond to carbamazepine, then clearly this is the treatment of choice. Doctors who have followed patients with TN for more than a decade have found the condition ebbs and floes, so it may be possible when using drugs to nudge the patient into another remission. When that occurs the drug can be decreased and perhaps stopped.

If the response to carbamazepine is only partial, other drugs also may be useful, including phenytoin (e.g., Dilantin) and baclofen (e.g., Lioresar).

Some neurosurgeons suggest that unpleasant side effects occur frequently with carbamazepine and that up to 20 to 30 percent of patients taking this drug need to stop it, which is surprising since the drug seems better tolerated when used to treat epilepsy.

Nonetheless, carbamazepine may produce undesirable sedation and other side effects, including in rare cases, blood disorders. For that reason patients who are taking it should undergo periodic blood tests.

Commonly used pain-killing drugs are of little use in treating TN. Carbamazepine, for example, is not an analgesic drug at all but an anticonvulsant that helps TN pain by reducing the sensitivity of the trigger zones.

Works Fast

Carbamazepine often helps dramatically and quickly—sometimes in as little as 4 to 24 hours. Generally, treatment starts with 100 to 200 mg doses of carbamazepine taken two or three times daily.

If this dose is well tolerated, the doctor should attempt to adjust the medication according to the severity of the pain. If the pain persists, the dosage should be increased; if the pain is well controlled, the dosage can be scaled back. It may be necessary to continue the carbamazepine at a maintenance level, such as 200 mg per day, in order to keep the patient pain-free.

Trigeminal Neuralgia (Tic Douloureux)

If symptoms persist while taking carbamazepine in adequate doses, add another drug to the regimen. Generally, baclofen is the choice, beginning with 10 mg daily and increasing to 60 to 80 mg daily in divided doses along with carbamazepine.

Rarely, if pain persists, a third drug—usually phenytoin—is added. By the time a three-drug treatment is reached though, it's time to consider referring the patient for surgery.

Other drugs such as sodium valproate (e.g., Depakene, Depakote, Epilim) and clonazepam (e.g., Klonopin, Rivotril) are sometimes used, but no formal studies have been done to document their effectiveness in treating TN.

The drug pimozide (ie. Orap) is another medication that has been offered for use in treating TN. In one study of 48 patients, pimozide was found to be superior to carbamazepine for pain relief. However, this antipsychotic drug can cause a variety of side effects that should be weighed carefully before prescribing it.

New Drug Being Tested

Yet another drug, oxcarbazepine (e.g., Trileptal), is currently being tested. Early studies of this drug, similar in makeup to carbamazepme, are showing an "excellent therapeutic response," according to a pair of European neurologists who are testing it. However, this drug so far is not available in the United States.

Two other researchers have reported some success using a cream containing capsaicin, the chemical that makes hot peppers hot. Six of 12 patients who rubbed this non-prescription cream on the painful area for several days got complete relief, while four others got partial relief. Two had no pain relief. Four of the 10 who were helped found their pain returned in three to five months, but after a second round of cream, the pain did not return for the remainder of the year.

Approximately 25 to 50 percent of TN patients eventually will fail on medical therapy and will need some form of neurosurgical treatment.

—by Dr. Donald J. Dalessio, TNA Medical Advisory Board

Dr. Dalessio is a neurologist at the Scripps Clinic and Research Foundation in La Jolla, California.

Section 21.3

Glycerol Can Be Shot of Relief for Persistent Pain

©1995 Trigeminal Neuralgia Association. Reprinted with permission.

Surgeries that attack trigeminal neuralgia by use of a needle through the cheek play an important role in relieving TN pain.

Due to their safety and less-invasive nature, these "percutaneous" procedures are often the first surgical choice for older patients and for those with other medical problems.

Although pain may be more likely to return after a percutaneous procedure than after an open-skull microvascular decompression surgery, these procedures are easily repeatable.

At the University of Pittsburgh, our first choice in percutaneous procedures is a "glycerol rhizotomy," a treatment that involves injecting glycerol around the trigeminal nerve. We prefer it to the two other commonly used percutaneous procedures—radio-frequency rhizotomy and balloon compression—due to its technical ease, lack of need for patient feedback and less chance of facial numbness.

A glycerol rhizotomy is performed with the patient awake but under sedation. The surgeon's aim is to insert a spinal needle through the cheek and into an opening at the base of the skull called the "foramen ovale." Just past that opening is the "trigeminal cistern," a small sac of spinal fluid that contains the trigeminal nerve.

With the patient lying down, the surgeon inserts the needle and uses X-ray guidance to direct it to the right spot. We then sit the patient up and confirm correct placement by injecting a contrast dye into the sac. This tells us the volume of the sac and also its shape.

Next, the dye is drained out and a solution of glycerol is injected into the sac. The needle is then withdrawn, and a small bandage is placed over the skin-puncture site.

The patient remains in the sitting position for the next two hours to prevent the glycerol from draining out of the cistern. The patient

Trigeminal Neuralgia (Tic Douloureux)

then returns to the ward and is either discharged home the same day or the following morning.

Some patients have a headache or discomfort around the eye for a few hours after the procedure, and a few have some short-lived nausea.

About 85 to 90 percent of patients have a good result—that is, significant relief from TN pain. In patients with multiple scleroses, the initial success rate is similar.

In half the patients who respond favorably, pain relief occurs the day of the procedure. In the other half, relief occurs gradually over several weeks—even as far out as one month afterward.

In our 10-year experience of 480 patients who had 620 glycerol rhizotomies, we found that 75 percent of patients were pain-free at an average follow-up of three years. If pain returns, either a new round of medication therapy or a repeat rhizotomy can be considered.

In an analysis of 55 patients with MS related trigeminal neuralgia, we found that complete pain relief with no further medication necessary was achieved in 60 percent of patients. Eight patients had satisfactory pain control but needed occasional medication, and 12 needed additional surgery. About 60 percent of the patients retained normal facial sensation after glycerol injection.

In our patient series, we have not observed any cases of anesthesia dolorosa which is a hard-to-treat potential complication involving numbness along with pain.

Recently, we and others have explored the use of Gamma Knife radio surgery in treating TN. The Gamma Knife is a device that precisely focuses irradiation on the trigeminal nerve as it first exits the brainstem.

The goal is to create a small controlled area of damage so as to disrupt pain signals from getting to the brain without causing numbness. The device has been used since the 1950s, mostly in treating brain tumors and brain blood-vessel malformations.

No Incision

This procedure involves fastening a frame to the patient's head that is needed to help direct the beams of radiation to the right area. There is no needle insertion, no incision of any kind and the procedure is done with the patient awake.

When the procedure is successful pain relief often comes within days and usually within four to six weeks.

Based on the results at five institutions, total relief was obtained in 12 of 19 patients in which the Gamma Knife was their first TN surgery. In cases of prior TN surgery, the Gamma Knife brought total relief to 12 of 31 patients and at least good results to 27 of the 31.

Reduction in facial sensation is uncommon in patients treated by this approach.

We initially used this technique for patients who had failed to gain relief from other surgeries. Recently, we and others have begun using it as the first surgical procedure in those who have medical problems that might make any other type of procedure hazardous.

Making the Choice

Any of the percutaneous procedures can provide pain relief and preserve facial sensation. Individual institutions recommend different procedures based on their own experience and results. Some prefer radio-frequency rhizotomy, in which the nerve is selectively damaged with an electrode, and others prefer balloon compression, in which the nerve is temporarily squeezed by a tiny balloon inflated at the end of an inserted catheter.

All of these procedures play an important role in the treatment of TN and have proved satisfying to many patients.

—by Dr. Douglas Kondziolka, Chief,
Stereotactic Functional Neurosurgery,
University of Pittsburgh

Trigeminal Neuralgia (Tic Douloureux)

Section 21.4

When Pain Returns after Surgery

©1995 Trigeminal Neuralgia Association. Reprinted with permission.

Sometimes TN pain stubbornly returns after surgery seemed to cure it.

Fortunately, the arsenal of TN treatments has grown to the point that if one method falls, there are others to fall back on, says Dr. John Alksne, chief of Neurological Surgery at the University of California in San Diego.

Alksne, a member of TNA's Medical Advisory Board, recently told the San Diego TNA support group that pain can even return after a microvascular decompression—the open-skull surgery in which the doctor aims to find and move a compressing blood vessel off the trigeminal nerve. Most doctors consider an MVD operation as offering the best chance of long-term pain relief without numbness.

"What we have found is that 90 percent of the cases of trigeminal neuralgia are due to a blood vessel right where the nerve enters the brain." Alksne says, "Where an artery is digging into the nerve actually damages the insulation of the nerve, and that sets up this 'static' within the nerve itself, which is what you perceive as pain."

According to reported results worldwide, MVDs relieve pain initially in more than nine of 10 cases. However, the data also show that within 10 years, the pain recurs in about 20 to 25 percent of those initial successes.

Alksne says there are several reasons why TN pain comes back. Sometimes it's because a surgeon moved one vessel out of the way only to have another one compress the nerve later. That happens because vessels elongate with age. In other cases, the cushion that surgeons insert to insulate the nerve from the offending vessel may fail. That's particularly true if the cushion material is a sliver of transplanted muscle, says Alksne.

"Some people in the past have used muscle, but over time the body absorbs it and it goes away ... then the vessel can fall back onto the nerve," he says.

Alksne says most surgeons today use bits of cotton-like Teflon felt as a cushion. Occasionally that implant falls out of place or is bumped out of place by elongating vessels. "You have to pack it in there so it doesn't dislodge," Alksne says.

In still other cases, MVDs can fail or pain can return because the compressing vessel has damaged the trigeminal nerve beyond repair. Alksne says if the nerve has become significantly scarred, it may never return to normal function even when the cause of the irritation is removed.

"My impression from the years I've been doing this is that the longer a person suffers with trigeminal neuralgia the greater the likelihood that damage inside the nerve is beyond repair," he says. "It's like if you have a rock in your shoe for 15 minutes and take it out you're great. If you have a rock in your shoe and you go on a 20-mile hike, you're going to have a sore on your foot that's going to take some time to heal. If you have a rock in your shoe for 10 years, that sore may never heal."

Alksne says when he gets a case of recurrent TN pain after surgery, he first reviews the pain history to make sure the patient really does have TN and not some other facial-pain syndrome mimicking TN pain.

If that checks out, he says he reviews the surgeon's notes from the patient's surgery to determine if an offending vessel might have been missed. If that's a good possibility he usually suggests a second MVD.

"If I'm convinced the person who did the operation did it the proper way, found a blood vessel and moved it and used Teflon, the chances that I am going to find something by going back in are very slim," Alksne says.

In that case, Alksne says he suggests that the patient first try a new round of medications—usually Tegretol. Often post-operation patients find their pain can be controlled by lower doses of Tegretol than they were taking before the operation.

If medication doesn't work, he usually suggests a balloon compression, his favorite of the three through-the-cheek surgeries designed to selectively damage the nerve. This surgery involves inflating a tiny balloon against the nerve for two to five minutes. The idea is to damage the nerve enough to stop pain signals from getting through to the brain without causing numbness.

*Trigeminal Neuralgia (*Tic Douloureux*)*

Another option is an injection of glycerol, an oily liquid that's toxic to nerve fibers, The third option is a radio-frequency rhizotomy, which uses a thin electrode inserted through the cheek to selectively burn the trigeminal nerve fibers. All three operations are repeatable.

If repeated surgery fails, there's always the option that surgeons used prior to the 1960s—cutting the nerve at the root. That ends TN pain but at the expense of permanent numbness.

—by George Weigel, TN Alert *Editor*

Chapter 22

Bell's Palsy: A Painful, Disfiguring Ailment

Most Recover Completely; Some Have Recurrences

Cathy M. was in her ninth month of pregnancy when she awakened with a toothache-like pain in her jaw that within hours spread to her ear. Thinking she had an abscessed tooth, she saw her dentist, who immediately referred her to an oral surgeon. But the surgeon's tests showed that it was not a tooth but more likely a facial nerve that was causing Cathy's pain.

By the next day, when she saw a neurologist, her eye was tearing uncontrollably and one side of her face had begun to feel numb and to droop. When she tried to smile, she looked like a split-faced clown: happy on one side, sad on the other.

The neurologist did a series of tests to be sure something far more serious like a brain tumor or stroke, was not the cause of Cathy's symptoms. Then he diagnosed Bell's palsy, an inflammation of a major facial nerve. A virus, probably Herpes simplex, which also causes cold sores, is strongly suspected as the cause of the inflammation.

Named for Sir Charles Bell, an early 19th-century Scottish physiologist who first described it, this frightening nerve ailment strikes about 40,000 Americans a year. One in 30 people develops it sometime over the course of a lifetime. And while 80 to 85 percent recover completely, 15 to 20 percent experience some degree of permanent nerve impairment. About 10 percent of all the victims suffer one or more recurrences.

©1993 *The New York Times*, July 28, 1993. Reprinted with permission.

Who Is Affected?

Bell's palsy can strike almost anyone at any age. But it disproportionately attacks pregnant women and people who have diabetes, influenza, a cold or some other upper respiratory ailment. People with a family history of the inflammation run a higher than average risk of developing it. Most cases occur after the age of 40, and are about equally distributed between men and women.

Its cause has never been clearly established, although studies have strongly suggested a virus. Viruses in the herpes family have a predilection for invading nerves and dwelling there permanently, which makes herpes the prime suspect. In at least one study, which involved 41 victims, all of the people with Bell's palsy had developed antibodies to Herpes simplex.

What may trigger an attack of Bell's palsy is also not known. For most people, its symptoms develop with alarming speed. However, a significant minority of patients reports that just before the attack, they had been exposed to a draft, perhaps from an air-conditioner or an open window near the bed. And often the draft was felt only on the affected side. For example, taxi drivers tend to get Bell's palsy on the left side of their faces, the side typically exposed to an open window.

Cathy's neurologist explained that for part of its route from the brain to the face, the involved nerve travels through a narrow, tortuous bony tunnel. If the nerve becomes inflamed and swollen, the pressure from its bony casing can cause it to stop functioning, and messages from the brain that control facial muscles no longer get through. Symptoms typically develop rapidly, and within 48 to 72 hours half the face can become paralyzed.

This results in a dramatic distortion of the face. On the affected side, the eye tears and the mouth drools; the eye may not close, even during sleep; the nose cannot twitch; the tongue cannot taste, and the corner of the mouth cannot turn up. It is almost as if the whole side of the face had been numbed by a dental anesthetic. Sometimes sounds are especially loud to the ear on the affected side and some patients have difficulty speaking and eating.

Treating Symptoms

Given these symptoms, it is easy to see why people with Bell's palsy often feel, as Cathy did, that they would like to hide under a rock until it goes away. Cathy was so distressed by her appearance, especially when she tried to smile, that she refused to be photographed with her new baby.

Bell's Palsy: A Painful, Disfiguring Ailment

There is no specific treatment for Bell's palsy, and the treatments that are used remain controversial. Some physicians prescribe a corticosteroid drug to reduce the inflammation and an analgesic to relieve the pain. But the steroid has never been proved to hasten recovery. Cathy, for one, was reluctant to take a steroid because she feared its possible effects on her unborn child.

With or without treatment, most patients begin to get significantly better within two weeks, and about 80 percent of patients recover completely within three months. However, the symptoms last much longer for some people, and, in a few cases—Cathy's might be among them—the symptoms may never completely disappear.

In patients whose eye muscles are affected, care must be taken to protect the delicate tissues of the eye against desiccation and debris. Outdoors, eyeglasses can help protect the eye from dust and particles. Artificial tears should be used repeatedly during the day, and an eye ointment should be used at night to prevent undue dryness, which could result in corneal ulcers. At night the eyelid may have to be manually or mechanically closed with tape or covered with a patch.

Physical therapy is often prescribed to stimulate the nerve and maintain tone in the affected muscles while the nerve is healing. Cathy, for example, was told to practice wiggling her nose, grinning and pouting with her mouth, raising her brow and blowing out her cheek; even when nothing seemed to be happening, the effort was thought to aid the muscles. Applications of heat for two five-minute periods a day followed by a gentle five minute facial massage are sometimes helpful.

Some physical therapists suggest electro-stimulation of the affected nerve. That approach has not been proved beneficial but, as Cathy put it, "at least it gives patients the feeling that something is being done to help."

For patients who are seriously debilitated by their condition or who fail to start recovering within months, neurologists may consider surgery to reduce the pressure on the nerve. However, this treatment also remains controversial and may not produce the desired result.

Even for those who recover fully, there remains the specter of a recurrence. For someone like Cathy, who, 19 months after her first attack, is concerned that she may never again have a completely normal face, there is a further concern that a subsequent pregnancy might trigger a second attack of the facial palsy.

One Inflamed Nerve Many Symptoms

Bell's palsy results from inflammation or irritation of a facial nerve. Depending on where the problem occurs, any or all of the organs served by the nerve may be affected.

- **Muscles**. All the muscles on each side of the face except those involved in chewing are controlled by one of the pair of facial nerves; the facial nerve is also called the seventh cranial nerve.

- **Glands and Sense**. The facial nerve also carries autonomic nerve fibers that control the salivary glands and tear glands, as well as sensory nerve fibers for the back two-thirds of the tongue.

- **Symptoms**. Numbness, pain, one-sided facial paralysis and distortion, tearing, drooling, inability to close the eye, hypersensitivity to sound in the affected ear and impairment of taste.

—by Jane E. Brody

Chapter 23

Fibromyalgia

Questions and Answers about Fibromyalgia

What is fibromyalgia?

Fibromyalgia is a chronic disorder characterized by widespread musculoskeletal pain, fatigue, and multiple tender points. "Tender points" refers to tenderness that occurs in precise, localized areas, particularly in the neck, spine, shoulders, and hips. People with this syndrome may also experience sleep disturbances, morning stiffness, irritable bowel syndrome, anxiety, and other symptoms.

How many people have fibromyalgia?

According to the American College of Rheumatology, fibromyalgia affects three to six million Americans. It primarily occurs in women of childbearing age, but children, the elderly, and men can also be affected.

What causes fibromyalgia?

Although the cause of fibromyalgia is unknown, researchers have several theories about causes or triggers of the disease. Some scientists believe that the syndrome may be caused by an injury or trauma.

National Institute of Arthritis and Musculoskeletal and Skin Diseases Office of Scientific and Health Communications October 1995.

This injury may affect the central nervous system. Fibromyalgia may be associated with changes in muscle metabolism, such as decreased blood flow, causing fatigue and decreased strength. Others believe the syndrome may be triggered by an infectious agent such as a virus in susceptible people, but no such agent has been identified.

How is fibromyalgia diagnosed?

Fibromyalgia is difficult to diagnose because many of the symptoms mimic those of other diseases. The physician reviews the patient's medical history and makes a diagnosis of fibromyalgia based on a history of chronic widespread pain that persists for more than three months. The American College of Rheumatology (ACR) has developed criteria for fibromyalgia that physicians can use in diagnosing the disease. According to ACR criteria, a person is considered to have fibromyalgia if he or she has widespread pain in combination with tenderness in at least 11 of 18 specific tender point sites.

How is fibromyalgia treated?

Treatment of fibromyalgia requires a comprehensive approach. The physician, physical therapist, and patient may all play an active role in the management of fibromyalgia. Studies have shown that aerobic exercise, such as swimming and walking, improves muscle fitness and reduces muscle pain and tenderness. Heat and massage may also give short-term relief. Antidepressant medications may help elevate mood, improve quality of sleep, and relax muscles. Fibromyalgia patients may benefit from a combination of exercise, medication, physical therapy, and relaxation.

What research is being conducted on fibromyalgia?

The NIAMS is sponsoring research that will increase understanding of the specific abnormalities that cause and accompany fibromyalgia with the hope of developing better ways to diagnose, treat, and prevent this disorder.

Recent NIAMS studies show that abnormally low levels of the hormone cortisol may be associated with fibromyalgia. At Brigham and Women's Hospital in Boston, Massachusetts, and at the University of Michigan Medical Center in Ann Arbor, researchers are studying regulation of the function of the adrenal gland (which makes cortisol) in fibromyalgia. People whose bodies make inadequate amounts of cortisol experience many of the same symptoms as people with fibromyalgia. It is hoped that these studies will increase understanding about fibromyalgia and may suggest new ways to treat the disorder.

Other NIAMS research studies are looking at different aspects of the disease. At the University of Alabama in Birmingham, researchers are concentrating on how specific brain structures are involved in the painful symptoms of fibromyalgia. Researchers at Vanderbilt University in Nashville, Tennessee, are using magnetic resonance imaging (MRI) and magnetic resonance spectroscopy (MRS) techniques to study patients with fibromyalgia. MRI and MRS are powerful tools that have been shown to be useful in evaluating muscle disorders and muscle performance. At the New York Medical College in Valhalla, scientists are investigating the causes of a post-Lyme disease syndrome as a model for fibromyalgia. Some patients develop a fibromyalgia-like condition following Lyme disease, an infectious disorder associated with arthritis and other symptoms.

NIAMS-supported research on fibromyalgia also includes several projects in the Institute's Multipurpose Arthritis and Musculoskeletal Diseases Centers. Researchers at these centers are studying individuals who do not seek medical care, but who meet the criteria for fibromyalgia. (Potential subjects are located through advertisements in local newspapers asking for volunteers with widespread pain or aching.) Other studies at the Centers are attempting to uncover better ways to manage the pain associated with the disease through behavioral interventions such as relaxation training.

The NIAMS supports and encourages outstanding basic and clinical research that increases the understanding of fibromyalgia. However, much more research needs to be done before fibromyalgia can be successfully treated or prevented.

The Federal Government, in collaboration with researchers, physicians, and private voluntary health organizations, is committed to research efforts that are directed to significantly improving the health of all Americans afflicted with fibromyalgia.

The NIAMS, a component of the National Institutes of Health, leads and coordinates the Federal biomedical effort in arthritis, musculoskeletal, bone, muscle, and skin diseases by conducting and supporting research projects, research training, clinical trials, and epidemiological studies, and by disseminating information on research initiatives and research results.

Chapter 24

Thoracic Outlet Syndrome

Description: Thoracic outlet syndrome consists of symptoms caused by compression of the nerves in the brachial plexus (nerves that pass into the arms from the neck) or blood vessels. Patients may have pain in the shoulder, arm, or hand, or in all three locations. The hand pain is often most severe in the fourth and fifth fingers. The pain is aggravated by the use of the arm, and "fatigue" of the arm is often prominent.

Treatment: The goals of treatment are two-fold: to correct postural abnormalities that might contribute to the compression, and to establish an exercise program to strengthen the shoulder muscles. Most often a conservative course of treatment is followed. If vascular or major neurological impairment is present, surgical decompression may be considered. However, only a small number of patients require surgery.

Prognosis: The prognosis for the majority of individuals who receive therapy for thoracic outlet syndrome is good.

Research: Within the NINDS research programs, thoracic outlet syndrome is addressed through research on pain. NINDS vigorously pursues a research program seeking new treatments for pain and

---

NIH Web Publication. National Institutes of Health, Bethesda, Maryland 20892. April 1996. National Institute of Neurological Disorders and Stroke. http://www.ninds.nih.gov/healinfo/disorder/thoracic/thoracic.htm#description Last Updated: May 20, 1997.

nerve damage with the ultimate goal of reversing cumulative trauma disorders such as thoracic outlet syndrome. NINDS has notified research investigators that it is seeking grant applications both in basic and clinical pain research.

These articles, available from a medical library, may provide more in-depth information on thoracic outlet syndrome:

Bonica, JJ. (ed). *The Management of Pain*, 2nd Edition, Lea & Febiger, Philadelphia (1990).

Cuetter, AC, and Bartoszek, DM. "The Thoracic Outlet Syndrome: Controversies, Overdiagnosis, Overtreatment, and Recommendations for Management." *Muscle and Nerve*, 12; 410-419 (May 1989).

Joynt, RJ. (ed). *Clinical Neurology*, 4 (1991).

Karas, SE. "Thoracic Outlet Syndrome." *Clinics in Sport Medicine*, 9:2; 297-310 (April 1990).

Sanders, RJ, and Haug, C. "Review of Arterial Thoracic Outlet Syndrome." *Surgery, Gynecology and Obstetrics*, 173; 415-425 (November 1991).

Schwartzman, RJ. "Brachial Plexus Traction Injuries." *Hand Clinics*, 7:3; 547-556 (August 1991).

Information may also be available from the following organizations:

National Rehabilitation Information Center
(NARIC)
Macro Systems-Suite 935
8455 Colesville Road
Silver Spring, MD 20910-3319
(301) 588-9284
(800) 346-2742
TTY (301) 495-5626
FAX (301) 587-1967
http://www.naric.com/naric

Thoracic Outlet Syndrome

American Chronic Pain Association
P.O. Box 850
Rocklin, CA 95677
(916) 632-0922

National Chronic Pain Outreach Association
7979 Old Georgetown Road
Suite 100
Bethesda, MD 20814-2429
(301) 652-4948

Chapter 25

Carpal Tunnel Syndrome and Other Repetitive Strain Injuries (RSIs)

Getting a Grip on Hand Problems

FDA Consumer, June 2, 1991

A trip to the supermarket or signing a paycheck didn't used to rank high on the list of 31-year-old Wanda Wood's concerns. But now, everyday chores like pumping gas and carrying groceries to the car are ordeals for her.

Wood can't hold a pen long enough to finish signing her check. She has trouble grasping a nozzle to fill her gasoline tank. And she can't grip her groceries to keep them from falling out of her hands.

"It's when a jar of tomato sauce cracks all over the pavement that I get real embarrassed," said Wood, a Richmond, Va., former postal worker. "It's pretty tough to handle when you're standing in a parking lot covered with red goo."

Like Wood, an increasing number of American workers are experiencing the sudden onset of one of several cumulative trauma disorders affecting the hands, according to James McGlothlin, Ph.D., a research hygienist at the National Institute for Occupational Safety and Health in Cincinnati. Doctors often call them repetitive strain injuries (RSIs).

FDA Consumer, June 2, 1991, and ©1995 Reprinted from October 1995 *Mayo Clinic Health Letter* Volume 13 Number 10 with permission of the Mayo Foundation for Medical Education and Research, Rochester, Minnesota 55905. For subscription information, please call 1-800-333-9038. Reprinted with permission.

RSI is a catch-all term used to refer to many painful conditions, such as trigger finger, nerve spasms, and carpal tunnel syndrome. They can cause stiffness, swelling, tingling, weakness, numbness, and, in some cases, irreversible nerve damage.

Carpal tunnel syndrome is the most frequently reported RSI, with 192 cases per 100,000 workers in 1989, according to the U.S. Public Health Service. It occurs when tissues on the palm side of the hand swell, compressing or entrapping the important median nerve, which runs through this area. Numbness and tingling usually start in the wrist, and can radiate down to the thumb and fingers, or up to the elbow. Many patients feel pins and needles when their wrist is tapped. Weakness occurs on effort. For example, patients may suddenly drop objects they are holding. A nerve conduction test, a recording of the electrical activity of the hand and arm muscles, is helpful in diagnosing this disorder.

Other RSIs include nerve spasm and "trigger finger." When nerve entrapment and the pressure caused by it occurs over a long period, the nerve can become irritated and go into spasms, stimulating muscle activity that eventually causes pain similar to severe muscle cramps.

When finger tendons, fibrous bands of tissue that connect muscle to bone, get irritated, they can grow nodules, which, at the points of attachment, get caught in the lubricating sheath that surrounds them. When this happens, the finger can become stuck; this condition is called trigger finger.

RSIs are self-limiting conditions that result from excessive use of the muscles and tendons of the hands, wrists and forearms. Meat cutters, auto workers, cashiers, journalists, keyboard operators, and others who spend long hours at repetitive chores are particularly vulnerable.

Wood used to spend long shifts operating a letter sorter, typing hours at a time at a computer keyboard to route the mail to its destination.

"My pain eventually became so severe that it worked its way from my fingers to my wrist to my elbow until it felt like a constant crook in my neck," she said.

Hopes for Help

Because the consequences of these disorders are so high, the goal of safety and health professionals across the country is to collect information on which to base decisions about the best ways to prevent and treat these illnesses.

Carpal Tunnel Syndrome and Other Repetitive Strain Injuries

But this is not an easy task. For example, some proposed treatments have not been substantiated by controlled clinical trials.

According to John Vanderveen, Ph.D., director of the Food and Drug Administration's division of nutrition, "We have from time to time dealt with claims for the use of nutrients to prevent or treat carpal tunnel syndrome, but could only find anecdotal reports."

He said, "It's difficult to do such studies because animal models are more tenuous to tease out pain and performance data from than humans. So right now we don't know if basic clinical research is likely to support such claims."

In addition to RSIs, various forms of arthritis can cause hand problems. Rheumatoid arthritis, for example, is a chronic, autoimmune disease affecting the entire musculoskeletal system. Osteoarthritis, a degenerative, "wear and tear" condition can also affect the hands. (See "Arthritis: Modern Treatment for that Old Pain in the Joints" in the July-August 1991 *FDA Consumer* and in Omnigraphics' *Arthritis Sourcebook*.)

Vanderveen said researchers are investigating the innovative use of omega-3 fatty acids, found in fish oils, to help suppress the disease by curtailing production of prostaglandins, a series of hormone-like substances associated with inflammation that occurs in arthritis. Vanderveen cautions that it's still premature at this time to think that these fatty acids will be therapeutic for many arthritis patients.

Today the best bet for RSI patients is to cope with the condition in ways similar to patients with arthritis. Such coping skills include protecting and caring for their joints and using OTC drugs such as aspirin or ibuprofen (Advil, Nuprin, Motrin IB) for mild to moderate symptoms or prescription NSAIDs (nonsteroidal anti-inflammatory drugs) for stronger anti-inflammatory relief.

A general practitioner can treat these disorders, in most patients, with either exercise, rest, aspirin, or NSAIDs, such as Motrin or Naprosyn. But if relief does not occur within a few weeks, the physician may refer the patient to a specialist.

Occupational therapists can also help patients with these disorders to practice "joint protection," according to Jan Chmela, director of Sheltering Arms Day Rehabilitation Program in Richmond, Va.

Chmela, herself an occupational therapist, said that patients can learn to use their hands in "non-deforming positions." For example, instead of grabbing a key with a thumb and twisting, patients can learn to turn a key with adaptive equipment. They can learn to use their largest joints for a job, rather than their smaller, more vulnerable ones, for opening a jar, for example. She advocates teaching patients to use their hands closest to their anatomical position, outstretched as much as possible instead of twisting and turning them, because bending the hands stresses the joints.

As with most other disorders, however, prevention, where possible, is the best cure.

The National Institute for Occupational Safety and Health is focusing research on ways to redesign the workplace to make RSIs less likely.

The agency's McGlothlin said, "We don't want to try and fit the worker to the job, but the job to the worker, and that can best be done through engineering controls so that both the worker and the company benefit."

For instance, he suggests adjustable-height tables to accommodate workers of different heights and builds. McGlothlin also stressed that employers must be sensitive to the extreme demands on many of their workers and allow for recovery time.

"There are more and more demands on people these days. Many work two jobs or through the night. Women in the workplace may also be raising families. Employees need time off to rest. In order for ideas that we've developed to succeed, there has to be a partnership between workers and their companies to make it a more productive and helpful workplace," he said.

Employers can also cut down on RSIs by providing their workers with chairs that give them better postural support and adjustable work stations that allow them to adjust their screen, keyboard and wrists.

Diagnosis Important

Forty-three-year-old Barbara McGhee, a public affairs specialist at a Virginia Department of Health and Human Services Social Security Administration office, was diagnosed with rheumatoid arthritis at age 19.

Over the years, her hand joints have become rigid and misshapen by chronic inflammation. Her hand dexterity is poor—just shuffling through the pages of a book is difficult.

When McGhee first heard the diagnosis, she said she refused to despair. "I went to the library and learned all I could about it." Because unrealistic expectations only make it that much harder on patients, McGhee said she "needed information so I could make some important decisions. I needed to learn what I would and would not be able to do."

"I realized my attribute was my high energy level and if I cultivated it, I could put it to good use." Twenty-four years later, she is unable to waterski or horseback ride or participate in other sports she used to adore, but she has nevertheless found her niche. McGhee not only holds down a full-time job, but also volunteers for her local chapter of the Arthritis Foundation and the Richmond Mayor's Commission for Disabilities.

McGhee said she only wishes that she hadn't waited five years from the onset of her problems to seek the help of a physician. She said she wonders if she had paid attention to her condition earlier whether she could have avoided having one wrist and one ankle replaced, and the other ankle fused.

Because aches and pains are commonplace, people with early morning stiffness, difficulty in movement, or tenderness in one or more joints sometimes do not realize that they may need to see a doctor.

But it's important that people whose symptoms last longer than several weeks see their physician immediately. For example, in some cases of moderate to severe carpal tunnel syndrome, early treatment can prevent significant permanent damage to nerves.

Hayes Willis, assistant professor of medicine, division of rheumatology, allergy and immunology at the Medical College of Virginia, explained that "damaged nerves just don't heal well."

He added that for both arthritis and RSIs, the earlier a diagnosis is made, the greater the likelihood of minimizing disability.

For More Information

For further information about repetitive strain injuries, call the National Institute for Occupational Safety and Health at (800) 356-4674.

For information and referral 24 hours a day about arthritis, call the Arthritis Foundation's National Hotline at (800) 283-7800. The hot line can provide local chapter numbers and brochures that address many of the physical, emotional and coping problems that arthritis patients can face. The impact of arthritis on the family, pain management, proper exercise, and up-to-date medication information is available.

— by Cheryl Platzman Weinstock

Cheryl Platzman Weinstock is a writer in Long Island, N.Y., who specializes in health and science issues.

Overuse Strain Injury

©1995 Reprinted from October 1995 *Mayo Clinic Health Letter* Volume 13 Number 10 with permission of the Mayo Foundation for Medical Education and Research, Rochester, Minnesota 55905. For subscription information, please call 1-800-333-9038. Reprinted with permission.

Common Conditions

Overuse strain injuries describe a variety of injuries to tendons and muscles. These four are among the most common:

- **Carpal tunnel syndrome.** The carpal tunnel is a passageway under the carpal ligament in your wrist that contains the median nerve and the tendons that bend your fingers. Overuse can cause swelling of the membrane linings (sheaths) surrounding the tendons. Swelling compresses the median nerve.

The result is numbness, tingling or pain starting in the wrist and moving down into your thumb and first three fingers or back toward your elbow. Symptoms may be worse at night.

Computer users like Wanda are the stereotype of people who get carpal tunnel syndrome. But it can affect people who spend long periods with their wrists in flexed or extended positions, especially if their movements include pinching or gripping.

People who work as grocery clerks, factory employees or mechanics may be prone to this injury. But hobbyists like Maria can develop carpal tunnel syndrome through activities such as playing certain musical instruments, needlework and canoeing. The combination of pressure and vibration such as using an electric drill, lawn mower or snowblower can also cause carpal tunnel syndrome.

- **Tennis elbow.** You don't have to spend time on the courts to have this condition. Any combination of rotating your wrist and using force—from playing golf to using a manual screwdriver—can cause a form of epicondylitis (ep-ih-konduh-LI-tis).

The pain begins near your elbow and may move toward the outside of your forearm. The actual injury may be tiny tears in the tendons that attach the muscles of your lower arm to your elbow.

Carpal Tunnel Syndrome and Other Repetitive Strain Injuries

- **Tendinitis**. The cause of an inflamed tendon near your wrist, elbow or shoulder is most often excessive exercise, beyond what you're used to. Repeated movements such as using a paintbrush above shoulder level contribute to this type of injury.

When tendinitis affects your shoulder, pain can cause you to limit range of motion. In turn, tendinitis can progress to a "frozen shoulder," in which ligaments and tendons near the joint continue to stiffen until the joint barely moves.

- **Triggerfinger**. A popping or catching sensation when you bend your finger is the source of the nickname for this type of tenosynovitis (ten-o-sin-o-VI-tis). However, tenosynovitis can also affect your wrist or shoulder.

When it occurs in your hand, tenosynovitis results from swelling of the tendon sheath in your finger or thumb, preventing the tendon from gliding easily through the membrane lining. Countless repetitions of the same hand movements can cause the inflammation.

Early Treatment Means Early Cure

Treating an overuse injury can be as easy as taking over-the-counter pain relievers and stopping for rest breaks at the first sign of pain. The further an injury progresses, the more aggressive the care.

To prevent an overuse injury from getting worse:

- **Treat the pain**. Apply heat or cold to ease the pain. As tolerated, take nonsteroidal anti-inflammatory drugs (NSAIDs) such as aspirin, ibuprofen and naproxen sodium.

- **Rest**. Don't keep pushing yourself in spite of your pain. Over use injuries usually heal if you stop the activity that's aggravating the condition. It may take several weeks for the pain to go away completely.

- **Immobilize the injured area**. One way to stop the pain is to wear a splint that prohibits the aggravating movement.

For carpal tunnel syndrome, you can purchase a splint that holds your wrist steady while allowing you to keep up with most of your regular tasks. Even if you don't need a splint all day, wearing a splint at night may help hold your wrist in a neutral position that relieves the pressure on your median nerve. If you have tennis elbow, a special pressure bandage purchased from a medical supply store and worn over your forearm can relieve symptoms.

If symptoms persist despite rest and self-care:

- **Talk to your doctor.** A prescription analgesic or antidepressant can help manage persistent pain. Your doctor may also want to exclude the possibility of other joint problems such as osteoarthritis.

- **Take advantage of physical therapy.** Cold and heat applications, ultrasound or electrical stimulation to block nerve pathways can relieve persistent pain and help restore normal muscle function.

  A physical therapist can also show you exercises and proper movements that can improve strength and flexibility. Learning simple range-of-motion activities can reduce the likelihood of tendinitis progressing to frozen shoulder.

- **Consider surgery a last resort.** A corticosteroid injection may relieve severe pain that doesn't respond to traditional treatments. In rare cases when it doesn't, you may need surgery.

  Carpal tunnel surgery involves dividing the carpal ligament to relieve pressure on the median nerve. Similarly, surgery for trigger finger relieves pressure by making an incision in the membrane, allowing the tendon to glide freely.

Prevention Is Simple Formula

The best cure for an overuse strain injury is to avoid initial injury:

- **Stretch.** Before beginning a repetitive task, stretch the muscles of your shoulders, arms and hands. Slowly bend your wrist back and forth. Or roll your shoulders in small, gentle rotations. Exercising can also prevent reinjury.

- **Adapt.** If you're using awkward movements or positions, find new equipment or approaches. For example, buy a table specially designed for comfortable use of your home computer.

Carpal Tunnel Syndrome and Other Repetitive Strain Injuries

- **Alternate**. Rotate repetitive tasks with other jobs.

- **Pace**. Take a break at least once an hour,

- **Stop**. You can avoid many overuse strain injuries by simply stopping at the first sign of pain.

Health Tips: Getting a Second Opinion

For minor health problems, second opinions are unnecessary. Plus, membership in a health maintenance organization or other health plan may require you to visit only certain physicians. But consider a second opinion if:

- **You're having elective major surgery**. Some insurance companies insist on a second opinion before many elective surgeries. When a second opinion isn't required, they don't always cover the cost. Ask your carrier first.

- **You question whether surgery is your only option**. Surgery to relieve back pain is frequently done. Yet conservative care such as medications and physical therapy often improve symptoms.

- **Your diagnosis is uncertain**. Ask your primary care physician for referral to a specialist. Most physicians welcome second opinions.

- **You're having trouble communicating**. Your diagnosis or treatment leaves you with questions, despite requests for a clear explanation.

- **You're not feeling better**. Your condition doesn't seem to be improving and your doctor doesn't have another approach.

- **You're solicited for an experimental study**. Your primary care physician can help alleviate concerns you may have about the protocol.

Chapter 26

Making a Stand Against Leg Cramps

Three a.m. I was awakened from what had been a typically uneventful sleep by a sharp, shooting and excruciating pain in my lower leg. My calf muscle had suddenly cramped, apparently when I stretched my leg while asleep. The muscle was pulled into a hard, tight cramp that refused to relax or ease on its own. It was as if I had lost all control over the muscle.

I rolled over, writhing in pain. I tried to rub the muscle, but the pain prevented my doing much except cussing and moaning. Even massaging the muscle did little right away to stop the spasm. Finally, all else having failed, I sat up, put my feet on the floor, and stood up, placing my weight on the cramped leg and foot.

Almost immediately the muscle began to relax. Taking a few steps further relieved the cramp. Within seconds, the pain that only moments before had virtually crippled me, was gone. My disposition markedly improved, and within a few minutes I was asleep.

Common Causes of Leg Cramps

Occasional leg cramps afflict millions of Americans, although no one knows exactly how often they occur or why. They may result from overexertion, certain medical conditions such as diabetes, or a reaction to medication, among other causes. Because leg cramps are usually symptoms of a disease or medical condition and rarely lead to more serious problems, little research has been done on them.

FDA Consumer, March 1988.

Thus, physicians do not know the precise physiological causes of muscle cramps, or why they seem to occur more often in the leg than other muscles, or why particular medications, most used primarily for other medical conditions, and home remedies seem to relieve them.

Perhaps the biggest unknown is why cramped muscles fail to relax. "Why someone who lifts weights and keeps the muscles contracted for a sustained time doesn't suffer a cramp or pain is beyond me," says Dr. Raymond Lipicky, director of the Food and Drug Administration's division of cardio-renal drugs. "A contraction is a contraction," he says, adding: "There is apparently something different about contractions that cause cramps, but nobody knows what."

What is known is that leg cramps seem to occur most commonly in athletes and others who exercise strenuously, in people who have reached middle age and beyond, and in those who suffer circulatory problems. They occur most often at night or when resting. Also, people who stand for long periods can suffer leg cramps. However painful at the moment, most leg cramps last no more than a few minutes and do not interfere with daily functioning.

In a few cases, however, leg cramps can cause a persistent, severe pain that may prevent sleeping, walking or other activities. Dr. Vincent Karusaitis, a medical review officer in FDA's division of oncology, says such cramps are "a sign that you should seek medical attention." In such severe cases, Karusaitis recommends a complete medical history and physical exam to find out what is causing the cramps. More on these cramps later.

Leg (and foot) muscles are not the only ones that cramp. People who write a lot using pen or pencil often get hand cramps, and those who play the cello or violin may get arm cramps.

Meanwhile, most leg cramps seem to occur for no apparent reason. "No physician can tell you why they happen," says Dr. Stanley Silverberg, a Chevy Chase, Md., cardiologist and vascular specialist. Silverberg explains the general process of how muscles cramp by likening the body's cell to an electrical battery. Both function, he says, by passing electrical charges across their surfaces.

Muscles contract when electrical impulses travel from the brain along the nerves and are transferred to muscle cells by special transmitters operating at the nerve-muscle junction. Most muscle contractions are voluntary, organized and controllable. A cramp or spasm occurs when the electrical impulses from the brain occur very rapidly, causing the muscle to contract in a sudden, disorganized and uncontrollable fashion.

Making a Stand Against Leg Cramps

In these cases, muscular activity is somehow related to changes in the balance of various body chemicals called electrolytes, such as potassium and sodium, at the nerve-muscle junction. Sweating a lot can alter the body's chemistry, changing sodium and potassium levels and ratios. An altered chemical balance can prevent the transmitters from functioning properly, perhaps by preventing the muscle from relaxing after contracting.

Such cramps may be an aftermath of overexercising or failing to properly stretch muscles before exerting them. Athletes have to prepare their muscles before running or playing a vigorous game, Karusaitis says, encouraging all who exercise to do the same. Cramps are particularly common among older or "weekend" athletes, who are less active and less likely to warm up first.

But athletes are not the only ones who over-exert muscles. It can happen to other people, too, especially normally inactive individuals. People who spend more time than usual in the garden, for example, may exercise their muscles more than they are used to and suffer leg cramps later. Again, those who are middle-aged or older are more likely to experience such cramps.

Here, weight can be a complicating factor, Karusaitis says. Being overweight can change body posture in ways that put extra pressure on leg muscles, leading to cramps. Similarly, the developing fetus in pregnant women can interfere with blood flow to and from the lower legs. Pregnant women are often advised to wear elastic stockings, especially before getting out of bed, to reduce swelling and cramps.

Additionally, some medications can alter chemical balances in the body that, in turn, can cause leg cramps. Patients taking diuretic drugs to control heart, blood pressure, and kidney disorders can suffer cramps. Diuretics remove electrolytes from the body, taking with them fluids, both needed for proper muscle function. Prednisone, a commonly prescribed hormonal drug used to treat cancer and other conditions, can affect potassium levels and cause leg cramps.

In the article "Making a Stand Against Leg Cramps" in the March 1988 *FDA Consumer*, it was mentioned that some drugs, such as diuretics, can cause chemical imbalances in the body that can, in turn, cause leg cramps. It was not made clear that the chemical that can sometimes be depleted by diuretics is potassium. Since the depletion of potassium depends on the diuretic used, patients taking diuretics should consult their doctors about the advisability of taking potassium supplements or adding to their diets foods rich in potassium, such as bananas and oranges.

Treatment

"The only way to really stop these kinds of leg cramps is to reduce the dosage [of electrolyte-affecting drugs]," says Dr. Frederick Smith, a Washington, D.C., physician. "But I prefer to prevent cramps with other medications."

One prescription drug that helps is Benadryl a widely prescribed medication. FDA has approved Benadryl as an antihistamine, for motion sickness, as a sleep aid, and for Parkinson's disease, but not for leg cramps. Physicians may prescribe a drug for uses beyond those approved by FDA, but on their own responsibility. Why Benadryl works for leg cramps is unknown, Smith says, but it does.

Another prescription drug is Valium, the popular tranquilizer. Yet a third is Flexeril. In all, Karusaitis says, about a half dozen prescription drugs are used to relax cramp-prone muscles. Most, such as Benadryl and Valium, were originally developed or are primarily prescribed for other medical conditions.

There are also several over-the-counter medications sold for leg cramps. Most are quinine-derived (as are some prescription drugs, such as Quinamm), and some contain vitamin E as well. Quinamm, once widely used in the United States to treat malaria (it still is in many countries), is a muscle relaxant. Patients on diuretics or with other chemical-balance problems can take sodium or calcium supplements, or eat foods rich in these nutrients (such as bananas and oranges).

Like most drugs, the quinine-based medications have side effects that patients and physicians should watch for. They can cause ringing in the ears and skin rashes, for example. Pregnant women are advised not to take these medications, nor should anyone take them for more than five days unless under the supervision of a physician.

In addition to prescription drugs, there are many simple home remedies that relieve leg cramps. Standing on the cramped leg and foot and walking around works by forcing the muscle in the direction against the cramp, which relaxes it. Home health guides often advise people to pull their toes forcefully yet smoothly up toward the knee, which similarly forces the muscle against the cramp.

Other home remedies include massaging the cramped muscle, applying heat to it, and wearing loose-fitting clothing to bed. Heating the muscle with a hot-water bottle or electric blanket, for example, increases blood flow to the leg, thus improving the electrolyte and other chemical balance needed for the muscle to function properly, Silverberg says.

Making a Stand Against Leg Cramps

For people who stand in the same position for much of the day, such as cashiers, Karusaitis recommends putting a spongy mat on the floor to cushion the legs. He also advises flexing the muscles periodically by moving about.

Leg Cramps Resulting from Serious Medical Conditions

Unfortunately, not all leg cramps are occasional or so easily treated. Some, in fact, result from serious medical conditions and can themselves make normal functioning difficult. In some cases, medical attention and treatment, beyond medications and home remedies, are required.

Some rare medical conditions can cause muscle cramps. One involves damage to the body's parathyroid glands during surgical removal of the nearby thyroid gland. The parathyroids secrete a hormone that increases the calcium content in the blood. Damage to them could result in insufficient calcium levels. But that is more likely to cause cramps in hand muscles than those of the leg.

One Israeli study has linked muscle cramps with liver disorders. By comparing healthy people with patients who had cirrhosis of the liver, researchers found that 88 percent of the latter had painful muscle cramps compared with 21 percent of healthy subjects. Dr. Fred Konikoff and Emanuel Theodor, the authors, conclude that "painful muscle cramps might be regarded as a symptom of liver cirrhosis."

A more common cause of leg cramps is varicose veins, Silverberg says. Varicose or abnormally swollen veins affect the interchange of fluids between the veins and muscles. Also, damaged valves in the veins can let blood leak back down the leg and into the muscles, causing cramps.

Other circulatory ailments, such as arteriosclerosis and arteritis, can likewise cause leg cramps. They result in narrowed leg arteries, thereby preventing an adequate supply of blood from reaching the muscles. People with these conditions often cannot walk long distances or for sustained periods without suffering pain and/or a cramp. Such symptoms, known collectively as intermittent claudication, are usually associated with cigarette smoking and high blood cholesterol levels.

"These are very special kinds of cramps caused by specific diseases," FDA's Lipicky says. "The cramp is caused by the muscle being asked to do too much work given the amount of oxygen and nutrients reaching it. The muscle contracts locally and [the contraction] is sustained."

Treatment

To prevent or treat these cramps, physicians often advise patients to rest or sit with their legs elevated. Some also prescribe Trental, a drug that can postpone or sometimes prevent the need for surgery, Lipicky says. Trental changes the outer layer of red blood cells so they can better squeeze through narrower openings in arteries, thus improving the flow of blood to muscles.

"That is only a little bit of increased blood supply," Lipicky says. "But that little bit of improvement can make the difference between being able to function and not." Indeed, studies show that people with arterial diseases can walk up to 50 percent longer after taking Trental.

Oftentimes, however, such circulatory disorders require surgical treatment. In recent years, that has meant bypass surgery (in which the clogged artery is replaced by another blood vessel), amputation (in the most severe cases), or balloon angioplasty.

In the latter, surgeons make an incision in the patient's leg and insert a probe into the blocked artery. The probe is then threaded through the artery to the site of the obstruction. There a tiny balloon is gently inflated to open the blocked vessel. Once the job is done, the balloon is collapsed and withdrawn.

While a significant advance over amputation or bypass surgery, balloon angioplasty is costly and cannot always be done. It cannot unclog totally blocked arteries, for example, nor can it be done on some older patients or those who have other health problems. And, although performed some 25,000 times a year, balloon angioplasty is reported only 56 percent to 84 percent successful.

A newer and still experimental surgical technique is thermal angioplasty. Similar in some respects to balloon angioplasty, it may one day supplement or replace the latter. Originally developed to unblock clogged heart arteries, hopefully replacing coronary bypass surgery and reducing the number of heart attacks, thermal angioplasty was approved by FDA for treating clogged leg arteries in January 1987. It has not been approved yet for treating coronary blockages.

The technique uses a specifically designed metal-tipped, fiber-optic probe that allows surgeons to aim a laser beam directly at the blockage within an artery, says Dr. Timothy Sanborn, a cardiologist at Mt. Sinai Hospital in New York City, and one of the technique's pioneers.

The laser vaporizes the blockage, thereby opening a hole in the clogged artery. Once the blockage is at least partially destroyed, surgeons can insert the balloon into the artery to open it more. Sanborn reports that thermal angioplasty is successful 80 percent to 90 percent of the time, depending on the degree of the blockage, how long the artery has been blocked, and how much calcium is present. When successful, though, patients are usually able to walk immediately with no pain or cramps. "They get right-away relief," he says.

First tested on laboratory animals in 1983 and people in 1985, thermal angioplasty is now being tried at 15 major medical centers in the United States and Europe, Sanborn says. For now, its use is limited to major arteries, but Sanborn hopes eventually that it will prove effective in smaller ones as well.

While intermittent claudication involves only large arteries, leg cramps can be caused by blood blockages in smaller ones, too. Diabetes, for example, can cause small arteries to become restricted, thereby cutting the blood flow through them, Lipicky says, but Trental can be prescribed.

Yet other medical conditions can cause leg cramps. Patients suffering from low calcium levels, which can be diagnosed easily by blood tests, can get leg cramps, as can patients on hemodialysis for end-stage renal disease. Why kidney disorders and hemodialysis should lead to leg cramps is unclear, Lipicky says, although it may be related to calcium or potassium levels in the body.

It should be pointed out that most people who suffer from arterial disorders, diabetes, or other medical conditions linked to leg cramps do not get them, or get them only occasionally. Similarly, only about 1 percent or 2 percent of those on diuretics get leg cramps. But since millions of people take the drugs, that can add up.

Because of their unpredictable nature and the fact that so little is known about them, leg cramps are a disconcerting problem. "As a doctor, I get frustrated by being unable to prevent leg cramps in my patients despite their frequency," says Smith. Those of us who experience occasional leg cramps get frustrated, too.

— by Jeffrey E. Cohn

Jeffrey E. Cohn is a free-lance writer in Washington, D.C. who often writes on health issues.

Chapter 27

Spinal Stenosis: A Subtle Source of Leg Pain

You may first notice an ache in your buttock, thigh and calf when you walk or stand. If you bend forward at your waist or sit for a few minutes, the pain passes.

These symptoms suggest spinal stenosis, a source of leg pain caused by narrowing of your spinal canal.

Symptoms of spinal stenosis are often subtle and similar to those associated with other causes of back and leg pain. Management usually involves conservative measures such as physical therapy. Yet spinal stenosis may be progressive and lead to disabling pain and limited activity that may warrant surgery.

Nerves under Pressure

Spinal stenosis typically affects adults after age 50. It can develop because of a congenital tendency. But spinal stenosis usually results from osteoarthritis.

Excessive use, previous injury or aging slowly deteriorates the protective tissue (cartilage) covering joint surfaces in your back. Discs between the bones in your back (vertebrae) become worn and spaces between bones narrow. Bony outgrowths called spurs (osteophytes) also develop.

©1995 Reprinted from September 1995 *Mayo Clinic Health Letter* with permission of the Mayo Foundation for Medical Education and Research, Rochester, Minnesota 55905. For subscription information, please call 1-800-333-9038. Reprinted with permission.

Pain Sourcebook

These changes can allow bones and soft tissues to fold inward into your spinal canal, compressing nerves.

As narrowing of your spinal canal progresses, one vertebra may slip forward on a lower vertebra in a condition called spondylolisthesis (spon-duh-lo-lis-THE-sis). Pressure may develop on spinal nerves that form the sciatic nerve. This nerve extends down each leg from your hip to your heel.

Pressure on these spinal nerves may cause pain to radiate from your lower back down your buttock to your lower leg. Numbness or weakness in your legs may eventually develop. Occasionally, nerves leading from your spine to your bladder and bowels can become compressed, reducing muscle control in these organs.

Bending forward at your waist or sitting relieves the pain because these positions increase the diameter of your spinal canal, reducing pressure on spinal nerves. In severe spinal stenosis, the pain persists regardless of your activity or position.

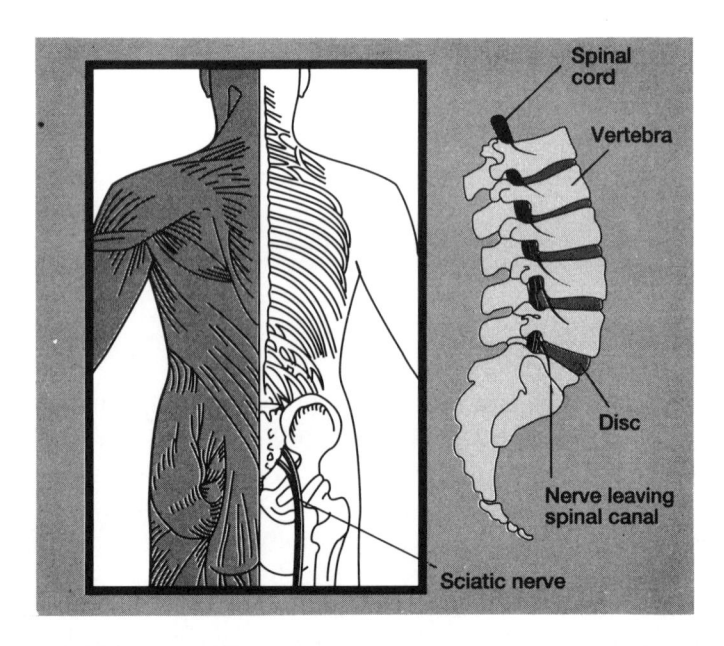

Figure 27.1. *The lower part of the back holds most of the body's weight. Even a minor problem with the bones, muscles, ligaments or tendons in this area can cause pain when a person stands, bends, or moves around. Less often, a problem with a disc can pinch or irritate a nerve from the spinal cord, causing pain that runs down the leg, below the knee called sciatica.*

Spinal Stenosis: A Subtle Source of Leg Pain

Sorting out the Pain

Your doctor may first perform tests to exclude other conditions that cause leg pain or numbness. Poor circulation through the arteries in your legs often mimics the pain caused by spinal stenosis. Herniation of a disc from its normal position between the bones in your back also can cause similar symptoms.

Pain from spinal stenosis tends to be more noticeable when walking downhill and persists while standing. Pain due to poor circulation is usually worse when walking uphill and subsides when standing.

If your doctor suspects spinal stenosis after an initial evaluation, computerized tomography, magnetic resonance imaging or X-ray after injection of a contrast material (myelography) can detect narrowing of your spinal canal.

Combining Treatments

Bed rest was once the mainstay of treatment for spinal stenosis. But as with the management of back pain, strict bed rest is recommended only for a few days if pain is severe. Prolonged bed rest can lead to loss of muscle tone.

For mild to moderate spinal stenosis, a combination of these approaches often works best:

- **Medication.** Nonsteroidal anti-inflammatory drugs and muscle relaxants prescribed by your doctor help manage chronic pain. For occasional pain, you may find relief with over-the-counter analgesics such as aspirin or acetaminophen.

- **Physical therapy.** For acute pain, applications of heat, cold or gentle massage performed by a physical therapist or other licensed professional may help. Once pain subsides, a physical therapist can design an exercise program to improve your flexibility, strengthen your back and abdominal muscles and correct your posture.

- **Back supports.** A support brace or corset worn around your lower back improves your posture. However, back supports are best used for short periods or only during back-straining activities. Long-term use can lead to muscle weakness in your back and abdomen.

- **Corticosteroids.** Injections may temporarily relieve the pain for some people. But they don't cure spinal stenosis.

When You May Need Surgery

Your doctor may recommend surgery if you have disabling pain, increasing weakness in your legs or reduced bladder or bowel control.

During laminectomy (lam-ih-NEK-tuh-me), your surgeon removes bones and soft tissues that protrude into your spinal canal or put pressure on your spinal nerves. If you also have spondylolisthesis, vertebrae in your lower back may be fused together using a bone graft and specialized screws or plates.

Laminectomy often improves or eliminates pain in your buttocks and legs. However, the surgery may not relieve low back pain caused by underlying conditions such as osteoarthritis.

The average hospital stay for a laminectomy is four to seven days. After three months, you can resume most of your daily activities with the exception of heavy physical labor. Recovery and rehabilitation may take longer if bone fusion was necessary.

Chapter 28

Knee Pain: Strong Enough to Stop the Pain

For women, especially, weak quadriceps can lead to painful misalignment.

Many runners and weekend athletes are familiar with a dull, achy pain behind or around their kneecaps; it occasionally comes on as a sharp, tweak when going up or down stairs. Patellofemoral pain syndrome is one of the most common reasons patients go to sports medicine specialists. Fortunately, a little rest along with some targeted strengthening exercises usually will overcome the problem.

You can get a feel–literally–for the problem by sitting down, placing your hand over a kneecap and straightening that leg. Notice how the kneecap glides back toward your palm in a natural groove. In some people, the kneecap rubs against the edges of this groove during exercise, leading to inflammation and pain. Doctors say misalignment causes microtrauma to the knee, and when excessive, can lead to overuse injury.

Faulty tracking has two main causes: unlucky anatomy (being knock-kneed) or having unbalanced quadricep strength that pulls the kneecap to the outside. Because women have wider hips, their quadriceps tug at the kneecap from an increased angle, compounding the problem.

Trying to run through this pain is foolish and can make a minor problem worse. It's better to reduce the inflammation by avoiding

---

©1997 St. Joseph Mercy–Oakland *SmartHealth*. Reprinted from the Spring 1997 issue of *Health Tips* with permission.

stressful activities, applying ice packs and taking nonsteroidal anti-inflammatory drugs such as aspirin. When the pain subsides, recurrence can be prevented by the exercises shown below.

Target Muscles That Keep the Kneecap on Track

These exercises may seem too simple to make a difference. But they are proven to be effective when performed daily. Before starting this exercise program, your knee pain should be controlled. Do each exercise in three sets of ten repetitions every day. Stop if you feel joint pain.

- **First, set your quadriceps.** Lying on your back, extend your toes, tighten your thigh muscles in the front of one leg and push down against the floor. Hold five seconds.

- **Second, add strength with straight leg raises.** With one leg bent, sit on the floor and lean back on your elbows. Extend your toes, straighten the other leg and lift it until both thighs are parallel. Hold five seconds and slowly lower to the floor.

- **Third, target the weakest quads with modified extensions.** Lie on the floor with a rolled towel under one knee so that the joint is about 6 inches from the floor. Straighten your leg and hold five seconds.

Avoid exercises that make knee pain worse: deep knee bends, full knee extensions (using the weight machine in gyms), running (especially on hills), deep-step stair-stepping, sports with quick side-to-side movements.

Chapter 29

Heel Pain: It's Usually a Symptom of Plantar Fasciitis

That first step out of bed in the morning really catches your attention—it feels just like someone poked you in the heel with a knife. But after walking for a few minutes, the pain slowly disappears.

Heel pain is very irritating, but rarely serious. Although it can result from a pinched nerve or a chronic condition, such as arthritis or bursitis, the most common cause is plantar fasciitis (PLAN-tur fas-e-I-tis).

Plantar fasciitis is an inflammation of the plantar fascia, the fibrous tissue that runs along the bottom of your foot and connects to your heel bone (calcaneus) and toes (see illustration).

The plantar fascia also acts as a bowstring for the arch of your foot to keep the arch from collapsing.

Treatment for plantar fasciitis involves simple steps to relieve the pain and inflammation. But don't expect a quick cure. It can take six months or longer before your heel is back to normal.

Stretching under Stress

A flattening of your arch or overuse can cause your plantar fascia to stretch and pull on your heel bone. That can result in microscopic tears in the fascia, inflammation, and a piercing pain or burning sensation.

©1996 Reprinted from July 1996 *Mayo Clinic Health Letter* with permission of the Mayo Foundation for Medical Education and Research, Rochester, Minnesota 55905. For subscription information, please call 1-800-333-9038. Reprinted with permission.

The pain usually develops gradually, but can come on suddenly and severely. It tends to be worse in the morning, when the fascia is stiff. Although both feet can be affected, it usually occurs in only one foot.

The pain generally goes away once your foot limbers up. But it can recur if you stand or sit for a long time. Climbing stairs or standing on your tiptoes can also produce pain.

In severe cases, your foot may hurt whenever you put pressure on it, making walking difficult.

You may also develop a bone spur that forms from tension on your heel bone. In most cases, the spur doesn't cause pain.

Common Causes

Plantar fasciitis can affect people of all ages. Factors that increase your risk include:

- **Age.** As you get older, your plantar fascia loses some of its elasticity and doesn't stretch as well. In addition, the fat pad covering your heel bone thins out and isn't able to absorb as much shock when you put weight on your foot. That places more stress on your heel bone and the tissues attached to it.

- **Weight-bearing activities.** Walking, jogging, lifting heavy objects and standing for long periods place added pressure on your feet. When performed regularly, they may stress your plantar fascia.

  Plantar fasciitis can also occur if you've been physically inactive and then plunge into a weight-bearing activity, such as playing golf or walking more than you're used to while vacationing.

- **Shoes.** Shoes with thin soles, poor arch support, that are too loose around your heels, lack shock absorbency, or are worn out can be harmful to your feet.

  In addition, regularly wearing high heels (greater than 2 inches) can shorten your Achilles' tendon, which attaches to your heel bone, and tighten your calf muscles. This increases the strain on your heels when you switch to a flatter shoe.

- **Weight.** Excess weight increases pressure on your feet.

Heel Pain: It's Usually a Symptom of Plantar Fasciitis

- **Poor biomechanics.** A flat foot, high-arched foot, or abnormalities in your gait may prevent your weight from being evenly distributed when you walk or run. This stresses your plantar fascia.

Treatment Steps

The goal of treatment is to heal the tears and decrease inflammation, as well as prevent the condition from recurring. Although you may find the slow course of healing frustrating, patience is important.

There are several steps you can take to relieve plantar fasciitis (see "Self-help steps that may relieve the pain"). But if these aren't effective, or you believe your condition is due to a foot abnormality, see your doctor. Treatment options include:

- **Custom orthotic devices.** If you have a foot deformity, a custom shoe insert from an orthopedist or podiatrist can compensate for the deformity and distribute pressure to your foot more evenly.

- **Night splints.** While you sleep, your plantar fascia relaxes and starts to heal in that position. When you bear weight on the foot, you can stretch and tear your fascia all over again. Splints worn at night keep tension on the tissue so it heals in a stretched position.

- **Ultrasound.** Deep heat may increase blood flow and promote healing.

- **Corticosteroids.** An injection in your heel can often help relieve the inflammation when other steps aren't successful. But multiple injections aren't recommended because they can weaken and rupture your plantar fascia, as well as shrink the fat pad covering your heel bone.

- **Surgery.** Doctors can detach your plantar fascia from your heel bone, but this is only recommended when all other treatments have failed. Side effects can include continued pain and weakening of your arch.

Additional options may be available in the future. Mayo Clinic and other medical centers are investigating a number of alternative therapies, including low-intensity laser treatments.

Stepping Away from the Pain

Heel pain can be frustrating, but it doesn't have to keep you from your daily routine or favorite exercise program. Most people are able to relieve the pain by following simple treatment recommendations and gradually working back into normal activities.

Maintaining a stretching program and continued attention to proper footwear may help prevent the condition from returning.

Chapter 30

No Strain, No Pain: The Bottom Line in Treating Hemorrhoids

Say the word hemorrhoids to just about anyone and they will either roll their eyes, moan or both. Invariably they will want to change the subject. According to the National Institutes of Health, about half the U.S. population over 50 have hemorrhoids.

"Hemorrhoids are one of the most common complaints a physician must evaluate," agrees Lee E. Smith, M.D., director of the division of colon and rectal surgery at the George Washington University Medical Center, Washington, D.C.

Common, but rarely a serious risk to health, hemorrhoids are the result of too much pressure on the hemorrhoidal veins in the rectum. The strain of constipation, diarrhea and pregnancy can cause the veins to swell. Other factors such as obesity and liver disease can also increase pressure and cause hemorrhoids.

There are two kinds of hemorrhoids—internal and external. Frequently, the only sign that internal hemorrhoids exist is bright red blood that appears on the surface of the stool, in the toilet bowl, or on the toilet paper. But, if the pressure and swelling continue, the hemorrhoidal veins may stretch out of shape, sometimes so much that they bulge through the anus to the outside of the body.

The veins around the anus can also become swollen, causing external hemorrhoids. These swollen veins bleed easily, either from straining or rubbing, and irritation from draining mucus may cause itching in the anal area. If blood clots form in these hemorrhoids, the pain can be severe.

FDA Consumer, June, 1991.

"If you see blood, it's probably hemorrhoids," says Smith. Hemorrhoids are the most common source of bleeding from the rectum and the anus. However, if the bleeding lasts for more than a couple of days, it's important to see a doctor for an exam. Smith stresses that a "thorough physical exam, not just talking about the symptoms" is essential.

"The unfortunate thing is every year I see somebody who has been seeing blood and they were treated as having hemorrhoids without really being examined, and they had a cancer," he says.

Treatment for hemorrhoids depends not only on the severity of the symptoms, but also on the patient's reaction to those symptoms.

"Hemorrhoids don't cause cancer; they're a nuisance," says Smith. "Rarely do they cause severe anemia and rarely do they cause something that is hazardous to health. If the patient doesn't mind, then let them live with the hemorrhoids."

Even though he's a surgeon, Smith considers surgery an option only after everything else has failed.

Relieving the Pressure

The first step in treating hemorrhoids is to relieve the pressure and straining. This can often be done by controlling constipation with a high-fiber diet, according to Barbara Frank, M.D., director of the division of gastroenterology at the Crozer-Chester Medical Center, Chester, Pa.

Eating the right amounts of bran (the outer coating of grains, available mainly as cereals), as well as fruits, vegetables, and whole grains results in a soft, bulky stool that is easily eliminated without strain or pressure on the hemorrhoidal veins.

"Bran is the cheapest way to go," says Smith, who also recommends bulk stool softeners (brand-name products include FiberCon, Metamucil, Citracil, and Serutan) as a way to relieve pressure and straining.

Lots to drink, as long as it isn't alcohol, which can actually cause dehydration, is also important for the regularity that can relieve hemorrhoids you already have and prevent new ones.

People should drink "several glasses [of liquid] a day, and it doesn't have to be just water," says Marilyn Stephenson, a registered dietitian with FDA's Center for Food Safety and Applied Nutrition. "Fruits and vegetables are high in fluids, too."

"Several" may seem a little too fluid an amount, but people's needs vary, sometimes daily, depending on things like the weather or exercise.

No Strain, No Pain: The Bottom Line in Treating Hemorrhoids

"Especially in hot weather, a glass [of water] every couple of hours is very reasonable," says Smith.

One thing to avoid when trying to relieve constipation is any laxative other than a stool softener, says Smith. Other laxatives frequently cause diarrhea, which can be just as rough on the hemorrhoidal veins as straining due to constipation, he explains.

Besides an improved diet, other simple steps to relieve the irritation some hemorrhoids cause include:

- warm soaks (sitz baths) three or four times a day
- cold packs
- good hygiene. (Be gentle about cleaning, though. Frank recommends using a soft, moist pad or even rinsing in the shower as an alternative to wiping.)

OTC Remedies

If necessary, there are several nonprescription drugs available that can help relieve certain symptoms of hemorrhoids. FDA's review of those drugs, published in August 1990, found 33 active ingredients safe and effective for protecting the skin, reducing swelling, or relieving discomfort, itching and inflammation. At the same time, however, FDA banned more than 30 other ingredients that have not been proven safe and effective.

Most of the approved ingredients are for external use on the skin, but some may also be used on mucous membranes just inside the rectum. The best drug depends on the particular individual's symptoms, and it may be advisable to consult a doctor or pharmacist about which one to buy, says William E. Gilbertson, director of FDA's division of over-the-counter drug evaluation.

No ingredients to relieve pain, soreness and burning were approved for internal use because there are no nerve endings inside the rectum.

Internal hemorrhoids "don't hurt and they don't itch," says Smith. "Pain means a fissure [break in the skin] or a thrombosed [blood-clot-filled] external hemorrhoid, but it doesn't mean internal hemorrhoid problems."

Manufacturers had until August 1991, when the FDA regulations went into effect, to reformulate products that contained ingredients for pain, soreness and burning or relabel with the statement "for external use only" and a warning not to put the product into the rectum.

In addition, nonprescription hemorrhoid remedy labels must include the statement "If condition worsens or does not improve within seven days, consult a doctor." Two other warnings—"Do not exceed the recommended daily dosage unless directed by a doctor" and "In case of bleeding, consult a doctor promptly"—must also be on the label.

Surgical Options

Occasionally, some form of surgery may be necessary to remove or destroy the hemorrhoid.

One of the most common surgical methods is rubber band ligation. A tiny rubber band-diameter one millimeter (about one-twenty-fifth of an inch)—is fitted onto a special gun-like device. When the trigger is pulled, the rubber band is forced onto the base of the hemorrhoid. Because there are no nerve endings in the rectum, no anesthesia is necessary.

It takes about a week for the strangled tissue to slough off and a scar to form. Rubber band ligation works best on first- and second-degree hemorrhoids.

Other surgical techniques for these less severe hemorrhoids include:

- **Infrared photocoagulation.** A specially designed device uses infrared light to create a small tissue-destroying burn around the base of the hemorrhoid.

- **Laser coagulation.** The laser causes a minor burn, which seals off the blood vessels. This results in the hemorrhoid being retained in a non-prolapsed position.

- **Sclerotherapy.** A solution (either quinine urea, sodium morrhuate, or phenol in oil) is injected into the hemorrhoid, which causes inflammation and eventual scarring that eliminates hemorrhoidal symptoms.

Third- and fourth-degree hemorrhoids may have to be surgically removed, either with traditional scalpels or with lasers.

Complications such as infection and incontinence are possible with all of these techniques.

External Hemorrhoids

Blood clots in external hemorrhoids are "like a black eye," says Smith. "Even if the patient does nothing, the clots will eventually disappear."

No Strain, No Pain: The Bottom Line in Treating Hemorrhoids

Treating the pain and irritation with sitz baths, bulk stool softeners, and pain medication may be all that's necessary, he says.

Sometimes, however, the clots are so painful the patient can't bear to wait, and traditional surgery to cut out the clots is necessary.

But even surgery is only a temporary solution. If a person's diet isn't improved, the hemorrhoid may return. And even in the best of cases, in the end, "hemorrhoids don't go away, they just get better," says Smith.

Preventing Constipation

A fiber-rich diet can help prevent constipation, which is important because the strain caused by constipation is how many hemorrhoid problems begin. Good sources of fiber include:

- potatoes
- beans-kidney, navy, lima, pinto
- whole-grain breads
- bran
- fresh fruits
- vegetables, especially asparagus, brussels sprouts, cabbage, carrots, cauliflower, corn, peas, kale, and parsnips.

It will also help to limit these low- or no-fiber foods:

- ice cream, soft drinks, cheese, white bread, and meat.

—by Dori Stehlin

Dori Stehlin is a staff writer for *FDA Consumer*.

Chapter 31

Painful Menstruation and Menstrual Cramps

Chapter Contents

Section 33.1—Facts about Dysmenorrhea 252
Section 33.2—Taming Menstrual Cramps 256

Section 33.1

Facts about Dysmenorrhea

Excerpts from NIH publication, Facts about Dysmenorrhea and Premenstrual Syndrome, 1983.

Dysmenorrhea (painful menstruation) can disable a woman for a few hours before or at the onset of her menstrual period and last for several hours or as long as two days. Pain may be severe and daily activities may have to be modified.

Hormones and the Normal Menstrual Cycle

Hormones play an important role in the proper functioning of the menstrual cycle. In studying menstrual disorders, scientists have tried to determine how menstruation occurs normally.

The onset of menstruation (menarche) is the dramatic marker of the change from girl to woman. Usually occurring between ages of ten and sixteen, the beginning of menstruation means that a young girl is developing the ability to bear children. At first the cycle may be irregular. Usually, a regular menstrual cycle is established by the end of the first year after menarche. Interrupted only for pregnancies or specific health problems, it continues month after month until a woman is in her forties or fifties when menstruation ceases (menopause). A typical cycle is about 28 days, but cycles varying from 24 to 30 days are not uncommon. Generally, a woman keeps to the established pattern although stress, illness or the use of oral contraceptives may alter her cycle temporarily.

During each cycle, the inner wall or lining (endometrium) of the uterus thickens to provide a suitable environment for a pregnancy. A mature egg (ovum) is released from one of the two ovaries in mid-cycle (ovulation) and remains in the reproductive tract for about three days. For a pregnancy to occur, the ovum must be fertilized by a sperm. If there is no pregnancy, the lining of the uterus breaks down and is discharged as the menstrual flow (menses) over the course of three to eight days.

Painful Menstruation and Menstrual Cramps

Although the reproductive organs are located in the body's pelvic area, the reproductive cycle is controlled by an area at the base of the brain containing the hypothalamus and the pituitary gland. The hypothalamus and the pituitary gland orchestrate menstrual cycle activities, sending "start" and "stop" signals each month to the ovaries and uterus.

On the first day of menstruation, hormone levels are low. But after one week and for most of the remaining cycle, *estrogens* are produced to promote ovulation and stimulate the development of the endometrium. During this time estrogens contribute to producing an appropriate environment in the reproductive organs for fertilization, implantation and nurturing of the early embryo. Estrogen production drops off a few days before the next cycle begins.

Progesterone, a hormone produced in large amounts during the latter half of the cycle, stimulates the development of the endometrium in preparation for a pregnancy. If there is no pregnancy, progesterone levels decrease and menstruation begins. If pregnancy occurs, production of progesterone continues throughout the nine months to help maintain the pregnancy.

Other hormone-like substances, prostaglandins, are also produced during the latter half of the cycle. Although the role of prostaglandins is not completely understood, they are believed to stimulate uterine contractions which are recognized as cramps during the menstrual period. The prostaglandins may be one of the possible factors that start labor.

Dysmenorrhea Explained

Many women experience some discomfort when a menstrual period begins. Most can manage daily routines and responsibilities because the discomfort is mild and brief in duration. For others, the discomfort is severe, lasts for hours, and is disabling. In a recent health survey of adolescent women, more than half reported pain during menstruation.

Dysmenorrhea is the medical term for painful menstruation. It is primarily caused by moderate to severe cramping of the uterus. Headache, backache, diarrhea and nausea are associated symptoms.

Dysmenorrhea usually does not begin until six to twelve months following menarche, when a woman's system has developed fully and ovulation occurs regularly. The disorder appears to affect young women and women who have not borne children more so than older women who have had children.

In the past, the young woman's complaints of pain were dismissed with the advice, "It's just part of being a woman. You'll get over it after you have a baby." There is a measure of truth in that latter statement because dysmenorrhea diminishes in many women after a full-term pregnancy. This may occur because uterine muscles are stretched during pregnancy. Another possible explanation is that uterine blood supply and muscle activity may be improved by the process of having a child.

Research Findings

Noting the similarity between menstrual cramps and mild labor pains, scientific investigation in the past had focused on the basic workings of uterine contractions. Prostaglandins were identified as one of the factors involved in causing contractions. These substances are secreted by the uterine lining and affect the smooth muscles of the uterus, thus assisting in the sloughing off of the lining during menstruation.

While attention was directed to this area of research, reports began to appear that oral contraceptive users seemed to have less menstrual problems than nonusers. One explanation given was that the decrease in menstrual flow associated with oral contraceptive use resulted in a reduction of prostaglandin concentration.

Other researchers, however, observed that oral contraceptives suppress ovulation, and in the absence of ovulation uterine production of prostaglandins is diminished. This observation, combined with the knowledge that prostaglandins stimulate uterine contractions, led researchers to conclude that an oversupply of prostaglandins is a likely cause of painful contractions of the uterus.

Although oral contraceptives seem effective in relieving dysmenorrhea, their side effects have prevented many women from using them. As a result, other substances were sought to lessen or inhibit prostaglandin production. Now, through research and careful testing, such products are available. These agents, previously developed for the treatment of arthritis, are similar to aspirin, but many times more potent.

Treatment Options

The first step in arriving at treatment for dysmenorrhea is a thorough pelvic examination. This can rule out certain medical conditions other than dysmenorrhea that can cause pelvic pain. At the time of

Painful Menstruation and Menstrual Cramps

the examination, other health factors and practices can also be discussed with the physician. For example, for some women reducing the amount of salt, caffeine and sugar in the diet, especially in the week before a period is due, often provides relief, as does moderate exercise and sufficient rest.

For a few women, menstrual disorders may stem from psychological problems and worries. Treating the psychological problems of these women often alleviates their menstrual problems. For most others who suffer dysmenorrhea, the source of their pain is the uterus, contracting too hard or too fast. Traditionally, analgesics and sedatives have been used to treat menstrual pain, although these drugs may affect a patient's normal activities, such as driving a car or taking an exam in school.

As a result of scientific research, new types of medication are available. For moderate to severe dysmenorrhea, drugs that prevent or lessen the production of prostaglandins in the first hours or day of the menstrual period have proved effective without serious side effects in about 75 percent of the patients. The drugs provide relief from pain by reducing the level of prostaglandins which in turn moderates the uterine contractions. Not all women can tolerate these drugs, however, especially those who have gastrointestinal problems.

Researchers continue to search for other possible causes of dysmenorrhea and to develop modes of treatment for women who are not helped by the present array of medications.

Section 33.2

Taming Menstrual Cramps

FDA Consumer, June 1991.

For many women "that time of the month" is one they'd rather forgo. More than half routinely experience some form of pain associated with menstruation, say doctors at the Mayo Clinic in Minnesota, and 1 in 10 suffers such severe dysmenorrhea—menstrual pain—she cannot function normally without taking medication.

Throughout history, women have tried to alleviate these menstrual discomforts themselves. But home remedies—teas, hot baths, heating pads, and such—offered only limited help. As recently as a decade ago, when there were far fewer products readily available for menstrual cramps than now, some doctors prescribed powerful prescription painkillers. Others, many women recall, told patients their problems would disappear as they grew older or after they had children.

But today, the pain associated with menstruation is taken more seriously, and there are new, highly effective treatments for it.

"Nearly all women—I would say 99.9 percent—should be able to function quite well during their periods with the menstrual treatments available now," says Charles H. Debrovner, M.D., a gynecologist in private practice and on the faculty of the New York University School of Medicine in New York City.

What's Causing the Pain?

There are two kinds of painful menses—primary and secondary dysmenorrhea—and it is very important to distinguish between them so both are treated properly, Debrovner stresses.

Primary dysmenorrhea usually starts within three years of the onset of menstruation and lasts one or two days each month. While this type of menstrual pain may lessen for some women as they grow older or after the birth of children, it also can continue until menopause.

Secondary dysmenorrhea is menstrual pain caused by disease such as pelvic inflammatory disease, endometriosis (abnormalities in the

Painful Menstruation and Menstrual Cramps

lining of the uterus), or uterine fibroids (nonmalignant growths). Endometriosis is a major cause of secondary dysmenorrhea. Pain from it usually starts later in life and worsens with time, according to Debrovner. Another hint that disease might be the cause of menstrual pain is if pain also occurs during intercourse or other parts of the cycle.

Primary dysmenorrhea is a result of the normal production of prostaglandins—chemical substances that are made by cells in the lining of the uterus. (Prostaglandins are also produced elsewhere throughout the body.) The lining of the uterus—which has built up and thickened during the early stages of the menstrual cycle—breaks up and is sloughed off at the end of the cycle and releases prostaglandins, explains Lisa Rarick, M.D., medical officer in FDA's division of metabolism and endocrine drug products.

The prostaglandins, in turn, make the uterus contract more strongly than at any other time of the cycle. They can even cause it to contract so much that the blood supply is cut off temporarily, depriving the uterine muscle of oxygen and thus causing pain. Women who suffer painful contractions may be producing excessive amounts of prostaglandins. Or, it may be that some women are just more sensitive to them, says Rarick.

The cramps themselves help push out the menstrual discharge. Because the cervical opening is often widened after childbirth or years of menstruation, cramps may lessen in severity later in life.

Most women describe their menstrual cramps as a dull aching or a pressure low in the abdomen. The pains may wax and wane, remain constant, or be so severe that they cause nausea, vomiting, diarrhea, backache, sweating, and an achiness that spreads to the hips, lower back, and thighs.

Inhibiting Prostaglandins

For many years, women had little help for these symptoms. Doctors recommended aspirin, heating pads, and hot baths. When those failed, they often prescribed painkillers such as Demerol or Tylenol with Codeine. These treatments were all aimed at the perception of pain rather than the cause of it. Even tranquilizers were sometimes used, according to Debrovner.

But the advent of pain relievers that impede the production of prostaglandins has made it possible to directly treat the cause of the cramps. Called NSAIDs, for nonsteroidal anti-inflammatory drugs, these medications have proven remarkably effective for many women.

Because NSAIDS inhibit synthesis of prostaglandins, and thereby the contractions of the uterus, they may actually reduce menstrual flow. Many of Debrovner's patients report shorter periods when they take the drugs at the first sign of pain. He recommends taking them as early as possible after the menstrual flow starts. Waiting too long may mean they won't be as effective.

The prostaglandin inhibitors can cause gastrointestinal distress, so most doctors also recommend they be taken with milk and food. Labeling on the OTC products contains this information.

While there are about a dozen prescription NSAIDs, three—ibuprofen (Motrin, Rufen, etc.), naproxen (Naprosyn), and mefenamic acid (Ponstel)—are now approved to treat menstrual cramps.

Over-the-counter Products

FDA approved ibuprofen for over-the-counter use in 1984. It now can be found as the active ingredient in several OTC medications, such as Advil, Nuprin, and Motrin IB. The OTC dose per pill is 200 milligrams. The recommended dose is one tablet every four to six hours (or two, if one does not work), not to exceed six in a 24-hour period. Prescription formulations come in dosages of 400 to 800 milligrams.

Aspirin—long a standard over-the-counter treatment for cramps—works as a prostaglandin inhibitor, although probably not so powerfully as the specific inhibitors such as ibuprofen. While aspirin is known to thin the blood and increase bleeding, it does not appear to have this effect on menstrual flow, according to Rarick.

Researchers are not sure if acetaminophen, an analgesic found in drugs such as Tylenol and Datril, works to prevent prostaglandin production. If it does, its effect appears to be milder than that of aspirin or other NSAIDs. Doctors say, however, that it can successfully treat the headache and backache that often accompany menstrual cramps.

Some OTC menstrual pain medications, such as Midol and Pamprin, contain a mix of ingredients that include an analgesic such as acetaminophen, a diuretic such as pamabrom, and an antihistamine such as pyrilamine maleate. Some newer formulations now use ibuprofen in place of more classic analgesics such as aspirin or acetaminophen. Midol 200 Advanced Cramp Formula, for example, contains ibuprofen as its active ingredient. Maximum Strength Midol Multi-Symptom Formula, however, contains acetaminophen as an analgesic. With the variety of ingredients now available, it's wise to read the label to make sure the product is the best one to treat your symptoms. If in doubt, consult your doctor.

Painful Menstruation and Menstrual Cramps

Other Treatments

Women who use oral contraceptives rarely suffer menstrual cramps, so some doctors prescribe them for women whose cramps are unrelieved by other treatments. Contraceptive pills disrupt the normal hormonal changes of the menstrual cycle, resulting in a thinner uterine lining and a decrease in production of prostaglandins. However, menstrual cramp relief is not considered by FDA to be a primary reason to use oral contraceptives; rather, it is included in the labeling as a secondary benefit.

Exercise, too, may be of some benefit, possibly because it raises levels of beta endorphins, chemicals in the brain associated with pain relief. With new knowledge, such as the possible roles of exercise and of prostaglandins in preventing cramps, most women can avoid suffering the monthly anguish of severe menstrual pain.

— by Ellen Hale

Part Five

Surgical Pain

Chapter 32

Acute Pain Management: Operative or Medical Procedures and Trauma

Foreword

Approximately 23.3 million operations were performed in 1989 in the United States, and most of these involved some form of pain management. Unfortunately, clinical surveys continue to indicate that routine orders for intramuscular injections of opioid as needed the standard practice in many clinical settings fail to relieve pain in about half of postoperative patients. Postoperative pain contributes to patient discomfort, longer recovery periods, and greater use of scarce health care resources and may compromise patient outcomes.

There is wide variation in the methods used to manage postoperative and other acute pain, ranging from no set strategy to a comprehensive team approach as advocated in this clinical practice guideline. This guideline sets forth procedures to minimize the incidence and severity of acute pain after surgical and medical procedures and pain associated with trauma in adults and children. It offers clinicians a coherent yet flexible approach to pain assessment and management for use in daily practice.

Although it is not practical or desirable to eliminate all postoperative and other acute pain, an aggressive approach to pain assessment and management can reduce such pain, increase patient

---

Extracted from NIH Publication No. 92-0032. Agency for Health Care Policy and Research (AHCPR). http://text.nlm.nih.gov/ftrs/pick?dbName=apmc&ftrsK=34191&cp=1&t=867859846&collect=ahcpr

comfort and satisfaction, and in some cases, contribute to improved patient outcomes and shorter hospital stays.

This clinical practice guideline was developed under the sponsorship of the Agency for Health Care Policy and Research (AHCPR), Public Health Service, U.S. Department of Health and Human Services. To develop the guideline, AHCPR convened an interdisciplinary expert panel made up of physicians, nurses, a pharmacist, a psychologist, a physical therapist, a patient/consumer, and an ethicist. The panel first undertook an extensive and interdisciplinary clinical review of current needs, therapeutic practices and principles, and emerging technologies for pain assessment and management. Second, the panel conducted a comprehensive review of the field to define the existing knowledge base and critically evaluate the assumptions and common wisdom in the field. Third, the panel initiated peer review of guideline drafts and field review with intended users in clinical sites. Comments from these reviews were assessed and used in developing the guideline.

This is the first edition of the Clinical Practice Guideline for Acute Pain Management: Operative or Medical Procedures and Trauma. Further editions will be produced as needed to reflect new research findings and experience with emerging technologies for pain assessment and relief.

Executive Summary

Clinical surveys continue to indicate that routine orders for intramuscular injections of opioid as needed fail to relieve pain in about half of postoperative patients. Recognition of the widespread inadequacy of pain management has prompted recent corrective efforts within multiple health care disciplines, including surgery, anesthesiology, and nursing, as well as pain management groups.

This Clinical Practice Guideline for Acute Pain Management: Operative or Medical Procedures and Trauma was commissioned by the Agency for Health Care Policy and Research (AHCPR). The guideline is designed to help clinicians, patients, and patients' families to understand the assessment and treatment of postoperative and other acute pain in both adults and children.

To develop the guideline, AHCPR convened an interdisciplinary panel of physicians, nurses, a pharmacist, a psychologist, a physical therapist, a patient/consumer, and an ethicist. The guideline development process included an extensive review of current needs, therapeutic practices and principles, and emerging technologies for postoperative pain control. All pertinent guidelines and standards were reviewed, opinions were

Acute Pain Management: Operative or Medical Procedures

obtained from external consultants, and testimony was received at an open forum held on November 20, 1990 in Washington, D.C.. An exhaustive literature search was conducted to define the knowledge base and critically evaluate the assumptions and common wisdom of the field. Although the review focused primarily on postoperative pain, literature on procedure-related and trauma pain was also considered. Drafts of the guideline were peer-reviewed and then tested in the field by intended users in various clinical sites.

The guideline has four major goals:

1. Reduce the incidence and severity of patients' acute postoperative or posttraumatic pain.
2. Educate patients about the need to communicate unrelieved pain so they can receive prompt evaluation and effective treatment.
3. Enhance patient comfort and satisfaction.
4. Contribute to fewer postoperative complications and, in some cases, shorter stays after surgical procedures.

Not all acute postoperative, procedural, or trauma-related pain can be eliminated, but several alternative approaches, when appropriately and attentively applied, prevent or relieve pain. The importance of effective pain management increases beyond patient satisfaction when additional benefits for the patient are realized, e.g., earlier mobilization, shortened hospital stay, and reduced costs.

This guideline addresses the care of patients with acute pain associated with operations, medical procedures, or trauma. All age groups are covered, from neonates to the elderly. It outlines the physiological basis of pain and summarizes clinical studies linking effective postoperative pain management with improved patient outcomes.

Because patients vary greatly in medical conditions and operations, responses to pain and interventions, and personal preferences, the guideline offers a flexible approach to management of acute pain that clinicians can adapt and use in daily practice.

The guideline emphasizes:

- A collaborative, interdisciplinary approach to pain control, including all members of the health care team and input from the patient and the patient's family, when appropriate;

- individualized proactive pain control plan developed preoperatively by patients and practitioners (since pain is easier to prevent than to bring under control, once it has begun);

- Assessment and frequent reassessment of the patient's pain;

- Use of both drug and non-drug therapies to control and/or prevent pain;

- A formal, institutional approach to management of acute pain, with clear lines of responsibility.

The guideline includes strategies for overall pain control as well as site-specific pain control and addresses issues related to special groups such as children and the elderly. Additionally, it contains analgesic dosage tables for adults and children, sample pain assessment tools, examples of non-drug interventions, and pre- and postoperative pain management flow charts.

Guideline development is a dynamic process, and new therapies and technologies are always emerging. This is the first edition of the Clinical Practice Guideline for Acute Pain Management. Further editions will be prepared to reflect new research findings and experience with emerging technologies for pain assessment and relief.

Introduction

This guideline addresses the care of patients with acute pain after operation, medical procedures, or trauma. It outlines the physiological basis for pain and cites clinical studies linking effective postoperative pain management with improved patient outcomes. The guideline also describes practices that can minimize or eliminate acute pain. Rigid prescriptions for postoperative pain control are inappropriate because patients vary greatly in the severity of their preexisting pain, medical conditions, and pain experiences; the extensiveness of pathology and associated operations; responses to interventions; personal preferences; and the settings in which they receive care. Instead, this guideline offers clinicians a coherent yet flexible approach to pain assessment and management in daily practice. This guideline has four major goals:

1. Reduce the incidence and severity of patients' postoperative or posttraumatic pain.
2. Educate patients about the need to communicate unrelieved pain so they can receive prompt evaluation and effective treatment.
3. Enhance patient comfort and satisfaction.

Acute Pain Management: Operative or Medical Procedures

4. Contribute to fewer postoperative complications and, in some cases, shorter stays after surgical procedures.

Need for Aggressive Postoperative Pain Control

Pain is an unpleasant sensory and emotional experience arising from actual or potential tissue damage or described in terms of such damage (International Association for the Study of Pain, 1979; Merskey, 1964). No matter how successful or how deftly conducted, operations produce tissue trauma and release potent mediators of inflammation and pain (Hargreaves, and Dionne, 1991).

Pain is just one response to the trauma of surgery, however. In addition to the major stress of surgical trauma and pain, the substances released from injured tissue evoke "stress hormone" responses in the patient. Such responses promote breakdown of body tissue; increase metabolic rate, blood clotting, and water retention; impair immune function; and trigger a "fight or flight" alarm reaction with autonomic features (e.g., rapid pulse) and negative emotions (Dinarello, 1984 ; Egdahl, 1959 ; Kehlet, 1982 ; Kehlet, Brandt, and Rem, 1980). Pain itself may lead to shallow breathing and cough suppression in an attempt to "splint" the injured site, followed by retained pulmonary secretions and pneumonia (Anscombe, and Buxton, 1958 ; Hewlett, and Branthwaite, 1975 ; Latimer, Dickman, Day, Gunn, and Schmidt, 1971 ; Marshall, and Wyche, 1972 ; Sydow, 1989). Unrelieved pain also may delay the return of normal gastric and bowel function in the postoperative patient (Wattwil, 1989).

The physiological and psychosocial risks associated with untreated pain are greatest in frail patients with other illnesses such as heart or lung disease, those undergoing major surgical procedures such as aortic surgery, and the very young or very old. Because of advances in surgical and anesthetic techniques, it is now common for such patients to undergo operations once dismissed as prohibitively risky.

Approximately 23.3 million operations were performed in the United States in 1989 (Peebles, and Schneidman, 1991), and most of these involved some form of pain management. Unfortunately, clinical surveys continue to show that routine orders for intramuscular injections of opioid "as needed" will leave more than half of postoperative patients with unrelieved pain due to under-medication (Marks, and Sachar, 1973 ; Donovan, Dillon, and McGuire, 1987; Oden, 1989; Sriwatanakul, Weis, Alloza, Kelvie, Weintraub, and Lasagna, 1983). In the past, postoperative pain was thought to be inevitable, a harmless though intense discomfort that the patient had to tolerate.

Unrelieved pain after surgery or trauma is often unhealthy; fortunately, it is preventable or controllable in an overwhelming majority of cases. Patients have a right to treatment that includes prevention or adequate relief of pain.

Recognition of the widespread inadequacy of pain management has prompted recent corrective efforts within multiple health care disciplines, including surgery (Kehlet, 1989a; Royal College of Surgeons, 1990), anesthesiology (Phillips, and Cousins, 1986; Ready, Oden, Chadwick, Bendetti, Rooke, Caplan, and Wild, 1988); nursing (Jacox, 1977; American Nurses Association, 1991), and pain management groups (National Health and Medical Research Council of Australia, 1988; American Pain Society, 1989; International Association for the Study of Pain, 1991). Although it is not practical or desirable to eliminate all postoperative pain, this clinical practice guideline sets forth procedures to minimize the incidence and severity of acute pain after surgical or medical procedures and trauma. The guideline is designed to help clinicians, patients, and patients' families understand the assessment and treatment of postoperative and other acute pain in both adults and children.

Health care is both a technical and an ethical enterprise. The ethical obligation to manage pain and relieve the patient's suffering is at the core of a health care professional's commitment. While medical treatments often involve risks and burdens, anything harmful to the patient, including postoperative pain, should be minimized or prevented if possible. The ethical importance of pain management is further increased when additional benefits for the patient are realized—earlier mobilization, shortened hospital stay, and reduced costs. If inadequate pain management results from a clinician's conflict between reducing pain and avoiding potential side effects and/or legal liability, achieving greater technical competence and knowledge of risks and benefits can help to reduce such conflicts.

Prevention Is Better than Treatment

Pain is dynamic. Without treatment, sensory input from injured tissue reaches spinal cord neurons and causes subsequent responses to be enhanced. Pain receptors in the periphery also become more sensitive after injury. Recent studies demonstrate long-lasting changes in cells within spinal cord pain pathways after a brief painful stimulus (Bullit, 1989; Fitzgerald, 1990; Hanley, 1988; Hunt, Pini, and Evan, 1987; Przewlocki, Haarmann, Nikolarakis, Herz, and Hollt, 1988). Such physiological studies confirm longstanding clinical impressions that

Acute Pain Management: Operative or Medical Procedures

established pain is more difficult to suppress (McQuay, 1989; Wall, 1988; Woolf, and Wall, 1986). The health care team should encourage patients to request pain medication before the pain becomes severe and difficult to control. Furthermore, the team should teach patients simple relaxation exercises to help decrease postoperative pain (Ceccio, 1984).

Aggressive pain prevention and control that occurs before, during, and after surgery can yield both short- and long-term benefits. In the very short term, for example, a patient's first request for analgesia after orthopedic surgery occurs later after operations performed with opioid premedication and intraoperative nerve blocks than after general anesthesia alone (McQuay, Carroll, and Moore, 1988). In the short term, patients who undergo cesarean section under epidural anesthesia request less postoperative pain medication in the next 3 days than patients who have general anesthesia (Hanson, Hanson, and Matousek, 1984). Also in the short term, postoperative patients able to self-medicate with small intravenous doses of opioids such as morphine metered out by a programmable infusion pump—patient controlled analgesia or PCA (Ferrante, Ostheimer, and Covino, 1990)—have less pain and are more satisfied with their pain relief. These patients tend to be discharged earlier from the hospital compared with those given the same drug on an "as-needed" basis (Guideline Report, in press; Bollish, Collins, Kirking, and Bartlett, 1985; Eisenach, Grice, and Dewan, 1988; Jackson, 1989; Wasylak, Abbott, English, and Jeans, 1990).

In the long term, after elective limb amputation for vascular insufficiency, patients who receive epidural analgesia before an operation are less likely to have chronic phantom limb pain, in contrast to those conventionally treated (Bach, Noreng, and Tjellden, 1988). Pilot studies such as these that show diverse benefits of aggressive pain treatment complement controlled clinical trials which indicate that postoperative morbidity and mortality decrease in high-risk populations such as the very young (Anand, Sippell, and Aynsley-Green, 1987) or very old (Egbert, Parks, Short, and Burnett, 1990) when postoperative care includes aggressive pain relief.

Much of the clinical research cited here is preliminary and needs to be confirmed by properly designed clinical trials. Yet, when considered with laboratory reports and well-documented under-treatment of pain in hospitalized patients, it is likely that routine provision of proactive, aggressive pain treatment will benefit large numbers of postoperative patients. To ensure these benefits, institutions must develop and use formal procedures to assess pain and employ patient-based feedback to gauge the effectiveness of pain control (American

Pain Society, 1990, 1991). The flow charts shown in Figures 30.1 and 30.2 indicate the points at which caregivers must make decisions about assessing and controlling patient pain.

Organization of the Guideline

To derive maximum benefit, clinicians should read the entire guideline. However, the guideline is organized so that users can go easily to those sections of immediate interest. Following a discussion of why clinicians should take an aggressive approach to prevention and control of postoperative pain, methods of pain assessment are described. Pharmacologic and non-pharmacologic methods of pain control are then presented for general control of postoperative pain, followed by discussion of pain control for specific operative sites and for specific types of patients. The final section discusses institutional responsibility for effective pain management. The original document includes appendixes containing a brief description of the methods used for scientific review and a table of scientific evidence for pain intervention, pain assessment tools, drug dosage tables for adults and children, and relaxation exercises. These have not been included here but can be accessed on-line at http://text.nlm.nih.gov/ftrs/pick?dbName=apmc&ftrsK=34191&cp=1&t=867859846&collect=ahcpr

Process of Pain Assessment and Reassessment

Pain is a complex, subjective response with several quantifiable features, including intensity, time course, quality, impact, and personal meaning. The reporting of pain is a social transaction between caregiver and patient. Therefore, successful assessment and control of postoperative pain depends in part on establishing a positive relationship between health care providers, patients, and (when appropriate) their families. Studies have shown that patients provided with information related to physiological coping (instruction in coughing, deep breathing, turning, and ambulation) reported less pain (Fortin, and Kirouac, 1976), were given fewer analgesics postoperatively (Fortin, and Kirouac, 1976; Voshall, 1980), and had shorter lengths of stay (Van Aernam, and Lindeman, 1971). Egbert, Battit, Welch, and Bartlett (1964) found that providing patients sensory information preoperatively (i.e., detailed descriptions of discomforts to be expected postoperatively) decreased pain, analgesic use, and length of stay. Still other researchers found that patients provided with procedural and sensory information as well as instructions related to physiological

Acute Pain Management: Operative or Medical Procedures

coping tended to receive fewer analgesics (Reading, 1982; Schmitt, and Wooldridge, 1973) and had shorter lengths of stay than patients who were given less complete information (Schmitt, and Wooldridge, 1973).

As noted in the flow charts (Figures 40.1 and 40.2), the subject of postoperative pain and its control is a critical part of the initial review of all relevant aspects of the planned procedure. The surgeon should discuss this with the patient and the family. In addition, pain assessment and management issues should be a part of the preoperative workups of the anesthesia and nursing staffs. Patients and their families should be informed that pain reports are valuable and important information, and also that pain may herald surgical complications that demand prompt diagnosis and therapy. To aid in planning and discussing pain control strategies with the patient, a member of the anesthesiology department should obtain a pain history during the preoperative visit. The pain history should include:

- Significant previous and/or ongoing instances of pain and its effect on the patient;
- Previously used methods for pain control that the patient has found either helpful or unhelpful;
- The patient's attitude toward and use of opioid, anxiolytic, or other medications, including any history of substance abuse;
- The patient's typical coping response for stress or pain, including more broadly, the presence or absence of psychiatric disorders such as depression, anxiety, or psychosis;
- Family expectations and beliefs concerning pain, stress, and postoperative course;
- Ways the patient describes or shows pain; and
- The patient's knowledge of, expectations about, and preferences for pain management methods and for receiving information about pain management.

Some patients fear over-medication (e.g., "They will medicate me into oblivion so that I won't be any trouble"). Others know from previous experience that they are prone to side effects of certain drugs (e.g., dysphoria or nausea). Patients who express fears or concerns related to previous analgesic effects may require a cautious approach to medication. Preoperative anxiety may indicate a concurrent medical condition such as substance abuse or withdrawal, hyperthyroidism, anxiety disorder, affective disorder, psychosis, or a medication side effect. Excessive preoperative anxiety should be assessed and a psychiatric or psychologic consultation considered to assist with perioperative management. When the preoperative assessment is complete (as noted in Figure 32.1), the health care team should develop a pain management plan in collaboration with the patient. When developing the pain management plan, clinicians must consider the relative risks, benefits, and costs of available pain control options. They also should attempt to correct patient misconceptions about the use of pharmacologic or non-pharmacologic strategies.

Once a pain management plan is in place, preoperative preparation of the patient and family is extremely important. Preoperative

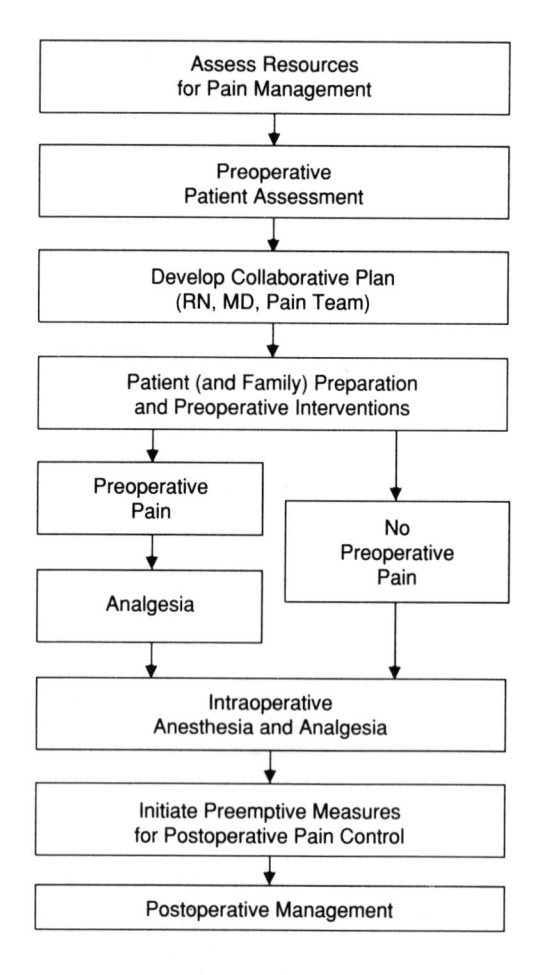

Figure 32.1. *Pain Treatment Flow Chart: Pre- and Intraoperative Phases*

Acute Pain Management: Operative or Medical Procedures

preparation of patients (and families, when appropriate) assists patients in understanding their responsibilities in pain management. To ensure that postoperative pain measurement is both valid and reliable, the staff should review the selected pain measurement tool—for example, a simple descriptive scale or a visual analog scale—with the patient before surgery. Pain assessment instruments are discussed below and samples are provided in appendix D of the original document. Similar instruments are provided in the chapter "Managing Cancer Pain" later in this sourcebook. The patient should be told how

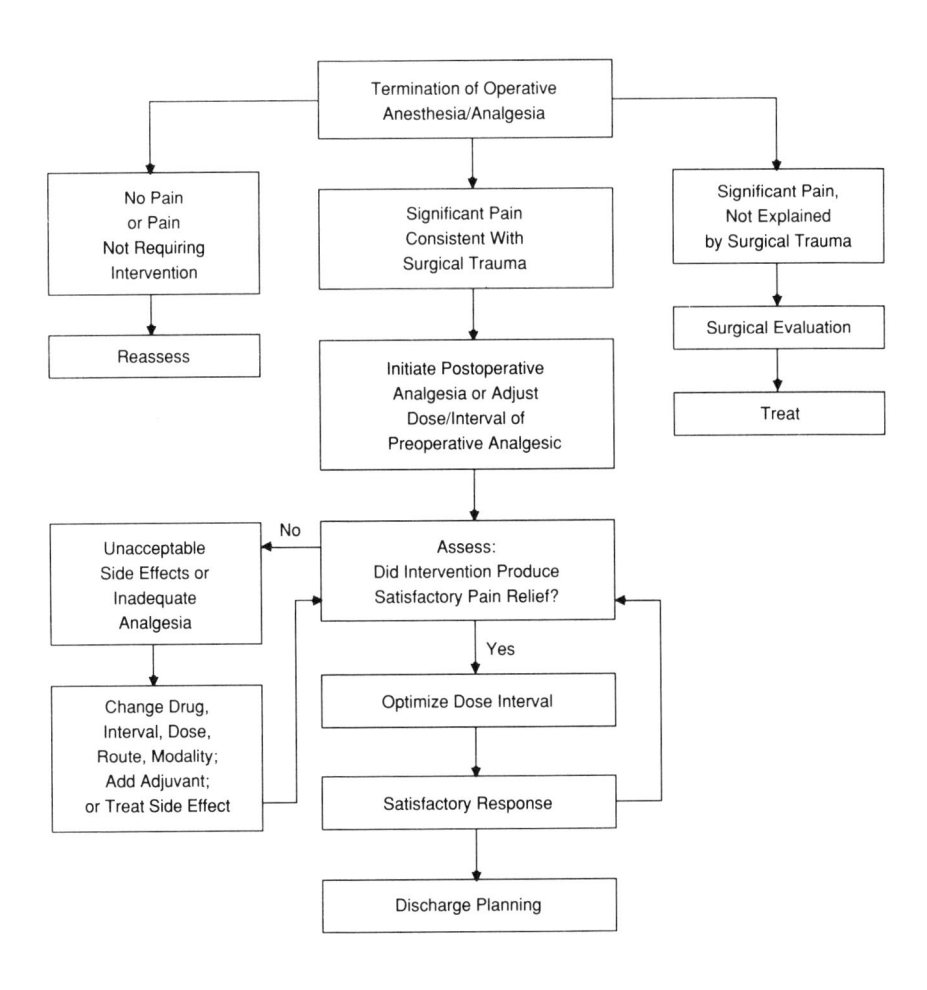

Figure 32.2. Pain Treatment Flow Chart: Postoperative Phase

frequently pain will be assessed and asked to select a measurement tool. A member of the health care team should advise the patient that a score above some predetermined criterion of the patient's choosing (e.g., a score of 3-4 on a 10-point scale) will result in a dose increment or other intervention. The patient's negotiation of this criterion is particularly important if the patient fears over-medication or intends to cope psychologically with the pain. Patient preferences should be supported.

Assessment of pain after surgery should be frequent and simple. Many different measurement tools are available, and several factors help determine the best choices (Chapman, and Syrjala, 1990). First, consider the patient's age; developmental status; physical, emotional, or cognitive condition; and preference. Second, consider the expertise, time, and effort available from the individual performing the assessment. Third, examine the institution's requirements for monitoring and documentation for quality assurance purposes. Based on these factors, each health care institution should educate staff in the proper and consistent use of a valid assessment tool(s) and establish its own quality assurance program for evaluation of postoperative pain assessment and management (American Pain Society, 1990, 1991; National Institutes of Health, 1987). For example, recording pain intensity on the bedside vital sign chart may be considered necessary to make the assessment easily accessible to members of the health care team. In addition, each institution should identify individuals responsible for postoperative pain assessment and control.

The single most reliable indicator of the existence and intensity of acute pain—and any resultant affective discomfort or distress—is the patient's self-report.

A comprehensive approach to postoperative pain assessment requires evaluation of:

1. patient perceptions;
2. physiological responses;
3. behavioral responses; and
4. cognitive attempts by the patient to manage pain.

Physiological responses such as heart rate, blood pressure, and respiratory rate provide critical information in the immediate postoperative period. Once the patient has recovered from anesthesia, the mainstay of pain assessment should be the patient's self-report to

Acute Pain Management: Operative or Medical Procedures

assess pain perceptions (including description, location, intensity/severity, and aggravating, and relieving factors) and cognitive response. Patient self-report is the single most reliable indicator of the existence and intensity of acute pain and any concomitant affective discomfort or distress (National Institutes of Health, 1987). Neither behavior nor vital signs can substitute for a self-report (Beyer, McGrath, and Berde, 1990). Patients may be experiencing excruciating pain even while smiling and using laughter as coping mechanisms (Fritz, 1988).

Samples of commonly used pain assessment tools are in appendix D of the original document. Similar instruments can be found in the chapter "Managing Cancer Pain" located later in this sourcebook. Three common self-report measurement tools useful for assessment of pain intensity and affective distress in adults and many children are: 1) a numerical rating scale (NRS); 2) a visual analog scale (VAS); and 3) an adjective rating scale (ARS). While many researchers prefer visual analog measures (Scott, and Huskisson, 1976; Sriwatanakul, Kelvie, Lasagna, Calimlim, Weis, and Mehta, 1983), each of these tools can be a valid and reliable instrument as long as end points and adjective descriptors are carefully selected (Gracely, and Wolskee, 1983; Houde, 1982; Sriwatanakul, Kelvie, and Lasagna, 1982).

In practical use, the visual analog scale is always presented graphically, usually with a 10-cm baseline and endpoint adjective descriptors. Patients place a mark on the line at a point that best represents their pain. The visual analog scale is scored by measuring the distance of a patient's mark from the zero. The numerical and adjective rating scales may be presented graphically or in other formats. For example, numerical rating scales are sometimes presented verbally, and adjective rating scales are presented as a list of pain descriptors. In a graphic format, scoring of the numerical and adjective rating scales may be the same as that described above for the visual analog scale, or they can be scored as numeric integers.

For each of these scales, the clinician should request the patient's self-report, not only with the patient at rest but also during routine activity such as coughing, deep breathing, or moving (e.g., turning in bed). Complaints of pain must be heeded. The patient should be observed for behaviors that often indicate pain, such as splinting the operative site, distorted posture, impaired mobility, insomnia, anxiety, attention seeking, and depression. Patient awareness of pain and the ability to control pain are important components of pain assessment. If pain behavior is observed or if the patient expresses feelings of inadequate control, a member of the health care team should discuss these with the patient and share this information with other members of the team. The management plan should then be revised as needed.

The clinician should document the patient's preferred tool for pain assessment and the goal for postoperative pain control as expressed by a score on a pain scale in the patient's chart as part of the pain history. Simply to record patient responses to the question "how is your pain?" invites misunderstanding or denial and hinders quantification. Pain should be assessed and documented:

1. preoperatively;
2. routinely at regular intervals postoperatively, as determined by the operation and severity of the pain (e.g., every 2 hours while awake for 1 day after surgery);
3. with each new report of pain; and
4. at a suitable interval after each analgesic intervention (e.g., 30 minutes after parenteral drug therapy, and 1 hour after oral analgesics).

Most important, the team should evaluate immediately each instance of unexpected intense pain, particularly if sudden or associated with oliguria or altered vital signs such as hypotension, tachycardia, or fever, and consider new diagnoses such as wound dehiscence, infection, or deep venous thrombosis.

Each instance of unexpected intense pain, particularly if sudden or associated with oliguria or altered vital signs such as hypotension, tachycardia, or fever, should be immediately evaluated to consider new diagnoses such as wound dehiscence, infection, or deep venous thrombosis.

Occasionally, apparent discrepancies between behaviors and a patient's self-report of pain may occur. For example, patients may describe pain as an 8 out of 10 on a pain scale while smiling and walking freely or as 2 out of 10 while tachycardic, splinting, and sweating. Discrepancies between behavior and a patient's self-report may result from excellent coping skills. The patient who uses distraction and relaxation techniques may engage in diversionary activities while still experiencing severe pain. Patients may deny severe pain for a variety of reasons, including fear of inadequate pain control or a perception that stoicism is expected or rewarded. Similarly, patients

Acute Pain Management: Operative or Medical Procedures

managed with as-needed analgesia may perceive that medication will be given only if the pain score is very high. Patients who perceive staff as inattentive to their concerns may use pain as a way to get help for other reasons.

When discussing pain assessment and control with patients, members of the health care team should emphasize the importance of a factual report, thereby avoiding both stoicism and exaggeration. Patients with anxiety or other concerns should rate their mood and emotional distress separately from their pain by using similar scales (see Pain Distress Scales). When discrepancies between behaviors and self-reports of pain occur, clinicians should address these differences with the patient. The team and the patient should then renegotiate the pain management plan.

Patients unable to communicate effectively with staff require special consideration for pain assessment, e.g., neonates and children, developmentally delayed persons, psychotic patients, patients with dementia, and non-English speaking patients. Children and cognitively impaired patients require simpler or modified pain measurement scales and assessment approaches (see section on pain in children). The staff should work with both the patient and parent or guardian pre- and postoperatively. Staff should endeavor to find a translator for the non-English speaking patient, at least once, to determine a convenient way to assess pain. Members of the health care team should attend to the preferences and needs of patients whose education or cultural tradition may impede effective communication. Certain cultures have strong beliefs about pain and its management, and these patients may hesitate to complain about unrelieved pain. Such beliefs and preferences should be determined and respected, if at all possible. In summary, health care providers should view good pain control as a source of pride and a major responsibility in quality care. Support personnel otherwise untrained in pain assessment should be encouraged to be "pain vigilant" and report to the health care team any patient discomfort, such as during transport or transfer to an x-ray table. At the institutional level, periodic evaluation studies should be conducted to monitor the effectiveness of pain assessment and management procedures. Without institutional support for an organized process by which pain is recognized, documented, assessed, and reassessed on a regular basis, staff efforts to treat pain may become sporadic and ineffectual. A pain care process relying on patients' or families' demands for analgesia "as needed" will produce intervals of inadequate pain control and worsen burdens of anxiety, loss of personal control, sleeplessness, and fatigue after surgery. Patients and their families should understand that pain relief is an important part of their health care, that information about options to control pain is available, and that they are welcome to discuss their preferences with the health care team. Patients should recognize that health professionals will elicit and respond quickly to their pain reports. Before a patient's discharge, those taking care of the patient should describe the interventions used to manage pain and assess their effectiveness. This review, while good practice for each patient, is especially important when initial management was unsuccessful and/or when side effects or other complications occurred.

Options to Prevent and Control Postoperative Pain

Patient education and reduction of any preexisting pain should occur before the operation. Because the goal of the treatment plan is to prevent significant postoperative pain from the outset, treatment alternatives, potential risks, dosage adjustments, and adjunctive therapies should be described to the patient and family. Teaching emphasizes what the patient is likely to experience postoperatively, including the specific method(s) of pain assessment, intervention(s) the staff will employ, and the level of patient participation required. Staff also should inform patients that it is easier to prevent pain than to "chase" or treat it once it has become established, and that communication of unrelieved pain is essential to its relief.

Pain control options include:

- Cognitive-behavioral interventions such as relaxation, distraction, and imagery; these can be taught preoperatively and can reduce pain, anxiety, and the amount of drugs needed for pain control;

- Systemic administration of nonsteroidal anti-inflammatory drugs (NSAIDs) or opioids using the traditional "as needed" schedule or around-the-clock administration (American Pain Society, 1989);

- Patient controlled analgesia (PCA), usually meaning self-medication with intravenous doses of an opioid; this can include other classes of drugs administered orally or by other routes;

- Spinal analgesia, usually by means of an epidural opioid and/or local anesthetic injected intermittently or infused continuously;

Acute Pain Management: Operative or Medical Procedures

- Intermittent or continuous local neural blockade (examples of the former include intercostal nerve blockade with local anesthetic or cryoprobe; the latter includes infusion of local anesthetic through an interpleural catheter);

- Physical agents such as massage or application of heat or cold; and

- Electroanalgesia such as transcutaneous electrical nerve stimulation (TENS).

A postoperative pain management plan might include several of these options.

A pamphlet, or "menu" of alternative strategies, can help focus discussion of these options between caregivers and the patient. The postoperative pain management plan should reflect coexisting and/or ongoing problems such as cancer-related pain or opioid tolerance. The plan should be consistent with the overall surgical and anesthetic plans. For example, an elixir form of analgesic is preferable to a tablet when painful or difficult swallowing is anticipated. Also, if the patient is to have an epidural catheter placed during surgery that could make postoperative pain control simpler or more effective, it should not be removed in the Post-Anesthesia Care Unit (PACU). Staff should note their plans for pre-, intra-, and postoperative pain management in the patient's chart so that other members of the care team can respond to patient questions and coordinate plans for rehabilitation and discharge.

Intraoperative management is often key to the success of postoperative pain control. If pain prevention and control are to be achieved through an epidural catheter, the catheter should be placed and its function verified preoperatively to assure its effective intra- and postoperative use. This is particularly true in patients whose position, body casts, or subsequent anticoagulation make postoperative catheter insertion problematic. The planned pre- and intraoperative use of opioids, and timing of the first postoperative opioid dose by the anesthesiologist, nurse anesthetist, surgeon, or PACU nurse are important in the postoperative care plan. Equally important are decisions during surgery on the concurrent use of local anesthetics (e.g., for intraoperative nerve blocks) and the nature of the surgical incision and placement of drains or tubes (e.g., chest, and nasogastric). If TENS is to be used for postoperative pain management, the electrodes may need to be placed intraoperatively. Finally, intraoperative placement of casts and splints to provide support and restrict postoperative movement may enhance other pain management efforts.

Pharmacologic Management

Pharmacologic management of mild to moderate postoperative pain should begin, unless there is a contraindication, with an NSAID. Moderately severe to severe pain normally should be treated initially with an opioid analgesic. After many relatively non-invasive surgical procedures, NSAIDs alone can achieve excellent pain control (Davie, Slawson, and Burt, 1982; Rosen, Absi, and Webster, 1985). NSAIDs decrease levels of inflammatory mediators generated at the site of tissue injury. Even when insufficient alone to control pain, NSAIDs have a significant opioid dose-sparing effect upon postoperative pain and can be useful in reducing opioid side effects (Guideline Report, in press; Hodsman, Burns, Blyth, Kenny, McArdle, and Rotman, 1987; Martens, 1982). The concurrent use of opioids and NSAIDs often provides more effective analgesia than either of the drug classes alone. Although it is likely that NSAIDs also act within the central nervous system, in contrast to opioids, they do not cause sedation or respiratory depression, nor do they interfere with bowel or bladder function. Acetaminophen does not affect platelet aggregation, nor does it provide peripheral anti-inflammatory activity. Some evidence exists that two salicylates do not affect platelet aggregation profoundly; these are salsalate (Estes, and Kaplan, 1980) and choline magnesium trisalicylate (Danesh, Saniabadi, Russell, and Lowe, 1987). All other NSAIDs appear to produce a risk of platelet dysfunction that may impair blood clotting and carry a small risk of gastrointestinal bleeding. At present, one NSAID (ketorolac) is approved by the Food and Drug Administration for parenteral use.

Opioid analgesics are the cornerstone of pharmacological postoperative pain management, especially for more extensive surgical procedures that cause moderate to severe pain. Other agents such as NSAIDs or single injections of local anesthetics may control mild to moderate pain after relatively minor procedures or reduce opioid dose requirements after more extensive operations when this is a goal (Guideline Report, in press; Egan, Herman, Doucette, Normand, and McLeod, 1988; Engberg, 1985a, 1985b; Kaplan, Miller, and Gallagher, 1975; Patel, Lanzafame, Williams, Mullen, and Hinshaw, 1983; Sabanathan, Mearns, Bickford-Smith, Eng, Berrisford, Bibby, and Majid, 1990; Toledo-Pereyra, and DeMeester, 1979). Even in the absence of preemptive efforts targeted at postoperative analgesia, adequate

Acute Pain Management: Operative or Medical Procedures

postoperative pain control can usually be achieved with opioid analgesics. When increasing doses of opioids are ineffective in controlling postoperative pain, a prompt search for residual pathology is indicated, and other diagnoses such as neuropathic pain should be considered.

Opioid tolerance or physiological dependence is unusual in short-term postoperative use in opioid naive patients. Likewise, psychologic dependence and addiction are extremely unlikely to develop after patients without prior drug abuse histories use opioids for acute pain (Porter, and Jick, 1980). Proper use of opioids involves selecting a particular drug and route of administration and judging: 1) suitable initial dose; 2) frequency of administration; 3) optimal doses of nonopioid analgesics, if these are also to be given; 4) incidence and severity of side effects; and 5) whether the analgesic will be given in an inpatient or ambulatory setting. Titration to achieve the desired therapeutic effect in the immediate postoperative period and to maintain that effect over time should be emphasized.

Opioids produce analgesia by binding to opioid receptors both within and outside the central nervous system. Opioid analgesics are classified as full agonists, partial agonists, or mixed agonist-antagonists, depending on the manner in which they interact with opioid receptors. Full agonists produce a maximal response within the cells to which they bind; partial agonists produce a lesser response, regardless of their concentration; and mixed agonist-antagonists activate one type of opioid receptor while simultaneously blocking another type. Several types and subtypes of such receptors exist. The most important receptor type for clinical analgesia is named "mu" because of its affinity for morphine. Other commonly used mu opioid agonists include hydromorphone, codeine, oxycodone and hydrocodone, methadone, levorphanol, and fentanyl. All mu opioid agonists have the potential to cause constipation, urinary retention, sedation, and respiratory depression and frequently also produce nausea or confusion. Mixed agonist-antagonists in clinical use include pentazocine [Talwin], butorphanol tartrate [Stadol], and nalbuphine hydrochloride [Nubain]; each of these blocks or is neutral at the mu opioid receptor while simultaneously activating a different type of opioid receptor termed "kappa." Patients receiving mu opioid agonists should not be given a mixed agonist-antagonist because doing so may precipitate a withdrawal syndrome and increase pain. Mixed agonist-antagonists and partial agonists may exhibit a ceiling effect not only with respect to respiratory depression (Nagashima, Karamanian, Malovany, Radnay, Ang, Koerner, and Foldes, 1976; Kallos, and Caruso, 1979) but also in regard to their analgesic activity. In the awake patient, there is a clinical ceiling analgesic effect even with morphine because side effects such as respiratory depression limit the dose that may be safely given. However, this does not limit the ability of clinicians to effectively increase the drug dose when the painful stimulus increases and respiratory status is monitored.

Meperidine [Demerol], a mu opioid analgesic, is commonly used for postoperative pain control. Meperidine is commonly under-dosed and administered too infrequently even by physicians aware of its pharmacokinetics (Marks, and Sachar, 1973). The common postoperative meperidine order of 75 mg parenterally every 4 hours as needed often is inadequate for several reasons. Meperidine produces clinical analgesia for only 2.5-3.5 hours, and a dose of 75 mg every 4 hours is equivalent to only 5-7.5 mg of morphine. Therefore, to obtain postoperative analgesia equal to that from 10 mg of morphine sulfate every 4 hours, a clinician would have to use 100-150 mg of meperidine every 3 hours. Because of its unique toxicity, meperidine is often contraindicated in patients with impaired renal function and those receiving antidepressants of the monamine oxidase inhibitor class (Wood, and Cousins, 1989). Normeperidine (6-N-desmethylmeperidine) is a toxic meperidine metabolite excreted through the kidney. In patients with normal renal function, Normeperidine has a half-life of 15 to 20 hours; this time is extended greatly in elderly individuals and patients with impaired renal function. Normeperidine is a cerebral irritant that can cause effects ranging from dysphoria and irritable mood to convulsions (Kaiko, Foley, Grabinski, Heidrich, Rogers, Inturissi, and Reidenberg, 1983; Szeto, Inturrisi, Houde, Saal, Cheigh, and Reidenberg, 1977). These effects have been observed even in young, otherwise healthy patients given sufficiently high doses of normeperidine postoperatively. Therefore, meperidine should be reserved for very brief courses in otherwise healthy patients who have demonstrated an unusual reaction (e.g., local histamine release at the infusion site) or allergic response during treatment with other opioids such as morphine or hydromorphone.

Titration of opioids should be based on the patient's analgesic response and side effects. Remember that patients vary greatly in their analgesic dose requirements and responses to opioid analgesics. Relative potency estimates provide a rational basis for selecting the appropriate starting dose to initiate analgesic therapy, changing the route of administration (e.g., from parenteral to oral), or when switching to another opioid. Dosage conversion factors based on relative potency estimates may differ somewhat between individual patients. When estimating the initial postoperative dose of an opioid analgesic, a clinician should consider whether patients have been receiving opioid analgesics preoperatively. In such patients, supplemental postoperative doses should be adjusted above the preoperative baseline requirement unless the operation itself is likely to remove the painful stimulus.

An "as-needed" order for opioid administration can result in prolonged delays while the nurse unlocks the controlled substances cabinet and prepares the drug for administration and until the drug takes effect. These delays can be eliminated by administering analgesics on a regular time schedule initially. For example, if the patient is likely to have pain requiring opioid analgesics for 48 hours following surgery, morphine could be ordered every 4 hours by the clock (not "as needed") for 36 hours. Once the duration of analgesic action is determined for a patient, the dosage frequency should be adjusted to prevent pain from recurring. Depending on patient preferences, the orders may be written so that the patient can refuse an analgesic if not in pain or forego it if asleep. However, as in dosing with other drugs that require a steady blood level to remain effective, interruption of an around-the-clock dosage schedule during the hours of sleep may cause the patient to be suddenly awakened by intense pain as blood analgesic levels decline.

It may be acceptable late in the postoperative course to give the same drug every 4 hours as requested. Switching from an around-the-clock to an as-needed dosage schedule later in the patient's course is one way to provide pain relief while minimizing the risk of adverse effects as the patient's analgesic dose requirement diminishes. As part of this schedule, a patient's pain should be assessed at regular intervals to determine the efficacy of the drug intervention, the presence of side effects, or the need for dosage adjustment or supplemental doses for breakthrough pain. Effective use of opioid analgesics should facilitate routine postoperative activities—e.g., coughing and deep breathing exercises, ambulation, and physical therapy (Alexander, Parikh, and Spence, 1973; Rawal, and Sjostrand, 1986; Wasylak, Abbott, English, and Jeans, 1990). The opioid should be withheld if the patient is sedated when awake or whenever there is respiratory depression (usually fewer than 10 breaths per minute).

Opioids may be administered by a variety of routes; oral dosing is usually the most convenient and least expensive route of administration. It is appropriate as soon as the patient can tolerate oral intake and is the mainstay of pain management in the ambulatory surgical population.

Preoperative intravenous or epidural access may be appropriate for postoperative management of severe pain, even when the oral route is available. Relatively few side effects will occur ordinarily, providing that these modalities are carefully managed by clinicians with appropriate expertise. Using potent analgesics or invasive techniques postoperatively, at a time when a patient's level of consciousness and physical function are returning to normal, requires careful titration and patient assessment.

Drug dosage, frequency, side effects, and risks differ even more noticeably between the intravenous and epidural routes than between the oral and intravenous routes. Clinicians not familiar with epidural opioid doses and pharmacokinetics must review the literature carefully before using that route. In addition, side effects (e.g., confusion, respiratory depression, hypotension, urinary retention, or pruritus) associated with opioids can be greater with intravenous and epidural administration and require ongoing assessment and monitoring. Other potential problems that dictate expert vigilance and followup during epidural analgesia include abscess development or anesthesia of a nerve root at the site of catheter tip. These routes of administration are best limited to specially trained staff who are knowledgeable and skilled in the management of patients receiving intravenous or epidural opioids, typically under the direction of an acute or postoperative pain treatment service.

Patient controlled analgesia is a safe method for postoperative pain management that many patients prefer to intermittent injections. Systemic PCA usually connotes intravenous drug administration, but it also can be subcutaneous or intramuscular. Few studies of the use of PCA drug delivery to the epidural space exist. A typical intravenous PCA prescription applicable to many contexts relies on a series of "loading" doses; for example, 3-5 mg of morphine, repeated every 5 minutes until the initial postoperative pain (if present) diminishes. A low-dose basal infusion (0.5-1 mg/hr) at night allows uninterrupted sleep. On-demand doses typically add 1 mg of morphine every 6 minutes, with a total hourly limit of 10 mg. Once the patient is able to take oral medications, an around-the-clock schedule of an oral opioid such as a codeine-acetaminophen combination is provided, and the basal infusion rate is discontinued. By observing the number of "on-demand" doses self-administered by the patient, the clinician can assess the adequacy of the oral medication and titrate it further, change to a stronger compound such as oxycodone with acetaminophen, or discontinue the PCA pump.

Acute Pain Management: Operative or Medical Procedures

Intravenous administration is the preferred route for postoperative opioid therapy when the patient cannot take oral medications. When intravenous access is problematic, sublingual and rectal routes should be considered as alternatives to traditional intramuscular or subcutaneous injections. All routes other than intravenous require a lag time for absorption of the drug into the circulation. In addition, repeated injections with associated pain and trauma may deter some patients, especially children, from requesting pain medication. Continuous administration of low doses of opioids intravenously or transdermally and intermittent delivery across the buccal mucosa are relatively new but apparently effective methods to administer opioids postoperatively. Further experience is needed to define the clinical roles of these innovative methods in relation to more well-established methods.

Patient controlled analgesia (PCA) is a safe method for postoperative pain management that many patients prefer to intermittent injections.

Opioids and local anesthetic agents interact favorably. Continuous administration into the epidural space of low concentrations of opioids in dilute solutions of local anesthetic provides excellent analgesia, while reducing the potential risks (e.g., respiratory depression or motor block) associated with equianalgesic concentrations of either agent administered singly. In a less technologically demanding approach, systemically administered opioids given pre-, intra-, or postoperatively augment the duration and effectiveness of local anesthetics given spinally or epidurally. Local anesthetics alone may be applied intermittently to specific nerves to interrupt pain pathways. For example, injecting local anesthetics around the intercostal nerves after thoracotomy significantly improves pulmonary function (Guideline Report, in press; Engberg, 1985b; Kaplan, Miller, and Gallagher, 1975; Toledo-Pereyra, and DeMeester, 1979). Catheters for continuous or repeated intermittent dosing of local anesthetic also have been employed postoperatively in the pleural space or adjacent to nerves such as the brachial plexus or cervical sympathetic ganglia. However, a clinical role for interpleural or perineural local anesthetics in the postoperative setting has not yet been defined.

Non-pharmacologic Management

Non-pharmacologic interventions can be classified as either cognitive-behavioral interventions or physical agents. Cognitive and behaviorally based approaches include several ways to help patients understand more about their pain and take an active part in its assessment and control. The goals of interventions classified as cognitive-behavioral therapies are to change patients' perceptions of pain, alter pain behavior, and provide patients with a greater sense of control over pain. The goals of interventions classified as physical agents or modalities are to provide comfort, correct physical dysfunction, alter physiological responses, and reduce fears associated with pain-related immobility or activity restriction. Non-pharmacologic approaches are intended to supplement, not substitute for, the pharmacologic or invasive techniques described above.

Non-pharmacologic interventions are appropriate for the patient who: 1) finds such interventions appealing; 2) expresses anxiety or fear, as long as the anxiety is not incapacitating or due to a medical or psychiatric condition that has a more specific treatment; 3) may benefit from avoiding or reducing drug therapy (e.g., history of adverse reactions, fear of or physiological reason to avoid over-sedation); 4) is likely to experience and need to cope with a prolonged interval of postoperative pain, particularly if punctuated by recurrent episodes of intense treatment-or procedure-related pain; or 5) has incomplete pain relief following appropriate pharmacologic interventions. Cognitive-behavioral approaches include preparatory information, simple relaxation, imagery, hypnosis, and biofeedback. Physical therapeutic agents and modalities include application of superficial heat or cold, massage, exercise, immobility, and electroanalgesia such as TENS therapy.

Giving a patient a detailed description of all medical procedures, expected postoperative discomfort, and instruction aimed at decreasing treatment- and mobility-related pain can decrease self-reported pain, analgesic use, and postoperative length of stay (Guideline Report, in press; Egbert, Battit, Welch, and Bartlett, 1964; Fortin, and Kirouac, 1976; Schmitt, and Wooldridge, 1973; Voshall, 1980). Patients should receive sufficient procedural and sensory information to satisfy their interest and enable them to assess, evaluate, and communicate postoperative pain. In addition, all preoperative patients should receive instruction emphasizing the importance of coughing, deep breathing, turning, and walking, along with suggestions on how to decrease physical discomforts from such activities. When fear or anxiety occur, it is important to assess psychological coping skills and provide practical suggestions for managing pain and maintaining a positive outlook. Patients who appear anxious or fearful before surgery, and others who express an interest in cognitive-behavioral strategies, should be assisted in selecting an intervention (e.g., simple

Acute Pain Management: Operative or Medical Procedures

relaxation or imagery) and taught how to use it. In some patients, particularly those with high levels of anxiety, too much information, or too many demanding decisions can exacerbate fear and pain (Johnson, Fuller, Endress, and Rice, 1978; Johnson, Rice, Fuller, and Endress, 1978). Psychiatric evaluation is appropriate for patients who manifest disabling or disruptive anxiety symptoms such as emotional instability, restlessness, inability to sleep, and dulled thinking.

Relaxation is the most widely evaluated cognitive-behavioral approach to postoperative pain management. Relaxation strategies, including simple relaxation (Horowitz, Fitzpatrick, and Flaherty, 1984; Lawlis, Selby, Hinnant, and McCoy, 1985; Levin, Malloy, and Hyman, 1987); imagery (Daake, and Gueldner, 1989; Horan, Laying, and Pursell, 1976); hypnosis (Kiefer, and Hospodarsky, 1980); biofeedback (Madden, Singer, Peck, and Nayman, 1978); and music-assisted relaxation (Locsin, 1981; Mullooly, Levin, and Feldman, 1988), have all shown some degree of effectiveness in reducing pain. Relaxation strategies and imagery techniques need not be complex to be effective. Relatively simple approaches such as the brief jaw relaxation procedure described on page 25 have been successful in decreasing self-reported pain and analgesic use (Flaherty, and Fitzpatrick, 1978; Wells, 1982). These strategies take only a few minutes to teach but require periodic reinforcement through encouragement and coaching. Supportive family members or audiotapes often can sustain patient skills. A relaxation strategy that can be used informally is music distraction. Both patients' personally preferred music (Locsin, 1981) and

Table 32.1. Examples of Non-pharmacologic Interventions for Postoperative Pain

Examples of Nonpharmacologic Interventions for Postoperative Pain

Cognitive-Behavioral

- education/instruction
- relaxation
- imagery
- music distraction
- biofeedback

Physical Agents

- applications of heat or cold
- massage, exercise, and immobilization
- transcutaneous electrical nerve stimulation

"easy listening" music (Mullooly, Levin, and Feldman, 1988) have significantly decreased postoperative pain in clinical studies. Patients who need repeated coaching may benefit from the use of a commercially prepared relaxation or music-assisted relaxation audiotape.

Other cognitive-behavioral strategies require greater professional involvement; these include complex imagery, hypnosis, biofeedback, and combined therapies. Such strategies are commonly applied when patients have chronic pain even before surgery.

Jaw Relaxation Instructions

- Let your lower jaw drop slightly, as though you were starting a small yawn.
- Keep your tongue quiet and resting on the bottom of your mouth.
- Let your lips get soft.
- Breathe slowly, evenly, and rhythmically: inhale, exhale, and rest.
- Allow yourself to stop forming words with your lips and stop thinking in words.

Reprinted with permission. McCaffery, M. and Beebe, A. (1989).*Pain: Clinical manual for nursing practice.* St. Louis: CV Mosby Company.

Although some data suggest that the use of complex imagery may reduce pain (Daake, and Gueldner, 1989; Horan, Laying, and Pursell, 1976), that biofeedback may lessen pain and operative site muscle tension (Madden, Singer, Peck, and Nayman, 1978; Moon, and Gibbs, 1984), and that interventions which combine imagery and relaxation may decrease pain (Mogan, Wells, and Robertson, 1985; Pickett, and Clum, 1982; Swinford, 1987), each requires specialized training and, for biofeedback, the use of special equipment. Findings from studies of hypnosis for control of postoperative pain are inconsistent (Daniels, 1976; John, and Parrino, 1983; Kiefer, and Hospodarsky, 1980 ; Snow, 1985). Insufficient research to demonstrate effectiveness in reducing postoperative pain and the need for special training or equipment preclude the recommendation of complex imagery, biofeedback, or hypnosis for routine postoperative pain control. This is not to say that patients who have a high level of preoperative anxiety, whose pain is severe and enduring, or who suffer recurrent episodes of procedure-related pain will not benefit from these strategies. However, for such patients a more comprehensive pain management program must include active involvement of professionals skilled in cognitive-behavioral therapy and psychological assessment.

Acute Pain Management: Operative or Medical Procedures

In addition to cognitive-behavioral interventions, several physical therapeutic methods can be used to manage pain (Lee, Itoh, Yang, and Eason, 1990). Commonly used physical agents include applications of heat and cold, massage, exercise, and rest or immobilization. Applications of heat or cold are used to alter pain threshold, reduce muscle spasm, and decrease congestion in an injured area. Applications of cold are used initially to decrease tissue injury response. Later, heat is used to facilitate clearance of tissue toxins and accumulated fluids. Massage and exercise are used to stretch and regain muscle and tendon length. Immobilization is used following many musculoskeletal procedures to provide rest and maintain the alignment necessary for proper healing. With the exception of applications of cold and immobilization, these interventions typically are not used following surgery unless complications occur or an extended postoperative course is expected. When physical modalities are used, it is often for a physiological goal other than pain relief. Of these modalities only cryotherapy (application of cold) has been evaluated in the literature (Cohn, Draeger, and Jackson, 1989; Lanham, Powell, and Hendrix, 1984; Rooney, Jain, McCormack, Bains, Martini, and Goldiner, 1986). Lanham and colleagues (1984) and Rooney and colleagues (1986) used cryotherapy in association with TENS therapy. There is insufficient evidence to suggest that cryotherapy alone is effective in reducing postoperative pain. Cryotherapy is different from cryoanalgesia (application of a cryoprobe to specific peripheral nerves), which has proven effective for post-thoracotomy pain (Guideline Report, in press).

TENS therapy is one physical modality for which there is some support. TENS therapy has been effective in reducing self-reported pain and analgesic use following abdominal surgery (Cooperman, Hall, Mikalacki, Hardy, and Sadar, 1977; Hargreaves, and Lander, 1989), orthopedic surgery (Jensen, Conn, Hazelrigg, and Hewett, 1985; Smith, Hutchins, and Hehenberger, 1983), thoracic surgery (Liu, Liao, and Lien, 1985; Rooney, Jain, McCormack, Bains, Martini, and Goldiner, 1986), mixed surgical procedures (Neary, 1981; Solomon, Viernstein, and Long, 1980; VanderArk and McGrath, 1975), and cesarean section (Davies, 1982; Smith, Guralnick, Gelfand, and Jeans, 1986). TENS therapy also has improved physical mobility following thoracic (Liu, Liao, and Lien, 1985; Warfield, Stein, and Frank, 1985) and orthopedic (Jensen, Conn, Hazelrigg, and Hewett, 1985; Smith, Hutchins, and Hehenberger, 1983) surgery. Both TENS therapy and sham TENS therapy (that is, application of electrodes without transmission of electric current) significantly reduced analgesic use and subjective reports of pain (Guideline Report, in press). No significant differences were found between TENS therapy and sham-TENS (Conn, Marshall, Yadav, Daly, and Jaffer, 1986; Hargreaves and Lander, 1989; Taylor, West, Simon, Skelton, and Rowlingson, 1983). Even though these findings suggest a placebo effect underlies the reduction of perceived pain and analgesic use during TENS therapy, beneficial effects do, in fact, result (Guideline Report, in press). The physical modalities of acupuncture and electroacupuncture also have been clinically evaluated in postoperative patients, with conflicting findings; no clear analgesic effect has been demonstrated (Evron, Schenker, Olshwang, Granat, and Magora, 1981; Facco, Manani, Angel, Vincenti, Tambuscio, Ceccherelli, Troletti, Ambrosio, and Giron, 1981; Hansson, and Ekblom, 1986; Wigram, Lewith, Machin, and Church, 1986).

How each patient's postoperative pain management program is designed and implemented will vary according to the type of medical facility and services available to support a pain management program. At the least, clinicians should be introduced to these methods so they recognize the benefits of cognitive-behavioral and physical interventions, know the indications for their use, and are able to provide information and counseling to patients. In addition, patients should have access to written information about available therapies, why and when to use them, and sources for self-management materials or professional consultations.

Catastrophic postoperative events are rarely, if ever, masked by any of the approaches to postoperative pain control previously described. Any sudden or unexplained change in pain intensity requires immediate evaluation by the surgeon. Likewise, a sudden increase in anxiety may signal cardiac or pulmonary decompensation and requires prompt medical or surgical assessment.

Process of Effective Pain Management

Postoperative pain management. As illustrated in the flow chart (Figure 32.2), the process of postoperative pain management is ongoing. Following intraoperative anesthesia and analgesia, postoperative pain assessment and management begin. Based on the preoperative plan, postoperative drug and non-drug interventions are initiated. Patients should be reassessed at frequent intervals (not less than every 2-4 hours for the first 24 hours) to determine the efficacy of the intervention in reducing pain. If the intervention is ineffective, additional causes of pain should be considered, the plan should then be reevaluated, and appropriate modifications should be made. Pharmacologic interventions should

Acute Pain Management: Operative or Medical Procedures

be titrated to achieve optimal pain control with minimal adverse effects. Ongoing reassessment ensures satisfactory pain relief with the most appropriate balance of drug and non-drug strategies.

Discharge planning. Inpatients, as well as ambulatory surgical patients, should be given a written pain management plan at discharge. Pertinent discharge instructions related to pain management include: specific drugs to be taken; frequency of drug administration; potential side effects of the medication; potential drug interactions; specific precautions to follow when taking the medication (e.g., physical activity limitations, dietary restrictions); and name of the person to notify about pain problems and other postoperative concerns.

Site-specific Pain Control

Even for a single operation, there may be great variability in the approach to postoperative pain management based on patient factors such as age, weight, ability to understand and cooperate with plans for care, coexisting medical and psychological problems, and idiosyncratic sensitivity to analgesics; intraoperative course, such as size and location of incisions or drain placement or anesthetic management; and institutional resources available for specialized treatment and monitoring in the particular setting.

Despite these variable factors, the clinician can still outline certain pain management options to present to an adult patient whose management is otherwise uncomplicated. Many aspects of pain control are shared between operations on different parts of the body. For practical reference, pain management options for various surgical procedures are presented according to region of the body rather than by the pathophysiological mechanisms involved. In all cases, however, preoperative psychological preparation and medication should be considered, and ongoing postoperative assessment and reassessment of pain should be routine. In this way, pain can be controlled effectively. Vigilance for changes in postoperative pain will trigger prompt searches for diagnostically significant causes of new pain.

Head and Neck Surgery

Dental surgery. The most common forms of dental surgery are brief and relatively non-invasive procedures often performed on an outpatient basis. A patient's anxiety is frequently disproportionate to the safety of the procedure; such a patient may benefit from behavioral or pharmacologic (anxiolytic) therapy. Mild pain associated with most forms of uncomplicated dental care such as simple tooth extractions, endodontic therapy, or scaling of the periodontal area or of a previously asymptomatic tooth is well managed by oral administration of an NSAID such as aspirin or ibuprofen. Preoperative administration of ibuprofen appears to delay the onset of postoperative pain and lessen its severity (Jackson, Moore, and Hargreaves, 1989). For patients unable to tolerate aspirin or ibuprofen, acetaminophen can provide an acceptable analgesic effect.

Dental procedures such as surgical removal of bony impactions and osseous periodontal surgery are more traumatic and typically produce intense and prolonged postoperative pain. The onset of such pain can be delayed by preoperative treatment with ibuprofen and/or application of a long-acting local anesthetic such as bupivacaine during the procedure.

Rarely, an intravascular or intraneural injection of local anesthetic in this context leads to bruising, bleeding, or systemic symptoms such as fainting, allergic reaction, or persistent pain due to direct nerve injury. When postoperative pain does emerge, it often requires the addition of an opioid to the nonsteroidal regimen. Codeine is frequently prescribed at a dosage of 30-60 mg every 4-6 hours. Increased analgesia—but also an increased number of opioid side effects such as nausea, constipation, sedation, and respiratory depression—follow dosage increases above this level. Alternative opioids include propoxyphene or oxycodone administered in doses that are equianalgesic to 30-60 mg of codeine.

Some operations on the oral cavity preclude the patient's taking oral medications postoperatively (e.g., wiring the mouth closed after an operation on a mandibular fracture). Alternative therapy should be based on the severity of the surgical procedure and expected pain associated with it, as well as the surroundings in which it will be managed. Formulations of NSAIDs such as rectal suppositories (indomethacin) or intramuscular injection (ketorolac) are now commonly available. Opioids may be administered by a variety of routes (intravenous, intramuscular, subcutaneous injection, transdermal, rectal) and schedules, including a patient controlled schedule. Cost-efficacy analyses of parenteral opioid administration for oral surgery are not sufficient to permit any clear recommendations. Pain that does not respond to these measures should prompt a search for infection, osteitis, peripheral nerve injury, or the emergence of psychological and behavioral changes consistent with the development of chronic pain syndrome.

Acute Pain Management: Operative or Medical Procedures

Radical head and neck surgery. These operative procedures commonly interfere with oral intake for prolonged periods postoperatively and may be combined with a feeding gastrostomy or jejunostomy. Airway patency is always a consideration in these patients, and a tracheostomy frequently is an integral part of the operation. The use of flap coverage or skin grafts further increases the number of potentially painful sites. Prolonged preoperative pain, radiotherapy, and chemotherapy are important preoperative modifiers of pain therapy. Thus, the very nature of the operative procedure may dictate alternate routes for pain therapy in patients who have undergone major head and neck ablative procedures that may interfere with a patient's ability to describe pain and his or her response to analgesic intervention.

Intraoperative positioning of the head and neck are critical. Protective padding and avoidance of extreme flexion, extension, and rotation may help obviate or minimize muscle spasm-induced pain after surgery. Foam cushion supports under the occiput can minimize decubitus, pressure-induced headache, palsies, and causalgia. Intraoperative traction on muscles and nerves should be started carefully and monitored during the operation to prevent reflex myalgias and causalgias. Painful swallowing after head and neck; ear, nose, and throat; and endocrine surgical procedures may require elixir (i.e., liquid) forms of pain medicine, a modified diet, including liquid or soft foods, and occasional use of topical anesthetics such as viscous lidocaine.

Postoperative pain is often short term and of moderate intensity. Within 1-3 days, parenteral and oral opioids can be discontinued or replaced with non-opioid analgesics (which may have to be delivered via gastrostomy or jejunostomy). The use of most NSAIDs may be contraindicated for such procedures as thyroidectomy and parathyroidectomy where postoperative hemorrhage and risk of airway obstruction are significant. In such cases, acetaminophen or "platelet-sparing" NSAIDs may be ordered.

Neurosurgery. Patients undergoing an operation on the central nervous system frequently show abnormal neurologic signs and symptoms that must be closely followed in the postoperative period. In addition, these patients may receive drugs designed to reduce cerebral edema or prevent seizures. A major dilemma in this clinical setting is the need to carefully monitor critical neurologic signs such as pupillary reflexes and the level of consciousness that may be affected by conventional opioid analgesics used for the relief of postoperative pain.

Ideally, postoperative pain control should not interfere with the ability to assess a patient's neurologic status, particularly the level of consciousness, or with assessment of motor and sensory function following spinal cord surgery. Therefore, the administration of opioids, benzodiazepines, and anxiolytics, in particular, is relatively contraindicated. However, the clinician must balance the need for analgesia with the requirement for appropriate neurologic monitoring.

The uncomplicated postcraniotomy patient typically has mild to moderate pain and is readily managed by a short period of parenteral medications followed by oral analgesics. Laminectomy and other spinal procedures usually are more painful than craniotomies. Ketorolac, a parenteral NSAID, may be considered in this setting because it has no effect on the level of consciousness or pupillary reflexes. As mentioned previously, the use of nonsteroidal analgesics may be contraindicated in some postoperative settings when the risk of coagulopathy or hemorrhage is high, the need to assess fever is important, or when the degree of pain is higher than the analgesic ceiling of the agent.

Epidural opioids and/or local anesthetics can minimize the need for systemic opioids and allow more accurate monitoring of brain-stem and cerebral function. However, a single dose of epidural morphine may produce significant blood concentrations (Max, Inturrisi, Kaiko, Grabinski, Li, and Foley, 1985) that in turn cause effects within the central nervous system. A recent study could not demonstrate a difference in neuropsychiatric functioning between patients receiving oral and epidural morphine (Sjogren, and Banning, 1989). Furthermore, motor and sensory dysfunction associated with epidural local anesthetics (which are often co-administered with opioids) may obscure important neurologic signs. Again, remember to balance the need for adequate analgesia while minimizing the confounding central nervous system effects of analgesics and anesthetics.

Chest and Chest Wall Surgery.

Thoracic surgery (non-cardiac). Operative sites within the thorax include the heart, esophagus, and lungs and somatically innervated structures such as the ribs, superficial chest wall, and breast. Preexisting disease of these organs (e.g., chronic obstructive pulmonary disease) or prior medical treatment (e.g., chemotherapy) are common. They contribute to postoperative morbidity through a variety of mechanisms, such as decreased pulmonary reserve. Drains and chest tubes can cause intense irritation and pain at entry sites or deeper. For this reason, NSAIDs such as indomethacin in suppository form are useful to reduce inflammation although they are rarely enough for complete pain relief and indeed are not approved by the Food and Drug Administration as simple analgesics.

Good evidence exists that aggressive pain control in the form of epidural analgesia or neural blockade with local anesthetics after thoracic surgery improves pulmonary function; however, at present there is insufficient evidence from randomized controlled trials (RCTs) to conclude that these forms of aggressive pain control after thoracic surgery hasten walking or reduce morbidity and length of hospital stay (Guideline Report, in press; Hasenbos, van Egmond, Gielen, and Crul, 1987; Kaplan, Miller, and Gallagher, 1975; Sabanthan, Mearns, Bickford Smith, Eng, Berrisford, Bibby, and Majid, 1990; Shulman, Sandler, Bradley, Young, and Brebner, 1984).

The greatest beneficial effects result from administration of opioids or a combination of opioid and local anesthetic in the thoracic epidural space. Reliance on a local anesthetic alone to secure postoperative epidural analgesia in the thoracic region carries possible side effects such as hypotension due to sympathetic blockade. Respiratory impairment because of somatic nerve block is another potential problem; therefore, intercostal nerve blocks are generally undesirable unless an opioid is contraindicated. Mixing a local anesthetic with an opioid produces better and more prolonged analgesia, but RCTs indicate that there is a tendency toward more side effects when an opioid is added to a local anesthetic, compared with the local anesthetic alone (Guideline Report, in press; Capogna, Celleno, Tagariello, and Loffreda-Mancinelli, 1988; Pybus, D'Bras, Goulding, Liberman, and Torda, 1983). An example of a coordinated approach to postoperative analgesia is the placement of an epidural catheter prior to induction of anesthesia, which is used to deliver local anesthesia, either alone or mixed with an opioid for intraoperative analgesia, and then left in place postoperatively for infusion of a dilute analgesic. As previously emphasized, monitoring and care of patients with epidural catheters and assessment of the optimal time for switching to oral analgesia are best accomplished by a specially trained team.

Direct injection of local anesthetics alone to block intercostal nerves has been done for years as a means to provide postoperative analgesia and improved pulmonary function after thoracotomy. Unfortunately, such analgesia lasts only 6 to 12 hours, so that a single injection rarely suffices for the entire postoperative period. A clinician can overcome the brief duration of intercostal anesthesia by administering interpleural local anesthetics. To accomplish this, a catheter is placed between the parietal and visceral pleura, and anesthetic is injected at 4- to 6-hour intervals or infused continuously to produce continuous analgesia across several dermatomes (Scott, Mogensen, Bigler, and Kehlet, 1989). As in all invasive techniques, this method requires skill in drug titration and vigilance for management of side effects such as pneumothorax.

The use of opioids to reduce postoperative pain after thoracotomy is well documented. Because of potential side effects, clinicians have tried to optimize delivery and closely match dose to need. In this context, PCA has resulted in incrementally improved analgesia, increased patient satisfaction, and tendencies towards improved pulmonary function and earlier recovery or discharge (Guideline Report, in press; Eisenach, Grice, and Dewan, 1988; Jackson, 1989; McGrath, Thurston, Wright, Preshaw, and Fermin, 1989; Wasylak, Abbott, English, and Jeans, 1990). One strategy to manage pain after thoracotomy is to deliver epidural analgesia to prevent pain and then switch to patient controlled intravenous analgesia if the epidural catheter ceases to function or is discontinued after several days on the ward.

A typical prescription for intravenous PCA in this setting relies first on a series of "loading" doses: for example, 3-5 mg of morphine, repeated every 5 minutes until the initial postoperative pain diminishes. A low-dose basal infusion at night (e.g., 0.5-1.0 mg/hr) allows uninterrupted sleep for the patient. On-demand doses typically add 0.5-1.5 mg of morphine every 6 minutes. PCA doses of opioid are valuable to supplement analgesia during respiratory therapy or ambulation, even after the patient is taking oral analgesics and especially while chest tubes are in place. The transition from intravenous PCA to oral opioids is accomplished as described above (p. 20). If adequate opioid analgesia yields undesired side effects, or if pain is not severe (e.g., when chest tubes are no longer in place), the patient can switch directly from epidural to oral analgesia using a combination of opioid and NSAID. Many opioid analgesics or mixtures are available in liquid form and are useful for patients unable to swallow tablets or capsules (e.g., after esophageal surgery).

Cardiac surgery. Most cardiac operations involve a median sternotomy and anesthetic induction using high doses of opioids (morphine at 1 mg/kg or another opioid at an equivalent dose). Because somatic nerves are not divided by the surgical incision, postoperative pain is usually less than after conventional thoracotomy, even when lower doses of opioids are given during surgery. For procedures that use intercostal incisions, such as implantation of automatic defibrillatory devices, methods of pain control need not differ from those of other

Acute Pain Management: Operative or Medical Procedures

thoracic operations. Close observation is essential to distinguish postoperative pain originating in the chest wall and pleura from cardiac pain, which may signal myocardial ischemia due to a tachyrhythmia or threatened infarction from inadequate revascularization.

Abdominal and Perineal Surgery

Upper abdominal surgery (includes cholecystectomy, aortic bypass). Although outside the thorax, operations on the upper abdomen such as cholecystectomy compromise pulmonary function. Other associated morbidity (that may lead to mortality) includes immobility, hypercoagulability, venous thrombosis, and increased myocardial oxygen consumption when pain leads to an increase in blood pressure or rapid heart rate. Patients who undergo major vascular surgery frequently have coexisting myocardial disease, wide swings in blood pressure as their major vessels are clamped and unclamped, and significant fluid shifts associated with blood loss and replacement. These patients are particularly at risk for postoperative myocardial infarctions and arrhythmias. For operations on the abdominal aorta, intraoperative epidural anesthesia is widely used and simplifies the transition to postoperative epidural analgesia through the same catheter.

Hormonal indexes of stress are reduced postoperatively in patients given epidural analgesia using a local anesthetic (e.g., 0.25 percent bupivacaine) such as after cholecystectomy. Yet even when pain is completely eliminated by this technique, these hormonal stress responses do not vanish (Analgesia and the metabolic, Normally, a minimum of 3 or 4 days will elapse postoperatively before oral analgesia is feasible following operations on the biliary system, stomach or intestine, or vasculature in the upper abdomen.

In preparing the patient for any upper abdominal operation, choices of pain management to be reviewed with the patient include: intramuscular or subcutaneous injection of an opioid as needed, a "round-the-clock" schedule of injections (or continuous infusion of opioid) to be withheld in the event of side effects such as respiratory depression or nausea, intravenous PCA, or epidural analgesia in the manner described for postthoracotomy pain. Each of these approaches carries its own risks and benefits, which depend on the health care team's knowledge, expertise, and ability to recognize and treat side effects and correct inadequate pain relief. Other techniques have been used for post-cholecystectomy pain, such as interpleural catheters or supplemental, long-acting local anesthetic blocks of the lower intercostal nerves and celiac plexus. These lie outside the range of most current clinical practice.

Lower abdominal and perineal surgery (includes abdominal hysterectomy, cesarean section, hernia repair, episiotomy, urological, and gynecological procedures, and hemorrhoidectomy). The pain management plan for the patient undergoing lower abdominal or perineal surgery is based on the same principles as those for patients undergoing upper abdominal procedures. On the other hand, analgesia to control pain of active labor must be approached with special expertise and caution in light of side effects that may impair fetal well-being (e.g., fetal respiratory depression after maternal opioids or maternal hypotension after epidural local anesthetic). Suppression of pain and surgical stress responses is more complete with epidural local anesthesia after lower abdominal surgery than after upper abdominal operations (Kehlet, 1989b). Presumably this is because pathways such as phrenic or thoracic somatosensory afferents are less easily blocked by epidural anesthesia. Many obstetrical or urological procedures (e.g., cystoscopy) routinely are performed using spinal or epidural anesthesia, and the addition of low doses of opioid to a local spinal anesthetic appears to lengthen the duration of analgesia observed after the local anesthetic effect has subsided (Capogna, Celleno, Tagariello, and Loffreda-Mancinelli, 1988; Chawla, Arora, Saksena, and Gode, 1989; Hanson, Hanson, and Matousek, 1984; Pybus, D'Bras, Goulding, Liberman, and Torda, 1983; Reay, Semple, Macrae, MacKenzie, and Grant, 1989). Pain after procedures on the anus is particularly severe and requires adjunctive measures such as stool softeners, dietary manipulation, and local anesthetic suppositories for control. Again, the precautions already outlined concerning spinal opioid use and the necessity for close monitoring apply. Goals of the postoperative pain management plan should include early ambulation. For obstetric procedures, opioid doses should be adjusted so as to produce minimum maternal and fetal sedation. Alternatively, if an epidural catheter has been placed for infusion of local anesthetic to control labor pain or to provide anesthesia for cesarean section, a dilute solution of local anesthetic may be infused through this catheter to control postoperative pain with little risk of sedating the nursing infant.

Musculoskeletal Surgery

Back surgery. Operations on the spine at any level are frequently done in patients who have experienced chronic pain. Such patients may have the typical complications of chronic pain: depression, anxiety, irritability, and if opioid analgesics were required preoperatively,

Acute Pain Management: Operative or Medical Procedures

a relative tolerance to opioid medications. All of these factors may complicate pain assessment and treatment in the postoperative period. In addition, the majority of procedures requiring a spinal operation are associated with paraspinal muscle spasm. In such cases, it is appropriate to add muscle relaxants to supplement conventional opioid therapy.

Operations on the spinal cord often involve laminectomy and bone grafting and may include opening the dura around the spinal cord. These procedures may limit the role of epidural and spinal delivery of pain medications. As with any neurologic procedure, postoperative patients require careful monitoring of neurologic functions, especially the assessment of sensory, motor, and autonomic functioning.

Surgery on extremities (orthopedic, vascular). Many common operations performed on extremities are elective and include total joint replacements. The high degree of morbidity related to venous thromboembolic complications must be considered. Pain control postoperatively should allow early ambulation and movement in the postoperative period. Supplementing conventional opioids with an epidural infusion of a local anesthetic may benefit these patients by decreasing the incidence of thromboembolism. Operations requiring a cast or other form of external fixation for stabilization demand frequent postoperative evaluation of circulation and neurologic functions. Pain therapy should not interfere with monitoring the patient.

Orthopedic or vascular procedures on an extremity may result in a compartment syndrome; this is usually associated with a period of ischemia or perhaps injury to the muscles of the lower extremity. It is manifested by intracompartmental swelling with loss of function, the earliest manifestation being loss of dorsiflexion of the foot and pain. Once again, this requires continuous observation; pain control measures should not mask this process. If not treated promptly by decompression, a compartment syndrome may result in chronic postischemic neuropathy.

The traumatic amputation is often associated with phantom limb pain. Evidence now exists that infusion of epidural local anesthetic prior to elective amputation for inoperative vascular disease can minimize this symptom (Bach, Noreng, and Tjellden, 1988); the applicability of these pilot data to treatment of other conditions or trauma remains to be defined.

The majority of operative procedures on extremities produce pain of moderate intensity usually controlled by early parenteral opioids supplemented by NSAIDs. Adding epidural analgesia is particularly attractive in terms of establishing early mobility and minimizing thromboembolic complications (Guideline Report, in press; Modig, Borg, Bagge, and Saldeen, 1983; Modig, Borg, Karlstrom, Maripuu, and Sahlstedt, 1983; Pettine, Wedel, Cabanela, and Weeks, 1989).

Soft Tissue Surgery

Surgical procedures involving local soft tissue resections usually obtain pain control with oral opioids. Many of these procedures are done on an ambulatory basis and require careful patient education prior to and immediately after the procedure. Anxiety because of the potential results of a small surgical biopsy (e.g., feared results of a breast biopsy) may demand adjuvant drug or non-drug therapy. Pre- and postoperative education and support by the surgeon and the health care team are supremely important.

Management of Postoperative and Procedural Pain in Infants, Children, and Adolescents

Much of the guideline thus far applies to both adults and children. The following section contains information specific to pain assessment and management in children. This section is not all-inclusive, and these recommendations should be used in conjunction with the entire guideline. This portion of the guideline, although based on a thorough review of the literature on procedure-induced and postoperative pain, is not a substitute for professional training and judgment. For further information, the clinician is referred to the bibliography and, when necessary, to experts for consultation.

Background

Children commonly experience postoperative pain. The incidence of moderate to severe pain in children in any health care setting is influenced by factors such as the child's medical condition, type of procedure performed, and attitudes of health care professionals toward pain management. In three studies on postoperative pain in children, the prevalence of moderate to severe pain varied from about 40 to 60 percent (Hester, Foster, Kristensen, and Bergstrom, 1989; Johnston, Jeans, Abbott, Grey-Donald, and Edgar, 1988; Mather, and Mackie, 1983).

Many children do not receive any opioid analgesics after surgical procedures, even though painful postoperative courses are expected

Acute Pain Management: Operative or Medical Procedures

(Beyer, DeGood, Ashley, and Russell, 1983; Eland, and Anderson, 1977; Foster, and Hester, 1990a, 1990b; Hester, Foster, Kristensen, and Bergstrom, 1989; Schechter, and Allen, 1986). Compared with adults undergoing similar procedures, less potent analgesic regimens usually are ordered for and given to children (Beyer, DeGood, Ashley, and Russell, 1983; Schechter, and Allen, 1986). When used, opioid doses and intervals of administration are often inadequate; when a physician's order includes a selection of one or more analgesics, the tendency is to choose the least potent drugs (Beyer, DeGood, Ashley, and Russell, 1983; Foster, and Hester, 1989, 1990a; Mather, and Mackie, 1983). In general, although children are less able than adults to articulate their treatment and medication needs, both opioid and non-opioid analgesics are commonly prescribed on an "as-needed" basis (Beyer, DeGood, Ashley, and Russell, 1983; Bush, Holmbeck, and Cockrell, 1989). This type of prescription (a) requires the child or the family to describe the presence of pain and the need for analgesia and (b) focuses on the treatment of emerging pain rather than aggressive treatment to prevent pain.

Infants, even when premature, experience pain in response to aversive stimuli (Anand, 1990; Anand, and Aynsley-Green, 1988; Anand, Sippell, and Ansley-Green, 1987; Fitzgerald, Millard, and MacIntosh, 1988, 1989; Fitzgerald, Shaw, and MacIntosh, 1988). However, infants often do not before or after major medical procedures (Franck, 1987). Although the majority of ventilated infants receive postoperative opioid analgesia (but often in less than adequate doses), non-ventilated infants often do not (Campbell, Reynolds, and Perkins, 1989 ; Purcell-Jones, Dormon, and Sumner, 1988; Schnurrer, Marvin, and Heimbach, 1985). A survey of the beliefs and practices of anesthesiologists in the United Kingdom revealed that, although the majority believed neonates experience pain, few provided opioid analgesics for postoperative pain (Purcell-Jones, Dormon, and Sumner, 1987). Discrepancies between beliefs and practices can occur for many reasons, but they have not been adequately explored.

Invasive and painful procedures are particularly distressing for children. Children often describe repeated invasive procedures as more distressing than any other aspect of illness or treatment (Eland, and Anderson, 1977; Fowler-Kerry, 1990; Jay, Ozolins, Elliott, and Caldwell, 1983; Weekes, and Savedra, 1988). Unlike adults, infants and young children may not understand the reason for procedures and may not participate actively in providing consent. Infants and young children also may not understand the time-limited nature of procedures. Although appropriate preparation and adequate analgesia for painful procedures are crucial for decreasing distress in children, these issues often are not addressed by health care providers, or they are approached haphazardly (Schechter, 1989).

Assessment

Pain is determined by many factors, including the medical condition, developmental level, emotional and cognitive state, personal concerns, meaning of pain, family issues and attitudes, culture, and environment. Caring for the child in pain requires frequent assessment and reassessment of the presence, amount, quality, and location of pain. It also means preventing or reducing anticipated pain and, when prevention is not possible, promptly alleviating pain. Because emotional distress accentuates the experience of pain, exploration of and intervention for possible sources of distress are necessary. For infants and children, the provider should recognize the potential for pain and pursue the possibility that a child is in pain. A knowledge of children, including their developmental level and their behavior, is necessary to adequately assess pain and distress.

Pediatric pain assessment includes a pain history, a search for diagnoses such as infection that could be increasing or causing pain, evaluation of the pain severity and location, and observation of the child and his or her responses to the environment. The inclusion of parents or guardians and other important family members is essential to pain assessment. Strategies for assessment should be tailored to the developmental level and personality of the child and to the context. Children who are developmentally delayed or retarded, learning disabled, emotionally disturbed, or non-English speaking require special assessment. Culturally determined beliefs about pain and medical care also should be considered. Getting to know the individual child is important for assessment and management of pain: obtaining a pain history and involving the parents in the child's care can optimize this process.

For infants and children, the provider should recognize the potential for pain or suspect that a child is in pain.

The pain history, obtained prior to or at admission, focuses on the language the child uses to describe pain (e.g., hurt, owie, booboo), previous pain experiences and coping strategies, how and to whom the child communicates pain, and the child's and the family's preferences to assess and treat pain (Hester, and Barcus, 1986).

Acute Pain Management: Operative or Medical Procedures

The provider, child, and family can then decide together on their approach to pain assessment and treatment.

Routine assessment and documentation of pain are critical for effective pain control. The frequency of assessment is tailored to the severity of the pain. For example, after a major surgical procedure, assessment reasonably could occur at least every 2 hours on the day of surgery and the first postoperative day and at least every 4 hours on subsequent days. More frequent assessment is necessary if the pain is poorly controlled despite treatment. Pain intensity and its response to analgesics should be recorded on the bedside chart just as vital signs are recorded for easy review by health care providers. Structured documentation on a bedside flow sheet may increase the frequency of assessment and provision of analgesia (Stevens, 1990). Assessment methods should be easy to administer or perform, and documentation forms should be readily accessible to health care providers for use in recording pain. If the child is old enough to participate in assessment, his or her ease in response is important for accurate measurement. Young children may not understand the relationship between pain assessment and pain relief; therefore, they may not respond to questions if they are anxious or in severe pain.

Methods for assessing pain. No one method to assess pain offers an error-free measure of the pediatric pain experience. Therefore, the use of more than one method of assessment may be helpful. Assessment tools should be appropriate for the child's age and cognitive development and for the context. A variety of assessment tools are available for all age groups; selection of appropriate tools depends on the psychometric adequacy of the tool as determined through estimates of reliability, validity, generalizability, and sensitivity. Several psychometrically sound and developmentally appropriate tools are available to assess pain for documentation on a bedside flow sheet.

As with adults, a self-report tool provides the most reliable and valid estimates of pain intensity, quality, and location. Self-reports can be used for developmentally normal children over the age of 4 (McGrath, 1990). Self-report tools for children over the age of 4 include the Oucher (Beyer, 1984), the Poker Chip Tool (Hester, 1979 ; Hester, Foster, and Kristensen, 1990), and a faces scale (McGrath, deVeber, and Hearn, 1985). Children over the age of 7 or 8 who understand the concept of order and number can use a numerical rating scale (McGrath, and Unruh, 1987), a horizontal word-graphic rating scale (Savedra, Tesler, Holzemer, and Ward, 1989), or a visual analog scale (Aradine, Beyer, and Tompkins, 1988). In a recent study,

958 well children and adolescents and 175 hospitalized children and adolescents rated the visual analog scale as the least preferred of five horizontal pain scales (Tesler, Savedra, Holzemer, Wilkie, Ward, and Paul, 1991). Reliability and validity for postoperative pain have been established for the Oucher, the Poker Chip Tool, and the horizontal word-graphic rating scale.

Children in pain or otherwise stressed may regress. For example, a child who before surgery uses a numerical scale appropriately may require a simpler scale after surgery. Similarly, children who are developmentally delayed or learning disabled may need assessment tools developed for younger children. If the child is unable or unwilling to respond, ratings can be obtained from the parents or health care providers. However, such ratings often underestimate moderate to severe pain and may overestimate lesser pain (Hester, Foster, Kristensen, and Bergstrom, 1989). To increase accuracy and consistency, ratings from parents and health care providers are obtained using the same tool as the child uses.

Observation of behavior is the primary assessment method for the nonverbal child and may be an adjunct to assessment for the verbal child. Such observations focus on vocalizations, verbalizations, facial expressions, motor responses, and activity. To obtain meaningful observations, the health care professional watches for and documents behaviors associated with distress. Several aspects of behavior should be observed. For example, a child may move easily in bed, guard the surgical site when moving, or be completely immobilized and resist movement.

Various scales based on behavioral observations have been designed for clinical use in infants and preverbal children (Barrier, Attia, Mayer, Amiel-Tison, and Shnider, 1989; Gauvain-Piquard, Rodary, Rezvani, and Lemerle, 1987; McGrath, Johnson, Goodman, Schillinger, Dunn, and Chapman, 1985). Although reliability and validity have not been well established, these scales offer a guide for observations of postoperative pain.

Use of behavioral observation to guide analgesia requires attention to the context of the child's behavior. For example, children cry not just in response to pain but also in response to fear, loneliness, and over- or understimulation. Thus, additional assessment is necessary when the source of a behavior is not evident, so that all sources of distress can receive appropriate intervention. Sleeping, watching television, or joking may be misinterpreted as indicators of no pain while the child may, in fact, be attempting to control pain. Behavioral responses may be absent or attenuated in circumstances where vocalization or movement increase pain or where

Acute Pain Management: Operative or Medical Procedures

intubation, use of paralyzing agents or sedatives, extreme illness, weakness, or depression impede vocalizations and movement. If care providers are unsure whether a behavior indicates pain, and if there is reason to suspect pain, an analgesic trial can be diagnostic as well as therapeutic.

Unstructured observations of how a child looks and acts may provide additional information about the presence and amount of pain. Documenting observations over time may reveal specific changes in behavior that serve as important pain indicators. For example, a child may be alert and talkative and then appear sullen and withdrawn. Such a change warrants further investigation since it may indicate the onset of or an increase in pain (Hester, and Foster, 1990).

Scales for assessing procedure-related pain have been developed. Assessment of facial expressions and the quality of crying have been used with infants [e.g., Neonatal Facial Coding System (Grunau, and Craig, 1987)]. The Procedure Behavior Rating Scale (Katz, Kellerman, and Siegel, 1980) and the Procedure Behavior Checklist (LeBaron, and Zeltzer, 1984) have been used with children. These tools are not applicable for routine postoperative use.

Physiologic indicators of pain and distress include heart rate, respiratory rate, blood pressure, and perspiration. However, these indicators are not specific for pain, and they vary among individual patients in pain. Therefore, the interpretation of physiological indicators should be done in the context of the clinical condition and in conjunction with other assessment methods.

Management

Pain is managed by the child, his or her parent(s), nurses, physicians, and other health care providers. Effective interaction is key to effective pain management. Although preferences of the child and the family deserve respect and careful consideration, the primary obligation of the health care provider is to ensure safe and competent care.

Children attempt to prevent or alleviate pain whether or not health care providers do so. When in pain, a child often prefers the use of medication and the presence of a parent (Adams, 1990; Hester, 1989; Savedra, Gibbons, Tesler, Ward, and Wegner, 1982). However, children may not be in control of these strategies. Specific methods initiated by children that may be helpful include: holding someone's hand, a stuffed toy, or favorite blanket; asking questions; using distraction; sleeping and resting; relaxing or using imagery; changing positions;

and engaging in humor. Seemingly simple interventions such as holding someone's hand can have powerful effects. Facilitation of the child's usual strategies for decreasing pain is important.

Although preferences of the child and the family deserve respect and careful consideration, the primary obligation of the health care provider is to ensure safe and competent care.

Management of pain related to procedures in hospitalized children. Diagnostic and therapeutic procedures are often associated with pain. A structured approach to pain management takes into consideration the type of procedure, anticipated range of pain, and individual factors such as age and condition.

Nonpainful procedures (e.g., computed tomographic scanning, magnetic resonance imaging, cast changes, and ultrasonic examination) often require a child to lie still. Preparatory education about the sensations and surroundings may decrease the child's distress and facilitate the procedure (Johnson, Kirchoff, and Endress, 1975). Non-drug approaches such as distraction and imagery may benefit the older child (Zeltzer, Altman, Cohen, LeBaron, Maunuksela, and Schechter, 1990). Sedation is appropriate in these situations, particularly if the child is under 6 years of age. Sedatives include oral chloral hydrate or pentobarbital. Pharmacologic sedation may result in the loss of the child's protective reflexes; therefore, children should be closely monitored even during "conscious sedation."

Painful procedures require a management plan that may include both drug and non-drug approaches. When planning the management of procedure-related pain and anxiety, a series of questions should be asked: 1) Why is the procedure being performed? 2) What is the expected intensity of pain? 3) What is the expected duration of pain? 4) What is the expected intensity of anxiety? 5) What is the expected duration of anxiety? 6) How often will the procedure be repeated? 7) How do the parents think the child will react? and 8) What are the child's and family's perceptions regarding the procedure? The following are general management principles for procedures:

- Treat anticipated procedure-related pain prophylactically.

- Ensure the competency of the person performing the procedure and the timeliness of the procedure (Zeltzer, Altman, Cohen, LeBaron, Maunuksela, and Schechter, 1990). Delays can escalate pain and anxiety. Children report that procedures are

Acute Pain Management: Operative or Medical Procedures

easier to tolerate if they know and trust the people doing them.

- Provide adequate and unhurried preparation of the child and family. Parental prediction of the child's response is highly correlated with the actual degree of distress (Fradet, McGrath, Kay, Adams, and Luke, 1990; Schechter, Bernstein, Beck, Hart, and Sherzer, 1991).

- Be attentive to environmental stimuli and the manner in which the child is handled. A room other than the child's room should be used whenever possible. Environmental factors, such as cold or crowded rooms or "beepers" on machines, can escalate distress (Fowler-Kerry, 1990; Hester, 1989).

- Allow parents to be with the child during the procedure. The presence of a parent may be a source of great comfort for the child (Bauchner, Waring, and Vinci, 1991; Shaw, and Routh, 1982). The parent's knowledge of the child can be invaluable. Parents should be educated, since they do not automatically know what to do, where to be, and what to say to help their child through the procedure.

- Tailor treatment options, both drug and non-drug, to the child's and the family's needs and preferences, to the procedure, and to the context. A child who undergoes a procedure as part of the treatment for a chronic or life-threatening disease has different needs from the child who has an occasional procedure as part of general well child care or for treatment of an acute but self-limited illness.

- If at all possible, administer pharmacologic agents by a route that is not painful (e.g., oral, transmucosal, or intravenous). If one or two doses of a parenteral agent are necessary and the child does not have intravenous access, a single injection may be preferable to multiple attempts at insertion of an intravenous catheter.

- Dovetail pharmacologic and non-pharmacologic options to complement one another.

- For repeated procedures, maximize treatment for the pain and anxiety of the first procedure to minimize anxiety before future procedures.

- Provide monitoring and resuscitative equipment if drugs are used for sedation. Facilities, equipment, and personnel to manage emergencies (e.g., vomiting, and anaphylaxis) should be immediately available.

- Manage preexisting pain optimally before beginning the procedure.

- After the procedure, review with the child and family their experiences and perceptions about the effectiveness of pain management strategies.

Pharmacologic Strategies for Procedural Pain

The needs of the individual child and the type of procedure to be performed shape the pharmacologic approach. As with assessment, the practitioner's expertise and experience with children are key to successful therapy. A pain-relieving agent, such as an opioid or a local anesthetic, is needed to reduce the pain. Anxiolytics and sedatives are used specifically to reduce anxiety before and during the procedure; if used alone, they may blunt the behavioral response without relieving the pain. When anxiety is present, pharmacologic anxiolysis can complement analgesia to decrease overall distress. The use of systemic analgesics and sedatives must be approached differently in the infant under 6 months of age (see section on Managing Postoperative Pain in Neonates, and Infants).

Agents that have a broad range of applicability include:

- **Local anesthetics:** These agents may be administered by local infiltration or topically. For topical use, a eutectic mixture of local anesthetics (EMLA) (Maunuksela, and Korpela, 1986) is promising but not yet available in the United States.

- **Opioids:** These drugs can be given via the intravenous, oral, or transmucosal route. The intravenous route has the advantage of rapid effect and ease of titration. Intravenous opioids can be given in increments (e.g., morphine at 0.03-0.05 mg/kg every 5 minutes) and titrated to analgesic effect. Oral opioids can be used when close and rapid titration to effect is not required.

- **Benzodiazepines:** These agents can be given either orally or intravenously. Like opioids, intravenous benzodiazepines are given in increments and titrated to sedative effect (Zeltzer, Altman, Cohen, LeBaron, Maunuksela, and Schechter, 1990). Unlike diazepam, midazolam does not cause pain and local sclerosis when given intravenously (Zeltzer, Altman, Cohen, LeBaron, Maunuksela, and Schechter, 1990). Benzodiazepines provide sedation, not analgesia, and hence they often are used with opioids for painful procedures. If the combination of opioid plus benzodiazepine is used, the risk of respiratory depression is increased.

- **Barbiturates:** These drugs provide excellent sedation. They have no analgesic effects and are used with analgesics for painful procedures. For most patients, the sedation persists for many hours after the procedure is completed (Zeltzer, Jay, and Fisher, 1989); rarely, some patients may have paradoxical reactions. As with benzodiazepines, close observation for respiratory depression is essential, particularly when the intravenous route is employed or if an opioid is co-administered.

NOTE: Exercise caution when using the mixture of meperidine (Demerol), promethazine (Phenergan), and chlorpromazine (Thorazine), also known as DPT. DPT—given intramuscularly—has commonly been used for painful procedures. The efficacy of this mixture is poor when compared with alternative approaches, and it has been associated with a high frequency of adverse effects (Nahata, Clotz, and Krogg, 1985). It is not recommended for general use and should be used only in exceptional circumstances.

Agents such as nitrous oxide and ketamine can be used if trained personnel and appropriate monitoring procedures are available (Zeltzer, Jay, and Fisher, 1989). General anesthesia is appropriate in certain situations (Zeltzer, Altman, Cohen, LeBaron, Maunuksela, and Schechter, 1990).

Monitoring conscious sedation for procedural pain. Skilled supervision is necessary whenever systemic pharmacologic agents are used for conscious sedation (i.e., the patient maintains a response to verbal, and physical stimuli). A health care provider not involved in performing the procedure or holding the child should monitor for conscious sedation including frequent assessment of heart rate, respiratory rate and effort, blood pressure, and level of consciousness. Continuous pulse oximetry to measure arterial oxygen saturation is strongly encouraged. Immediate accessibility of resuscitative drugs and equipment and the presence of at least one health professional trained in advanced life support are necessary. After completion of the procedure, monitoring should continue until the child is fully awake and has resumed the former level of function.

Deep sedation (i.e., the patient is not responsive to verbal or physical stimuli) is equivalent to general anesthesia and should be performed only under controlled circumstances by a professional trained in its use and skilled in pediatric airway management and pediatric basic life support. Reference to specific published guidelines is recommended (American Academy of Pediatrics, 1985; American Academy of Pediatrics, in press). To quote from the latter guideline, "The caveat that loss of consciousness should be unlikely is a particularly important aspect of the definition of conscious sedation, and the drugs and techniques used should carry a margin of safety wide enough to render unintended loss of consciousness highly unlikely. Since the patient who receives conscious sedation may progress into a state of deep sedation and obtundation, the practitioner should be prepared to increase the level of vigilance corresponding to that necessary for deep sedation."

Hospitalized children undergo procedures that include lumbar punctures, chest tube insertions, bone marrow aspirates and biopsies, cardiac catheterization, circumcisions, and burn dressing changes. General principles for the management of procedural pain and distress can be applied to all painful procedures:

- Most hospitalized children undergo minor invasive procedures, such as heelsticks and fingersticks, injections, venipunctures, and insertion of intravenous catheters. Such procedures, even though categorized as "minor," can be a major source of distress for sick or hospitalized children. The hospitalized child benefits from predictability as to time and frequency and "clustering" of procedures, with an identified block of time when no procedures are to be performed, barring emergencies. Intramuscular and subcutaneous routes should be avoided unless necessary for proper administration (e.g., immunizations).

- Non-drug strategies are effective for pain and anxiety associated with minor procedures. Providing emotional support, eliciting concerns, and providing information and age-appropriate choices are crucial. Infants can benefit from sensorimotor interventions (i.e., using a pacifier, and using verbal or tactile strategies) (Campos,

1989; Field, and Goldson, 1984; Triplett, and Arneson, 1979). A variety of strategies have been studied in older children. The child and family can be prepared in several ways, such as provision of preparatory sensation information (Siegel, and Peterson, 1980, 1981); empathetic preparation (Fernald, and Corry, 1981); and a multimodality approach using stories, art, and play (Fassler, 1985). Other potentially effective cognitive-behavioral strategies include distraction techniques such as music (Fowler-Kerry, and Lander, 1987; Ryan, 1989); coping skills (Siegel, and Peterson, 1980, 1981); hypnosis (Andolsek, and Novik, 1980; Olness, 1981; Zeltzer, and LeBaron, 1982); play therapy (Ellerton, Caty, and Ritchie, 1985); and thought-stopping (Ross, 1984). Physical agents include TENS therapy (Eland, 1989) and counterirritants such as ice (Zeltzer, Altman, Cohen, LeBaron, Maunuksela, and Schechter, 1990). One or more non-pharmacologic intervention in addition to preparation can be chosen by the health care team, family, and child. Choice should be based on the child's preference, personality, and coping style.

For lumbar punctures, local anesthetics are used for all age groups, although efficacy in infants is controversial. Systemic drugs that alter mental status cannot be used in acute medical illnesses, such as meningitis, where observation of the level of consciousness is crucial to treatment. In situations where such monitoring is not necessary, younger children and many older ones benefit from a benzodiazepine. Supplementation with opioids is helpful for some cases, especially when difficulty in performing the procedure is anticipated. Children over 5 years of age who have learned and can effectively use cognitive and behavioral coping skills may prefer not to use sedatives or opioids (Zeltzer, Altman, Cohen, LeBaron, Maunuksela, and Schechter, 1990).

Management strategies for bone marrow aspirations and biopsies include use of either general anesthesia or conscious sedation using benzodiazepines and opioids, along with local anesthesia. Adequate time is necessary for the local anesthetic agent to have full effect.

Non-pharmacologic methods with demonstrated efficacy for lumbar punctures and bone marrow aspirates and biopsies include hypnosis (Zeltzer, and LeBaron, 1982); thought-stopping (Ross, 1984); and a multidimensional psychological intervention that includes a breathing exercise, reinforcement, imagery, behavioral rehearsal, and filmed modeling (Jay, Elliott, Ozolins, Olson, and Pruitt, 1985). Additionally, the strategies described for minor invasive procedures can be used for lumbar punctures and bone marrow aspirates and biopsies.

The management of pain associated with circumcision is controversial. Circumcision often has a religious context, and the religious beliefs of the family should be respected. Pain associated with circumcision can be managed with a penile block (Maxwell, Yaster, Wetzel, and Niebyl, 1987). However, recent evidence suggests that topical anesthesia may be a safe and effective option (Andersen, 1989; Tree-Trakarn, Pirayavaraporn, and Lertakyamanee, 1987).

Pain Related to Burn Dressing Changes

Burn dressing changes in the child with burns severe enough to require hospitalization are approached in a multidisciplinary fashion, using drug and non-drug strategies. Pain and anxiety coexist in these situations and must be assessed and managed concurrently using opioids and benzodiazepines, respectively. Depending on the child and the level of anxiety, an opioid may be administered alone or used with a benzodiazepine. Since undertreatment of the pain can escalate anxiety, optimal pain control is necessary. Dressing changes occur repeatedly, and tolerance to opioids and benzodiazepines can develop, necessitating higher doses. For efficacy, doses should be increased as needed and titrated according to the response obtained during the previous procedure. The child also may have ongoing pain from the burns in addition to the pain and anxiety of the burn dressing changes. If the ongoing pain is not treated, the child's anxiety during the dressing changes may make it difficult to manage, even with significant doses of opioids and sedatives. Initial regimens for pain management may include a continuous infusion or around-the-clock intermittent doses of an opioid and additional bolus doses of an opioid and a benzodiazepine before the burn dressing changes. For extensive debridement procedures, conscious sedation may not be adequate; general anesthesia may be required.

A variety of non-pharmacologic approaches are effective adjuvants. These include hypnosis (Bernstein, 1963); a multimodal approach involving distraction, relaxation, imagery, and positive reinforcement (Elliott and Olson, 1983); and cartoon viewing with positive reinforcement (Kelley, Jarvie, Middlebrook, McNeer, and Drabman, 1984). Children as young as 18 months do better during burn dressing changes if their participation and control are maximized (Kavanagh, 1983a, 1983b). For example, a child can help to remove his or her own dressings and call for a "time-out" if necessary. Dressing changes are performed in a treatment room or similar place, so that the child can consider his or her room as a safe place. The time and environment

Acute Pain Management: Operative or Medical Procedures

for the dressing change should be predictable to the child. The situation causing the burns may be one that produces emotional distress for the child (e.g., burns sustained as a result of the child playing with fire or disobeying rules), and the developing body image of the child may be threatened by the burns. Psychiatric and psychologic intervention should be provided when necessary. Discharge planning initiated soon after admission can help relieve anxiety and increase compliance with the therapeutic regimen, particularly for children with burns on more than 30 percent of the body surface area (Quay, and Alexander, 1983).

Management of Pain Associated with Surgical Procedures

Management of surgical pain involves three phases: preoperative, intraoperative, and postoperative.

Preoperative management. Individual or group psychological preparation with or without home preparation (Ferguson, 1979; McGrath, 1979; Visintainer, and Wolfer, 1975; Wolfer, and Visintainer, 1979) may decrease pain, anxiety, and distress before and after the operation. Parental presence during the induction of anesthesia decreases postoperative pain and reduces adverse psychological sequelae (Hannallah, and Rosales, 1983; Johnston, Bevan, Haig, Kirnon, and Tousignant, 1988; Schofield, and White, 1989). Preoperative medication should be given painlessly. For example, a child with intravenous access can receive medication by that route; alternative routes for the child without intravenous access include oral, rectal, and transmucosal administration.

Intraoperative management. Adequate analgesia for pre-term and fullterm infants significantly reduces surgical stress and postoperative morbidity (Anand, Brown, Causon, Christofides, Bloom, and Aynsley-Green, 1985; Anand, and Hickey, 1987). This finding directly challenges the previous practice of providing minimal intraoperative anesthesia for infants based on concerns about the respiratory and hemodynamic side effects of opioids. High dose opioid anesthesia appears to be well tolerated, even in critically ill infants, provided it is used in a carefully monitored setting by skilled anesthesiologists (Collins, Koren, Crean, Klein, Roy, and MacLeod, 1985; Yaster, 1987).

Other intraoperative techniques that may help to reduce, delay, or prevent postoperative pain include epidural blockade with opioids and/or local anesthetics and local anesthetic infiltrated into the wound or applied to block a peripheral nerve. These approaches should be limited to personnel qualified in these anesthetic techniques. Children who receive intraoperative epidural opioids require careful monitoring after the procedure; this method should be used only in settings where such monitoring is available.

Postoperative management. Drug therapies are the most important aspect of pain management. Non-drug techniques to reduce postoperative pain are useful adjuncts; the approaches are similar to those described for procedural pain: relaxation, distraction, the presence of a parent or a special toy or blanket, and cognitive preparation for anticipated events (Hester, 1989). Physical methods, such as positioning with blanket rolls for support and the use of heat or ice, also can be helpful. Pacifiers, swaddling, and a calming environment may be helpful for infants (Campos, 1989; Field, and Goldson, 1984).

Drug therapy for postoperative pain depends on the child's age, medical condition, type of surgery, and expected postoperative course. Pain after minor surgery, such as herniorrhaphy or tonsillectomy, usually can be managed with acetaminophen with or without codeine when the oral route is available. Often children are sent home on the day of surgery after such procedures; thus, parental instruction in pain control is important (Gedaly-Duff, and Ziebarth, 1991).

For major surgery, such as abdominal, thoracic, urologic, or orthopedic procedures, parenteral opioids are the mainstay of pain management. These drugs can be administered systemically or spinally, depending on individual needs. NSAIDs are useful in certain situations. Intravenous administration of NSAIDs is currently being studied in children; these and other agents may be used more widely in the future.

Some health care professionals are concerned about the potential for psychological dependence and addiction when using opioids for pain control in children. In adults, the risk of addiction after use of opioids for pain relief is small. Although studies of the risks in children are lacking, no known aspect of childhood development or physiology increases the risk of physiologic or psychologic vulnerability to chemical dependence.

Several issues are pertinent to opioid administration:

- **Route:** In the immediate postoperative period, systemic opioids are delivered by either the intravenous or epidural routes. Intramuscular injections are painful and frightening to children; many children would rather have pain than a "shot" (Eland, and

Acute Pain Management: Operative or Medical Procedures

Anderson, 1977). Since an intravenous catheter is required for hydration after major surgery, this route is always available. After the child is able to take medication by mouth, an oral opioid can be given with a non-opioid analgesic.

- **Schedule:** Intermittent boluses of opioids can be provided on an around-the-clock basis, using a dose of about 0.1 mg/kg of morphine or its analgesic equivalent. Dose intervals are the same as those recommended for adults. Continuous infusion of morphine (0.02-0.04 mg/kg/hr) for children over 6 months of age has been well studied (Bray, 1983; Hendrickson, Myre, Johnson, Matlak, Black, and Sullivan, 1990; Lynn, Opheim, and Tyler, 1984). Continuous infusion avoids the extreme variations that may occur with intermittent intravenous doses. "Rescue" doses for breakthrough or poorly controlled pain can be offered at regular intervals to patients receiving a continuous infusion. Because of wide variability in the opioid dose needed for adequate analgesia, no matter which route and schedule of administration is employed, pain and side effects (particularly respiratory depression) should be reassessed at frequent intervals and the dose and interval adjusted for the best pain relief.

- **Agent:** As in adults, morphine is the standard. Fentanyl may be preferable when cardiovascular stability is an issue and patients are closely monitored and/or intubated. Meperidine should be used only in exceptional circumstances. (See related discussion on pages 18 and 19.)

- **Patient controlled analgesia:** PCA provides safe and effective analgesia in children as young as 7 years of age (Berde, Lehn, Yee, Sethna, and Russo, 1991). This approach is appropriate for older children and adolescents, since it offers an element of developmentally appropriate control. The addition of a basal infusion may provide better analgesia without increasing the total dose of opioid (Berde, Lehn, Yee, Sethna, and Russo, 1991). Children and young adolescents may benefit from reminders to "push the button for pain" in the immediate postoperative period. Regular assessment and reassessment of pain and side effects, with adjustment of the PCA parameters as indicated, is necessary with PCA. Education of the patient and the family are key to the success of this approach. PCA must be supervised by professionals trained in its use.

- **Side effects:** The pharmacologic approach to managing side effects in children is similar to that in adults. However, young verbal children may have difficulty communicating subjective symptoms, like pruritus, nausea, and dysphoria; the pre-verbal child may show only generalized discomfort. Assessment of side effects occurs with assessment of pain relief. If an infant or pre-verbal child becomes increasingly restless or irritable despite an increased opioid dose, treatment of presumed side effects or a change to an alternative opioid can be considered.

- **Monitoring:** Regular assessment of vital signs and level of consciousness is necessary when parenteral opioids are used for managing postoperative pain. Because of wide inter- and intraindividual variations in the response to opioids, an occasional child will have an adverse reaction despite even the most careful titration of doses and intervals. The use of cardiorespiratory monitors is controversial, and professional judgment is required. In any case, machines cannot substitute for skilled and frequent assessment and observation by the health care provider.

Regional Analgesia

Regional analgesia is now widely used for infants and children and may be particularly applicable for young infants as well. Hemodynamic and respiratory effects of major regional analgesia in infants appear minimal (Meignier, Souron, and LeNeel, 1983). The proper use of infusions or intermittent doses of epidural opioids and/or local anesthetics requires expertise and close monitoring, at least equal to that needed for infants receiving systemic opioids. An acute or postoperative pain service is usually necessary to provide the expertise and vigilance required.

Continuous epidural analgesia is effective for thoracic, abdominal, urologic, and orthopedic procedures (Hendrickson, Myre, Johnson, Matlak, Black, and Sullivan, 1990). Epidural infusions can be administered caudally (especially in children under 6 months of age) or via lumbar or thoracic epidural catheters in older children. Solutions infused into the epidural space are similar to but often more dilute than those applied in adults. Other regional techniques available to children include interpleural continuous infusions, brachial plexus infusions, lumbar sympathetic catheter infusions, and peripheral nerve blockade such as penile blocks.

Acute Pain Management: Operative or Medical Procedures

Managing Postoperative Pain in Neonates and Infants

Young infants, especially premature infants or those who have neurologic abnormalities or pulmonary disease, are susceptible to apnea and respiratory depression when systemic opioids are used (Way, Costley, and Way, 1965; Purcell-Jones, Dormon, and Sumner, 1987). Metabolism is altered so that the elimination half-life is prolonged, and the blood-brain barrier is more permeable (Collins, Koren, Crean, Klein, Roy, and MacLeod, 1985; Koehntop, Rodman, Brundage, Hegland, and Buckley, 1986; Koren, Butt, Chinyanga, Soldin, and Pape, 1985; Lynn, and Slattery, 1987). Thus, the adequate management of pain in this age group requires special consideration and expertise.

Clearly, neonates and infants experience pain, and adequate analgesia after surgery is necessary for both physiologic and ethical reasons. Institutions in which major surgery on neonates and infants is performed should provide training for personnel in the effective and safe administration of analgesia for children in this age group, as well as the technologic capability to provide appropriate monitoring. Several aspects of care should be noted.

Age. Some evidence suggests that the clearance of opioids increases rapidly over the first few weeks of life, and approaches adult rates by 1 to 2 months of age (Hertzka, Gauntlett, Fisher, and Spellman, 1989 ; Koren, Butt, Chinyanga, Soldin, and Pape, 1985; Lynn, and Slattery, 1987). Because the available data are based on small numbers of infants, most practitioners reduce the initial dose and use intensive monitoring for infants up to about 6 months of age; this age is arbitrary and based on a cautious interpretation of the literature. It is reasonable to continue intensive monitoring up to about 1 year of age, as extreme sedation and decreased effort of respiration may be more difficult to assess in this age group than in older children.

Dosing and schedules. Although further investigation is necessary, apnea and respiratory depression appear to be dose related (Koren, Butt, Chinyanga, Soldin, and Pape, 1985). For non-ventilated infants under 6 months of age, the initial opioid dose, calculated in milligrams per kilogram, should be about one-fourth to one-third of the dose recommended for older infants and children. For example, morphine could be used at a dose of 0.03 mg/kg instead of the traditional 0.1 mg/kg. Careful assessment is necessary after any dose, so that the optimal dose and interval of administration can be determined from clinical parameters (e.g., when pain breaks through, and whether the infant appears comfortable after the dose). Many infants have inadequate pain relief after the initial small dose and require upward titration, sometimes to doses used for older children. Continuous infusions can be used, but a reduced dose is again necessary.

Clearly, neonates and infants experience pain, and adequate analgesia after surgery is necessary for both physiologic and ethical reasons.

Regional analgesia. Regional analgesia for neonates and young infants is as previously described for older infants and children.

Monitoring. Close monitoring of heart and respiratory rates, respiratory effort, blood pressure, and responsiveness to stimuli is mandatory. Frequent or continuous assessment of arterial oxygen saturation using pulse oximetry is a valuable adjunct to close clinical observation. Serum levels of opioids may increase many hours after a one-time intramuscular or subcutaneous dose, presumably due to late release from tissue stores. Thus, monitoring is continued for 24 hours after an opioid dose (Koehntop, Rodman, Brundage, Hegland, and Buckley, 1986).

Non-opioid analgesics. These analgesics (e.g., acetaminophen) can be safely administered to neonates and infants without concern for hepatotoxicity when given for short courses at the recommended doses (Berde, 1989, 1991). Acetaminophen can be given rectally or orally to augment analgesia.

Responsibility for Effective Pain Relief in Children

A formal and structured institutional review of pain management is as necessary for children as for adults. It begins with affirming the rights of all children in any institution to receive the best level of pain relief that can be provided safely. The available methods of pain management should be appropriate for the medical conditions of the children and the surgical procedures that are performed. Recommendations in this guideline (see Responsibility for Effective Pain Relief, page 71) apply to children as well as adults. Patient and family feedback is necessary to ascertain and ensure the adequacy of pain management in children of all ages.

Acute Pain Management: Operative or Medical Procedures

An environment centered on the child is necessary for adequate communication and assessment and to decrease the emotional distress of hospitalization. In addition to a staff experienced in caring for children, a child-centered environment lets parents participate in child care and provides adequate toys and age-appropriate activities.

Critical Questions Regarding the Adequacy of Pain Management Strategies

Knowledge of children—developmentally, behaviorally, and physiologically—is necessary for optimal assessment and treatment. Children are likely to talk less about pain than adults. Thus, the burden of vigilance for pain rests with the health care provider. The following questions focus on decision points of pain management. These questions serve as a guide for the health care provider to optimize pain management. Some children, however, will present with pain that is difficult to manage. In these situations, consultation is recommended.

Children are likely to talk less about pain than adults. Thus, the burden of vigilance for pain rests with the health care provider.

Critical questions to consider before and during pharmacologic management include:

- Have the child and parent(s) been asked about their previous experiences with pain and their preferences for use of analgesics?
- Is the child being adequately assessed at appropriate intervals?
- Are analgesics ordered for prevention and relief of pain?
- Is the analgesic strong enough for the pain expected or the pain being experienced?
- Is the timing of drug administration appropriate for the pain expected or experienced?
- Is the route of administration appropriate (preferably oral or intravenous) for the child?
- Is the child adequately monitored for the occurrence of side effects?
- Are side effects appropriately managed?
- Has the analgesic regimen provided adequate comfort and satisfaction from the child's or parents' perspective?

Parallel questions regarding non-pharmacologic strategies include:

- Have the child and parent(s) been asked about their experience with and preferences for a given strategy?
- Is the strategy appropriate for the child's developmental level, condition, and type of pain?
- Is the timing of the strategy sufficient to optimize its effects?
- Is the strategy adequately effective in preventing or alleviating the child's pain?
- Are the child and parent(s) satisfied with the strategy for prevention or relief of pain?
- Are the treatable sources of emotional distress for the child being addressed?

Other Patients with Special Needs

Elderly Patients

Elderly patients present several pain management problems. First, relatively little attention has been paid to the topic of geriatric pain control in medical or nursing texts (Ferrell, 1991). This is ironic because elderly people often suffer acute and chronic painful diseases, have multiple diseases, and take many medications (From the NIH, 1979). They may have more than one source of pain and an increased risk for drug-drug as well as drug-disease interactions (Kane, Ouslander, and Abrass, 1989). It has been estimated from population studies that the prevalence of pain is two-fold higher in those over age 60 (250 per thousand) compared with those under 60 (125 per thousand) (Crook, Rideout, and Browne, 1984). Among institutionalized elderly, the prevalence may be over 70 percent (Ferrell, Ferrell, and Osterweil, 1990). Indeed, more than 80 percent of elderly people suffer various forms of arthritis, and most will have acute pain at some time (Davis, 1988). Many elective or emergent operations are performed in the elderly to correct orthopedic problems (e.g., fractures, degenerative joint disease). Acute and/or postoperative severe pain related to cancer and its treatment are also more common in the elderly (Foley, 1985). Other acutely painful conditions that affect the elderly disproportionately include herpes zoster, temporal arteritis, polymyalgia rheumatica, and atherosclerotic peripheral vascular disease (From the NIH, 1979).

Second, pain assessment may present unique problems in elderly patients. They often report pain very differently from younger patients

Acute Pain Management: Operative or Medical Procedures

due to physiologic as well as psychological and cultural changes associated with aging (Fordyce, 1978). Institutionalized elderly are often stoic about pain (Foley, 1985). Age-associated changes in acute pain perception have long been of interest. Elderly patients often demonstrate altered presentations of common illnesses including "silent" myocardial infarctions and "painless" intra- abdominal emergencies (Bayer, Chada, Farag, and Pathy, 1986; Bender, 1989). Whether these clinical observations are the result of age-associated changes in pain perception remains to be explained. The widespread belief among clinicians that aging results in increased pain thresholds may be a myth. A variety of experiments using heat, pressure, or electrical current have not disclosed a trend regarding age-associated changes in either pain threshold or tolerance. It should be noted that the clinical relevance of these studies remains questionable, since experimentally induced pain may not be analogous to clinically experienced pain (Harkins, Kwentus, and Price, 1984).

Cognitive impairment, delirium (common among acutely ill frail elderly), and dementia (occurring in as many as 50 percent of institutionalized elderly) represent serious barriers to pain assessment for which no solution exists in the literature. Whether behavioral observations (e.g., agitation, restlessness, groaning) are sensitive and specific for pain assessment among the demented elderly remains to be shown. Traditional approaches, including the use of visual analog scales, verbal descriptor scales, and numerical scales, have not been psychometrically established in this population. Moreover, a high prevalence of visual, hearing, and motor impairments in the elderly may impede the universal use of such scales by clinicians. Preliminary reports from ongoing work among the nursing home population suggest that many patients with moderate to severe cognitive impairment are able to report acute pain reliably at the moment or when prompted, although pain recall and integration of pain experience over time may be less reliable. If these early observations prove correct, pain assessment among this population may require frequent monitoring. Monitoring may have major implications for quality assurance, quality of care, and quality of life among this large population of elderly people (Ferrell, and Ferrell, personal communication: Work in progress on the epidemiology of pain among community nursing homes, July 1991).

Third, elderly people, especially the frail and old-old (those over 85) are at particular risk for both under- and over-treatment. Unfortunately, few studies of analgesic dosage requirements are performed in the elderly, and most studies have systematically excluded all potential subjects over 65. Age-related observations are extremely variable among elderly people. Indeed, the variance in measurements of most physiologic and pharmacologic parameters increases with age in cross-sectional studies (Kane, Ouslander, and Abrass, 1989). Age-related changes in pharmacokinetics and pharmacodynamics contribute to a variety of adverse drug effects that have been reported in the elderly.

The widespread belief among clinicians that aging results in increased pain thresholds may be a myth.

Non-opioid analgesic drugs, including NSAIDs and acetaminophen, are effective and appropriate for a variety of pain complaints in the elderly. However, it is recognized that the risk for gastric and renal toxicity from NSAIDs is increased among elderly patients, and unusual drug reactions including cognitive impairment, constipation, and headaches are also more common in the elderly population (Roth, 1989). If gastric ulceration is a particular concern, co-administration of misoprostol or use of "platelet-sparing" NSAIDs should be considered as a way to lessen the risk of gastrointestinal bleeding.

Opioid analgesic drugs are effective for the management of acute pain in most elderly patients. Cheyne-Stokes breathing patterns are not unusual during sleep in the elderly and need not prompt discontinuation of opioid analgesia unless such analgesia clearly is associated with unacceptable degrees of arterial oxygen desaturation (< 85 percent). PCA has been shown in at least one study to be safe and effective for postoperative pain relief among selected patients (Egbert, Parks, Short, and Burnett, 1990). If PCA is used, careful titration of dosage is necessary to avoid undesirable effects due to drug accumulation or from a decrease in the arousal effect as painful stimuli subside later in the patient's course. Elderly people are more sensitive to the analgesic effects of opioid drugs as they experience a higher peak and longer duration of pain relief (Bellville, Forrest, Miller, and Brown, 1971; Kaiko, 1980; Kaiko, Wallenstein, Rogers, Grabinski, and Houde, 1982). They are also more sensitive to sedation and respiratory depression probably as a result of altered distribution and excretion of the drugs. This is especially true in opioid-naive patients. Caution is required in the use of longer acting drugs such as methadone for this reason (Ferrell, 1991).

Elderly people, in general, have increased fat-to-lean body mass ratios and reduced glomerular filtration rates (Kane, Ouslander, and Abrass, 1989). Opioids produce cognitive and neuropsychiatric

Acute Pain Management: Operative or Medical Procedures

dysfunction through poorly defined mechanisms that in part include the accumulation of biologically active metabolites such as morphine-6-glucuronide or normeperidine (Wood, and Cousins, 1989). Opioid dosage titration should take account of not only analgesic effects but also side effects that extend beyond cognitive impairment. These side effects may include urinary retention that looms as a larger threat in elderly males with prostatic hypertrophy, constipation and intestinal obstruction, respiratory depression, or exacerbation of Parkinson's disease. The management of nausea using phenothiazines or antihistamines is fraught with problems, because elderly people are exquisitely sensitive to anticholinergic side effects including delirium, bladder and bowel dysfunction, and movement disorders (Ferrell, 1991).

Local anesthetic infusions may result in cognitive impairment if significant blood levels are reached. Yet prior to that point, orthostatic hypotension may result from sympathetic blockade and clumsiness may ensue from partial motor or sensory anesthesia. Thus, appropriate precautions should be taken, such as help with ambulation or the use of side rails at night.

Finally, attitudes among health care professionals, the lay public, and patients themselves may impede appropriate care. Many members of all three groups consider acute and chronic pain a part of normal aging (Ferrell, Ferrell, and Osterweil, 1990; Ferrell, 1991).

Patients Who Are Known or Suspected Substance Abusers

Management of acute pain in the substance abuser is a difficult but increasingly common clinical problem. Substance abusers experience traumatic injuries (see section on Patients with Shock, Trauma, and Burns) and a variety of health problems more often than the general population. Often during their postoperative care issues arise that prompt the staff to request consultation with specialized "pain teams." For example, the question of possible withdrawal from preexisting opioid use may be raised because sympathetic nervous system stimulation (restlessness, tachycardia, sleeplessness) may be caused by either under-treated pain or opioid abstinence. The related issue of risk of development of substance abuse behaviors in opioid-naive patients given opioid analgesics postoperatively appears to be small based on survey data by Porter and Jick (1980), who found that only four such instances of iatrogenic drug abuse occurred in approximately 12,000 patients screened through the Boston Collaborative Drug Study.

A variety of reports, increasingly frequent in number, have addressed the difficult questions surrounding postoperative opioid use in substance abusers, and several recommendations have recently emerged from reviews of this literature (Portenoy, and Payne, in press). First, every effort should be made to define the mechanism of the pain and to treat the primary problem. Infection, tissue ischemia, or a new surgical diagnosis in the postoperative period may require specific measures such as antibiotic therapy, fasciotomy, or re-operation rather than an increase in the opioid dose. Attention to the primary cause of pain symptoms may reduce greatly the requirement for and negotiations about opioid analgesics.

Second, clinicians should distinguish between the temporal characteristics of the abuse behavior. For example, a distant history of substance abuse might predispose to re-emergence of substance abuse behaviors with the stress of surgery and postoperative pain but may not require treatment approaches different from those appropriate for non-addicted patients. The implications are different for patients with a recent history of active drug abuse who may require higher than usual starting doses of opioids and who may not have acquired an ability to set limits on their drug use.

Third, one should follow relevant pharmacological principles of opioid use. For example, treatment with an opioid agonist-antagonist should not be started in the patient who enters tolerant to opioid agonists such as methadone. Mixed agonist-antagonists may precipitate withdrawal if given in this setting. Loading doses of opioids will be required in normal patients as well as in substance abusers to reduce the intensity of postoperative pain to acceptable levels. PCA is being used with increasing frequency for many patients, including known substance abusers. This mode of opioid delivery can be utilized safely in substance abusers when appropriate lockout intervals and hourly dosage limits are programmed, and when the device is "tamper-resistant," so that the patient cannot reprogram the pump or remove any drug. If used for an opioid-tolerant patient, PCA doses must be increased to achieve the same analgesic effect as for opioid-naive or non-addicted patients.

Fourth, just as for other patients, non-opioid therapies should be given concomitantly with or even to replace opioids. Such therapies include NSAIDs, local anesthetic solutions given via catheter into the epidural space or surrounding peripheral nerves, cryoanalgesia, TENS, and non-drug therapies. Appropriate use of non-opioid therapies frequently will reduce the dosage requirement for opioid analgesia.

Fifth, specific drug abuse behavior in the postoperative patient should be recognized and dealt with firmly. Such behavior includes

Acute Pain Management: Operative or Medical Procedures

tampering with PCA machines (or other drug delivery devices), hoarding of oral doses of opioid analgesics, or attempting to self-inject the melted contents of capsules or siphoned infusion solutions. At that point, limits of analgesic dosages and expected patient behavior should be made clear to the patient in a frank discussion that also considers the medical, ethical, and legal consequences to the patient and physician if drug abuse behaviors continue. For the most part, security measures already in place (locked closets, and inventory checks each nursing shift, anti-tamper features on PCA machines) will frustrate such attempts. A toxicological screen may be ordered on an inpatient's urine or blood specimens to confirm or exclude a diagnosis of surreptitious drug use (e.g., cocaine administration).

In the outpatient setting, clear instructions (preferably written out and copied into the patient's record) should be offered regarding doses and frequency of medication and the number of days the prescription is expected to last. The addition of a random urine testing procedure to outpatient medication contracts should be considered in all outpatients with a known history of substance abuse who are given opioid analgesics for pain. Opioid medications should be prescribed only by one physician, and attempts to circumvent this restriction or to falsify prescriptions should not be tolerated. The claim of needing additional medication to make up for lost or stolen controlled substances should be accompanied by documentation that the patient has reported this to the police.

Sixth, caregivers should set limits to avoid excessive negotiation about drug selections or choices. For example, it is not appropriate to depart from an institutional policy for morphine use for postoperative analgesia just because of a substance abuser's request for meperidine, as long as the patient has no history of adverse reaction to morphine. Once every effort has been made by clinicians to adjust a patient's opioid regimen in light of the extent and site of the operation, the patient's prior tolerance to opioids, and clinical response to initial analgesic titration, it is not unreasonable to adhere to this regimen with few, if any, changes. When possible, the treatment plan should include clear criteria (e.g., number of days postoperatively, ability to ambulate) by which opioid doses will be tapered and stopped. Within such a treatment plan, requests for higher dosage by a patient who can walk easily or spends much of the time resting comfortably may appropriately be denied. Consultation should be obtained with appropriate services early in a difficult patient's course. Consultation should help develop a unified multidisciplinary plan that includes, usually, psychiatric, psychological, and substance abuse expertise. Medical input can be obtained beyond the scope of the immediate caretakers to evaluate these and other problematic behaviors. Medical and/or neurologic input can be valuable when assessing neurologic symptoms such as seizures in patients who have recently discontinued alcohol or barbiturate use.

These guidelines will aid the clinician in distinguishing "drug seeking" behaviors from "pain avoidance" behaviors. Often patients who are under-treated for pain and who voice displeasure are labeled as "addicts." This phenomenon has been called "pseudo-addiction" (Weissman and Haddox, 1989). Careful and objective assessment and reassessment of the postoperative patient with an active or previous substance abuse history will minimize the chance of a clinician being "duped" into providing inappropriate opioids but still provide the patient with legitimate pain complaints the opportunity to obtain meaningful and safe pain relief with opioids.

Patients with Concurrent Medical Conditions

Postoperative pain frequently must be treated in patients who have concurrent medical conditions for which they are taking one or more medications. The medical condition per se or the medications taken for it may influence the choice of analgesic and its dosage. These medical conditions are frequently chronic, and it may not be possible to discontinue problematic medications because of surgery. The most common medications or classes of medications that produce clinically significant drug interactions with opioid analgesics include alcohol and any central nervous system depressants, phenytoin, and monoamine oxidase inhibitors. Drugs whose primary site of action lies outside the central nervous system (e.g., antibiotics such as rifampin) also may interact with opioid analgesics.

Coexisting conditions themselves influence the type and doses of opioid analgesics and the relative risks of pain treatment in the postoperative period. For example, patients with chronic pain who have been treated recently with opioids (e.g., patients with cancer, and sickle cell disease) will usually require higher-than-the-recommended starting doses to overcome opioid tolerance. Coagulopathy, neutropenia, and sepsis may contraindicate the use of epidural catheters or other regional anesthetic techniques in which the risks of bleeding or "seeding" of infection are increased.

Drug pharmacokinetics may change following surgery because of changes in drug absorption and distribution caused by alterations in cardiac output, venous capacitance, extravascular fluid shifts ("third

Acute Pain Management: Operative or Medical Procedures

spacing"), and changes in protein binding. Fever and sepsis in the postoperative period may affect drug disposition, as do shock, trauma, and burns. In addition, patients may not attain clinically effective plasma concentrations of opioids following intramuscular and subcutaneous injections due to pharmacokinetic alterations.

The major factor to consider in selecting analgesics for patients with concurrent medical conditions is whether the disorder produces either hepatic or renal impairment. Most analgesics are metabolized by the liver or kidney, so that any impairment of function in these organs influences the pharmacokinetics of the analgesic. The net result can be drug accumulation. Therefore, caution is essential when using opioids in patients with altered hepatic or renal function. Morphine is metabolized in the liver, and the parent compound, along with the metabolites, is excreted through the kidney. Acute or chronic hepatic failure (e.g., viral hepatitis or cirrhosis) appears to lower plasma clearance of morphine, prolong the terminal elimination half-life, and increase oral bioavailability (Hasselstrom, Eriksson, Persson, Rane, Svensson, and Sawa, 1990). Even mild renal failure, such as that associated with a decline in glomerular filtration rate with aging, can impede excretion of the metabolites of many opioids, resulting in clinically significant narcosis and respiratory depression (Sear, Hand, Moore, and McQuay, 1989). Physiological alterations during surgery (e.g., changes in regional blood flow to the liver or kidneys, hepatic enzyme activity, enterohepatic circulation, or hormonal responses) may also alter drug metabolism and excretion. Meperidine, pentazocine, and propoxyphene have increased bioavailability, prolonged half-lives, and decreased systemic clearance and thus accumulate in hepatic and renal dysfunction. Doses of these drugs must be decreased appropriately. In contrast, the disposition and elimination of methadone are not significantly altered in patients with chronic liver disease.

Renal excretion is a major route of elimination for pharmacologically active opioid metabolites: norpropoxyphene, normeperidine, morphine-6-glucuronide, and dihydrocodeine. Elimination is decreased in patients with renal failure, and doses must be lowered or given less frequently.

For individual patients, it is difficult to predict the degree of impairment of metabolism or excretion of the most commonly used analgesics from either the clinical condition or laboratory indicators of hepatic or renal function because many factors impinge on clinical response. A lowered initial dose, careful titration of the opioid to desired effect, and ongoing monitoring of clinical response, level of consciousness, and respiratory effort are indicated. Continuous infusions and opioid administration around-the-clock at conventional intervals can result in accumulation of the parent compound or clinically active metabolites. To avoid under-treatment of pain during as-needed dosage schedules, the patient can be assessed at regular intervals, and if stable, a dose of opioid can be offered. PCA does not necessarily protect against accumulation of opioids and respiratory depression (Covington, Gonsalves-Ebrahim, Currie, Shepard, and Pippenger, 1988). In renal failure, especially, a decreased dose and prolonged lockout interval may be required. Non-opioid analgesics are often contraindicated in patients with hepatic or renal dysfunction.

Other diseases that may influence the control of postoperative pain include psychiatric illnesses requiring tricyclic antidepressants and monoamine oxidase inhibitors for treatment; neurologic disorders; pulmonary diseases; and acute and chronic infections.

Patients with respiratory insufficiency and those with chronic obstructive pulmonary disease, cystic fibrosis, and neuromuscular disorders affecting respiratory effort (e.g., muscular dystrophy, myasthenia gravis) are vulnerable to the respiratory depressant effects of opioids. However, when a patient splints his or her respiratory effort because of uncontrolled pain, that also can impair gas exchange. Therefore, careful planning is required to provide effective and safe postoperative analgesia. Unless specific contraindications exist, the use of non-opioid analgesics can be optimized in this group of patients.

However, severe postoperative pain may not be adequately controlled with just these agents. Epidural opioids have a lesser effect on pulmonary function than do systemic opioids (Bromage, Campoersi, and Chestnut, 1980). Other regional anesthetic techniques can also be applied in this setting as a way to lower the dosage of systemic opioids required for satisfactory postoperative analgesia. If epidural analgesia cannot be used, small doses of opioids given frequently, continuous infusion, or PCA may provide smoother control of pain with less impact on respiratory effort at the time of peak effect. Whichever method is used to administer systemic opioids, a low initial dose is recommended; later doses can then be titrated to the desired effect. Appropriate monitoring of respiratory rate and effort and adequacy of gas exchange is necessary. Oximetry may be useful in selected cases.

Neurologic disorders can influence postoperative pain management if they: 1) produce weakness of the respiratory muscles (e.g., amyotrophic lateral sclerosis, poliomyelitis); 2) impair alertness and mental function so that the sedative effects of opioids are exaggerated, and pain cannot

Acute Pain Management: Operative or Medical Procedures

be assessed easily; and 3) cause seizures requiring use of chronic anticonvulsant medications that may interact with analgesics. The first two circumstances have been addressed in the discussion above and other sections of this Guideline. Phenytoin, a very commonly used anticonvulsant, increases the biotransformation of meperidine, causing faster elimination and necessitating increased doses of this analgesic (Foley, and Inturrisi, 1987).

Patients with psychiatric illnesses taking anxiolytics or other psychoactive drugs must be carefully evaluated for drug interactions between the psychotropic and pain medications they take. Because both opioids and psychotropic drugs generally have sedative effects, it is not uncommon for these effects to be additive when the drugs are combined. Further, the tricyclic antidepressants, clomipramine and amitriptyline, may increase morphine levels as measured by an increase in bioavailability and the half-life of morphine (Ventafridda, Ripamonti, DeConno, Bianchi, Pazzuconi, and Panerai, 1987). Of particular importance is avoiding meperidine in patients receiving monoamine oxidase inhibitors. Severe adverse reactions, including death through mechanisms that mimic malignant hyperthermia, have been reported when these drugs have been used together (Armstrong, and Bersten, 1986; Foley, and Inturrisi, 1987).

Patients treated with drugs for cardiovascular and metabolic disease frequently must continue their drugs throughout the intra- and postoperative period. Fortunately, severe interactions between these drugs and opioids are unlikely.

Alcoholics who must have surgical procedures should be maintained on benzodiazepines or alcohol throughout the intra- and postoperative period to prevent a withdrawal reaction or delirium tremens.

Clinicians must remain aware that patients in the categories discussed in this section may not respond as expected to medications administered for symptom control following surgery. Careful assessment and reassessment of patients' responses to analgesics and dose titration to response are always necessary. The concomitant use of nonpharmacological treatments as adjunctive therapy of postoperative pain is also strongly recommended.

Patients with Shock, Trauma, and Burns

Victims of injury frequently present in a state of cardiovascular or respiratory instability that mandates immediate life-saving procedures (e.g., endotracheal intubation, defibrillation, cut-down, and chest tube insertion) without analgesia. The trauma patient is usually young (58.4

percent), frequently male (72.8 percent), and commonly (51.2 percent) has used alcohol or drugs prior to injury (Soderstrom, Trifillis, Shankar, Clark, and Cowley, 1988).

Beecher (1959) was the first to point out the difficulties in providing analgesia via the intramuscular route following a significant burn or injury. He noted the variability in absorption from site to site and prolonged absorption times in soldiers with shock. He also provided the basis for modern-day pain control after burns or injuries by suggesting the exclusive use of the intravenous route. Most authorities now recommend incremental small intravenous doses of an opioid analgesic (morphine) carefully titrated to cardiovascular and respiratory stability. Concern for cardiorespiratory instability is particularly important in the first hour after injury. Any analgesic therapy also must allow for continuous monitoring of neurologic status after a head injury and neurovascular status after limb injury.

Once the patient is resuscitated and requires definitive surgical procedures, analgesia should be provided as outlined in this guideline for the various operative sites. The use of NSAIDs in the trauma patient remains controversial. They are undoubtedly of value in the patient with minor trauma, but the risk of excessive bleeding and gastric stress ulcers may prohibit their use following closed head injury, burn injury, or other multisystem injuries. When not contraindicated by sepsis, coagulopathy, or cardiorespiratory instability, the use of regional anesthetic approaches may be beneficial as described earlier for particular operative sites. For example, discomfort and splinting due to flail chest injury may improve with epidural analgesia, and borderline perfusion of an injured limb can increase with a sympathetic blockade by an epidural local anesthetic. On the other hand, surgical evaluation must always take priority over analgesic titration in the face of sudden increases in pain (e.g., extremity swelling) or somnolence (e.g., from an expanding subdural hematoma).

The serious burn injury will require very special pain control after the initial resuscitation. The myth that "third degree burns don't hurt" unfortunately still serves as a basis for widespread institutional denial of pain assessment and treatment for burned patients (Atchison, Osgood, Carr, and Szyfelbein, 1991). Pain control is essentially absent from current reviews of burn management, scientific programs of national burn associations, or funding agendas of the Federal government or major private burn treatment organizations, much as pediatric pain and cancer pain were a decade ago. In reality, after a brief (hours-long) period of endogenous analgesia evoked by the stress of immediate burn injury, pain is often severe and intermittently excruciating for months during burn

Acute Pain Management: Operative or Medical Procedures

dressing changes, skin grafts, reconstructive surgery, or other interventions related to needs for prolonged ventilation or intravascular access. Nonviable, insensate tissue is always surrounded by regenerating areas from which pain may arise, considering that viable perfused tissue typically forms the inner margin of an excision. Altered pharmacokinetics and pharmacodynamics in the burn patient, who may be intubated, splinted, and unable to articulate pain, further combine to render pain management an individualized challenge. The almost universal presence of hypotension and vasodilation with or without sepsis generally precludes the use of spinal or epidural routes for pain control until the burn wound is closed. While some authors have described analgesic regimens for burn dressing changes that call for non-narcotic analgesics, such as ketamine or nitrous oxide, these approaches are best reserved for unusual or refractory instances because of side effects such as dysphoria (Dripps, Eckenhoff, and Vandam, 1982) or bone marrow depression (Skacel, Hewlett, Lewis, Lamb, Nunn, and Chanarin, 1983), respectively. More typically, high doses of opioids are required to bring pain under control. Even then, there may be pain that is relatively refractory to opioid use, particularly if the burn site is deep or extensive. A morphine infusion alone is inadequate to produce anesthesia, such as for operative procedures or prolonged ventilation, since awareness often persists. Recent clinical studies suggest that damage to underlying nerves may account for the opioid-resistant quality of pain after severe burns (Choiniere, Melzack, and Papillon, 1991; Atchison, Osgood, Carr, and Szyfelbein, 1991), and that the continuous infusion of low doses of lidocaine—known to lessen neuropathic pain in other settings—may be a useful analgesic option in patients with burns (Jonsson, Cassuto, and Hanson, 1991). For these reasons, and also because fear and anxiety are an almost universal response to burn injury and trauma of any kind, sedatives such as benzodiazepines are useful to supplement opioid analgesics. In addition, cognitive-behavioral strategies such as relaxation, imagery, and hypnosis have been described by burn survivors as very helpful. The large full-thickness burn with its consequences of pain, separation from family and job, and (frequently) disfigurement, is usually accompanied by depression that may require drugs and, in turn, influence analgesic effects.

Patients Who Have Procedures Outside of the Operating Room

Thousands of patients undergo painful procedures each day outside of operating rooms in emergency departments, clinics, wards, and intensive care units. Analgesia issues outside the operating room also broadly apply to patients who have ambulatory surgical procedures, after which same-day discharge is expected. In any of the above settings, many procedures can be safely performed under local infiltration or regional anesthesia or by adopting behavioral, non-drug strategies, but systemic analgesia is often required to provide optimal pain control.

Only when immediate treatment of cardiorespiratory instability is required, or if a competent patient declines treatment, should analgesia be withheld for a painful procedure. The presence of a condition that could eventually result in cardiovascular, hemodynamic, neurologic, or pulmonary instability (e.g., femur fracture, pneumothorax, skull fracture) is not an absolute contraindication to systemic analgesia, although careful titration and monitoring must be provided. Though pain control may not be needed for certain procedures (e.g., diagnostic computerized imaging, intravenous pyelogram, or ultrasound examination), providing analgesia is likely to enhance the accuracy of these studies by reducing patient writhing or restlessness because of pain.

No anesthetic or analgesic agent should be used unless the clinician understands the proper technique of administration, dosage, contraindications, side effects, and treatment of overdose. As described earlier, the intravenous route is the preferred delivery mode because of its rapid onset and easy and reliable dosing. Using an intravenous route sidesteps the pain and the unpredictable absorption, onset, and duration of action associated with intramuscular or subcutaneous injections. An intravenous cannula may be placed painlessly following intradermal injection of 1 ml of 1-2 percent lidocaine through a 27-30 gauge needle. Most often, intravenous titration of an opioid like morphine, with observation for 5-10 minutes between doses, will provide safe and adequate analgesia. Intravenous morphine doses may range from 1 to 10 mg depending on the age, weight, pain intensity, opioid tolerance, and nature of the procedure to be done. Dose titration must be continued throughout the procedure, since pain may break through, for example, during reduction of a joint or vigorous probing of an abscess.

Contraindications to opioid analgesia include altered sensorium, lung disease, pregnancy near term, or an inability to monitor and manage side effects such as respiratory depression in the setting where care is given. Since respiratory depression is strongly correlated with the degree of sedation, stimulation of the patient as well as the administration of small doses of naloxone (e.g., 0.04 mg), may

Acute Pain Management: Operative or Medical Procedures

be adequate to reverse mild degrees of hypoventilation. Of course, assisted ventilation by bag and mask, or (ultimately) endotracheal intubation and repetitive naloxone dosing, may be required to reverse more severe degrees of respiratory depression. If such respiratory depression does occur, the patient should be observed until well after the naloxone effect has worn off (usually after 1 hour). Nausea, bradycardia, and hypotension are other side effects to watch for in the clinic, ward, or emergency department.

Other opioids may be used in place of morphine. Meperidine is suitable for brief, titrated dosing but not for prolonged use. Fentanyl may be used in small doses (25 [mu]g increments in the above example) but carries a higher risk than morphine or meperidine of inducing chest wall rigidity that must be immediately managed by administering a quick-onset muscle relaxant and supporting ventilation. Apart from chest wall rigidity, any opioid may trigger an acute Parkinson's-like syndrome particularly in the elderly or in patients with Parkinson's disease under medical therapy. Some mixed agonist-antagonists have the advantage that they produce lesser degrees of biliary or ureteral smooth muscle spasm, but they also may precipitate a withdrawal syndrome in patients habituated to opioid agonists such as methadone or heroin (or in other patients taking opioids for chronic pain).

No anesthetic or analgesic agent should be used unless the clinician understands the proper technique of administration, dosage, contraindications, side effects, and treatment of overdose.

NSAIDs currently have a limited role in the management of pain during brief, painful procedures, but two other non-narcotic agents have proven useful when administered in monitored settings by trained personnel. Intravenous ketamine has a rapid onset of action and produces a state of conscious sedation in which patients respond to verbal commands and maintain airway reflexes but experience analgesia. Possible side effects include dysphoria, tachycardia, increased salivary and tracheal secretions, and myocardial ischemia in patients with preexisting cardiac disease. Inhalation of a nitrous oxide:oxygen mixture can provide prompt anxiolysis and moderate analgesia. As a precaution, the patient should breathe through a face mask that he or she is holding, so that the mask will drop away if the patient becomes somnolent. Appropriate precautions should be taken to prevent environmental contamination with nitrous oxide (i.e., scavenging system), to avoid the possible inhalation of pure nitrous oxide without oxygen, and to withhold nitrous oxide in cases of altered sensorium, entrapped air such as pneumothorax or pulmonary blebs, bowel obstruction, air embolism, chronic pulmonary disease, or suspected decompression sickness.

Benzodiazepines may be valuable adjuncts to opioids in this setting. Although they lack analgesic properties for treatment of pain due to acute tissue injury, benzodiazepines diminish skeletal muscle spasm (e.g., during orthopedic reduction), reduce anxiety, and in higher doses, provide amnesia. Co-administration of an opioid and a benzodiazepine carries a substantially higher risk of inducing respiratory depression than administration of either drug individually, so particular vigilance is necessary. Typically, in a 70-kg adult, midazolam is used in incremental doses of 1 mg intravenously. Other agents such as phenothiazines (as antiemetics) or antihistamines (because of their weak sedative, and analgesic properties) are useful in individual cases.

Regardless of the analgesic or adjuvant given, patients should be monitored closely according to institutional standards. Such standards may include continuous observation of the electrocardiogram, frequent recording of heart rate, blood pressure, and respiratory rate, and pulse oximetry. Considering the risks associated with opioid, benzodiazepine, and other analgesic use, patients should not be left unattended between successive doses of these agents and should be watched for at least 30 minutes after the completion of outpatient procedures for which intravenous analgesia has been provided. In a transient care setting, patients should not be discharged until they are awake and can converse and ambulate. Once discharged they should be accompanied by an adult for at least two half-lives of the agents used (e.g., at least 6 hours for morphine) and should be advised not to drive an automobile or operate dangerous machinery until it is likely that all medication effects are resolved (usually 24-48 hours). Documentation of monitoring during the procedure, observation prior to discharge, and discharge instructions should be part of the patient's permanent record.

At any site where painful procedures may be performed, equipment should be available to promptly treat any untoward effects of the analgesics selected. Apart from monitoring devices, such equipment includes supplemental oxygen, devices to maintain airway patency (e.g., oral, and nasal airways, face masks, endotracheal tubes, laryngoscopes, and a bag-valve device), suction, drugs for resuscitation (e.g., atropine, naloxone), and a defibrillator. Most important, there must be present on site a physician or other provider skilled in resuscitation, particularly airway management.

Acute Pain Management: Operative or Medical Procedures

Responsibility for Effective Pain Relief

Optimal application of pain control methods depends on cooperation between different members of the health care team throughout the patient's course of treatment. To ensure that this process occurs effectively, formal means must be developed and used within each institution to assess pain and to obtain patient feedback to gauge the adequacy of its control (American Pain Society, 1990, 1991; National Institutes of Health, 1987).

The institutional process of acute pain management begins with an affirmation that patients should have access to the best level of pain relief that may safely be provided. Each institution should develop the resources necessary to provide the best and most modern pain relief appropriate to its patients.

In any setting, the quality of pain control will be influenced by the availability of a pain management program and the training, expertise, and experience of its members.

In any setting, the quality of pain control will be influenced by the availability of a pain management program and the training, expertise, and experience of its members. There is wide variation among institutions in size, complexity, volume of surgical procedures, and differing patient populations; therefore, different pain management programs are suitable. In all cases, responsibility for this care should be assigned to those most knowledgeable, experienced, interested, and available to deal with patients' needs in a timely fashion.

Risks associated with sophisticated options for effective pain relief, such as epidural analgesia or PCA, are minimized by encouraging their application in an organized, methodical fashion with frequent followup and titration. It is logical to assign responsibility for effective pain relief under such circumstances to experts working in dedicated groups. The sense of security present in many hospitals where such dedicated groups are active should not seduce other providers into offering sophisticated pain relief options beyond the institutional resources to manage them vigilantly. Patient controlled or epidural analgesia, or even conventional analgesia given by injection, are all potentially lethal. Death can occur if dosages are not titrated, drug interactions not watched for, and patients not monitored for side effects like respiratory depression. In this sense, analgesics should be prescribed with no less care and expertise than other medications such as digitalis or insulin. In settings where pain management teams are not feasible (e.g., surgicenters, primary care clinics, or nursing homes), less sophisticated options may be appropriate, yet responsibility for effective pain control should still be assigned to designated, accountable individuals. Only if institutions recognize the importance of effective pain control and assign responsibility to interested individuals or groups can the quality of care in this area be at its best.

The key items to be considered when developing an institutional quality assurance program to monitor the provision of pain relief are:

- Patient comfort and satisfaction with pain management.
- The range and appropriateness of options available within a particular institution.
- How those options can best be applied.
- Minimizing side effects and complications related to pain control.

Implementation of this guideline requires more than quality assurance procedures: interdisciplinary, interprovider collaboration should occur. Three elements are essential for interdisciplinary collaboration: a common purpose, diverse professional skills and contributions, and effective coordinating and communicating processes. For nurses, physicians, and others treating acute pain, the common purpose is relief of patients' pain. The purpose should be explicit, and a commitment to this goal should be elicited from every provider who can influence the patient's pain. Each health professional's diverse and complementary skills and contributions should be recognized and used toward meeting the common goal of pain relief. Knowledgeable and talented providers with a common purpose may not achieve effective pain control without effective communication and coordination. The following elements will help ensure successful collaboration:

- Clarity among professionals about what they can and will contribute (such as, who will coordinate pain management—primary nurse, and attending physician or specialized pain control team?; can consultants write prescriptions or orders?).

- Decision making that reflects input from the patient and family (when appropriate), such as providing when feasible a menu of pain control choices that includes pharmacologic and non-pharmacologic means.

- Contingency planning, such as orders to avert or treat possible drug side effects like constipation, nausea, or urinary retention;

Acute Pain Management: Operative or Medical Procedures

a range of analgesic doses to deal with varying pain intensity; post-discharge followup of acute pain problems such as phantom pain; and clear coverage for off-shifts or weekends.

- Regular meetings (e.g., daily rounds) of all providers (as many, and as interdisciplinary as possible) at mutually convenient times to maximize communication and information sharing.

In addition to the above clinical communications, interpersonal issues of power, leadership, and conflict can hamper efforts to relieve pain. An ability to analyze these situations, as well as interpersonal competence in leadership and conflict resolution, are vital for building teams and keeping them focused on their shared purpose of relieving pain.

Summary

Summary recommendations 1-5 and 7, below, should be implemented in every hospital where operations are performed on inpatients. The Acute Pain Management Guideline Panel recommends that any hospital in which abdominal or thoracic operations are routinely performed offer patients postoperative regional anesthetic, epidural or intrathecal opioids, PCA infusions, and other interventions requiring a similar level of expertise, under the supervision of an acute pain service as described in summary recommendation 6, below. For pain management to be effective, each hospital must designate who or which department will be responsible for all of the required activities.

There are a number of alternative approaches to preventing or relieving postoperative pain, many of which can give good results if attentively applied. The following elements, however, apply to most cases and might serve as a focus for assessing the results of these guidelines:

1. Promise patients attentive analgesic care. Patients should be informed before surgery, verbally and in printed format, that effective pain relief is an important part of their treatment, that talking about unrelieved pain is essential, and that health professionals will respond quickly to their reports of pain. It should be made clear to patients and families, however, that the total absence of any postoperative discomfort is normally not a realistic or even a desirable goal.

2. Chart and display assessment of pain and relief. A simple assessment of pain intensity and pain relief should be recorded on the bedside vital sign chart or a similar record that encourages easy, regular review by members of the health care team and is incorporated in the patient's permanent record. The intensity of pain should be assessed and documented at regular intervals (depending on the severity of pain) and with each new report of pain. The degree of pain relief should be determined after each pain management intervention, once a sufficient time has elapsed for the treatment to reach peak effect. A simple, valid measure of intensity and relief should be selected by each clinical unit. For children, age-appropriate measures should be used.

3. Define pain and relief levels to trigger a review. Each institution should identify pain intensity and pain relief levels that will elicit a review of the current pain therapy, documentation of the proposed modifications in treatment, and subsequent review of its efficacy. This process of treatment review and followup should include participation by physicians and nurses involved in the patient's care.

4. Survey patient satisfaction. At regular intervals defined by the clinical unit and quality assurance committee, each clinical unit should assess a randomly selected sample of patients who have had surgery within 72 hours. Patients should be asked their current pain intensity, the worst pain intensity in the past 24 hours, the degree of relief obtained from pain management interventions, satisfaction with relief, and their satisfaction with the staff's responsiveness.

5. Analgesic drug treatment should comply with several basic principles:

    - Non-opioid "peripherally acting" analgesics. Unless contraindicated, every patient should receive an around-the-clock postoperative regimen of an NSAID. For patients unable to take medications by mouth, it may be necessary to use the parenteral or rectal route.

    - Opioid analgesics. Analgesic orders should allow for the great variation in individual opioid requirements, including

Acute Pain Management: Operative or Medical Procedures

a regularly scheduled dose and "rescue" doses for instances in which the usual regimen is insufficient.

6. Specialized analgesic technologies, including systemic or intraspinal, continuous or intermittent opioid administration or patient controlled dosing, local anesthetic infusion, and inhalational analgesia (e.g., nitrous oxide) should be governed by policies and standard procedures that define the acceptable level of patient monitoring and appropriate roles and limits of practice for all groups of health care providers involved. The policy should include definitions of physician and nurse accountability, physician and nurse responsibility to the patient, and the role of pharmacy.

7. Non-pharmacological interventions: Cognitive and behaviorally based interventions include a number of methods to help patients understand more about their pain and to take an active part in its assessment and control. These interventions are intended to supplement, not replace, pharmacological interventions. Staff should give patients information about these interventions and support patients in using them.

8. Monitor the efficacy of pain treatment: Periodically review pain treatment procedures as defined in summary recommendations 1-4 above, using the institution's quality assurance procedures.

References

Adams, J. (1990). A methodological study of pain assessment in Anglo and Hispanic children with cancer. In Tyler, D., & Krane, E. (Eds.), Advances in pain research and therapy: Pediatric pain (vol. 15, pp. 43-52). New York: Raven Press.

Alexander, J.I., Parikh, R.K., & Spence, A.A. (1973). Postoperative analgesia and lung function: A comparison of narcotic analgesic regimens. British Journal of Anaesthesia, 45, 346-352.

American Academy of Pediatrics. (1985). Guidelines for the elective use of conscious sedation, deep sedation, and general anesthesia in pediatric patients. Pediatrics, 76, 317-321.

American Academy of Pediatrics. (In press). Guidelines for monitoring and management of pediatric patients during and following sedation for diagnostic and therapeutic procedures. Pediatrics.

American Nurses Association. (1991). Position statement on the registered nurses' (RN) role in the management of patients receiving I.V. conscious sedation for short-term therapeutic, diagnostic, or surgical procedures. Kansas City: American Nurses Association.

American Pain Society. (1989). Principles of analgesic use in the treatment of acute pain and chronic cancer pain: A concise guide to medical practice (2nd ed.). Skokie, IL: American Pain Society.

American Pain Society, Committee on Quality Assurance Standards. (1990). Standards for monitoring quality of analgesic treatment of acute pain and cancer pain. Oncology Nursing Forum, 17, 952-954.

American Pain Society quality assurance standards for relief of acute pain and cancer pain. (1991). In Bond, M.R., Charlton, J.E., & Woolf C.J. (Eds.), Proceedings of the 6th World Congress on Pain. Amsterdam, NY: Elsevier Science Publications.

Analgesia and the metabolic response to surgery (Editorial). Analgesia and the metabolic response to surgery (Editorial). (1985). Lancet, 1, 1018-1019.

Anand, K. (1990). The biology of pain perception in newborn infants. In Tyler, D., & Krane, E. (Eds.), Advances in pain research and therapy: Pediatric pain (vol. 15, pp. 113-122). New York: Raven Press.

Anand, K.J., & Aynsley-Green, A. (1988). Measuring the severity of surgical stress in newborn infants. Journal of Pediatric Surgery, 23, 297-305.

Anand, K.J., Brown, M.J., Causon, R.C., Christofides, N.D., Bloom, S.R., & Aynsley-Green, A. (1985). Can the human neonate mount an endocrine and metabolic response to surgery? Journal of Pediatric Surgery, 20, 41-48.

Anand, K.J., & Hickey, P. (1987). Pain and its effects in the human neonate and fetus. New England Journal of Medicine, 317, 1321-1329.

Anand, K.J., Sippell, W.G., & Aynsley-Green, A. (1987). Randomized trial of fentanyl anaesthesia in preterm babies undergoing surgery: Effects on the stress response. [Published erratum appears in Lancet 1987 Jan 24, 1, 234.] Lancet, 1, 62-66.

Andersen, K.H. (1989). A new method of analgesia for relief of circumcision pain. Anaesthesia, 44, 118-120.

Andolsek, K., & Novik, B. (1980). Use of hypnosis with children. Journal of Family Practice, 10, 503-507.

Acute Pain Management: Operative or Medical Procedures

Anscombe, A.R., & Buxton, R.J. (1958). Effect of abdominal operations on total lung capacity and its subdivisions. British Medical Journal, 2, 84-87.

Aradine, C.R., Beyer, J.E., & Tompkins, J.M. (1988). Children's pain perception before and after analgesia: A study of instrument construct validity and related issues. Journal of Pediatric Nursing, 3, 11-23.

Armstrong, P.J., & Bersten, A. (1986). Normeperidine toxicity. Anesthesia and Analgesia, 65, 536-538.

Atchison, N.E., Osgood, P.F., Carr, D.B., & Szyfelbein, S.K. (1991). Pain during burn dressing change in children: Relationship to burn area, depth, and analgesic regimens. Pain, 47, 41-46.

Bach, S., Noreng, M.F., & Tjellden, N.U. (1988). Phantom limb pain in amputees during the first 12 months following limb amputation, after preoperative lumbar epidural blockade. Pain, 33, 297-301.

Barrier, G., Attia, J., Mayer, M.N., Amiel-Tison, C., & Shnider, S.M. (1989). Measurement of post-operative pain and narcotic administration in infants using a new clinical scoring system. Intensive Care Medicine, 15, Suppl. 1, S37-S39.

Bauchner, H., Waring, C., & Vinci, R. (1991). Parental presence during procedures in an emergency room: Results from 50 observations. Pediatrics, 87, 544-548.

Bayer, A.J., Chada, J.S., Farag, R.R., & Pathy, M.S. (1986). Changing presentations of myocardial infarctions with increasing old age. Journal of the American Geriatric Society, 34, 263-266.

Beecher, H.K. (1959). Measurement of subjective responses: Quantitative effects of drugs. New York: Oxford University Press.

Bellville, W.J., Forrest, W.H., Miller, E., & Brown, B.W. Jr. (1971). Influence of age on pain relief from analgesics. A study of postoperative patients. Journal of the American Medical Association, 217, 1835-1841.

Bender, J.S. (1989). Approach to the acute abdomen. Medical Clinics of North America, 73, 1413-1422.

Berde, C.B. (1989). Pediatric postoperative pain management. Pediatric Clinics of North America, 36, 921-940.

Berde, C.B. (1991). Pediatric analgesic trials. In Max, M.B., Portenoy, R.K., & Laska, E.M. (Eds.), Advances in pain research and therapy: The design of analgesic clinical trials (vol. 18, pp. 445-455). New York: Raven Press.

Berde, C.B., Lehn, B.M., Yee, J.D., Sethna, N.F., & Russo, D. (1991). Patient-controlled analgesia in children and adolescents: A randomized, prospective comparison with intramuscular administration of morphine for postoperative analgesia. Journal of Pediatrics, 118, 460-466.

Bernstein, N. (1963). Management of burned children with the aid of hypnosis. Journal of Child Psychology and Psychiatry, 4, 93-98.

Beyer, J.E. (1984). The Oucher: A user's manual and technical report. [Available from: Judith Beyer, University of Colorado, Denver, CO 80262.]

Beyer, J.E., DeGood, D.E., Ashley, L.C., & Russell, G.A. (1983). Patterns of postoperative analgesic use with adults and children following cardiac surgery. Pain, 17, 71-81.

Beyer, J.E., McGrath, P.J., & Berde, C.V. (1990). Discordance between self-report and behavioral pain measures in children age 3-7 years after surgery. Journal of Pain and Symptom Management, 5, 350-356.

Bollish, S.J., Collins, C.L., Kirking, D.M., & Bartlett, R.H. (1985). Efficacy of patient-controlled versus conventional analgesia for postoperative pain. Clinical Pharmacy, 4, 48-52.

Bray, R.J. (1983). Postoperative analgesia provided by morphine infusion in children. Anaesthesia, 38, 1075-1078.

Bromage, P.R., Campoersi, E., & Chestnut, D. (1980). Epidural narcotics for postoperative analgesia. Anesthesia and Analgesia, 59, 473-480.

Bullit, E. (1989). Induction of c-fos-like protein within the lumbar spinal cord and thalamus of the rat following peripheral stimulation. Brain Research, 493, 391-397.

Bush, J.P., Holmbeck, G.N., & Cockrell, J.L. (1989). Patterns of PRN analgesic drug administration in children following elective surgery. Journal of Pediatric Psychology, 14, 433-448.

Campbell, N.N., Reynolds, G.J., & Perkins, G. (1989). Postoperative analgesia in neonates: An Australia-wide survey. Anaesthesia and Intensive Care, 17, 487-499.

Campos, R.G. (1989). Soothing pain-elicited distress in infants with swaddling and pacifiers. Child Development, 60, 781-792.

Capogna, G., Celleno, D., Tagariello, V., & Loffreda-Mancinelli, C. (1988). Capogna, G., Celleno, D., Tagariello, V., & Loffreda-Mancinelli, C. (1988). Intrathecal buprenorphine for postoperative analgesia in the elderly patient. Anaesthesia, 43, 128-130.

Ceccio, C.M. (1984). Postoperative pain relief through relaxation in elderly patients with fractured hips. Orthopedic Nursing, 3, 11-19.

Chapman, C.R., & Syrjala, K.L. (1990). Measurement of pain. In Bonica, J.J. (Ed.), The management of pain (2nd ed., vol. 1, pp. 580-594). Philadelphia: Lea & Febiger.

Chawla, R., Arora, M.K., Saksena, R., & Gode, G.R. (1989). Efficacy and dose-response of intrathecal pentazocine for postoperative pain relief. Indian Journal of Medical Research, 90, 220-223.

Choiniere, M., Melzack, R., & Papillon, J. (1991). Pain and paresthesia in patients with healed burns: An exploratory study. Journal of Pain and Symptom Management, 6, 437-444.

Cohn, B.T., Draeger, R.I., & Jackson, D.W. (1989). The effects of cold therapy in the postoperative management of pain in patients undergoing anterior cruciate ligament reconstruction. American Journal of Sports Medicine, 17, 344-349.

Collins, C., Koren, G., Crean, P., Klein, J., Roy, W.L., & MacLeod, S.M. (1985). Collins, C., Koren, G., Crean, P., Klein, J., Roy, W.L., & MacLeod, S.M. (1985). Fentanyl pharmacokinetics and hemodynamic effects in preterm infants during ligation of patent ductus arteriosus. Anesthesia and Analgesia, 64, 1078-1080.

Conn, I.G., Marshall, A.H., Yadav, S.N., Daly, J.C., & Jaffer, M. (1986). Conn, I.G., Marshall, A.H., Yadav, S.N., Daly, J.C., & Jaffer, M. (1986). Transcutaneous electrical nerve stimulation following appendicectomy: The placebo effect. Annals of the Royal College of Surgeons of England, 68, 191-192.

Cooperman, A.M., Hall, B., Mikalacki, K., Hardy, R., & Sadar, E. (1977). Use of transcutaneous electrical stimulation in the control of postoperative pain. American Journal of Surgery, 133, 185-187.

Covington, E.C., Gonsalves-Ebrahim, L., Currie, K.O., Shepard, K.V., & Pippenger, C.E. (1988). Severe respiratory depression from patient-controlled analgesia in renal failure. Psychosomatics, 30, 226-228.

Crook, J., Rideout, E., & Browne, G. (1984). The prevalence of pain complaints in a general population. Pain, 18, 299-314.

Daake, D.R., & Gueldner, S.H. (1989). Imagery instruction and the control of postsurgical pain. Applied Nursing Research, 2, 114-120.

Danesh, B.J., Saniabadi, A.R., Russell, R.I., & Lowe, G.D. (1987). Therapeutic potential of choline magnesium trisalicylate as an alternative to aspirin for patients with bleeding tendencies. Scottish Medical Journal, 32, 167-168.

Daniels, L.K. (1976). The treatment of acute anxiety and postoperative gingival pain by hypnosis and covert conditioning: A case report. American Journal of Clinical Hypnosis, 19, 116-119.

Davie, I.T., Slawson, K.B., & Burt, R.A. (1982). A double-blind comparison of parenteral morphine, placebo, and oral fenoprofen in management of postoperative pain. Anesthesia and Analgesia, 61, 1002-1005.

Davies, J.R. (1982). Ineffective transcutaneous nerve stimulation following epidura anaesthesia. Anaesthesia, 37, 453-457.

Davis, M.A. (1988). Epidemiology of osteoarthritis. Clinics in Geriatric Medicine, 4, 241-255.

Dinarello, C. (1984). Interleukin-1. Reviews of Infectious Diseases, 6, 51-95.

Donovan, M., Dillon, P., & McGuire, L. (1987). Incidence and characteristics of pain in a sample of medical-surgical inpatients. Pain, 30, 69-78.

Dripps, R.D., Eckenhoff, J.E., & Vandam, L.D. (1982). Introduction to anesthesia: The principles of safe practice. Philadelphia:, W.B. Saunders.

Egan, T.M., Herman, S.J., Doucette, E.J., Normand, S.L., & McLeod, R.S. (1988). A randomized, controlled trial to determine the effectiveness of fascial infiltration of bupivacaine in preventing respiratory complications after elective abdominal surgery. Surgery, 104, 734-740.

Egbert, A.M., Parks, L.H., Short, L.M., & Burnett, M.L. (1990). Randomized trial of postoperative patient controlled analgesia vs intramuscular narcotics in frail elderly men. Archives of Internal Medicine, 150, 1897-1903.

Egbert, L.D., Battit, G.E., Welch, C.E., & Bartlett, M.K. (1964). Reduction of postoperative pain by encouragement and instruction of patients. New England Journal of Medicine, 270, 825-827.

Egdahl, G. (1959). Pituitary-adrenal response following trauma to the isolated leg. Surgery, 46, 9-21.

Eisenach, J.C., Grice, S.C., & Dewan, D.M. (1988). Patient-controlled analgesia following cesarean section: A comparison with epidural and intramuscular narcotics. Anesthesiology, 68, 444-448.

Eland, J.M. (1989). The effectiveness of transcutaneous electrical nerve stimulation (TENS) with children experiencing cancer pain. In Funk, S.G., Tornquist, E.M., Champagne, M.T., Copp, L.A., & Wiese, R.A. (Eds.), Key aspects of comfort: Management of pain, fatigue, and nausea (pp. 87-100). New York: Springer.

Eland, J.M., & Anderson, J.E. (1977). The experience of pain in children. In Jacox, A.K. (Ed.) Pain: A source book for nurses and other health professionals (pp. 453-473). Boston: Little, Brown.

Ellerton, M., Caty, S., & Ritchie, J. (1985). Helping young children master intrusive procedures through play. Children's Health Care, 13, 167-173.

Elliott, C.H., & Olson, R.A. (1983). The management of children's distress in response to painful medical treatment for burn injuries. Behavioral Research and Therapy, 21, 675-683.

Engberg, G. (1985a). Factors influencing the respiratory capacity after upper abdominal surgery. Acta Anaesthesiologica Scandinavica, 29, 434-445.

Engberg, G. (1985b). Respiratory performance after upper abdominal surgery: A comparison of pain relief with intercostal blocks and centrally acting analgesics. Acta Anaesthesiologica Scandinavica, 29, 427-433.

Estes, D., & Kaplan, K. (1980). Lack of platelet effect with the aspirin analog, salsalate. Arthritis and Rheumatism, 23, 1301-1307.

Evron, S., Schenker, J.G., Olshwang, D., Granat, M., & Magora, F. (1981). Postoperative analgesia by percutaneous electrical stimulation in gynecology and obstetrics. European Journal of Obstetrics, Gynecology, and Reproductive Biology, 12, 305-313.

Facco, E., Manani, G., Angel, A., Vincenti, E., Tambuscio, B., Ceccherelli, F., Troletti, G., Ambrosio, F., & Giron, G.P. (1981). Comparison study between acupuncture and pentazocine analgesic and respiratory post-operative effects. American Journal of Chinese Medicine, 9, 225-235.

Fassler, D. (1985). The fear of needles in children. American Journal of Orthopsychiatry, 55, 371-377.

Ferguson, B.F. (1979). Preparing young children for hospitalization: A comparison of two methods. Pediatrics, 64, 656-664.

Fernald, C., & Corry, J. (1981). Empathic versus directive preparation of children for needles. Child Health Care, 10, 44-47.

Ferrante, F.M., Ostheimer, G.W., & Covino, B.G. (Eds.). (1990). Patient-controlled analgesia. Chicago: Blackwell.

Ferrell, B.A. (1991). Pain management in elderly people. Journal of the American Geriatric Society, 39, 64-73.

Ferrell, B.A., Ferrell, B.R., & Osterweil, D. (1990). Pain in the nursing home. Journal of the American Geriatric Society, 38, 409-414.

Field, T., & Goldson, E. (1984). Pacifying effects of nonnutritive sucking on term and preterm neonates during heelstick procedures. Pediatrics, 74, 1012-1015.

Fitzgerald, M. (1990). C-fos and changing the face of pain. Trends in Neurosciences, 13, 439-440.

Fitzgerald, M., Millard, C., & McIntosh, N. (1988). Hyperalgesia in premature infants. Lancet, 1, 292.

Fitzgerald, M., Millard, C., & MacIntosh, N. (1989). Cutaneous hypersensitivity following peripheral tissue damage in newborn infants and its reversal with topical anesthesia. Pain, 39, 31-36.

Fitzgerald, M., Shaw, A., & MacIntosh, N. (1988). Postnatal development of the cutaneous flexor reflex: Comparative study of preterm infants and newborn rat pups. Developmental Medicine and Child Neurology, 30, 520-526.

Flaherty, G.G., & Fitzpatrick, J.J. (1978). Relaxation technique to increase comfort level of postoperative patients: A preliminary study. Nursing Research, 27, 352-355.

Foley, K.M. (1985). The treatment of cancer pain. New England Journal of Medicine, 313, 84-95.

Foley, K.M., & Inturrisi, C.E. (1987). Analgesic drug therapy in cancer pain: Principles and practice. Medical Clinics of North America, 71, 207-232.

Fordyce, W.E. (1978). Evaluating and managing chronic pain. Geriatrics, 33, 59-62.

Fortin, F., & Kirouac, S. (1976). A randomized controlled trial of preoperative patient education. International Journal of Nursing Studies, 13, 11-24.

Foster, R., & Hester, N. (1989). The relationship between assessment and pharmacologic intervention for pain in children. In Funk, S.G., Tornquist, E.M., Champagne, M.T., Copp, L.A., & Wiese, R.A. (Eds.), Key aspects of comfort: Management of pain, fatigue, and nausea (pp. 72-79). New York: Springer.

Foster, R.L., & Hester, N.O. (1990a). Administration of analgesics for children's pain. Pain, Suppl. 5, S27.

Foster, R.L., & Hester, N.O. (1990b). The relationship between pain ratings and pharmacologic interventions for children in pain. In Tyler, D.& Krane, E. (Eds.), Advances in pain research and therapy: Pediatric pain (vol. 15, pp. 31-36). New York: Raven Press.

Fowler-Kerry, S. (1990). Adolescent oncology survivors' recollection of pain. In Tyler, D., & Krane, E. (Eds.), Advances in pain research and therapy: Pediatric pain (vol. 15, pp. 365-371). New York: Raven Press.

Acute Pain Management: Operative or Medical Procedures

Fowler-Kerry, S., & Lander, J.R. (1987). Management of injection pain in children. Pain, 30, 169-175.

Fradet, C., McGrath, P.J., Kay, J., Adams, S., & Luke, B. (1990). A prospective survey of reactions to blood tests by children and adolescents. Pain, 40, 53-60.

Franck, L.S. (1987). A national survey of the assessment and treatment of pain and agitation in the neonatal intensive care unit. Journal of Obstetric, Gynecologic, and Neonatal Nursing, 16, 387-393.

Fritz, D.J. (1988). Noninvasive pain control methods used by cancer outpatients (meeting abstract). Oncology Nursing Forum, Suppl. 108.

From the NIH. (1979). Pain in the elderly: Patterns change with age. Journal of the American Medical Association, 241, 2191-2192.

Gauvain-Piquard, A., Rodary, C., Rezvani, A., & Lemerle, J. (1987). Pain in children aged 2-6 years: A new observational rating scale elaborated in a pediatric oncology unit; A preliminary report. Pain, 31, 177-188.

Gedaly-Duff, V., & Ziebarth, D. (1991). Mothers' management of surgical pain in preschool children [abstract of paper presented at the Second International Symposium on Pediatric Pain]. Journal of Pain and Symptom Management, 6, 147.

Gracely, R.H., & Wolskee, P.J. (1983). Semantic functional measurement of pain: Integrating perception and language. Pain, 15, 389-398.

Grunau, R.V.E., & Craig, K.D. (1987). Pain expression in neonates: Facial action and cry. Pain, 28, 395-410.

Guideline report. Acute pain management: Operative or medical procedures and trauma (AHCPR Pub. No. 92-0022). (In press). Rockville, Md: Agency for Health Care Policy and Research.

Hanley, M.R. (1988). Proto-oncogenes in the nervous system. Neuron, 1, 175-182.

Hannallah, R.S., & Rosales, J.K. (1983). Experience with parents' presence during anaesthesia induction in children. Canadian Anaesthetists' society Journal, 30, 286-289.

Hanson, A.L., Hanson, B., & Matousek, M. (1984). Epidural anesthesia for cesarean section. The effect of morphine-bupivacaine administered epidurally for intra- and postoperative pain relief. Acta Obstetrica Gynecologica Scandinavica, 63, 135-140.

Hansson, P., & Ekblom, A. (1986). Influence of stimulus frequency and probe size on vibration-induced alleviation of acute orofacial pain. Applied Neurophysiology, 49, 155-165.

Hargreaves, A., & Lander, J. (1989). Use of transcutaneous electrical nerve stimulation for postoperative pain. Nursing Research, 38, 159-161.

Hargreaves, K.M., & Dionne, R.A. (1991). Evaluating endogenous mediators of pain and analgesia in clinical studies. In Max, M., Portenoy, R., & Laska, E. (Eds.), Advances in pain research and therapy. The design of analgesic clinical trials (vol. 19, pp. 579-598). New York: Raven Press.

Harkins, S.W., Kwentus, J., & Price, D.D. (1984). Pain and the elderly. In Benedetti, C., Chapman, C., & Moricca, G. (Eds.), Advances in pain research and therapy. Recent advances in the management of pain (vol. 7, pp. 103-121). New York: Raven Press.

Hasenbos, M., van Egmond, J., Gielen, M., & Crul, J.F. (1987). Post-operative analgesia by high thoracic epidural versus intramuscular nicomorphine after thoracotomy. Part III. The effects of pre- and post-operative analgesia on morbidity. Acta Anaesthesiologica Scandinavica, 31, 608-615.

Hasselstrom, Eriksson, S., Persson A., Rane, A., Svensson, J.O., & Sawa, J. (1990). The metabolism and bioavailability of morphine in patients with severe liver cirrhosis. British Journal of Clinical Pharmacology, 29, 289-297.

Hendrickson, M., Myre, L., Johnson, D.G., Matlak, M.E., Black, R.E., & Sullivan, J.J. (1990). Postoperative analgesia in children: A prospective study of intermittent intramuscular injections versus continuous intravenous infusion of morphine. Journal of Pediatric Surgery, 25, 185-191.

Hertzka, R., Gauntlett, I., Fisher, D., & Spellman, M. (1989). Fentanyl-induced ventilatory depression: Effects of age. Anesthesiology, 70, 213-218.

Hester, N.K.O. (1979). The preoperational child's reaction to immunization. Nursing Research, 28, 250-255.

Hester, N.O. (1989). Comforting the child in pain. In Funk, S.G., Tornquist, E.M., Champagne, M.T., Copp, L.A., & Wiese, R.A. (Eds.), Key aspects of comfort: Management of pain, fatigue, and nausea (pp. 290-298). New York: Springer.

Hester, N.O., & Barcus, C.S. (1986). Assessment and management of pain in children. Pediatrics: Nursing Update, 1, 1-8.

Hester, N.O., & Foster, R.L. (1990). Cues nurses and parents use in making judgments about children's pain. Pain, Suppl. 5, S31.

Hester, N. O., Foster, R. L., & Kristensen, K. (1990). Measurement of pain in children: Generalizability and validity of the Pain

Ladder and the Poker Chip tool. In Tyler, D.C., & Krane, E.J. (Eds.), Advances in pain research and therapy: Pediatric pain (vol. 15, pp. 79-84). New York: Raven Press.

Hester, N.O., Foster, R., Kristensen, K., & Bergstrom, L. (1989). Measurement of children's pain by children, parents, and nurses: Psychometric and clinical issues related to the poker chip tool and the pain ladder. Generalizability of procedures assessing pain in children: Final report. Research funded by NIH, National Center for Nursing Research under Grant Number NR01382. [Available from, N.O. Hester, Center for Nursing Research, School of Nursing, University of Colorado, Denver, CO 80262.]

Hewlett, A.M., & Branthwaite, M.A. (1975). Postoperative pulmonary function. British Journal of Anaesthesia, 47, 102-107.

Hodsman, N.B., Burns, J., Blyth, A., Kenny, G.N., McArdle, C.S., & Rotman, H. (1987). The morphine sparing effects of diclofenac sodium following abdominal surgery. Anaesthesia, 42, 1005-1008.

Horan, J.J., Laying, F.C., & Pursell, C.H. (1976). Preliminary study of effects of in vivo emotive imagery on dental discomfort. Perceptual and Motor Skills, 42, 105-106.

Horowitz, B.F., Fitzpatrick, J.J., & Flaherty, G.G. (1984). Relaxation techniques for pain relief after open heart surgery. Dimensions in Critical Care Nursing, 3, 364-371.

Houde, R.W. (1982). Methods for measuring clinical pain in humans. Acta Anaesthesiologica Scandinavica, 74 (Suppl), 25-29.

Hunt, S.P., Pini, A., & Evan, G. (1987). Induction of c-fos-like protein in spinal cord neurons following sensory stimulation. Nature, 328, 632-634.

International Association for the Study of Pain. (1979). Pain terms: A list with definitions and notes on usage. Pain, 6, 249.

International Association for the Study of Pain. (In press). Report of the task force on acute pain management.

Jackson, D. (1989). A study of pain management: Patient controlled analgesia versus intramuscular analgesia. Journal of Intravenous Nursing, 12, 42-51.

Jackson, D.L., Moore, P.A., & Hargreaves, K.M. (1989). Pre-operative nonsteroidal anti-inflammatory medication for the prevention of postoperative dental pain. Journal of the American Dental Association, 119, 641-647.

Jacox, A.K. (Ed.). (1977). Pain: A sourcebook for nurses and other health professionals. Boston: Little, Brown.

Jay, S.M., Elliot, C., Ozolins, M., Olson, R., & Pruitt, S. (1985). Behavioral management of children's distress during painful medical procedures. Behavioral Research and Therapy, 23, 513-520.

Jay, S.M., Ozolins, M., Elliott, C.H., & Caldwell, S. (1983). Assessment of children's distress during painful medical procedures. Health Psychology, 2, 133-147.

Jensen, J.E., Conn, R.R., Hazelrigg, G., & Hewett, J.E. (1985). The use of transcutaneous neural stimulation and isokinetic testing in arthroscopic knee surgery. American Journal of Sports Medicine, 13, 27-33.

John, M.E.Jr., & Parrino, J.P. John, M.E. Jr., & Parrino, J.P. (1983). Practical hypnotic suggestion in ophthalmic surgery. American Journal of Ophthalmology, 96, 540-542.

Johnson, J., Fuller, S., Endress, P., & Rice, V. (1978). Altering patients' responses to surgery: An extension and replication. Research in Nursing and Health, 1, 111-121.

Johnson, J., Rice, V., Fuller, S., & Endress, P. (1978). Sensory information, instruction in a coping strategy, and recovery from surgery. Research in Nursing and Health, 1, 4-17.

Johnson, J.E., Kirchoff, K., & Endress, M.P. (1975). Altering children's distress behavior during orthopedic cast removal. Nursing Research, 24, 404-410.

Johnston, C.C., Bevan, J.C., Haig, M.J., Kirnon, V., & Tousignant, G. (1988). Johnston, C.C., Bevan, J.C., Haig, M.J., Kirnon, V., & Tousignant, G. (1988). Parental presence during anesthesia induction. Association of Operating Room Nurses Journal, 47, 187-194.

Johnston, C.C., Jeans, M.E., Abbott, F.V., Grey-Donald, K., & Edgar, L. (1988). A survey of pain in hospitalized children: Preliminary results [abstract, p. 80]. In Tyler, D., & Krane, E. (Chairs), Proceedings of the 1st International Symposium on Pediatric Pain. New York: Raven Press.

Jonsson, A., Cassuto, J., & Hanson, B. (1991). Inhibition of burn pain by intravenous lignocaine infusion. Lancet, 338, 151-152.

Kaiko, R.F. (1980). Age and morphine analgesia in cancer patients with post-operative pain. Clinical Pharmacology Therapeutics, 28, 823-826.

Kaiko, R.F., Foley, K.M., Grabinski, P.Y., Heidrich, G., Rogers, A.G., Inturissi, C.E., & Reidenberg, M.M. (1983). Central nervous system excitatory effects of meperidine in cancer patients. Annals of Neurology, 13, 180-185.

Acute Pain Management: Operative or Medical Procedures

Kaiko, R.F., Wallenstein, S.L., Rogers, A.G., Grabinski, P.Y., & Houde, R.W. (1982). Narcotics in the elderly. Medical Clinics of North America, 66, 1079-1089.

Kallos, T., & Caruso, F.S. (1979). Respiratory effects of butorphanol and pethidine. Anaesthesia, 34, 633-637.

Kane, R.L., Ouslander, J.G., & Abrass, I.B. (Eds.). (1989). Essentials of clinical geriatrics (2nd ed.). New York: McGraw-Hill.

Kaplan, J.A., Miller, E.D. Jr., & Gallagher, E.G. Kaplan, J.A., Miller, E.D. Jr., & Gallagher, E.G. Jr. (1975). Postoperative analgesia for thoracotomy patients. Anesthesia and Analgesia, 54, 773-777.

Katz, E.R., Kellerman, J., & Siegel, S.E. (1980). Behavioral distress in children with cancer undergoing medical procedures: Developmental considerations. Journal of Consulting and Clinical Psychology, 48, 356-365.

Kavanagh, C. (1983a). A new approach to dressing change in the severely burned child and its effects on burn-related psychopathology. Heart and Lung, 12, 612-619.

Kavanagh, C. (1983b). Psychological intervention with the severely burned child: Report of an experimental comparison of two approaches and their effects on psychological sequelae. Journal of the American Academy of Child Psychiatry, 22, 145-156.

Kehlet, H. (1982). The endocrine-metabolic response to postoperative pain. Acta Anaesthesiologica Scandinavica, 74 (Suppl), 173-175.

Kehlet, H. (1989a). Postoperative pain. In Committee on Pre- and Postoperative Care, American College of Surgeons, Care of the surgical patient (vol. 1, pp. 3-12). New York: Scientific American Medicine.

Kehlet, H. (1989b). Surgical stress: The role of pain and analgesia. British Journal of Anaesthesia, 63, 189-195.

Kehlet, H., Brandt, M.R., & Rem, J. (1980). Role of neurogenic stimuli in mediating the endocrine-metabolic response to surgery. Journal of Parenteral & Enteral Nutrition, 4, 152-156.

Kelley, M.L., Jarvie, G.J., Middlebrook, J.L., McNeer, M.F., & Drabman, R.S. (1984). Decreasing burned children's pain behavior: Impacting the trauma of hydrotherapy. Journal of Applied Behavioral Analysis, 17, 147-158.

Kiefer, R.C., & Hospodarsky, J. (1980). The use of hypnotic technique in anesthesia to decrease postoperative meperidine requirements. Journal of the American Osteopathic Association, 79, 693-695.

Koehntop, D., Rodman, J., Brundage, D., Hegland, M., & Buckley, J. (1986). Pharmacokinetics of fentanyl in neonates. Anesthesia and Analgesia, 65, 227-232.

Koren, G., Butt, W., Chinyanga, H., Soldin, S., & Pape, K. (1985). Postoperative morphine infusion in newborn infants: Assessment of disposition characteristics and safety. Journal of Pediatrics, 107, 963-967.

Lanham, R.H. Jr., Powell, S., & Hendrix, B.E. Lanham, R.H. Jr., Powell, S., & Hendrix, B.E. (1984). Efficacy of hypothermia and transcutaneous electrical nerve stimulation in podiatric surgery. Journal of Foot Surgery, 23, 152-158.

Latimer, R.G., Dickman, M., Day, W.C., Gunn, M.L., & Schmidt, C.D. (1971). Ventilatory patterns and pulmonary complications after upper abdominal surgery determined by preoperative and postoperative computerized spirometry and blood gas analysis. American Journal of Surgery, 122, 622-632.

Lawlis, G.F., Selby, D., Hinnant, D., & McCoy, C.E. (1985). Reduction of postoperative pain parameters by presurgical relaxation instructions for spinal pain patients. Spine, 10, 649-651.

LeBaron, S., & Zeltzer, L. (1984). Assessment of acute pain and anxiety in children and adolescents by self-reports, observer reports, and a behavior checklist. Journal of Consulting and Clinical Psychology, 52, 729-738.

Lee, M., Itoh, M., Yang, G.W., & Eason, A.L. (1990). Physical therapy and rehabilitation medicine. In Bonica, J.J. (Ed.), The management of pain (2nd ed., vol. 2, pp. 1769-1788). Philadelphia: Lea & Febiger.

Levin, R.F., Malloy, G.B., & Hyman, R.B. (1987). Nursing management of postoperative pain: Use of relaxation techniques with female cholecystectomy patients. Journal of Advanced Nursing, 12, 463-472.

Liu, Y.C., Liao, W.S., & Lien, I.N. (1985). Effect of transcutaneous electrical nerve stimulation for post-thoracotomic pain. Journal of the Formosan Medical Association, 84, 801-809.

Locsin, R.G. (1981). The effect of music on the pain of selected postoperative patients. Journal of Advanced Nursing, 6, 19-25.

Lynn, A.M., Opheim, K.E., & Tyler, D.C. (1984). Morphine infusion after pediatric cardiac surgery. Critical Care Medicine, 12, 863-866.

Lynn, A.M., & Slattery, J.T. (1987). Morphine pharmacokinetics in early infancy. Anesthesiology, 66, 136-139.

Madden, C., Singer, G., Peck, C., & Nayman, J. (1978). The effect of EMG biofeedback in postoperative pain following abdominal surgery. Anaesthesia and Intensive Care, 6, 333-336.

Marks, R.M., & Sachar, E.J. (1973). Undertreatment of medical inpatients with narcotic analgesics. Annals of Internal Medicine, 78, 173-181.

Marshall, B.E., & Wyche, M.Q. Jr. Marshall, B.E.,& Wyche, M.Q. Jr. (1972). Hypoxemia during and after anesthesia. Anesthesiology, 37, 178-209.

Martens, M. (1982). A significant decrease of narcotic drug dosage after orthopaedic surgery. A double-blind study with naproxen. Acta Orthopaedica Belgica, 48, 900-906.

Mather, L., & Mackie, J. (1983). The incidence of postoperative pain in children. Pain, 15, 271-282.

Maunuksela, E.L., & Korpela, R. (1986). Double-blind evaluation of a lignocaine-prilocaine cream (EMLA) in children. British Journal of Anaesthesia, 58, 1242-1245.

Max, M.B., Inturrisi, C.E., Kaiko, R.F., Grabinski, P.Y., Li, C.H., & Foley, K.M. (1985). Epidural and intrathecal opiates: Cerebrospinal fluid and plasma profiles in patients with chronic cancer pain. Clinical Pharmacology and Therapeutics, 38, 631-641.

Maxwell, L., Yaster, M., Wetzel, R., & Niebyl, J. (1987). Penile nerve block for newborn circumcision. Obstetrics and Gynecology, 70, 415-419.

McCaffery, M., & Beebe, A. (1989). Pain: Clinical manual for nursing practice. St. Louis:, C.V. Mosby.

McGrath, D., Thurston, N., Wright, D., Preshaw, R., & Fermin, P. (1989). Comparison of one technique of patient-controlled postoperative analgesia with intramuscular meperidine. Pain, 37, 265-270.

McGrath, M.M. (1979). Group preparation of pediatric surgical patients. Image, 11, 52-62.

McGrath, P.A. (1990). Pain in children: Nature, assessment, and treatment. New York: Guilford Press.

McGrath, P.A., de Veber, L.L., & Hearn, M.T. (1985). Multidimensional pain assessment in children. In Fields, H.L., Dubner, R., & Cervero, F. (Eds.), Proceedings of the Fourth World Conference on Pain. Advances in pain research and therapy (vol. 9, pp. 387-393). New York: Raven Press.

McGrath, P.J., Johnson, G., Goodman, J.T., Schillinger, J., Dunn, J., & Chapman, J. (1985). CHEOPS: A behavioral scale for rating postoperative pain in children. In Fields, H.L., Dubner, R., & Cervero, F. (Eds.), Proceedings of the Fourth World Conference on Pain. Advances in pain research and therapy (vol. 9, pp. 395-402). New York: Raven Press.

McGrath, P.J., & Unruh, A.M. (1987). Pain in children and adolescents. Amsterdam: Elsevier.

McQuay, H. (1989). Opioids in chronic pain. British Journal of Anaesthesia, 63, 213-226.

McQuay, H.J., Carroll, D., & Moore, R.A. (1988). Postoperative orthopaedic pain: The effect of opiate premedication and local anaesthetic blocks. Pain, 33, 291-295.

Meignier, M., Souron, R.,& LeNeel, J.C. (1983). Postoperative dorsal epidural analgesia in the child with respiratory disabilities. Anesthesiology, 59, 473-475.

Merskey, H. (1964). An investigation of pain in psychological illness. D.M. Thesis, Oxford.

Modig, J., Borg, T., Bagge, L., & Saldeen, T. (1983). Role of extradural and of general anaesthesia in fibrinolysis and coagulation after total hip replacement. British Journal of Anaesthesia, 55, 625-629.

Modig, J., Borg, T., Karlstrom, G., Maripuu, E., & Sahlstedt, B. (1983). Thromboembolism after total hip replacement: Role of epidural and general anesthesia. Anesthesia and Analgesia, 62, 174-180.

Mogan, J., Wells, N., & Robertson, E. (1985). Effects of preoperative teaching on postoperative pain: A replication and expansion. International Journal of Nursing Studies, 22, 267-280.

Moon, M.H., & Gibbs, J.M. (1984). The control of postoperative pain by EMG biofeedback in patients undergoing hysterectomy. New Zealand Medical Journal, 97, 643-646.

Mullooly, V.M., Levin, R.F., & Feldman, H.R. (1988). Music for postoperative pain and anxiety. Journal of the NY State Nurses Association, 19, 4-7.

Nagashima, H., Karamanian, A., Malovany, R., Radnay, P., Ang, M., Koerner, S., & Foldes, F.F. (1976). Respiratory and circulatory effects of intravenous butorphanol and morphine. Clinical Pharmacology and Therapeutics, 19, 738-745.

Nahata, M., Clotz, M., & Krogg, E. (1985). Adverse effects of meperidine, promethazine, and chlorpromazine for sedation in pediatric patients. Clinical Pediatrics, 24, 558-560.

National Health and Medical Research Council [Australia]. National Health and Medical Research Council [Australia]. (1988). Management of severe pain. Canberra, Australia: National Health and Medical Research Council.

National Institutes of Health. (1987). The integrated approach to the management of pain. Journal of Pain and Symptom Management, 2, 35-44.

Acute Pain Management: Operative or Medical Procedures

Neary, J. (1981). Transcutaneous electrical nerve stimulation for the relief of post-incisional surgical pain. Journal of the American Association of Nurse Anesthetists, 149, 151-155.

Oden, R. (1989). Acute postoperative pain: Incidence, severity, and the etiology of inadequate treatment. Anesthesiology Clinics of North America, 7, 1-15.

Olness, K. (1981). Imagery (self-hypnosis) as adjunct therapy in childhood cancer: Clinical experience with 25 patients. The American Journal of Pediatric Hematology/Oncology, 3, 313-321.

Patel, J.M., Lanzafame, R.J., Williams, J.S., Mullen, B.V., & Hinshaw, J.R. (1983). The effect of incisional infiltration of bupivacaine hydrochloride upon pulmonary functions, atelectasis, and narcotic need following elective cholecystectomy. Surgery, Gynecology and Obstetrics, 157, 338-340.

Peebles, R.J., & Schneidman, D.S. (1991). Socio-Economic Factbook for Surgery, 1991-92. Chicago: American College of Surgeons.

Pettine, K.A., Wedel, D.J., Cabanela, M.E., & Weeks, J.L. (1989). The use of epidural bupivacaine following total knee arthroplasty. Orthopedic Review, 18, 894-901.

Phillips, G.D., & Cousins, M.J. (1986). Practical decision making. In Cousins, J.M. & Phillips, G.D. (Eds.), Acute pain management (pp. 275-290). New York: Churchill Livingstone.

Pickett, C., & Clum, G.A. (1982). Comparative treatment strategies and their interaction with locus of control in the reduction of postsurgical pain and anxiety. Journal of Consulting and Clinical Psychology, 50, 439-441.

Portenoy, R.K., & Payne, R. (In press). Acute and chronic pain. In Lowinson, J.H., Ruit, P., Milman, R., & Langvod, J. (Eds.), Comprehensive textbook of substance abuse. Baltimore: Williams and Wilkins.

Porter, J., & Jick, H. (1980). Addiction rare in patients treated with narcotics [letter]. New England Journal of Medicine, 302, 123.

Przewlocki, R., Haarmann, I., Nikolarakis, K., Herz, A., & Hollt, V. (1988). Prodynorphin gene expression in spinal cord is enhanced after traumatic injury in the rat. Brain Research, 464, 37-41.

Purcell-Jones, G., Dormon, F., & Sumner, E. (1987). The use of opioids in neonates. A retrospective study of 933 cases. Anaesthesia, 42, 1316-1320.

Purcell-Jones, G., Dormon, F., & Sumner, E. (1988). Paediatric anaesthetists' perceptions of neonatal and infant pain. Pain, 33, 181-187.

Pybus, D.A., D'Bras, B.E., Goulding, G., Liberman, H., & Torda, T.A. (1983). Postoperative analgesia for haemorrhoid surgery. Anaesthesia and Intensive Care, 11, 27-30.

Quay, N.B., & Alexander, L.L. (1983). Preparation of burned children and their families for discharge. The Journal of Burn Care and Rehabilitation, 4, 288-290.

Rawal, N., & Sjostrand, U.H. (1986). Clinical application of epidural and intrathecal opioids for pain management. International Anesthesiology Clinics, 24, 43-57.

Reading, A.E. (1982). The effects of psychological preparation on pain and recovery after minor gynecological surgery: A preliminary report. Journal of Clinical Psychology, 38, 504-512.

Ready, L.B., Oden, R., Chadwick, H.S., Bendetti, C., Rooke, G.A., Caplan, R., & Wild, L.M. (1988). Development of an anesthesiology-based postoperative pain service. Anesthesiology, 68, 100-106.

Reay, B.A., Semple, A.J., Macrae, W.A., MacKenzie, N., & Grant, I.S. (1989). Low-dose intrathecal diamorphine analgesia following major orthopaedic surgery. British Journal of Anaesthesia, 62, 248-252.

Rooney, S.M., Jain, S., McCormack, P., Bains, M., Martini, N., & Goldiner, P. (1986). A comparison of pulmonary function tests for postthoracotomy pain using cryoanalgesia and transcutaneous nerve stimulation. The Annals of Thoracic Surgery, 41, 204-207.

Rosen, H., Absi, E.G., & Webster, J.A. (1985). Suprofen compared to dextropropoxyphene hydrochloride and paracetamol (Cosalgesic) after extraction of wisdom teeth under general anesthesia. Anaesthesia, 40, 639-641.

Ross, D.M. (1984). Thought-stopping: A coping strategy for impending feared events. Issues in Comprehensive Pediatric Nursing, 7, 83-89.

Roth, S.H. (1989). Merits and liabilities of NSAID therapy. Rheumatic Diseases Clinics of North America, 15, 479-498.

Royal College of Surgeons of England, the College of Anesthetists. (1990). Report of the Working Party on Pain After Surgery. London: Royal College of Surgeons.

Ryan, E. (1989). The effect of musical distraction on pain in hospitalized school-aged children. In Funk, W., Tournquist, E., Champagne, M., Copp, L., & Wiese, R. (Eds.), Key aspects of comfort: Management of pain, fatigue, and nausea (pp. 101-104). New York: Springer.

Sabanathan, S., Mearns, A.J., Bickford Smith, P.J., Eng, J., Berrisford, R.G., Bibby, S.R., & Majid, M.R. (1990). Efficacy of continuous extrapleural intercostal nerve block on post-thoracotomy pain and pulmonary mechanics. British Journal of Surgery, 77, 221-225.

Savedra, M., Gibbons, P., Tesler, M., Ward, J., & Wegner, C. (1982). How do children describe pain? A tentative assessment. Pain, 14, 95-104.

Savedra, M.C., Tesler, M.D., Holzemer, W.L., & Ward, J.A. (1989). Adolescent Pediatric Pain Tool (APPT) preliminary user's manual. San Francisco: University of California. [Available from, M.C. Savedra, UCSF School of Nursing, San Francisco, CA 94143-0606.]

Schechter, N.L. (1989). The undertreatment of pain in children: An overview. Pediatric Clinics of North America, 36, 781-794.

Schechter, N.L., & Allen, D.A. (1986). Physician's attitudes toward pain in children. Journal of Developmental and Behavioral Pediatrics, 7, 350-354.

Schechter, N.L., Bernstein, B.A., Beck, A., Hart, L., & Sherzer, L. (1991). Individual differences in children's response to pain: Role of temperament and parental characteristics. Pediatrics, 87, 171-177.

Schmitt, F., & Wooldridge, P.J. (1973). Psychological preparation of surgical patients. Nursing Research, 22, 108-116.

Schnurrer, J.A., Marvin, J.A., & Heimbach, D.M. (1985). Evaluation of pediatric pain medications. Journal of Burn Care and Rehabilitation, 6, 105-107.

Schofield, N., & White, J. (1989). Interrelations among children, parents, premedication, and anaesthetists in paediatric day stay surgery. British Medical Journal, 299, 1371-1375.

Scott, J., & Huskisson, E.C. (1976). Graphic representation of pain. Pain, 2, 175-184.

Scott, N.B., Mogensen, T., Bigler, D., & Kehlet, H. (1989). Comparison of the effects of continuous intrapleural vs epidural administration of 0.5 percent bupivacaine on pain, metabolic response and pulmonary function following cholecystectomy. Acta Anaesthesiologica Scandinavica, 33, 535-539.

Sear, J.W., Hand, C.W., Moore, R.A., & McQuay, H.J. (1989). Studies on morphine disposition: Influence of renal failure on the kinetics of morphine and its metabolites. British Journal of Anaesthesia, 62, 28-32.

Shaw, E., & Routh, D. (1982). Effect of mothers' presence on children's reaction to aversive procedures. Journal of Pediatric Psychology, 7, 33-42.

Shulman, M., Sandler, A.N., Bradley, J.W., Young, P.S., & Brebner, J. (1984). Postthoracotomy pain and pulmonary function following epidural and systemic morphine. Anesthesiology, 61, 569-575.

Siegel, L., & Peterson, L. (1980). Stress reduction in young dental patients through coping skills and sensory information. Journal of Consulting and Clinical Psychology, 48, 785-787.

Siegel, L., & Peterson, L. (1981). Maintenance effects of coping skills and sensory information on young children's response to repeated dental procedures. Behavior Therapy, 12, 530-535.

Sjogren, P., & Banning, A. (1989). Pain, sedation, and reaction time during long-term treatment of cancer patients with oral and epidural opioids. Pain, 39, 5-11.

Skacel, P.O., Hewlett, A.M., Lewis, J.D., Lamb, M., Nunn, J.F., & Chanarin, I. (1983). Studies on the haemopoetic toxicity of nitrous oxide in man. British Journal of Haematology, 53, 189-200.

Smith, C.M., Guralnick, M.S., Gelfand, M.M., & Jeans, M.E. (1986). The effects of transcutaneous electrical nerve stimulation on post-cesarean pain. Pain, 27, 181-193.

Smith, M.J., Hutchins, R.C.,& Hehenberger, D. (1983). Transcutaneous neural stimulation use in postoperative knee rehabilitation. American Journal of Sports Medicine, 11, 75-82.

Snow, B.R. (1985). The use of hypnosis in the management of preoperative anxiety and postoperative pain in a patient undergoing laminectomy. Bulletin of the Hospital for Joint Disease Orthopaedic Institute, 45, 143-149.

Soderstrom, C.A., Trifillis, A.L., Shankar, B.S., Clark, W.E., & Cowley, R.A. (1988). Marijuana and alcohol use among 1023 trauma patients. A prospective study. Archives of Surgery, 123, 733-777.

Solomon, R., Viernstein, M., & Long, D. (1980). Reduction of postoperative pain and narcotic use by transcutaneous electrical nerve stimulation. Surgery, 87, 142-146.

Sriwatanakul, K., Kelvie, W., & Lasagna, L. (1982). The quantification of pain: An analysis of words used to describe pain and analgesia in clinical trials. Clinical Pharmacology and Therapeutics, 32, 143-148.

Sriwatanakul, K., Kelvie, W., Lasagna, L., Calimlim, J., Weis, O., & Mehta, G. (1983). Studies with different types of visual analog scales for measurement of pain. Clinical Pharmacology and Therapeutics, 34, 234-239.

Sriwatanakul, K., Weis, O.F., Alloza, J.L., Kelvie, W., Weintraub, M., & Lasagna, L. (1983). Analysis of narcotic usage in the treatment of postoperative pain. Journal of the American Medical Association, 250, 926-929.

Stevens, B. (1990). Development and testing of a pediatric pain management sheet. Pediatric Nursing, 16, 543-548.

Swinford, P. (1987). Relaxation and positive imagery for the surgical patient: A research study. Perioperative Nursing Quarterly, 3, 9-16.

Sydow, F.W. (1989). The influence of anesthesia and postoperative analgesic management on lung function. Acta Chiurgica Scandinavica, 550 (Suppl), 159-165.

Syrjala, K.L. (1990). Relaxation techniques. In Bonica, J.J. (Ed.), The management of pain (vol. 2, pp. 1742-1750). Philadelphia: Lea & Febiger.

Szeto, H., Inturrisi, C., Houde, R., Saal, S., Cheigh, J., & Reidenberg, M.M. (1977). Accumulation of normeperidine, an active metabolite of meperidine, in patients with renal failure of cancer. Annals of Internal Medicine, 86, 738-741.

Taylor, A.G., West, B.A., Simon, B., Skelton, J., & Rowlingson, J.C. (1983). How effective is TENS for acute pain? American Journal of Nursing, 83, 1171-1174.

Tesler, M.D., Savedra, M.C., Holzemer, W.L., Wilkie, D.J., Ward, J.A., & Paul, S.M. (1991). The word-graphic rating scale as a measure of children's and adolescents' pain intensity. Research in Nursing and Health, 14, 361-371.

Toledo-Pereyra, L.H., & DeMeester, T.R. (1979). Prospective randomized evaluation of intrathoracic intercostal nerve block with bupivacaine on postoperative ventilatory function. The Annals of Thoracic Surgery, 27, 203-205.

Tree-Trakarn, T., Pirayavaraporn, S., & Lertakyamanee, J. (1987). Topical analgesia for relief of post-circumcision pain. Anesthesiology, 67, 395-399.

Triplett, J.L., & Arneson, S.W. (1979). The use of verbal and tactile comfort to alleviate distress in young hospitalized children. Research in Nursing and Health, 2, 17-23.

Van Aernam, B., & Lindeman, C. (1971). Nursing intervention with the presurgical patient: The effects of structured and unstructured preoperative teaching. Nursing Research, 20, 319-332.

VanderArk, G., & McGrath, K. (1975). Transcutaneous electrical stimulation in treatment of postoperative pain. The American Journal of Surgery, 130, 338-340.

Ventafridda, V., Ripamonti, C., DeConno, F., Bianchi, M., Pazzuconi, F., & Panerai, A.E. (1987). Antidepressants increase bioavailability of morphine in cancer patients (Letter to the Editor). Lancet, 1, 1204.

Visintainer, M., & Wolfer, J. (1975). Psychological preparation for surgical pediatric patients: The effects on children's and parents'stress responses and adjustment. Pediatrics, 56, 187-202.

Voshall, B. (1980). The effects of preoperative teaching on postoperative pain. Topics in Clinical Nursing, 2, 39-43.

Wall, P.D. (1988). The prevention of postoperative pain. Pain, 33, 289-290.

Warfield, C., Stein, J., & Frank, H. (1985). The effect of transcutaneous electrical nerve stimulation on pain after thoracotomy. The Annals of Thoracic Surgery, 39, 462-465.

Wasylak, T.J., Abbott, F.V., English, M.J., & Jeans, M.E. (1990). Reduction of post-operative morbidity following patient-controlled morphine. Canadian Journal of Anaesthesia, 37, 726-731.

Wattwil, M. (1989). Postoperative pain relief and gastrointestinal motility. Acta Chiurgica Scandinavica, 550 (Suppl), 140-145.

Way, W.L., Costley, E.C., & Way, E.L. (1965). Respiratory sensitivity of the newborn infant to meperidine and morphine. Clinical Pharmacology and Therapeutics, 6, 454-461.

Weekes, D., & Savedra, M. (1988). Adolescent cancer: Coping with treatment-related pain. Journal of Pediatric Nursing, 3, 318-328.

Weissman, D.E., & Haddox, J.D. (1989). Opioid pseudoaddiction: An iatrogenic syndrome. Pain, 36, 363-366.

Wells, N. (1982). The effect of relaxation on postoperative muscle tension and pain. Nursing Research, 31, 236-238.

Wigram, J.R., Lewith, G.T., Machin, D., & Church, J.J. (1986). Electroacupuncture for postoperative pain. Physiotherapy Practice, 2, 83-88.

Wolfer, J., & Visintainer, M. (1979). Prehospital psychological preparation for tonsillectomy patients: Effects on children's and parents' adjustment. Pediatrics, 64, 646-655.

Wood, M.M., & Cousins, M.J. (1989). Iatrogenic neurotoxicity in cancer patients. Pain, 39, 1-3.

Woolf, C.J., & Wall, P.D. (1986). Morphine-sensitive and morphine-insensitive actions of C-fibre input on the rat spinal cord. Neuroscience Letters, 64, 221-225.

Yaster, M. (1987). The dose response of fentanyl in neonatal anesthesia. Anesthesiology, 66, 433-435.

Acute Pain Management: Operative or Medical Procedures

Zeltzer, L.K., Altman, A., Cohen, D., LeBaron, S., Maunuksela, E.L., & Schechter, N.L. (1990). American Academy of Pediatrics: Report of the Subcommittee on Management of Pain Associated with Procedures in Children with Cancer. Pediatrics, 86, Suppl. 5, 826-831.

Zeltzer, L.K., Jay, S.M., & Fisher, D.M. (1989). The management of pain associated with pediatric procedures. Pediatric Clinics of North America, 36, 941-964.

Zeltzer, L., & LeBaron, S. (1982). Hypnosis and nonhypnotic techniques for reduction of pain and anxiety during painful procedures in children and adolescents with cancer. Journal of Pediatrics, 101, 1032-1035.

Glossary

General Terms

AHCPR: Agency for Health Care Policy and Research; Federal agency established in 1989.

Best evidence synthesis: Evidence based on the best evidence principle as used in law, in which the same evidence that would be essential in one case might be disregarded in a second case because better evidence becomes available.

Case study design: A nonexperimental study that extensively explores a single unit (a unit may be a person, family, or group) or a very small number of units.

Descriptive study: A nonexperimental study in which variables or subject characteristics are examined as they naturally occur for the purpose of describing or comparing samples or examining relationships among a set of variables.

Experimental study: (Randomized controlled trial or randomized clinical trial) An experiment that uses random assignment to create treatment and control groups so that changes can be inferred or attributed to the experimental treatment.

Meta-analysis: The process of combining the results of several related studies to obtain more reliable conclusions.

Peer review: Evaluation of the present guideline document by an interdisciplinary panel of experts using the Institute of Medicine (Field and Lohr, 1990) attributes of clinical practice guidelines as evaluation criteria.

Pilot review: Review and testing of the present guideline by clinicians to evaluate aspects of the guideline such as clarity, clinical applicability, flexibility, resource utilization, training needs, and cost of guideline implementation. Review of a consumer version of the present guideline by consumers and clinicians to evaluate its clarity, usefulness, flexibility, and accuracy.

Quasi-experimental study: (Includes nonrandomized controlled trial or nonrandomized clinical trial) A design that does not use random assignment to create treatment and control groups but uses other methods to control validity threats so that changes can be inferred or attributed to the experimental treatment.

Scientific review: An exhaustive literature search to define and critically evaluate the knowledge base for pain assessment and interventions.

Pain Physiology

Anxiolysis: Sedation or hypnosis used to reduce anxiety, agitation, or tension.

Neuropathic pain: Pain that arises from a damaged nerve.

Nociception: The process of pain transmission; usually relating to a receptive neuron for painful sensations.

Pain: An unpleasant sensory and emotional experience associated with actual or potential tissue damage or described in terms of such damage.

Pain threshold level: The level of intensity at which pain becomes appreciable or perceptible.

Non-pharmacologic Management

Acupuncture: The piercing of specific body sites with needles to produce pain relief.

Counterirritant: An agent that is applied to produce irritation at one site so as to decrease perception of pain at the same or a distant site.

Cryoanalgesia: The destruction of peripheral nerves by extreme cold to achieve prolonged pain relief.

Cryotherapy: The therapeutic use of cold to reduce discomfort, limit progression of tissue edema, or break a cycle of muscle spasm.

Patient education: Providing the patient with an explanation of perioperative procedures, expected postoperative sensations, and instruction to help decrease mobility-related discomfort.

Relaxation methods: A variety of techniques to help decrease anxiety and muscle tension; these may include imagery, distraction, and progressive muscle relaxation.

Acute Pain Management: Operative or Medical Procedures

Tactile strategies: Strategies that provide comfort through the sense of touch, such as stroking or massage.

TENS (transcutaneous electrical nerve stimulation): A method of producing electroanalgesia through electrodes applied to the skin.

Pain Assessment

Conscious sedation: "Light sedation" during which the patient retains airway reflexes and responses to verbal stimuli.

Oximetry: Determination of the oxygen saturation of arterial blood, typically by means of an external probe applied around a finger or toe.

Paradoxical reaction: A response (e.g., to a drug) that is the opposite of the usual response, such as agitation produced in a individual patient by a drug normally considered to be a sedative.

Pharmacologic Management

EMLA (eutectic mixture of local anesthetic): An ointment that contains local anesthetics so that topical application causes local anesthesia without the need for injection.

Epidural: Situated within the spinal canal, on or outside the dura mater (tough membrane surrounding the spinal cord); synonyms are "extradural" and "peridural."

Equianalgesic: Having equal pain killing effect; for example, morphine sulfate 10 mg intramuscular is generally used for opioid analgesic comparisons.

Interpleural: Situated between the membrane surrounding the lungs and the membrane lining the thoracic cavity.

Intrathecal: Within a sheath (e.g., cerebrospinal fluid that is contained within the dura mater).

Local nerve block: Infiltration of a local anesthetic around a peripheral nerve so as to produce anesthesia in the area supplied by the nerve.

Mixed opioid agonist-antagonist: A compound that has an affinity for two or more types of opioid receptors and blocks opioid effects on one receptor type while producing opioid effects on a second receptor type.

NSAID (nonsteroidal anti-inflammatory drug): Aspirin-like drug that reduces pain and inflammation arising from injured tissue.

Opioid agonist: Any morphine-like compound that produces bodily effects including pain relief, sedation, constipation, and respiratory depression.

Opioid partial agonist: A compound that has an affinity for and stimulates physiological activity at the same cell receptors as opioid agonists but that produces only a partial (i.e., submaximal) bodily response.

PCA (patient controlled analgesia): Self-administration of an analgesic by a patient instructed in doing so; usually refers to self-dosing with intravenous opioid (e.g., morphine) administered by means of a programmable pump.

Peridural: Synonym for epidural and extradural.

Perineural: Surrounding a nerve.

References

Cook, T.D. & Campbell, D.T. (1979). *Quasi-experimentation: Design and analysis issues for field settings*. Chicago: Rand McNally College Publishing Co.

Field, M.D. & Loh, K.N. (Eds.). (1990). *Clinical practice guidelines: Directions for a new program*. Committee to Advise the Public Health Service on Clinical Practice Guidelines, Institute of Medicine. Washington: National Academy Press.

International Association for the Study of Pain. (1979). *Pain terms: A list with definitions and notes on usage*. Pain, 6, 249.

Appendix A: Methods Used to Develop Clinical Practice Guideline

Three processes were used for the development of the guideline. First was an extensive interdisciplinary clinical review of current needs, therapeutic practices and principles, and emerging technologies for postoperative pain control. This process included review of all pertinent guidelines and standards, receipt of information and opinion from external consultants, a commissioned paper on the ethical aspects of postoperative pain management, an open forum to receive input from concerned parties, and extensive discussion among the panel members.

The second process was a comprehensive review of published research on management of acute postoperative pain and, to a lesser extent, pain associated with trauma and procedure-induced pain. The panel determined that the review should include research related to

Acute Pain Management: Operative or Medical Procedures

pain assessment and both pharmacologic and non-pharmacologic treatments. The panel was particularly interested in the effects of the interventions on pain, complications, patient satisfaction, length of stay, and treatment costs.

Articles selected for review were (1) published empirical studies of pain in adults and children after elective and nonelective surgery, pain associated with diagnostic and treatment procedures, and pain associated with post-traumatic injuries and burns; (2) research based articles on measurement and assessment of pain; (3) pain management guidelines; and (4) review articles.

Articles excluded from review included: reports of animal studies and surgical interventions outside the scope of interventions accessible to specialized pain treatment teams or primary caregivers, studies of chronic benign or malignant pain except when also relevant to postoperative or procedural pain, studies comparing within-class analgesic potencies, descriptions of basic pain mechanisms except where specific clinical interventions were tested, editorials and commentaries, discussions of the etiology of pain, studies written in non-English languages, discussions of psychological characteristics, and pure dose-efficacy studies.

The literature review was done at sites in Boston (Harvard University and Massachusetts General Hospital), Baltimore (University of Maryland and The Johns Hopkins University), and Denver (University of Colorado). A group at the School of Public Health, Harvard University performed meta-analyses of drug and TENS studies. Non-drug studies were reviewed at the Baltimore and Denver sites.

The search strategy was developed in conjunction with the National Library of Medicine (NLM). Twelve databases were searched, producing a list of approximately 2,400 drug citations and 2,750 non-drug citations; additional citations were retrieved through other sources, for example another 4,314 non-drug and pain assessment citations and 42 drug citations were obtained from bibliographies of review articles, annotated bibliographies, and the like. From these, approximately 600 drug studies and 500 non-drug articles were reviewed and coded for analysis. Using a best evidence synthesis, the research relevant to particular aspects of pain management was summarized and analyzed. Best- evidence synthesis is based on the best-evidence principle as used in law, in which the same evidence that would be essential in one case might be disregarded in another because better evidence is available (Slavin, 1986). When possible, meta-analyses were performed on the randomized controlled trials. The evidence used for recommendations regarding various interventions in adults is summarized in appendix B (Summary Table of Scientific Evidence for Interventions to Manage Pain in Adults). The table includes the intervention, the type of evidence, and comments regarding use of the intervention.

The third process was peer review of drafts of the guideline and pilot review with intended users. Thirty-three experts in various aspects of pain management reviewed and commented on an early draft of the guideline, using as a framework for their evaluation the attributes of clinical practice guidelines developed by the Institute of Medicine (IOM) of the National Academy of Sciences (Field and Lohr, 1990). Nine additional experts in pain management or practice guideline development reviewed a later draft, using the IOM attributes of guidelines and methods suggested by the Agency for Health Care Policy and Research (AHCPR). Nine additional experts in pain management in children reviewed the section of the guideline on neonates, infants, and children. Pilot review of a later draft was done with physicians, nurses, and others (n = 151) involved in pain management at 15 clinical sites. They reviewed and commented on the clarity, clinical applicability, flexibility, resources or training needed to implement the guideline, and cost implications of the guideline if implemented. A consumer version was developed and tested in clinical sites with 54 patients and 62 nurses and physicians, who reviewed it for clarity and accuracy.

Health policy issues related to ethical, economic, and legal aspects of postoperative pain management were addressed by the panel in several ways. A paper was commissioned on the ethical aspects of postoperative pain management, and the legal implications of pain management were addressed through the limited information available in the literature.

The entire process was anchored by an interdisciplinary panel of experts who used an integrated approach to synthesize the scientific evidence with the knowledge of experts to develop the guideline. Prior to printing of this guidance, drug dosage tables were reviewed by the U.S. Food and Drug Administration. The panel recommends that the guideline be updated 2 years after its publication.

References

Field, M.D. & Lohr, K.N. (Eds). (1990). *Clinical Practice Guidelines: Directions for a New Program*. Committee to Advise the Public Health Service on Clinical Practice Guidelines, Institute of Medicine. Washington: National Academy Press.

Slavin, R.E. (1986). Best-evidence synthesis: An alternative to meta-analytic and traditional reviews. *Educational Researcher*, 15, 5-11.

Appendix B: Summary Table of Scientific Evidence for Interventions to Manage Pain in Adults

Type of Evidence Key

[Applies to Table 32.2 and Table 32.3 on pages 368-370]

Ia: Evidence obtained from meta-analysis of randomized controlled trials.
b: Evidence obtained from at least one randomized controlled trial.

IIa: Evidence obtained from at least one well-designed controlled study without randomization.
b: Evidence obtained from at least one other type of well-designed quasi-experimental study.

III: Evidence obtained from well-designed non-experimental studies, such as comparative studies, correlational studies, and case studies.

IV: Evidence obtained from expert committee reports or opinions and/or clinical experiences of respected authorities.

Table 32.2.B1. Pharmacologic Interventions

Intervention[1]		Type of Evidence[2]	Comments
NSAIDs	Oral (alone)	Ib, IV	Effective for mild to moderate pain. Begin preoperatively. Relatively contraindicated in patients with renal disease and risk of or actual coagulopathy. May mask fever.
	Oral (adjunct to opioid)	Ia, IV	Potentiating effect resulting in opioid sparing. Begin pre-op. Cautions as above.
	Parenteral (ketorolac)	Ib, IV	Effective for moderate to severe pain. Expensive. Useful where opioids contraindicated, especially to avoid respiratory depression and sedation. Advance to opioid.
Opioids	Oral	IV	As effective as parenteral in appropriate doses. Use as soon as oral medication tolerated. Route of choice.
	Intra-muscular	Ib, IV	Has been the standard parenteral route, but injections painful and absorption unreliable. Hence, avoid this route when possible.
	Sub-cutaneous	Ib, IV	Preferable to intramuscular when a low-volume continuous infusion is needed and intravenous access is difficult to maintain. Injections painful and absorption unreliable. Avoid this route for long-term repetitive dosing.
	Intravenous	Ib, IV	Parenteral route of choice after major surgery. Suitable for titrated bolus or continuous administration (including PCA), but requires monitoring. Significant risk of respiratory depression with inappropriate dosing.

Acute Pain Management: Operative or Medical Procedures

Intervention[1]		Type of Evidence[2]	Comments
Opioids	PCA (systemic)	Ia, IV	Intravenous or subcutaneous routes recommended. Good steady level of analgesia. Popular with patients but requires special infusion pumps and staff education. See cautions about opioids above.
	Epidural & intrathecal	Ia, IV	When suitable, provides good analgesia. Significant risk of respiratory depression, sometimes delayed in onset. Requires careful monitoring. Use of infusion pumps requires additional equipment and staff education. Expensive if infusion pumps are employed.
Local anesthetics	Epidural & intrathecal	Ia, IV	Limited indications. Effective regional analgesia. Opioid sparing. Addition of opioid to local anesthetic may improve analgesia. Risks of hypotension, weakness, numbness. Requires careful monitoring. Use of infusion pump requires additional equipment and staff education.
	Peripheral nerve block	Ia, IV	Limited indications and duration of action. Effective regional analgesia. Opioid sparing.

1. Selected references are included in this Clinical Practice Guideline. More complete references are available; see Acute Pain Management Guideline Panel. *Acute Pain Management: Operative or Medical Procedures and Trauma. Guideline Report*. AHCPR Pub. No. 92-0022. Rockville, MD: Agency for Health Care Policy and Research, Public Health Service, U.S. Department of Health and Human Services. In press.

2. See type of evidence key on page 367.

Table 32.3.B2. *Non-pharmacologic Interventions. [Type of Evidence Key is on page 367.]*

Intervention[1]		Type of Evidence[2]	Comments
Simple relaxation (begin preoperatively)	Jaw relaxation Progressive muscle relaxation Simple imagery	Ia, IIa, IIb, IV	Effective in reducing mild to moderate pain and as an adjunct to analgesic drugs for severe pain. Use when patients express an interest in relaxation. Requires 3-5 minutes of staff time for instructions.
	Music	Ib, IIa, IV	Both patient-preferred and "easy listening" music are effective in reducing mild to moderate pain.
Complex relaxation (begin preoperatively)	Biofeedback	Ib, IIa, IIb, IV	Effective in reducing mild to moderate pain and operative site muscle tension. Requires skilled personnel and special equipment.
	Imagery	Ib, IIa, IV	Effective for reduction of mild to moderate pain. Requires skilled personnel.
Education/instruction (begin preoperatively)		Ia, IIa, IIb, IV	Effective for reduction of pain. Should include sensory and procedural information and instruction aimed at reducing activity related pain. Requires 5-15 minutes of staff time.
TENS		Ia, IIa, III, IV	Effective in reducing pain and improving physical function. Requires skilled personnel and special equipment. May be useful as an adjunct to drug therapy.

Acute Pain Management: Operative or Medical Procedures

Notes to Table 32.3.

1. Selected references are included in this Clinical Practice Guideline. For more complete references, see: Acute Pain Management Guideline Panel. *Acute Pain Management: Operative or Medical Procedures and Trauma. Guideline Report.* AHCPR Pub. No. 92-0022. Rockville, MD: Agency for Health Care Policy and Research, Public Health Service, U.S. Department of Health and Human Services. In press.

2. Insufficient scientific evidence is available to provide specific recommendations regarding the use of hypnosis, acupuncture, and other physical modalities for relief of postoperative pain.

Appendix C: Dosage Tables for Adult and Pediatric Patients

Table 32.4.C1. Dosing Data for NSAIDs

Drug	Usual adult dose	Usual pediatric dose [1]	Comments
Oral NSAIDs			
Acetaminophen	650–975 mg q 4 hr	10–15 mg/kg q 4 hr	Acetaminophen lacks the peripheral anti-inflammatory activity of other NSAIDs
Aspirin	650–975 mg q 4 hr	10–15 mg/kg q 4 hr [2]	The standard against which other NSAIDs are compared. Inhibits platelet aggregation; may cause postoperative bleeding
Choline magnesium trisalicylate (Trilisate)	1000–1500 mg bid	25 mg/kg bid	May have minimal antiplatelet activity; also available as oral liquid
Diflunisal (Dolobid)	1000 mg initial dose followed by 500 mg q 12 hr		
Etodolac (Lodine)	200–400 mg q 6–8 hr		
Fenoprofen calcium (Nalfon)	200 mg q 4–6 hr		
Ibuprofen (Motrin, others)	400 mg q 4–6 hr	10 mg/kg q 6–8 hr	Available as several brand names and as generic; also available as oral suspension
Ketoprofen (Orudis)	25–75 mg q 6–8 hr		
Magnesium salicylate	650 mg q 4 hr		Many brands and generic forms available

Acute Pain Management: Operative or Medical Procedures

Drug	Usual adult dose	Usual pediatric dose[1]	Comments
Oral NSAIDs			
Meclofenamate sodium (Meclomen)	50 mg q 4–6 hr		
Mefenamic acid (Ponstel)	250 mg q 6 hr		
Naproxen (Naprosyn)	500 mg initial dose followed by 250 mg q 6–8 hr	5 mg/kg q 12 hr	Also available as oral liquid
Naproxen sodium (Anaprox)	550 mg initial dose followed by 275 mg q 6–8 hr		
Salsalate (Disalcid, others)	500 mg q 4 hr		May have minimal antiplatelet activity
Sodium salicylate	325–650 mg q 3–4 hr		Available in generic form from several distributors

Drug	Usual adult dose	Usual pediatric dose[1]	Comments
Parenteral NSAID			
Ketorolac	30 or 60 mg IM initial dose followed by 15 or 30 mg q 6 hr Oral dose following IM dosage: 10 mg q 6–8 hr		Intramuscular dose not to exceed 5 days

Note: Only the above NSAIDs have FDA approval for use as simple analgesics, but clinical experience has been gained with other drugs as well.

1. Drug recommendations are limited to NSAIDs where pediatric dosing experience is available.
2. Contraindicated in presence of fever or other evidence of viral illness.

Table 32.5.C2. Dosing Data for Opioid Analgesics

Drug	Approximate equianalgesic oral dose	Approximate equianalgesic parenteral dose
Opioid Agonist		
Morphine[2]	30 mg q 3–4 hr (around-the-clock dosing)	10 mg q 3–4 hr
	60 mg q 3–4 hr (single dose or intermittent dosing)	
Codeine[3]	130 mg q 3–4 hr	75 mg q 3–4 hr
Hydromophone[2] (Dilaudid)	7.5 mg q 3–4 hr	1.5 mg q 3–4 hr
Hydrocodone (in Lorcet, Lortab, Vicodin, others)	30 mg q 3–4 hr	Not available
Levorphanol (Levo-Dromoran)	4 mg q 6–8 hr	2 mg q 6–8 hr
Meperidine (Demerol)	300 mg q 2–3 hr	100 mg q 3 hr
Methadone (Dolophine, others)	20 mg q 6–8 hr	10 mg q 6–8 hr
Oxycodone (Roxicodone, also in Percocet, Percodan, Tylox, others)	30 mg q 3–4 hr	Not available
Oxymorphone[2] (Numorphan)	Not available	1 mg q 3–4 hr
Opioid Agonist-Antagonist and Partial Agonist		
Buprenorphine (Buprenex)	Not available	0.3–0.4 mg q 6–8 hr
Butorphanol (Stadol)	Not available	2 mg q 3–4 hr
Nalbuphine (Nubain)	Not available	10 mg q 3–4 hr
Pentazocine (Talwin, others)	150 mg q 3–4 hr	60 mg q 3–4 hr

Note: Published tables vary in the suggested doses that are equianalgesic to morphine. Clinical response is the criterion that must be applied for each patient; titration to clinical response is necessary. Because there is not complete cross tolerance among these drugs, it is usually necessary to use a lower than equianalgesic dose when changing drugs and to retitrate to response.

Caution: Recommended doses do not apply to patients with renal or hepatic insufficiency or other conditions affecting drug metabolism and kinetics.

[1] **Caution:** Doses listed for patients with body weight less than 50 kg cannot be used as initial starting doses in babies less than 6 months of age. Consult the *Clinical Practice Guideline for Acute Pain Management: Operative or Medical Procedures and Trauma* section on management of pain in neonates for recommendations.

Acute Pain Management: Operative or Medical Procedures

Recommended starting dose (adults more than 50 kg body weight) oral	parenteral	Recommended starting dose (children and adults less than 50 kg body weight)[1] oral	parenteral
30 mg q 3–4 hr	10 mg q 3–4 hr	0.3 mg/kg q 3–4 hr	0.1 mg/kg q 3–4 hr
60 mg q 3–4 hr	60 mg q 2 hr (intramuscular/ subcutaneous)	1 mg/kg q 3–4 hr[4]	Not recommended
6 mg q 3–4 hr	1.5 mg q 3–4 hr	0.06 mg/kg q 3–4 hr	0.015 mg/kg q 3–4 hr
10 mg q 3–4 hr	Not available	0.2 mg/kg q 3–4 hr[4]	Not available
4 mg q 6–8 hr	2 mg q 6–8 hr	0.04 mg/kg q 6–8 hr	0.02 mg/kg q 6–8 hr
Not recommended	100 mg q 3 hr	Not recommended	0.75 mg/kg q 2–3 hr
20 mg q 6–8 hr	10 mg q 6–8 hr	0.2 mg/kg q 6–8 hr	0.1 mg/kg q 6–8 hr
10 mg q 3–4 hr	Not available	0.2 mg/kg q 3–4 hr[4]	Not available
Not available	1 mg q 3-4 hr	Not recommended	Not recommended
Not available	0.4 mg q 6–8 hr	Not available	0.004 mg/kg q 6–8 hr
Not available	2 mg q 3–4 hr	Not available	Not recommended
Not available	10 mg q 3–4 hr	Not available	0.1 mg/kg q 3–4 hr
50 mg q 4–6 hr	Not recommended	Not recommended	Not recommended

[2] For morphine, hydromorphone, and oxymorphone, rectal administration is an alternate route for patients unable to take oral medications, but equianalgesic doses may differ from oral and parenteral doses because of pharmacokinetic differences.

[3] **Caution:** Codeine doses above 65 mg often are not appropriate due to diminishing incremental analgesia with increasing doses but continually increasing constipation and other side effects.

[4] **Caution:** Doses of aspirin and acetaminophen in combination opioid/NSAID preparations must also be adjusted to the patient's body weight.

Appendix D: *Pain Assessment Tools*

Examples of Pain Intensity and Pain Distress Scales

Simple Descriptive Pain Intensity Scale*

|—————|—————|—————|—————|—————|
No pain / Mild pain / Moderate pain / Severe pain / Very severe pain / Worst possible pain

0 - 10 Numeric Pain Intensity Scale*

0 1 2 3 4 5 6 7 8 9 10
No pain — Moderate pain — Worst possible pain

Visual Analog Scale (VAS)**

No pain ——————————————— Pain as bad as it could possibly be

*If used as a graphic rating scale, a 10-cm baseline is recommended.
**A 10-cm baseline is recommended for VAS scales.

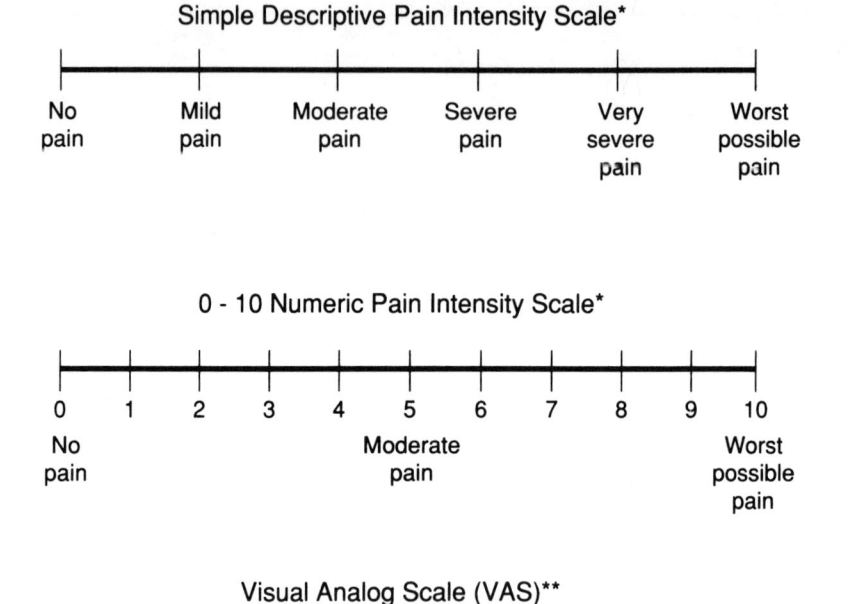

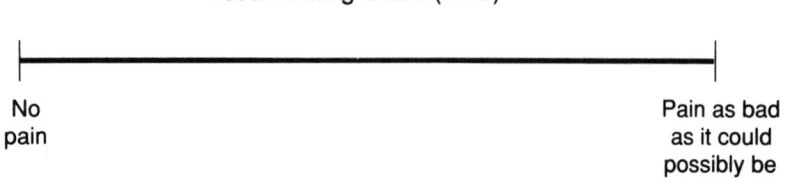

Figure 32.3. *Pain Intensity Scales*

Acute Pain Management: Operative or Medical Procedures

Simple Descriptive Pain Distress Scale*

None — Annoying — Uncomfortable — Dreadful — Horrible — Agonizing

0 - 10 Numeric Pain Distress Scale*

0 1 2 3 4 5 6 7 8 9 10
No pain   Distressing pain   Unbearable pain

Visual Analog Scale (VAS)**

No distress — Unbearable distress

*If used as a graphic rating scale, a 10-cm baseline is recommended.
**A 10-cm baseline is recommended for VAS scales.

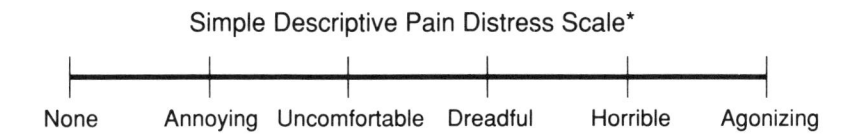

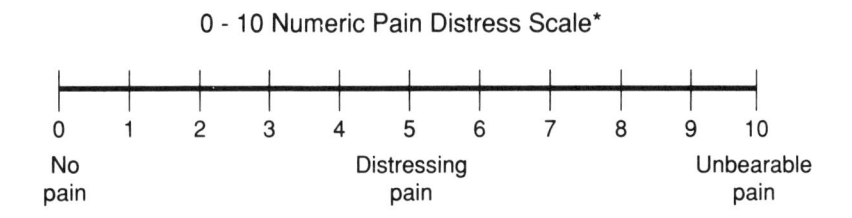

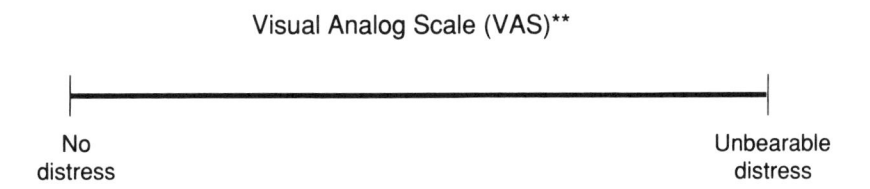

Figure 32.4. D1 Pain Distress Scales

Figure 32.5.D2. Initial Pain Assessment Tool

Date _____

Patient's Name _____ Age _____ Room _____

Diagnosis _____ Physician _____

Nurse _____

I. Location: Patient or nurse mark drawing.

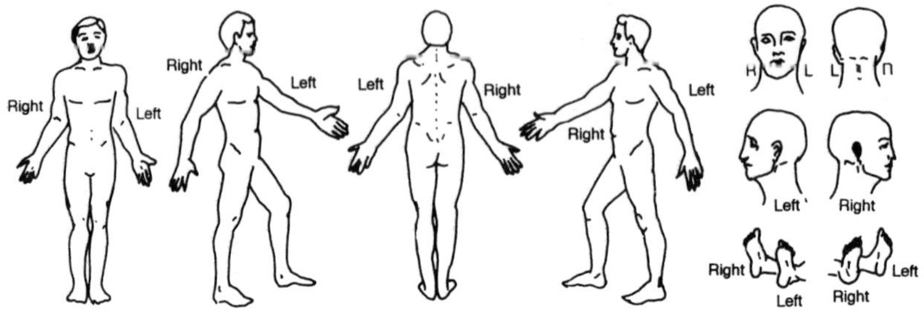

II. Intensity: Patient rates the pain. Scale used _____
   Present: _____
   Worst pain gets: _____
   Best pain gets: _____
   Acceptable level of pain: _____

III. Quality: (Use patient's own words, e.g. prick, ache, burn, throb, pull, sharp) _____

IV. Onset, duration variations, rhythms: _____

V. Manner of expressing pain: _____

VI. What relieves the pain? _____

VII. What causes or increases the pain? _____

VIII. Effects of pain: (Note decreased function, decreased quality of life.)
   Accompanying symptoms (e.g. nausea) _____
   Sleep _____
   Appetite _____
   Physical activity _____
   Relationship with others (e.g. irritability) _____
   Emotions (e.g. anger, suicidal, crying) _____
   Concentration _____
   Other _____

IX. Other comments: _____

X. Plan: _____

■ May be duplicated for use in clinical practice. Used with permission from McCaffery, M. and Beeebe, A. *Pain: Clinical Manual for Nursing Practice.* (1989), St. Louis: C.V. Mosby

Acute Pain Management: Operative or Medical Procedures

Figure 32.6.D3. Flow Sheet—Pain

Patient _____ Date _____

* Pain rating scale used _____

Purpose: to evaluate the safety and effectiveness of the analgesic(s).

Analgesic(s) prescribed: _____

Time	Pain rating	Analgesic	R	P	BP	Level of arousal	Other†	Plan & comments

* *Pain rating*: A number of different scales may be used. Indicate which scale is used and use the same one each time. For example, 0-10 (0 = no pain, 10 = worst pain).

† *Possibilities for other columns*: bowel function, activities, nausea and vomiting, other pain relief measures. Identify the side effects of greatest concern to patient, family, physician, and nurses.

■ May be duplicated for use in clinical practice. Used with permission from McCaffery, M. and Beeebe, A. *Pain: Clinical Manual for Nursing Practice*. (1989). St. Louis: C.V. Mosby

Other assessment tools are included in the original text including "Pain History for Pediatric Patients," "Poker Chip Tool Instructions (English and Spanish)," "Word-Graphic Rating Scale," and "Pain Interview for Pediatric Patients."

Appendix E: Relaxation Exercises

Example 1: Deep Breath/Tense, Exhale/Relax, Yawn for Quick Relaxation

1. Clench your fists; breathe in deeply and hold it a moment.
2. Breathe out slowly and go limp as a rag doll.
3. Start yawning.

Additional points: Yawning becomes spontaneous. It is also contagious, so others may begin yawning and relaxing too.

Example 2: Slow Rhythmic Breathing for Relaxation

1. Breathe in slowly and deeply.
2. As you breathe out slowly, feel yourself beginning to relax; feel the tension leaving your body.
3. Now breathe in and out slowly and regularly, at whatever rate is comfortable for you. You may wish to try abdominal breathing. If you do not know how to do abdominal breathing, ask your nurse for help.
4. To help you focus on your breathing and breathe slowly and rhythmically: Breathe in as you say silently to yourself, "in, two, three." Breathe out as you say silently to yourself, "out, two, three," or each time you breathe out, say silently to yourself a word such as peace or relax.
5. You may imagine that you are doing this in a place you have found very calming and relaxing for you, such as lying in the sun at the beach.
6. Do steps 1 through 4 only once or repeat steps 3 and 4 for up to 20 minutes.
7. End with a slow deep breath. As you breathe out say to yourself "I feel alert and relaxed."

Additional points: If you intend to do this for more than a few seconds, try to get in a comfortable position in a quiet environment, you may close your eyes or focus on an object. This technique has the advantage of being very adaptable in that it may be used for only a few seconds or for up to 20 minutes.

Acute Pain Management: Operative or Medical Procedures

Example 3: Peaceful Past

Something may have happened to you a while ago that brought you peace and comfort. You may be able to draw on that past experience to bring you peace or comfort now. Think about these questions:

1. Can you remember any situation, even when you were a child, when you felt calm, peaceful, secure, hopeful, comfortable?
2. Have you ever daydreamed about something peaceful? What were you thinking of?
3. Do you get a dreamy feeling when you listen to music? Do you have any favorite music?
4. Do you have any favorite poetry that you find uplifting or reassuring?
5. Have you ever been religiously active? Do you have favorite readings, hymns, or prayers? Even if you haven't heard or thought of them for many years, childhood religious experiences may still be very soothing.

Additional points: Very likely some of the things you think of in answer to these questions can be recorded for you, such as your favorite music or a prayer. Then you can listen to the tape whenever you wish. Or, if your memory is strong, you may simply close your eyes and recall the events or words.

Adapted with permission from McCaffery, M. & Beebe, A. (1989). *Pain: Clinical manual for nursing practice*. St. Louis: CV Mosby.

Chapter 33

Pains Following an Amputation

An amputation, like any surgical procedure, will cause postoperative pain. However, most people describe the amputation pain as being less than what they expected.

You may have a **patient controlled analgesia machine** (PCA) when you return to your room. This machine allows you to control the amount of pain medication you receive. If you don't have a PCA, other pain medicine will be available upon request from your nurse.

Phantom Sensations

Nearly every amputee experiences the sensation that the amputated part is still present. You may have feelings of tingling, itching, or movement where your arm or leg used to be. Phantom sensations may occur immediately after surgery or any time thereafter. A variety of factors can stimulate these sensations—pressure applied to the residual limb, yawning, or even weather changes. Sometimes the sensation may feel like it is moving closer to the site of the amputation, and then soon disappear completely. While phantom sensations are different for everyone, they usually present no problems.

Phantom Pain

In addition to phantom sensations, some people experience various types of pain in the missing limb. Phantom pain is often described

©1991 Department of Prosthetics & Orthotics, Duke University Medical Center. Reprinted with permission.

as fleeting episodes of sharp, squeezing, burning, or "electric shock" sensations either within the residual limb or the missing limb.

While the causes of phantom pain are not clearly understood, some factors are thought to contribute to it—for instance, the presence of persistent pain in the affected limb prior to the amputation. Residual limb complications (like infection) and emotional distress may also trigger episodes of phantom pain.

Because phantom pain occurs unpredictably, it is important to let your physician or nurse know if you are experiencing it so that they can recommend ways to manage it. Gentle massages, certain medications, the application of warmth, or an electrical stimulation unit placed on the skin are among the methods used to help relieve phantom pain. Most occurrences of phantom pain disappear within a few weeks after surgery.

Common Feelings after Surgery: An Emotional Whirlwind!

Having an amputation is difficult for anyone at any age. Losing a limb can threaten your feelings of self-worth and your physical capabilities. Most new amputees are filled with feelings and questions concerning:

- **Appearance:** "What will I look like?"...with or without the prosthesis.
- **Physical Abilities:** "What will I be able to do?"
- **Social Acceptance:** "What will other people think about me?"
- **Finances:** "How can I afford all this?"...related to the cost of health care, the prosthesis, and employment changes.

In addition to all these concerns, losing a limb creates a variety of grief responses. People experience feelings of numbness and disbelief—"I can't believe this is really happening to me!" Some feel anger and resentment—"Why ME?" Others feel extreme sadness over the loss and fear the uncertainty of their future. All of these emotions are normal responses to having an amputation. It is important for you and/or your family members to talk about these feelings and concerns with someone (your physician, nurse, social worker, or minister) who can help you sort through them.

Receiving detailed explanations and having your questions answered about the surgery and rehabilitation process will also enable you to regain a sense of emotional balance and begin your life as an amputee.

Chapter 34

Anesthesia: Safer and More Choices

General Anesthesia: Advances Increase Safety

"What if I don't wake up?"

That's a common fear for anyone facing surgery that requires general anesthesia.

But it's a fear with little basis in fact. Serious complications almost never occur in the absence of a pre-existing medical problem. Experts estimate it's safer to have general anesthesia than to ride in a car.

Anesthesia is 10 times safer than it was in the 1970s—100 times safer than in 1955. Fast-acting medications, new monitoring devices plus higher safety standards for their use are credited with reducing complications and accidental deaths during general anesthesia.

Newer Fast-acting Drugs

The type of anesthesia you receive during surgery depends on the procedure and your general health. Some reactions to certain anesthetics are hereditary and may also determine the type of drug used.

Anesthetics are delivered by inhaling the drugs through a mask or by intravenous injection. The drugs circulate throughout your

---

©1995 Reprinted from March 1995 *Mayo Clinic Health Letter* with permission of Mayo Foundation for Medical Education and Research, Rochester, Minnesota 55905. For subscription information, please call 1-800-333-9038. Reprinted with permission.

bloodstream to all areas of your body, including your brain, and cause loss of consciousness.

Anesthetics also control pain and relax muscles by interfering with transmitters in your nervous system.

Traditionally, general anesthetics had unpleasant side effects such as nausea or vomiting after surgery. As outpatient surgery has evolved, new anesthesia drugs have appeared that act faster and are less likely to cause nausea and prolonged drowsiness.

Some newer drugs allow members of the anesthesia team to more accurately adjust the doses of the drugs throughout the procedure. This means you awaken sooner after surgery with less residual effect of the anesthetics.

Better Safety Checks

Within the last decade, the American Society of Anesthesiologists has set a variety of standards for practice. The standards include a requirement that qualified members of the anesthesia team be present throughout a procedure involving use of anesthesia.

Standards also specify continually monitoring oxygen levels, breathing, circulation, heart rate, blood pressure, temperature and anesthetic administration throughout a procedure.

Standards extend to the use of new equipment that monitors your heart and breathing during anesthesia. The monitoring equipment must also pass standards of reliability. Most machines have safety devices to detect mechanical error and monitor medication dosages.

Two new monitoring devices help ensure you get adequate oxygen during anesthesia. Their use has played a major role in making surgery safer:

- **Fingertip readings**. By transmitting a special light through a small device attached to your finger, a pulse oximeter measures and records the amount of oxygen in your blood on a beat-by-beat basis. If your oxygen level drops too low, an alarm sounds.

- **Breath-by-breath monitor.** An end-tidal capnograph measures, analyzes and displays the amount of carbon dioxide in each breath. The display alerts members of the anesthesia team of unexpected changes in breathing.

Anesthesia: Safer and More Choices

Options to "Going Under"

Some operations are best done while you're awake. These include minor surgery or procedures where the doctor may want to monitor your conscious responses.

Two types of anesthesia allow you to stay awake during surgery:

- **Local anesthesia.** You may be most familiar with this type of anesthesia from visits to your dentist. An injection under your skin numbs the site of the operation so you won't feel any pain. You're conscious during the operation and the anesthesia is usually short-lived.

  A catheter may be placed in a vein to give you fluid, sedatives or other medications as needed.

- **Regional anesthesia.** Used to numb just one region of your body, these anesthetics don't cause unconsciousness or significantly affect heart and lung function.

  Spinal, epidural and caudal anesthesia involve injection of a local anesthetic near the spinal cord. They're often used for operations such as hernia repair, pelvic operations and leg and hip surgery.

  Doctors numb arms and legs by injecting a local anesthetic into areas where major nerves pass. Typically, major nerve blocks are used for hand, arm or foot surgery.

  Regional anesthesia also helps control pain after surgery.

Chapter 35

Calming Fears, Easing Pain: Children's Anesthesia Is Tricky

At the age of two, Russ Irvin of Woodbridge, Va., knew what scrub masks and surgical bonnets meant—pain. Diagnosed with a brain tumor as an infant, the child had already endured four surgeries and numerous tests. When he needed a neural shunt removed in the spring of 1989, a nurse and doctor, both wearing scrubs, came to carry him to the operating room.

"He was fine on my lap until he saw them coming," says his mother, Liz Irvin. "He started crying and clinging to me. That was the time I lucked out and got a sensitive anesthesiologist. They gave him a shot, and they let me hold Russ until he was groggy. Other times, they had taken him off crying."

To a small child, pain and fear are inseparable. Relieving both safely with medication can be very tricky. Children often need to be sedated not just to relieve pain, but to hold them still for tedious procedures like drilling cavities or collecting blood samples.

Too much of a drug can harm a child. Too little doesn't work. Too often, there's not much room in between. Pediatric sedation is the subject of growing debate and research in the medical community.

Until recently, there were no anesthetics or sedatives specifically approved by the Food and Drug Administration for use in children. Physicians commonly use adult drugs "off label," a practice that is legal and often necessary in pediatrics. But since doses for children aren't listed on the labels, anesthesiologists rely on their own knowledge and experience to mix drugs for young patients.

FDA Consumer, October 1994.

"There's a whole host of cocktails out there with no FDA approval for children and no testing in children," says Edward D. Miller Jr., M.D., an anesthesiologist at Columbia University and chairman of FDA's advisory committee on anesthetic and life-support drugs.

In an ongoing effort to stimulate research for pediatric drugs, last March the committee met to discuss the issue of pediatric sedation. Miller and other experts met in Rockville, Md., to hear from parents pleading for better and safer pain medications, and from physicians knowledgeable about pediatric sedation.

During the meeting, the committee discussed the drug Oralet (fentanyl). Approved in October 1993 but not yet on the market at press time, Oralet is the first narcotic ever tested in and approved specifically for children.

It is approved for calming children before surgery. Because Oralet is administered by mouth in a hardened candy-like mass on top of a stick, it has acquired the nickname "narcotic lollipop." But it is a far cry from candy.

Oralet contains the powerful narcotic fentanyl, a drug commonly marketed as a skin patch called Duragesic and in several injectable brands. What kids like best about Oralet is that it doesn't require a shot—the most dreaded part of any hospital visit.

But opponents of Oralet fear it will be abused or misused by physicians and doctors, possibly leading to accidental death. Advocates say Oralet will be very useful in easing children's anxiety without needles.

"There is no reason to hurt children any more than we need to," says Charles Cote, M.D., a proponent of Oralet and an anesthesiologist at Children's Memorial Hospital in Chicago and Northwestern University Medical School.

Lack of Research

Research in children's pain relief lags behind that for adults. Side effects from each drug aren't consistently reported, and no one can say for certain what a child's risks are from most painkillers and anesthetics.

As recently as the mid-1980s, some physicians thought infants couldn't feel pain as well as adults because their nervous systems were underdeveloped. Even today some doctors use little or no pain medication because they fear it is unsafe for young children, or that older children might become addicted to it. Plus, they reason, children heal quickly anyway.

Liz Irvin remembers how her son's doctor removed a central venous tube (for delivering chemotherapy to a main vein near his heart) without anesthesia when he was an infant. She recalls, "the surgeon said a baby couldn't feel pain." When Russ was four years old, the same surgeon planned to remove a stomach tube without medication, so his mother mixed Tylenol and Valium for him at home.

"I cleared it with his oncologist first," she says. "It seemed to help." Few parents feel compelled to go to such extremes. But it's difficult to watch a child undergo a painful procedure without any relief.

Research has shown that children are often undermedicated. A study in 1968 showed that only 15 percent of children in a hospital's intensive care unit received any type of narcotic for pain, and only 3 percent received pain medicine after surgery. A 1992 study reported that infants received less than half the number of doses of pain medication that adults did after open heart surgery.

One problem is that children can't describe their pain in words that nurses and doctors understand. Instead, they express it through crying, facial expression, and body movements. Heart rate and breathing also increase when a child is in pain.

Another reason children may be undermedicated is the fear that strong drugs will suppress their breathing. Indeed, FDA has received reports—though rare—of deaths in otherwise healthy children from doses of anesthesia and painkillers.

"Nobody really knows the absolute risk. It's just something you have to be wary of," says Robert Bedford, M.D., an anesthesiologist and medical officer on FDA's pilot drug evaluation staff. The overall risk of a child's dying from anesthesia is estimated to be 1 in 10,000, he says. Doctors recognize the risk to be greater for young children, and much greater for newborn and premature babies, but there are no definite statistics on those risks.

According to FDA's Spontaneous Reporting System (SRS), which collects information on serious reactions to drugs, from 1968 to 1993, there were 133 cases of serious reactions among children who were sedated before undergoing medical procedures or receiving anesthesia.

The reports included a 4-year-old girl who died of drugs given to calm her for a dental procedure, and a 2-year-old boy who died of sedatives given to calm him for a CAT (computed axial tomography) scan.

Because the SRS is voluntary, the data collected cannot be used to determine the absolute risks of any drug. What the SRS can do is signal potential problems.

Calming Helps

The most dangerous time during anesthesia administration is just as the patient is going to sleep. If a frightened toddler is crying hysterically and gagging on a runny nose, it makes anesthesia more risky, Bedford says.

"If you can sedate kids in advance, then they don't seem to care as much what's going on," he says. That's the advantage of Oralet. "Kids doze off, then the doctor can whisk them away for a nice smooth anesthetic induction."

One alternative to Oralet is an oral sedative called Versed (midazolam). Although not approved for use in children, Versed is commonly used to calm them before surgery. Physicians dilute the drug with Tylenol syrup, which is cherry-flavored and a favorite among youngsters.

But some doctors argue that anxiety relief should first be tried without drugs.

"Perioperative stress is a psychological thing, not a painful thing," says Allen J Hinkle, M.D., an anesthesiologist at Dartmouth Medical School and opponent of Oralet.

He urges taking extra time with a child, explaining the procedure if possible, and having a parent come into the operating room, holding the child on his or her lap if necessary. Only when those attempts don't work does he advocate a sedative before anesthesia.

"My experience is that parents like [the drug-free approach] and will do it again," says Hinkle.

Promoting Research

Nevertheless, pediatric drugs are often necessary, and FDA is actively encouraging drug companies to do more research on their products for use in children. The agency has held symposiums, published guidelines on pain relief, and urged drug manufacturers to test new drugs, including those for anesthesia and sedation, in children.

Companies have been hesitant to test pain medications on children for fear of causing harm, says Miller, and parents often dislike entering their children in drug trials. Plus, he says, there's little economic incentive for drug manufacturers to conduct extra tests on drugs if a product is already on the market.

Even so, Miller predicts there will likely be more testing in children in the future.

As for Oralet, few other drugs have been subjected to as stringent a regulated introduction to the market, according to Curtis Wright, M.D., acting director of FDA's pilot drug evaluation staff.

For one year after the drug enters the market, Oralet will only be available in children's hospitals and university teaching hospitals, where the manufacturer can track any side effects. Any child sucking an Oralet

Calming Fears, Easing Pain: Children's Anesthesia Is Tricky

will be watched carefully by a health-care professional and monitored electronically with a pulse oximeter, a device that measures pulse and oxygen levels through the fingertip. After a year, FDA will reevaluate the drug's distribution plan and decide whether it can be used safely in general hospitals.

FDA has been very cautious with the drug, Wright says, holding extra meetings with pediatric anesthesiology experts, and supervising the drug's labeling, advertising and introduction plan.

"The concern with Oralet is that physicians would not identify it as an anesthetic, but as a way to manage pain before a well-baby exam," says Wright.

Fentanyl, the narcotic in Oralet, can cause death if misused. For example, a 17 year-old boy died after having his wisdom teeth out because his dentist gave him a high dose of fentanyl in a Duragesic skin patch to use at home.

Duragesic is approved only for long-term chronic pain, and is not recommended for pain after surgery. The boy's mother testified before FDA that she feared Oralet, too, would be misused with tragic results.

Still another concern about Oralet is its so-called "lollipop" dosage and raspberry flavor.

"By associating a child's popular item like the lollipop with the euphoria of narcotics, we are indeed sending a confusing message to our children," Hinkle warned in a letter to FDA.

"That's something you worry about," says Wright, "but we've made medicine taste like candy for years." Consider cherry-flavored cough drops and Tylenol, or sweet orange-flavored baby aspirin, for example. Even Mary Poppins used a spoonful of sugar to help the medicine go down.

"We all realize the dangers of this drug," says Miller. "But we know about the dangers of many drugs, and we do all we can to make them safe."

"We have prepared as many safeguards for Oralet as any drug ever put out. If physicians will follow those safeguards and use common sense, this will be a very safe drug."

Facing Anesthesia

When a child is facing surgery or a medical procedure requiring sedation, there are a few things parents can do beforehand to help it go smoothly.

First, try to find a doctor, nurse or technician who is patient and understanding with children.

"It really boils down to the patience of the technician," says Jim Kitterman of Damascus, Md., whose 7-year-old son, Ben, was treated for cancer as a preschooler.

"It makes a world of difference if they're patient and understanding with kids," Kitterman says, "even in something as simple as drawing blood."

Parents can also educate themselves about their child's treatment. Liz Irvin discovered, and now demands, newer stomach tubes for her son that aren't painful to replace.

Physicians say it's best to find a hospital where the staff is thoroughly knowledgeable about pediatrics, such as a children's hospital. Then, talk with the anesthesiologist about any procedure that requires sedation.

"Anesthesia is very safe today, and problems are rare," says Miller. "There have been major improvements in monitoring drugs, training doctors, and in the drugs themselves," he adds. "Parents should not worry."

Where's the Boo-boo?

Very young children usually cannot verbalize their pain. Even those old enough to talk have difficulty explaining where it hurts, and whether it's a sharp pain or a dull ache. Infants, especially premature ones, may not always cry when in pain, instead lying quietly as they suffer.

Much research has been done on assessing pain in children, and a few useful methods have evolved. One method is showing the child a scale of faces, progressing from a crying face (severe pain) to a smiling face (no pain). Children as young as three can point to the one that shows how much they hurt.

Other studies have used drawing, number scales, and dolls to help children describe their pain and its location in ways that adults can understand.

No matter the method, children almost always rate their pain higher than doctors or nurses do. And studies have shown that parents almost always assess their child's pain more accurately than do medical personnel.

—by Rebecca D. Williams

Rebecca D. Williams is a writer in Oak Ridge, Tenn.

Part Six

Cancer Pain

Chapter 36

Cancer Pain: What Is It? How Do I Talk About It?

Introduction

Having cancer does not always mean having pain. Pain is hardly ever a symptom of early cancer. And even patients with advanced cancer do not always have pain. But if pain does occur, there are many ways to relieve or reduce it. This chapter should help you understand some of the methods available for pain control. It can guide you so that you can take an active part in choosing the methods you wish to use if you do have pain.

Reminders to check with your doctor, nurse, or pharmacist about certain aspects of pain relief appear throughout this chapter. Yet many other people may be able to help: physical therapists, occupational therapists, social workers, members of the clergy, and family members and friends. Cancer pain almost always can be relieved or controlled. You have a right to ask those caring for you to help you control your pain as much as possible.

Defining Pain

What is pain?

Pain is a sensation that hurts. It may cause discomfort or distress or agony It may be steady or throbbing. It may be stabbing, aching, or pinching. However you feel pain, only you can describe it or define

Extracted from NCI/American Cancer Society Pub No. 92-200M-4518: DHHS Agency for Health Care Policy and Research AHCPR Pub No. 94-0593.

it. Because pain is so individual, your pain cannot be "checked out" by anyone else.

Pain may be acute or chronic. Acute pain is severe and lasts a relatively short time. It is usually a signal that body tissue is being injured in some way, and the pain generally disappears when the injury heals. Chronic pain may range from mild to severe, and it is present to some degree for long periods of time.

What causes pain in people with cancer?

Cancer patients may have pain for a variety of reasons. It may be due to the effects of the cancer itself, or it could result from treatment methods. For example, after surgery a person feels pain as a result of operation itself. Or the pain could be unrelated to the cancer: a muscle sprain, a toothache, or a headache.

Remember that not all people with cancer have pain. And those who do are not in pain all the time.

Cancer pain may depend on the type of cancer, the stage (extent) of the disease, and your pain threshold (or tolerance for pain). Cancer pain that lasts a few days or longer may result from:

- The tumor causing pressure on organs, nerves, or bone.
- Poor blood circulation because the cancer has blocked blood vessels.
- Blockage of an organ or tube in the body.
- Metastasis, cancer cells that have spread to other sites in the body.
- Infection or inflammation.
- Side effects from chemotherapy, radiation therapy, or surgery.
- Stiffness from inactivity.
- Psychological responses to illness such as tension, depression, or anxiety.

Whatever the cause, pain can be relieved.

What can be done for cancer pain?

The best way to manage pain is to treat its cause. Whenever possible, the cause of the pain is treated by removing the tumor or decreasing its size. To do this, your doctor may recommend surgery, radiation therapy, or chemotherapy. When none of these procedures can be done, or when the cause of the pain is not known, pain-relief methods are used. This chapter describes many methods for controlling

Cancer Pain: What Is It? How Do I Talk About It?

pain. They include pain medicines, operations on nerves, nerve blocks, physical therapy, and techniques such as relaxation, distraction, and imagery. Only you and your doctor and nurse, who know where your pain is, how bad it is, the kind of cancer you have, and your general health, can decide which methods might be best for you.

What do I tell those caring for me about my pain?

If you are feeling pain, you need to be able to describe it to those who are trained to help you. Some people find pain very hard to explain. Try to use words that will help others understand what you are feeling. Your doctor and others who are caring for you need to know:

- Where do you feel your pain?
- When did it begin?
- What does it feel like? Sharp? Dull? Throbbing? Steady?
- How bad is it?
- Does it prevent you from doing your daily activities? Which ones?
- What relieves your pain?
- What makes it worse?
- What have you tried for pain relief? What helped? What did not help?
- What have you done in the past to relieve other kinds of pain?
- Is your pain constant? If not, how many times a day (or week) does it occur?
- How long does it last each time?

Pain has different effects on different people. The chart below may help you describe the effects that pain has on you. You may want to add other effects that you notice when you're in pain. Be sure that those who are caring for you know about them.

Don't hesitate to talk about your pain to those who can help you. You have a right to the best pain control you can get. Relieving your pain means you can continue to do the everyday things that are important to you. Remember, only you know what you are feeling.

Some of the effects of pain

Symptoms accompanying your pain:

Nausea
Headache
Dizziness

Weakness
Drowsiness
Constipation
Diarrhea
Perspiration

Ability to sleep:

Good
Fitful
Can't sleep

Desire to eat:

Good
Some
Little
Can't eat

Emotional effects:

Fear
Anger
Depression
Crying
Mood swings
Irritability
Suicidal feelings

Lifestyle changes:

Work
Recreation
Interpersonal relationships
Ability to get around
Self-care activities

How can I describe how bad or intense the pain is?

Understanding how bad your pain is helps your doctor decide how to treat it. You can rate how much pain you are feeling by using a pain scale like the one below. Try to assign a number from 0 to 5 to your pain level. If you have no pain, use a 0. A 5 means the pain is as bad

Cancer Pain: What Is It? How Do I Talk About It?

as it can be. As the numbers get larger, they stand for pain that is gradually getting worse.

You may wish to make up your own pain scale using numbers from 0 to 10 or even 0 to 100. Be sure to let others know what pain scale you are using: for example, "My pain is a 7 on a scale of 0 to 10."

You can use a rating scale to answer:

- How bad is your pain at its worst?
- How bad is your pain most of the time?
- How bad is your pain at its least?
- How does your pain change with treatment?
  From _____ to _____.

    0= No pain
    1= Discomfort
    2= Mild pain
    3= Distress
    4= Severe pain
    5 = The worst pain you can imagine

How can I remember all the details about the pain I have, and what I do to relieve it?

You may find it helpful to keep a record or a diary about your pain and what you try for pain relief. The record helps you and those who are caring for you understand more about your pain, the effects it has on you, and what works best to ease your pain. Items that should be included are:

- The number from your rating scale that describes your pain before and after using a pain-relief measure.
- The time you take pain medicine.
- Any activity that seems to be affected by the pain or that increases or decreases the pain.
- Any activity that you cannot do because of the pain.
- The name of the pain medicine you take and the dose.
- How long the pain medicine works.
- Any pain-relief methods other than medicine you use such as rest, relaxation techniques, distraction, skin stimulation, or imagery.

Can anxiety or depression cause pain?

No, but these feelings can make the pain seem worse. People often have an emotional reaction to pain. You may feel worried, depressed, or easily discouraged when you are in pain. Some people feel hopeless or helpless. Others feel alone or embarrassed, inadequate or angry, frightened or frantic.

People with cancer have many reasons for feeling anxious or depressed even when they are not in pain. Try to talk about your feelings with your doctors, nurses, family members, friends, a member of the clergy, or other cancer patients. Talking with family members is often helpful, even though this might be hard for you to do at first.

In some communities, cancer patients meet informally to talk about their feelings and share how they have coped with this disease. Just understanding that others feel the same way as you do might help you deal with having cancer. For information about support services in your area contact your local Unit of the American Cancer Society, the Visiting Nurses Association, the Cancer Information Service at 1-800-4-CANCER (1-800-422-6237), or someone from a hospice, if one is located in your area.

If you feel that these informal ways to lessen your anxiety or depression are not helpful, you may wish to talk with a counselor, a mental health professional who is skilled at dealing with such problems. Your doctor or nurse may be able to help you find a counselor who is specially trained to help people with chronic illnesses. The social services department at your local hospital is another source of information about people who can help you deal with anxiety and depression.

Another option is to ask your doctor about medication. Sometimes, medicine such as antidepressants or tranquilizers can be helpful. Some of these medicines relieve pain in addition to their antidepressant effects.

How does fatigue affect my pain?

Fatigue can make it harder for you to deal with pain. When you are tired, you may not be able to cope with the pain as well as when you are rested. Many people notice that pain seems to get worse as they get tired. Lack of sleep can increase your pain. Be sure to tell your doctor or nurse if you have not been sleeping well because of pain or worry.

What is phantom limb pain?

If you have had an arm or leg removed by surgery, you may still feel pain or other unpleasant sensations as if they were coming from the absent limb. Doctors are not sure why it occurs, but phantom limb pain is real; it is not imaginary. This also can occur if you have had a breast removed; you may have a sensation of pain in the missing breast.

No single pain-relief method controls phantom limb pain in all patients all the time. Many methods have been used to treat this type of pain, including pain medicine, physical therapy, and nerve stimulation. If you are having phantom pain, ask your doctor, nurse, or pharmacist about how you might relieve it.

Relief of Pain

How is cancer pain treated?

When treating cancer pain, the doctor will usually try to treat the cause of the pain first. Surgery, chemotherapy, or radiation therapy may be used to shrink tumors.

There are several ways to relieve pain:

- **With medicine, also called "pharmacological pain relief."** You should ask your doctor, pharmacist, or nurse for advice before you take any medicine for pain. Medicines are safe when they are used properly. You can buy some effective pain relievers without a prescription. For others, a prescription from your doctor is necessary.

- **Without medicine, sometimes called "non-invasive measures."** These usually have very few side effects, and they can be combined with medicines. Methods may include skin stimulation and techniques such as distraction, relaxation, and imagery.

- **Nerve blocks, or "neurological pain relief."** Blocking the pain messages that are sent by nerves to the brain (with surgery or injection of local anesthetic into the nerve) can sometimes be used when nothing else works to relieve pain.

- **Radiation therapy** is often used to relieve pain that is due to cancer that has spread to other sites in the body (metastasis).

There is no one best way to relieve pain, but something usually can be found to help every patient.

Are there any general guidelines for relieving pain?

It is important to try to prevent the pain before it starts or gets worse by using some pain-relief method on a regular schedule. If pain begins, don't wait for it to get worse before doing something about it.

Learn which methods of pain relief work best for you. Vary and combine pain-relief methods. For instance, you might use a relaxation method at the same time you take medicine for the pain.

Know yourself and what you can do. Often when people are rested and alert, they can use a method that demands attention and energy. When tired, they may need to use a method that requires less effort. For example, try distraction when you are rested and alert; use hot or cold packs when you are tired.

Be open-minded and keep trying. You may find that some things that sound as if they could not possibly work might be helpful. Be willing to try different methods. Keep a record of what makes you feel better and what doesn't help.

Try each method more than once. If it doesn't work the first time, try it a few more times before you give up. Keep in mind that what doesn't work one day may work the next. Also, you might need help in figuring out the best way to use a certain technique. But don't get discouraged if a certain method does not work for you. People are different, and not all the methods will work for everyone.

Most important, always ask yourself: "Which is more bothersome, the pain or the method of making it go away? Does pain relief allow me to do what is important to me and those I care about?"

What should I do if my pain is not relieved and my doctor says nothing more can be done for me?

Cancer pain almost always can be substantially lessened or relieved. However, no one doctor can know everything about all medical problems. If you are in pain and your doctor has nothing more to offer, ask to see a pain specialist. Pain specialists may be oncologists, anesthesiologists, neurosurgeons, other doctors, nurses, or pharmacists. A pain control team may also include psychologists and social workers.

If you have difficulty locating a pain program or specialist, contact a cancer center, a hospice, or the oncology department at your local hospital or a medical center. The following sources can provide names of pain specialists, pain clinics, or programs in your area:

Cancer Pain: What Is It? How Do I Talk About It?

The Cancer Information Service (CIS). Supported by the National Cancer Institute, is a nationwide telephone service that answers questions from cancer patients and their families, health care professionals, and the public. At the CIS, health information specialists provide information and publications on all aspects of cancer, including pain control. They can give you information about clinical trials (research studies) that are open to patients and that test new and promising treatments for cancer and cancer pain. They also may know about cancer-related services in local areas. By dialing 1-800-4-CANCER (1-800-422-6237), you will reach a CIS office serving your area. A trained staff member will answer your questions and listen to your concerns. Spanish-speaking staff members are available.

The American Cancer Society (ACS). ACS is a national nonprofit organization whose programs include research, education, patient services, and rehabilitation. Every state has a chartered Division of the ACS. In addition, there are more than 3,500 local ACS Units (offices) in the United States and Puerto Rico. Local ACS Units are another source of information about pain specialists in your area. The local Units are listed in your telephone directory. For more information, call the ACS at 1-800-ACS-2345.

Information about pain specialists is also available from:

American Academy of Pain Medicine
5700 Old Orchard Road
Skokie, IL 60077
(708) 966-9510

American Pain Society
5700 Old Orchard Road
Skokie, IL 60077
(708) 966-5595

American Society of Anesthesiologists
Pain Therapy Committee
515 Busse Highway
Park Ridge, IL 60068
(708) 825-5586

International Association for the Study of Pain
909 N.E. 43rd Street,
Suite 306
Seattle, WA 98105
(206) 547-6409

National Chronic Pain Outreach Association
7979 Old Georgetown Road
Suite 100
Bethesda, MD 20814-2429
(301) 652-4948

A listing of facilities with accredited pain programs is available from:

Commission on Accreditation of Rehabilitation Facilities
101 North Wilmot Road,
Suite 500
Tucson, AZ 85711
(602) 748-1212

Chapter 37

Relieving Cancer Pain with Medicines

How to Relieve Pain with Medicines

NOTE: If your doctor has said you should take medicines to relieve your pain, the information that follows will help you understand how to take them safely and effectively. Before taking any medicine, talk with your doctor, nurse, or pharmacist. Tell them about any other medications you take. Ask if it is safe to drink alcoholic beverages if you are taking pain medicine. Try to identify the cause of your pain. Remember, your pain may not always be caused by your cancer.

What medicines are used to relieve pain?

Medicines that relieve pain are called **analgesics**. Analgesics act on the nervous system to relieve pain without causing loss of consciousness. Analgesics provide only temporary pain relief because they do not affect the cause of the pain. There are two types of analgesics:

- **Nonprescription** or over-the-counter (OTC) pain relievers for mild and moderate pain.

- **Prescription pain relievers** for moderate to severe pain.

Extracted from NCI/American Cancer Society Pub No. 92-200M-4518: DHHS Agency for Health Care Policy and Research AHCPR Pub No. 94-0593.

How are medicines best used to relieve pain?

Preventing pain from starting or getting worse is the best way to control it. Some people call this **"staying on top of the pain."** It may mean you can use lower doses of a pain reliever than if you wait until the pain gets bad. Don't be afraid to admit that you have pain.

Different pain medicines take different lengths of time to work. This is called **"onset of action."** For some medicine, it is only a few minutes. For others, it is several hours. If you wait too long to take pain medicine, your pain may get worse before the medicine helps. Some pain medicine must even be taken for several days or weeks before you get the best relief.

If you are in some pain all the time, your pain medicine should be taken regularly. It's important to follow the directions on the label. They may say, "Take one or two tablets three or four times a day for pain." Or the directions may tell you to take the medicine every 4 to 6 hours. You may be able to control your pain with a mild pain reliever if you take it as directed instead of once in a while. Check with your doctor, nurse, or pharmacist if the labeled dose does not help your pain.

Sometimes people with pain think that they should wait as long as they can before taking medicine. This is not the way to control your pain. The pain may get worse if you wait, and it may then take longer for your medicine to give you relief. Waiting also may mean that larger doses or a stronger medicine will be needed to help your pain.

When I take medicine, the pain goes away, but it comes back quickly. Why?

The length of time that a pain relief medicine works is called the **"duration of action."** It varies among the different kinds of pain medicines. It is also different for different people.

Pain relief also depends on how much you take—the dose—and how often you take it, the frequency. If the pain relief that you get is wearing off before you are supposed to take the next dose, be sure to tell your doctor or nurse. Ask if you may take the medicine more often or in larger doses to keep the pain under control.

If the analgesic you are taking does not seem to lessen or stop the pain, ask if you can try a different one.

Relieving Cancer Pain with Medicines

How should I take my pain medicine?

Most pain medicines are taken by mouth, usually as a tablet or capsule. Sometimes they are called caplets or gelcaps. Take your medicine with a large glass of water or other liquid, unless your doctor tells you otherwise. Do not take your medicine with alcoholic beverages. If you have trouble swallowing tablets, ask your doctor or nurse about taking liquid pain medicine.

Pain medicine also can be injected under the skin or into a muscle or vein. Some pain medicine is available in suppository form. The easiest way to take pain medicine is by mouth, but shots or suppositories can be used if you have nausea or problems with swallowing. A skin patch that gradually releases pain medicine into the body is also available.

What should I do if I have side effects from pain medicine?

Stop taking the medicine if you notice a rash, wheezing, or shortness of breath. Let your doctor know right away.

You need to tell your doctor or nurse if you are having such side effects as indigestion, nausea, dizziness, headache, constipation, or drowsiness. If you want to stop taking a medicine because of these side effects, discuss it with your doctor, nurse, or pharmacist first.

Are the same pain medicines used for children with cancer as for adults?

Yes, but usually smaller doses are used. The dose must be adjusted carefully depending on the age and size of the child.

If you are taking care of a child with cancer, you should talk with the doctor (usually a **pediatric oncologist**, a doctor who specializes in treating children with cancer), nurse, or other health professional caring for the child about the best method of pain relief.

Can I take nonprescription medications for colds or other problems while I'm taking pain medications?

When you are taking medicine for pain, ask your doctor, nurse, or pharmacist about taking any other medications.

Many cold pills and other over-the-counter (nonprescription) medicine can be taken along with analgesics and there are no harmful effects. However, some combination cold medicines contain pain relievers and it may be necessary to lower the dose of your pain medicine.

Many combination medicines for colds, menstrual pain, headaches, and joint or muscle aches contain aspirin. Cancer patients are usually told to avoid aspirin, especially if they recently have been on chemotherapy.

Over-the-counter medicines for allergies may cause you to feel drowsy. Some pain medicine can also cause sleepiness. Taking them together can make it dangerous to drive or to operate machinery.

Before you take any nonprescription medicine, it's a good idea to read the label and seek the advice of a health professional if there's anything you don't understand.

Nonprescription Pain Relievers

What are nonprescription pain relievers?

Nonprescription pain relievers are analgesics that can be bought without a doctor's order (prescription). Sometimes they are called **"over-the-counter"** pain remedies. They include aspirin (Bufferin, Ascriptin, Ecotrin,) acetaminophen (Anacin-3, Tylenol, Datril,) and ibuprofen (Advil, Motrin, Nuprin). Many nonprescription pain relievers have different names, but if you check the labels, nearly all contain one of these three medicines. They are effective for relief of mild and moderate pain.

> **NOTE:** The brand names that appear in this book are listed for information only. No endorsement by Omnigraphics, NCI or ACS is implied.

What's the difference between a brand name drug and a generic drug?

Drugs are complex substances, and they may have as many as three different names: chemical, generic, and brand. Chemical names are long and difficult to pronounce. The US Food and Drug Administration approves the generic, shortened names by which drugs are usually known. Drug companies give their products brand names. For example N-(4-hydroxyphenyl) acetamide is the chemical name for acetaminophen, which is the generic name for Tylenol. Many nonprescription and prescription pain relievers are available under both generic and brand names. Your doctor or pharmacist can tell you the generic name.

Generic products tend to be less expensive than brand-name drugs and usually are just as effective. However, because of differences in manufacturing methods, medicines with the same generic name produced by different companies may differ in the way they are absorbed by the body. For this reason, your doctor may prefer that you take a brand-name drug. You might want to ask your doctor or pharmacist if you can use a less expensive medication. Pharmacies are careful to obtain high-quality generic products, so it is sometimes possible to make substitutions.

Are aspirin, acetaminophen, and ibuprofen different?

Yes. Each is a different chemical. They all have similar pain-relieving effects, but they have some important differences:

- Aspirin and ibuprofen reduce inflammation; acetaminophen does not.
- Aspirin and ibuprofen are often used to reduce the pain of swollen joints and other inflamed areas; acetaminophen is not.
- Aspirin and ibuprofen can irritate the stomach. Sometimes they even cause stomach bleeding. Acetaminophen does not have this effect.
- Aspirin and ibuprofen can affect blood clotting and may cause bleeding. Acetaminophen has no effect on blood clotting.
- When aspirin is used to treat children with viral diseases such as the flu or chickenpox, it may cause Reye's syndrome, a rare brain and liver disease. Acetaminophen and ibuprofen do not cause Reye's syndrome.
- Ibuprofen can make existing kidney problems worse. In normal doses, aspirin and acetaminophen usually do not injure the kidneys.

Are there reasons I should not take aspirin?

Although aspirin is a very common medicine, it should not be used by everyone. Before you take aspirin in any form, ask your doctor or nurse if there is any reason for you not to take it.

Some people have conditions that may be made worse by aspirin or by any product that contains aspirin. In general, aspirin should be avoided by people who:

- Are on anticancer drugs that may cause bleeding.
- Are on steroid medicines (such as prednisone).
- Will have surgery within a week.
- Are allergic to aspirin.

- Are taking blood-thinning medicine (anticoagulants such as Coumadin).
- Have stomach ulcers or a history of ulcers, gout, or bleeding disorders.
- Are taking prescription drugs for arthritis.
- Are taking oral medicines for diabetes or gout.

Be careful about mixing aspirin with alcohol; taking aspirin and drinking alcohol on an empty stomach can cause stomach upset and internal bleeding.

Is there aspirin in any other medicine?

Yes. If your doctor does not want you to take aspirin, be sure to read labels carefully. Many nonprescription products contain **"hidden" aspirin**. For example, aspirin is in Excedrin (a pain reliever), Coricidin (a cold or allergy medicine), and Alka-Seltzer (an antacid).

Some prescription pain relievers, such as Percodan and Empirin Compound with Codeine, also contain aspirin. If you are not sure if your prescription contains aspirin, ask your pharmacist.

What are the side effects from aspirin?

The most common side effect from aspirin is stomach upset or indigestion. Taking aspirin with food lessens the chance of this side effect. If aspirin upsets your stomach, you can use buffered aspirin or coated aspirin. Ask your pharmacist to tell you which aspirin products are less likely to upset your stomach.

When some people take aspirin for long periods of time they may notice:

- Ringing in the ears or hearing loss.
- Unusual sweating.
- Headache, dizziness, dimness of vision, confusion, fever, or drowsiness.
- Rapid breathing and rapid heartbeat.
- Thirst, nausea, vomiting, or diarrhea.

If you notice these symptoms, check with your doctor right away.

Aspirin also can cause internal bleeding, which usually is painless. If your stools become darker than normal or you notice unusual bruising, tell your doctor or nurse. These can be signs of internal bleeding.

Relieving Cancer Pain with Medicines

Are there side effects from acetaminophen or ibuprofen?

People rarely have any side effects from the usual dose of acetaminophen. However, liver or kidney damage may result from using large doses of this drug every day for a long time or drinking large amounts of alcohol with the usual dose.

Serious side effects from ibuprofen are uncommon. Some people notice that it upsets the stomach. When it is used for long periods of time or when it is used by patients taking steroid medications, there is an increased risk of stomach bleeding. If you have kidney problems, ibuprofen may make them worse. And because it may interfere with the ability of blood to clot, it may be dangerous for patients with low platelet counts.

How many aspirin or acetaminophen tablets can I take at one time, and how many can I take during an entire day? What about ibuprofen?

The doses of these pain relievers are different for different people. Some people get the best pain relief when they take a small dose every 3 hours. Other people may find that a larger dose taken less frequently works for them. You should not take a larger dose than the label tells you without first checking with your doctor, nurse, or pharmacist.

Aspirin: The usual safe dose of aspirin for adults is two or three tablets (325 mg or 5 grains each) taken three or four times a day. A total of eight adult aspirins a day usually does not produce any major side effects. Many adults can safely take a total of 12 tablets a day. Any dose higher than 12 a day, however, should be taken only with your doctor's or nurse's advice.

Acetaminophen: The usual safe dose of acetaminophen for adults is 2 or 3 tablets (325 mg or 5 grains each) taken three or four times a day, for a total of 8 to 12 tablets a day. Extra-strength forms, such as extra-strength Tylenol are equal to 1 1/2 regular tablets (500 mg or 7 1/2 grains each); you should take no more than 8 of these tablets in 24 hours.

Ibuprofen: The usual dose of ibuprofen for adults is 1 tablet (200 mg each) every 4 to 6 hours. You should not take more than 6 tablets in 24 hours. Larger doses should only be taken if they are prescribed by your doctor.

How long does it take these medicines to work, and how long does pain relief last?

The effect of aspirin begins 30 to 60 minutes after you take it. (Coated aspirin may need 1 1/2 to 8 hours to work.) The pain-relieving action of one dose usually lasts about 4 hours but may last up to 12 hours.

Acetaminophen relieves pain within 10 to 60 minutes of taking it. Its effect may last up to 6 hours.

Ibuprofen begins to relieve pain in 1 to 2 hours and lasts from 5 to 10 hours. You may need to take ibuprofen for 2 to 3 days before you get the most pain relief.

There are so many nonprescription pain relievers available. What are the differences among them?

Drugstore shelves are filled with many pain remedies. Each one is advertised to be better and faster acting than the others. But nearly all nonprescription pain relievers rely on aspirin, acetaminophen, or ibuprofen for pain relief. Some brands also contain substances called additives. Common ones include the following:

- Buffers (e.g., magnesium carbonate, aluminum hydroxide) to decrease stomach upset.
- Caffeine to act as a stimulant and lessen pain.
- Antihistamines (e.g., diphenhydramine, pyrilamine) to help you relax or sleep.

Combination products have some disadvantages. The additives can produce undesirable effects. For example, antihistamines sometimes cause drowsiness. You may find this acceptable at bedtime, but it could be a problem during the day or while driving. In addition, additives tend to increase the cost of nonprescription pain relievers. They also can change the action of other medicines you may be taking.

Plain aspirin, acetaminophen, or ibuprofen are probably as effective as any combination product. But if you find that a brand with certain additives is a better pain reliever for you, ask your doctor, nurse, or pharmacist if the additives are safe for you. If you have any questions about the drugs contained in your nonprescription analgesics, ask your doctor, nurse, or pharmacist.

Relieving Cancer Pain with Medicines

Why should I take nonprescription medicines for my pain? Aren't there stronger, more effective pain relievers?

In many cases, the nonprescription medicines are all you will need to relieve your pain, especially if you stay on top of the pain by taking them on a regular, preventive basis. These medicines are stronger analgesics than most people realize.

Certain doses of prescription pain relievers given by mouth are no more effective than two or three regular tablets of aspirin, acetaminophen, or ibuprofen. Research has shown that for most people the usual dose of nonprescription pain relievers provides as much pain relief as prescription medications such as codeine or Darvon.

If you get pain relief from nonprescription medicines, you do not need to take prescription pain relievers. For most people, nonprescription pain relievers have fewer side effects than prescription pain relievers.

Can I take nonprescription pain relievers if my doctor has also prescribed stronger analgesics?

You should discuss this question with your doctor or nurse. Many people who need prescription analgesics also can benefit from continuing to take regular doses of aspirin, acetaminophen, or ibuprofen. The nonprescription analgesics and the stronger prescription medicines relieve pain in different ways. When you take both of them, your pain is attacked on two different levels. Aspirin, acetaminophen, or ibuprofen taken four times a day might help reduce the amount of stronger pain reliever you need.

Some prescription pain tablets contain aspirin or acetaminophen. Ask your pharmacist or doctor how much aspirin or acetaminophen, if any, is in your prescription. A nurse, doctor, or pharmacist can help you figure out how much aspirin or acetaminophen you can safely add.

Prescription Pain Relievers

What are the different kinds of prescription pain relievers?

For many years, the most widely used prescription pain relievers have been narcotics. Narcotics are drugs that relieve pain and cause drowsiness or sleep. In addition, they all have similar side effects. Historically, these drugs came from the opium poppy. They are also called opioids or opiates. Today, many narcotics are synthetic, that is, they are chemicals manufactured by drug companies.

Frequently used opioid pain relievers include the following:

- codeine
- hydromorphone (Dilaudid)
- levorphanol (Levo-Dromoran)
- methadone (Dolophine)
- morphine
- oxycodone (in Percodan)
- oxymorphone (Numorphan)

You can get these pain relievers only with a doctor's written prescription. They may be taken by mouth (**orally, or PO**), by injection (**intramuscularly, or IM**), through a vein (**intravenously, or IV**), or by rectal suppository. There are also other methods of giving pain medicines for more continuous pain relief. Not all narcotics are available in each of these forms.

Another group of prescription pain relievers is similar to ibuprofen (in large doses, ibuprofen requires a prescription). They are called **nonsteroidal anti-inflammatory drugs (NSAIDs)**. Included in this group of pain relievers are Motrin, Naprosyn, Nalfon, and Trilisate. They are useful for moderate to severe pain. They may be especially helpful in treating the pain of bone metastasis. Because NSAIDs are not narcotics, their use does not result in **drug tolerance** or physical dependence.

These drugs are used alone or with nonprescription pain relievers to treat moderate to severe pain. Some are more effective than others in relieving severe pain.

How do I decide which pain medications to use?

This is not something you should decide alone. Discuss this with your doctor, nurse, or pharmacist before you use any drugs for pain. Medications that worked for you in the past or that helped a friend or relative may not be right for you at this time. **Never take someone else's medicine!**

Only one doctor should prescribe your pain medicine. If a consulting doctor changes your medicine, be sure the two doctors discuss your treatment. Otherwise, you may take too much or too little.

Let your doctor or nurse know whether your pain medication gives you relief. Work together to find the medication or pain-relief program that is best for you. Remember, your need for pain medicine may change as your cancer treatment changes.

Relieving Cancer Pain with Medicines

It is important to record the name and amount of pain medication you take. You can then give precise information to the doctor or nurse about its effect on your pain.

Will I become addicted if I use narcotics for pain relief?

No. **Narcotic addiction** is defined as dependence on the regular use of narcotics to satisfy physical, emotional, and psychological needs rather than for medical reasons. Pain relief is a medical reason for taking narcotics. Therefore, if you take narcotics to relieve your pain, you are not an "addict," no matter how much or how often you take narcotic medicines. If you and your doctor decide that narcotics are a proper choice for your pain relief, use them as directed.

Addiction is a very common fear of people who take narcotics for pain relief. Narcotic addiction is an emotionally charged subject. You may hear people use the term "addiction" very loosely without understanding exactly what it means, the compulsive use of habit-forming drugs for their pleasurable effects.

Drug addiction in cancer patients is rare. Generally, when narcotics are used under proper medical supervision the chance of addiction is very small. Most patients who take narcotics for pain relief can stop taking these drugs if their pain can be controlled by other means. It is important to remember that if narcotics are the only effective way to relieve pain, the patient's comfort is more important than any possibility of addiction.

If you take narcotics for several weeks or more, be prepared for someone to express a concern about addiction. Most people with prolonged pain who take narcotics have faced this problem. Remind yourself that other people's concerns about addiction are often due to lack of information.

If you have concerns about addiction, share them with those who are caring for you. These fears should not prevent you from using narcotics to effectively relieve your pain.

What is drug tolerance?

When certain drugs are taken regularly for a length of time, the body doesn't respond to them as well as it once did, and the drugs at a fixed dose become less effective. Larger or more frequent doses must be taken to obtain the effect that was achieved with the original dose. People who take narcotics for pain control sometimes find that over time they will need to take larger doses. This either may be due to an increase in the pain or the development of drug tolerance. Increasing the doses of narcotics to relieve increasing pain or to overcome drug tolerance is not addiction.

Can taking narcotics be dangerous?

All medicines can be dangerous if they are not taken properly. The risks of improperly taking narcotics include overdose, drug interactions, and accidents resulting from drowsiness.

Overdose: Too large a dose of a narcotic may cause breathing to slow down or stop (respiratory depression). Doses required for good pain relief are rarely, if ever, large enough to cause death. Doctors carefully adjust the doses of narcotic pain relievers so that pain is relieved with little effect on breathing. You may have heard of addicts dying from narcotic overdose. This usually is due to taking the narcotic with other drugs that interact with it, or to taking a much higher dose than would be necessary for pain relief, or to impurities in illegally obtained narcotics. The first sign of narcotic overdose is a feeling of unusual sleepiness or difficulty in waking up. If you have either of these problems, someone should contact your doctor or nurse as soon as possible.

Drug Interactions: Combinations of narcotics, alcohol, and tranquilizers can be dangerous. If you drink alcohol or if you take tranquilizers, sleeping aids, antidepressants, antihistamines, or any other drugs that make you sleepy, tell your doctor how much and how often. Even small doses might cause problems. The use of alcohol or any of these drugs with narcotics can lead to overdose symptoms such as weakness, difficulty in breathing, confusion, anxiety, or more severe drowsiness or dizziness. These drug interactions may result in unconsciousness and death. Tell your doctor about any medicine or combination of medicines that makes you drowsy or sleepy.

Accidents: Narcotics often cause drowsiness or dizziness. If you are aware of this, you can be extra careful to avoid accidents. Sometimes it may be unsafe for you to drive a car or even to walk up or down stairs. Avoid operating equipment such as saws or drills or performing activities that require alertness. Be aware of the effect narcotics have on you so that you can take necessary precautions.

How much narcotic pain reliever is safe for me to take?

The amount of pain reliever you take should be determined by your doctor. Analgesics affect different people in different ways. A very

Relieving Cancer Pain with Medicines

small dose may be effective for you, while someone else may need to take a much larger dose to obtain pain relief.

You need to ask these questions:

- How much should I take? How often?
- If my pain is not relieved, can I take more? If the dose should be increased, by how much? Must I call the doctor before increasing the dose?
- What if I forget to take it or take it late?

Your doctor will try to prescribe the amount of narcotic that will be both safe for you and effective for your pain.

Take the medicine as your doctor or nurse has prescribed but tell them at once if your pain is not controlled or if you have severe side effects such as extreme drowsiness or difficulty in breathing. If you do not need as much narcotic as has been prescribed, your doctor or nurse will tell you how to reduce the dose or frequency.

What if the medicine that has been recommended doesn't relieve my pain?

Tell your doctor or nurse as soon as you can if you are not getting effective pain relief. Don't wait for your next appointment! They need to know:

- How much, if any, pain relief you get.
- How long the pain is relieved.
- Any side effects that occur or do not occur, especially drowsiness.
- How pain interferes with your normal activities such as sleep, work, eating, or sex.

With your doctor's help, you can usually get good pain relief. When the medicine does not give you enough pain relief, the doctor may increase the dose or the frequency or prescribe a different drug. Some narcotics are stronger than others, and you may need a stronger one to control your pain.

If your pain relief is not lasting long enough, ask your doctor about long-acting forms of medicine. Morphine is now available in a tablet form that releases it over a long period of time (MS Contin or Roxanol SR).

You may have developed drug tolerance if you have taken narcotics for a long time. As a result, doses that may have been too large for you a few weeks before may be safe now. The desired effect is pain relief with as few side effects as possible, regardless of the size of the dose.

Some doctors are reluctant to prescribe large enough doses or stronger narcotics for pain control. However, with careful medical observation, the doses of strong narcotics (by mouth or injection) can be safely raised enough to ease severe pain. Do not increase the dose of your pain medicine on your own.

Remember, you are the best judge of whether your pain is relieved. If you still have pain and your doctor does not seem to be aware of other alternatives, ask to see a specialist in cancer pain management.

What are the side effects of narcotics?

Although not everyone has side effects from narcotics, some of the more common ones are drowsiness, constipation, and nausea and vomiting.

Some people also might experience dizziness, mental effects (nightmares, confusion, hallucinations), a moderate decrease in rate and depth of breathing, or difficulty in urinating.

You should always discuss side effects with your doctor or nurse. Side effects from narcotic pain relievers can usually be handled successfully.

What can I do about drowsiness?

At first, narcotics cause some drowsiness in most people, but this usually goes away after a few days. If the narcotic is giving you pain relief for the first time in a long time, your drowsiness might be the result of the decrease in pain, allowing you much needed rest. This kind of drowsiness will go away after you "catch up" on your sleep. Drowsiness will also lessen as your body gets used to the medicine. Call your doctor or nurse if you feel you are too drowsy for your normal activities after you have been taking the medicine for a week.

If you are drowsy, be very careful to avoid situations in which you might hurt yourself as a result of not being alert, such as cooking, climbing stairs, or driving. Here are some ways to handle drowsiness:

- Wait a few days and see if it disappears.

- Check to see if there are other reasons for the drowsiness. Are you taking other medicines that can also cause drowsiness?

- Ask the doctor if you can take a smaller dose more frequently.

- If the narcotic is not relieving the pain, the pain itself may be wearing you out. In this case, better pain relief may result in

Relieving Cancer Pain with Medicines

less drowsiness. Ask your doctor what you can do to get better pain relief.

- Sometimes a small decrease in the dose of a narcotic will still give you pain relief but no drowsiness. If drowsiness is severe, you may be taking more narcotic than you need. Ask your doctor about lowering the amount you are presently taking.

- Ask your doctor if you can take a mild stimulant such as caffeine, or your doctor can prescribe a stimulant such as dextroamphetamine (Dexedrine) or methylphenidate (Ritalin).

- If drowsiness is severe or if it suddenly occurs after you have been taking narcotics for a while, notify your doctor or nurse right away.

What can I do about constipation?

Narcotics cause constipation in most people. The stool does not move along the intestinal tract as fast as usual and becomes hard because more water is absorbed. Your doctor will probably prescribe a stool softener and a laxative.

After checking with your doctor or nurse, you can try the following:

- Eat foods high in fiber or roughage such as uncooked fruits and vegetables and whole grain breads and cereals. Adding 1 or 2 tablespoons of unprocessed bran to your food adds bulk and stimulates bowel movements. Keeping a shaker of bran handy at mealtimes makes it easy to sprinkle on foods. A dietitian can suggest other ways to add fiber to your diet.

- Drink plenty of liquids. Eight to ten 8-ounce glasses of fluid each day will help keep your stools soft.

- Exercise as much as you are able.

- Eat foods that have helped relieve constipation in the past.

- Try to use the toilet or bedside commode when you have a bowel movement, even if that is the only time you get out of bed.

- Plan your bowel movements for the same time each day, if possible. Set aside time for sitting on the toilet or commode, preferably after a meal. Have a hot drink about half an hour before your planned time for a bowel movement.

- If you have difficulty eating enough bran or other foods high in fiber, check with your doctor, nurse, or pharmacist about using a bulk laxative, such as Metamucil.

Be sure to check with your doctor or nurse before taking any laxative or stool softener on your own.

What can I do for nausea and vomiting?

Nausea and vomiting caused by narcotics usually will disappear after a few days of taking the medicine. The following suggestions may be helpful:

- If your nausea occurs mainly when you are walking around (as opposed to being in bed), remain in bed for an hour or so after you take your medicine. This type of nausea is like motion sickness. Sometimes the doctor will tell you to use medicines (such as Bonine or Dramamine) that can be bought without a prescription to counteract this type of nausea. Do not take these medicines without checking with your doctor, nurse, or pharmacist.
- If pain itself is the cause of the nausea, using narcotics to relieve the pain usually makes this nausea go away.
- Medicine (such as Compazine, or Torecan by mouth or by rectal suppositories) can sometimes be prescribed.
- Ask your doctor or nurse if some other medical condition or other medications you are taking such as steroids, anticancer drugs, or aspirin might be causing your nausea.

Some people mistakenly think they are allergic to narcotics if the narcotic causes nausea. Nausea and vomiting alone usually are not allergic responses. But nausea and vomiting accompanied by a rash or itching may be an allergic reaction. If this occurs, stop taking the drug and notify your doctor at once.

I've heard that some people who stop taking narcotics have withdrawal effects. Is this true?

You should not stop taking narcotic pain relievers suddenly. People who stop taking narcotic medicine usually are taken off the drug gradually so that any withdrawal symptoms will be mild or scarcely noticeable. If you stop taking narcotics suddenly and develop a flu-like illness, excessive perspiration, diarrhea, or any other unusual reaction, tell your doctor or nurse. These symptoms can be treated and tend to disappear in a few days to a few weeks.

If my pain becomes severe, will I need shots for pain relief?

Probably not. Intramuscular injections or "shots" are rarely used for relieving cancer pain. Narcotic rectal suppositories can be effective, and new methods of giving narcotic pain relievers have been developed. Long-acting morphine tablets are now available, and some narcotics provide quick pain relief when they are given under the tongue (sublingually). One narcotic drug, fentanyl, is now available as a skin patch which continuously releases the medicine through the skin for 48 to 72 hours.

If you and your doctor have not been able to find a way to get good pain control with medicine you take by mouth, some kinds of pain medicine can be given intravenously. You may want to ask about patient-controlled analgesia. With this method, a portable computerized pump containing the medicine is attached to a needle that is placed in a vein. Whenever pain relief is needed, the patient presses a button on the pump that delivers a preset dose of pain medicine into the vein.

A new simple, safe, and effective method of pain control is called continuous subcutaneous infusion. A small electronic pump dispenses the drug automatically through a small needle placed under the skin. Another way of treating cancer pain is to inject pain medicine into the spinal cord (intrathecal) or into the space around the spinal cord (epidural).

Your doctor or a pain specialist can give you more information about these advances in pain treatment.

Is it true that severe pain can only be relieved by heroin?

No. That is not true. Some newspaper and magazine articles have suggested that heroin is the only way to relieve severe pain, but the reported success with heroin was due more to how the drug was given (in a preventive way) than to the effects of the drug itself. Strong narcotics such as morphine and Dilaudid usually can relieve very severe pain. In fact, the body converts heroin to morphine.

Heroin is available in England and has been used there to treat pain in cancer patients. However, even in England morphine now is being used routinely because it has been shown to be just as effective as heroin. In the United States, heroin is not legally available.

What other prescription medicines are used to relieve cancer pain?

Several different classes of drugs can be used along with (or instead of) narcotics to relieve cancer pain. They may have their own pain-relieving action or they may increase the pain-relieving activity of narcotics. Others lessen the side effects of narcotic pain relievers. The following classes of non-narcotic drugs might be prescribed by your doctor to help you get the best pain relief:

- Antidepressants such as Elavil, Tofranil, or Sinequan are used to treat the pain that results from surgery, radiation therapy, or chemotherapy.

- Antihistamines such as Vistaril or Atarax relieve pain, help control nausea, and help patients sleep.

- Antianxiety drugs such as Xanax or Ativan may be used to treat muscle spasms that often go along with severe pain. In addition they are helpful for treating the anxiety that some cancer patients feel.

- Dextroamphetamine (Dexadrine) increases the pain-relieving action of narcotic pain relievers and also reduces the drowsiness they cause.

- Anticonvulsants such as Tegretol or Klonopin are helpful for pain from nerve injury caused by the cancer or cancer therapy.

- Steroids such as prednisone or Decadron are useful for some kinds of both chronic and acute cancer pain.

- NSAIDs such as Motrin decrease inflammation and lessen post-surgical pain and the pain from bone metastases.

Chapter 38

Relieving Cancer Pain without Medicines

How To Relieve Pain Without Medicine

What are some of the ways I can relieve pain without taking medicine?

For some people, pain can be relieved without using medicine. They use relaxation, imagery, distraction, and skin stimulation. You may need the help of health professionals to learn to do these for yourself. Friends or family members can help with some of them. The techniques are also useful along with pain medicines.

Information about non-drug treatments for pain also may be available at a local hospice, cancer treatment center, or hospital pain clinic.

How does relaxation work?

Relaxation relieves pain or keeps it from getting worse by reducing tension in the muscles. It can help you fall asleep, give you more energy, make you less tired, reduce your anxiety, and make other pain relief methods work better. Some people, for instance, find that taking a pain medicine or using a cold or hot pack works faster and better when they relax at the same time.

Extracted from NCI/American Cancer Society Pub No. 92-200M-4518: DHHS Agency for Health Care Policy and Research AHCPR Pub No. 94-0593; McCaffery and Beebe, 1989. Adapted and reprinted with permission.

Are there any basic guidelines for using relaxation techniques?

The following suggestions may help:

- Understand that your ability to relax may vary from time to time and that relaxation cannot be forced.
- Remember that it may take up to two weeks of practice to feel the first results of relaxation.
- Try several relaxation methods until you find one that works for you.
- Stick with the same method so that it becomes easy and routine for you. Use it regularly for at least 5 to 10 minutes twice a day.
- Check for tension throughout the day by noticing tightness in each part of your body from head to foot. Relax any tense muscles. You may use a quick technique such as inhale/tense, exhale/relax, described below.
- If you have any lung problems, check with your doctor before using any relaxation technique that requires deep breathing.

Is there any special position I should be in when I am doing relaxation exercises?

Relaxation may be done sitting up or lying down. Choose a quiet place whenever possible. Close your eyes. Do not cross your arms and legs because that may cut off circulation and cause numbness or tingling. If you are lying down, be sure you are comfortable. Put a small pillow under your neck and under your knees or use a low stool to support your lower legs.

How do I use relaxation?

There are many methods. Here are some for you to try:

Visual concentration and rhythmic massage:

- Open your eyes and stare at an object, or close your eyes and think of a peaceful, calm scene.
- With the palm of your hand, massage near the area of pain in a circular, firm manner. Avoid red, raw, swollen, or tender areas. You may wish to ask a family member or friend to do this for you.

Relieving Cancer Pain without Medicines

Inhale/tense, exhale/relax:

- Breathe in (inhale) deeply. At the same time, tense your muscles or a group of muscles. For example, you can squeeze your eyes shut, frown, clench your teeth, make a fist, stiffen your arms and legs, or draw up your arms and legs as tightly as you can.
- Hold your breath and keep your muscles tense for a second or two.
- Let go! Breathe out (exhale) and let your body go limp.

Slow rhythmic breathing:

- Stare at an object or close your eyes and concentrate on your breathing or on a peaceful scene.
- Take a slow, deep breath and, as you breathe in, tense your muscles (such as your arms).
- As you breathe out, relax your muscles and feel the tension draining.
- Now remain relaxed and begin breathing slowly and comfortably, concentrating on your breathing, taking about 9 to 12 breaths a minute. Do not breathe too deeply.
- To maintain a slow, even rhythm as you breathe out, you can say silently to yourself, "In, one, two; out, one, two." It may be helpful at first if someone counts out loud for you. If you ever feel out of breath, take a deep breath and then continue the slow breathing exercise. Each time you breathe out, feel yourself relaxing and going limp. If some muscles are not relaxed such as your shoulders, tense them as you breathe in and relax them as you breathe out. You need to do this only once or twice for each specific muscle group.
- Continue slow, rhythmic breathing for a few seconds up to 10 minutes, depending on your need.
- To end your slow rhythmic breathing, count silently and slowly from one to three. Open your eyes. Say silently to yourself: "I feel alert and relaxed." Begin moving about slowly.

Other methods you can add to slow rhythmic breathing:

- Imagery (see below for ideas).
- Listen to slow, familiar music through an earphone or headset.

- Progressive relaxation of body parts. Once you are breathing slowly and comfortably, you may relax different body parts, starting with your feet and working up to your head. Think of words such as limp, heavy, light, warm, or floating. Each time you breathe out, you can focus on a particular area of the body and feel it relaxing. Try to imagine that the tension is draining from that area. For example, as you breathe out, feel your feet and ankles relaxing; the next time you breathe out, feel your calves and knees relaxing, and so on up your body.

Relaxation tapes:

Ask your doctor or nurse to recommend commercially available relaxation tapes. These tape recordings provide step-by-step instructions in relaxation techniques.

Will I have any problems with using relaxation techniques?

Some people who have used relaxation for pain relief have reported the following problems and solutions to them:

- Relaxation may be difficult to use with severe pain. If you have this problem, use a quick and easy relaxation method such as visual concentration with rhythmic massage or breathe in/tense, breathe out/relax.
- You may have a feeling of "suffocation." If so, take a deep breath.
- Sometimes breathing too deeply for a while can cause shortness of breath. If this is your problem, take shallow breaths and/or breathe more slowly.
- You may fall asleep. If you do not wish to fall asleep, sit in a hard chair while doing the relaxation exercise or set a timer or alarm.
- You might get feelings of depression or withdrawal. Sometimes being relaxed makes you aware of problems you have been worrying about subconsciously. If this happens, talk to someone who can help you sort out your feelings. If you have trouble using these methods, ask your doctor or nurse to refer you to a therapist who is experienced in relaxation techniques. Do not continue any relaxation technique that increases your pain, makes you feel uneasy, or causes any unpleasant effects.

Relieving Cancer Pain without Medicines

What is biofeedback?

With the help of special machines, people can learn to control certain body functions such as heart rate, blood pressure, and muscle tension. Biofeedback is sometimes used to help people learn to relax. Cancer patients can use biofeedback techniques to reduce anxiety and help them cope with their pain. Biofeedback usually is used with other pain-relief methods.

What is imagery, and how does it work?

Imagery is using your imagination to create mental pictures or situations. The way imagery relieves pain is not completely understood. Imagery can be thought of as a deliberate daydream that uses all of your senses—sight, touch, hearing, smell, and taste. Some people believe that imagery is a form of self-hypnosis.

Certain images may reduce your pain both during imagery and for hours afterward. If you must stay in bed or can't go out of the house, you may find that imagery helps reduce the closed-in feeling; you can imagine and revisit favorite spots in your mind. Imagery can help you relax, relieve boredom, decrease anxiety, and help you sleep.

How do I use the technique of imagery?

Usually, imagery for pain relief is done with the eyes closed. A relaxation technique may be used first. The image can be something such as a ball of healing energy or a picture drawn in your mind of yourself as a person without pain (for example, imagine that you are cutting wires that transmit pain signals from each part of your body to your brain).

Here is an exercise with the first image: **the ball of energy**. It is a variation of the technique credited to Dr. David Bresler at the Pain Control Unit, University of California, Los Angeles (UCLA).

- Close your eyes. Breathe slowly and feel yourself relax.

- Concentrate on your breathing. Breathe slowly and comfortably from your abdomen. As you breathe in, say silently and slowly to yourself. "In, one, two." As you breathe out, say: "Out, one, two." Breathe in this slow rhythm for a few minutes.

- Imagine a ball of healing energy forming in your lungs or on your chest. It may be like a white light. It can be vague. It does not have to be vivid. Imagine this ball forming, taking shape.

- When you are ready, imagine that the air you breathe in blows this healing ball of energy to the area of your pain. Once there, the ball heals and relaxes you.
- When you breathe out, imagine the air blows the ball away from your body. As it goes, the ball takes your pain with it. (Be careful: Do not blow as you breathe out; breathe out naturally.)
- Repeat the last two steps each time you breathe in and out.
- You may imagine that the ball gets bigger and bigger as it takes more and more discomfort away from your body.
- To end the imagery, count slowly to three, breathe in deeply, open your eyes, and say silently to yourself: "I feel alert and relaxed." Begin moving about slowly.

Are there any problems with using imagery?

The problems are similar to the ones that may occur with relaxation techniques.

What is distraction, and how does it work?

Distraction means turning your attention to something other than the pain. Many people use this method without realizing it when they watch television or listen to the radio to "take their minds off" the pain.

Distraction may work better than medicine if pain is sudden and intense or if it is brief, lasting only 5 to 45 minutes.

Distraction is useful when you are waiting for pain medicine to start working. If pain is mild, you may be able to distract yourself for hours.

Some people think that a person who can be distracted from pain does not have severe pain. This is not necessarily true. Distraction can be a powerful way of temporarily relieving even the most intense pain.

How can I use distraction?

Any activity that occupies your attention can be used for distraction. If you enjoy working with your hands, crafts such as needlework, model building, or painting may be useful. Losing yourself in a good book might divert your mind from the pain. Going to a movie or watching television are also good distraction methods. Slow, rhythmic breathing can be used for distraction as well as relaxation.

You may find it helpful to listen to rather fast music through a headset or earphones. To help keep your attention on the music, tap

Relieving Cancer Pain without Medicines

out the rhythm. You can adjust the volume to match the intensity of pain, making it louder for very severe pain. This technique does not require much energy, so it may be very useful when you are tired.

Are there any drawbacks to using distraction for pain relief?

After using a distraction technique, some people report that they are tired, irritable, and feel more pain. Some also find that other people do not believe they are in pain if distraction provides pain relief. If these are problems for you, you may not wish to use distraction or you may simply be careful about which distraction methods you use and when you use them.

What is skin stimulation, and how does it work to relieve pain?

Skin stimulation is the use of pressure, friction, temperature change, or chemical substances to excite the nerve endings in the skin. Scientists believe that the same nerve pathways transmit the sensations of pain, heat, cold, and pressure to the brain. When the skin is stimulated so that pressure, warmth, or cold is felt, pain sensation is lessened or blocked. Skin stimulation also alters the flow of blood to the affected area. Sometimes skin stimulation will get rid of the pain, or the pain will be less during the stimulation and for hours after it is finished.

NOTE: If you are having radiation therapy, check with your doctor or nurse before using skin stimulation. You should not apply ointments, salves, or liniments to the treatment area, and you should not use heat or extreme cold on treated areas.

Where is skin stimulation done?

Skin stimulation is done either on or near the area of pain. You also can use skin stimulation on the side of the body opposite to the pain. For example, you might stimulate the left knee to decrease pain in the right knee. Stimulating the skin in areas away from the pain can be used to increase relaxation and may relieve pain.

What is used to stimulate the skin?

Massage, pressure, vibration, heat, cold, and menthol preparations are used for skin stimulation.

How do I use massage for pain relief?

For pain relief, massage is most effective when using slow, steady, circular motions. You can massage over or near the area of pain with just your bare hand or with any substance that feels good such as talcum powder, warm oil, or hand lotion. Depending upon where your pain is located, you may do it yourself or ask a family member or friend to give you a massage. Remember, having someone give you a foot rub, back rub, or hand rub can be very relaxing and may relieve pain. Some people find brushing or stroking lightly more comforting than deep massage. Use whatever works best for you.

NOTE: *If you are having radiation therapy, avoid massage in the treatment area.*

How do I use pressure?

Pressure can be applied with the entire hand, the heel of the hand, the fingertip or the knuckle, the ball of the thumb, or by using one or both hands to encircle your arm or leg. You can experiment by applying pressure for about 10 seconds to various areas over or near your pain to see if it helps. You can also feel around your pain and outward to see if you can find "trigger points," small areas under the skin that are especially sensitive or that trigger pain. Pressure is usually most effective if it is applied as firmly as possible without causing pain. You can use pressure for up to about 1 minute. This often will relieve pain for several minutes to several hours after the pressure is released.

How do I use vibration?

Vibration over or near the area of pain may bring temporary relief. For example, the scalp attachment of a hand-held vibrator often relieves a headache. For low back pain, a long, slender battery-operated vibrator placed at the small of the back may be helpful. You may use a vibrating device such as a small battery-operated vibrator, a hand-held electric vibrator, a large heat-massage electric pad, or a bed vibrator.

Which is better for relieving pain-cold or heat?

As for any of the techniques described, you should use what works best for you. Heat often relieves sore muscles; cold lessens pain sensations by numbing the affected area. Many people with prolonged

Relieving Cancer Pain without Medicines

pain use only heat and have never given cold a try. Some people find that cold relieves pain faster, and relief may last longer.

What are some comfortable and convenient ways to use cold or heat?

For cold, try gel packs that are sealed in plastic and remain soft and flexible even at freezing temperatures. Gel packs are available at drugstores and medical supply stores. They are reusable and can be kept in the freezer when not in use. Wrap the pack with a layer of towels so that it is comfortable for you. An ice pack or ice cubes wrapped in a towel can be just as effective.

To use heat for pain relief, a heating pad that generates its own moisture (Hydrocolater) is convenient. Gel packs heated in hot water, hot water bottles, a hot, moist towel, a regular heating pad, or a hot bath or shower can also be used to apply heat. For aching joints, such as elbows and knees, you can wrap the joint in lightweight plastic wrap (tape the plastic to itself). This retains body heat and moisture.

NOTE: *Do not use heat or cold over any area receiving radiation therapy.*

What are menthol preparations?

Many menthol preparations are available for pain relief. There are creams, lotions, liniments, or gels that contain menthol. Brands include Ben-Gay, Icy Hot, Mineral Ice, and Heet. When they are rubbed into the skin, they increase blood circulation to the affected area and produce a warm (sometimes cool) soothing feeling that lasts for several hours.

How do I use menthol preparations?

First, test your skin by rubbing a small amount of the menthol preparation in a circle about 1 inch in diameter in the area of pain (or the area to be stimulated). This will let you know whether the menthol is uncomfortable to you or irritates your skin. If the menthol does not create a problem, rub some more into the area. The sensation caused by the menthol gradually increases and remains up to several hours. To increase the intensity and duration of the menthol sensation, you can open your skin pores with heat (e.g., shower, sun) or wrap a plastic sheet over the area after the menthol application. (Don't use a heating pad because it may cause a burn.) If you're afraid others will find the odor offensive, you can use the menthol product when you are alone, or perhaps in the evening or through the night.

NOTE: *Many menthol preparations contain an ingredient similar to aspirin. A small amount of this aspirin-like substance is absorbed through the skin. If you have been told not to take aspirin, do not use these preparations until you check with your doctor.*

What precautions should I take if I use skin stimulation?

Heat and cold can easily damage your skin. It is easy to burn the skin with hot water from the tap or with settings too high on the heating pad. Extreme cold can also burn your skin.

- Never use a heating pad on bare skin.
- Never go to sleep for the night with the heating pad on.
- Be very careful while using a heating pad if you are taking drugs or medicines that make you sleepy or if you do not have much feeling in the area.
- Limit heat or cold application to 5 to 10 minutes.
- Do not use heat or cold over any area where your circulation or sensation is poor.
- If you start to shiver when using cold, stop using it right away.
- Do not use cold so intense or for so long that the cold itself causes pain.
- Do not use heat over a new injury because heat can increase bleeding. Wait at least 24 hours.
- Do not rub menthol preparations over broken skin, a skin rash, or mucous membranes (such as inside your mouth or around your rectum). Make sure you do not get the menthol in your eyes.
- Avoid massage and vibration over red, raw, tender, or swollen areas.
- If skin stimulation increases your pain, stop using it.
- As noted earlier, if you are undergoing (or have undergone) radiation treatments, do not use any skin stimulation method without first checking with your doctor or nurse.

Other Methods of Pain Relief

Are there any operations to relieve pain?

Yes. Pain cannot be felt if the nerve pathways that relay pain impulses to the brain are interrupted. To block these pathways, a neurosurgeon may cut a nerve close to the spinal cord (rhizotomy) or cut bundles of nerves in the spinal cord itself (cordotomy).

When the nerves that transmit pain are destroyed, the sensations of pressure and temperature can no longer be felt. Therefore, after these operations, patients are more likely to injure the affected area because they no longer have the protective reflexes of pain, pressure, or temperature.

What are nerve blocks?

When certain substances are injected into or around a nerve, that nerve is no longer able to transmit pain. A local anesthetic, which may be combined with cortisone, provides temporary pain relief. For longer lasting pain relief, phenol or alcohol can be injected. A nerve block may cause muscle paralysis. Loss of all feeling in the affected area is a frequent side effect of a nerve block.

What is transcutaneous electric nerve stimulation (TENS)?

This is a technique in which mild electric currents are applied to selected areas of the skin by a small power pack connected to two electrodes. The sensation is described as a buzzing, tingling, or tapping feeling. The small electric impulses seem to interfere with pain sensations. The current can be adjusted so that the sensation is pleasant and relieves the pain. Pain relief lasts beyond the time that the current is applied. Your doctor or a physical therapist can tell you where to get a TENS unit.

Can alcohol help relieve my pain?

Drinking alcohol sometimes can provide pain relief, increase appetite, reduce anxiety, and help you sleep. Drinking small amounts of alcoholic beverages with meals or in the evening may be beneficial for you. Ask your doctor's advice before you start using alcohol, because it is dangerous to combine alcohol with certain pain-relieving drugs.

Will marijuana relieve my pain?

No. The pain-relieving effects of marijuana are not consistent. Marijuana has been reported to reduce anxiety or control nausea so that the person in pain feels better. However, some cancer patients have reported that smoking marijuana increased their pain. At this time, marijuana is not legally available.

What about acupuncture for pain relief?

In acupuncture, special needles are inserted into the body at certain points and at various depths and angles. Particular groups of acupuncture points are believed to control specific areas of pain sensation. The procedure has been used as an anesthetic in China and elsewhere to treat many types of pain, but its usefulness for cancer patients has not been proven. Most doctors believe that it is not harmful as long as the needles are sterile. Acupuncture should not be used for patients who are getting chemotherapy because of the danger of increased bleeding where the needles are placed.

Can hypnosis help?

No one knows how hypnosis works to control pain. Hypnosis is a trance-like state that can be brought on by a person trained in special techniques. During hypnosis, a person is very receptive to suggestions made by the hypnotist. To relieve pain, the hypnotist may suggest that pain will be gone when the person "wakes up." Some cancer patients have learned methods of self-hypnosis that they use to control pain. However, it's hard to predict when hypnosis will work for pain relief.

Treating Cancer Pain in the Elderly

Like other adults, elderly patients require comprehensive assessment and aggressive management of cancer pain. However, older patients are at risk for under treatment of pain because of underestimation of their sensitivity to pain, the expectation that they tolerate pain well, and misconceptions about their ability to benefit from the use of opioids. Issues in assessing and treating cancer pain in older patients include:

Relieving Cancer Pain without Medicines

- **Multiple chronic diseases and sources of pain.** Complex medication regimens place them at increased risk for drug-drug and drug-disease interactions.

- **Visual, hearing, motor, and cognitive impairments.** The use of simple descriptive, numeric, and visual analog pain assessment instruments may be impeded. Cognitively impaired patients may require simpler scales and more frequent pain assessment.

- **NSAID side effects.** Although effective alone or as adjuncts to opioids, NSAIDs are more likely to cause gastric and renal toxicity and other drug reactions such as cognitive impairment, constipation, and headaches in older patients. Alternative NSAIDs (e.g., choline magnesium trisalicylate) or co-administration of misoprostol should be considered to reduce gastric toxicity.

- **Opioid effectiveness.** Older persons tend to be more sensitive to the analgesic effects of opioids. The peak opioid effect is higher and the duration of pain relief is longer.

- **Patient-controlled analgesia.** Slower drug clearance and increased sensitivity to undesirable drug effects (e.g., cognitive impairment) indicate the need for cautious initial dosing and subsequent titration and monitoring.

- **Alternative routes of administration.** Although useful for patients who have nausea or vomiting, the rectal route may be inappropriate for elderly or infirm patients who are physically unable to place the suppository in the rectum.

- **Postoperative pain control.** Following surgery, surgeons and other health care team members should maintain frequent direct contact with the elderly patient to reassess the quality of pain management.

- **Change of setting.** Reassessment of pain management and appropriate changes should be made whenever the elderly patient moves (e.g., from hospital to home or nursing home).

Relaxation Exercises

Source: McCaffery and Beebe, 1989. Adapted and reprinted with permission.

Exercise 1. *Slow Rhythmic Breathing for Relaxation*

1. Breathe in slowly and deeply.
2. As you breathe out slowly, feel yourself beginning to relax; feel the tension leaving your body.
3. Now breathe in and out slowly and regularly, at whatever rate is comfortable for you. You may wish to try abdominal breathing.
4. To help you focus on your breathing and breathe slowly and rhythmically: (a) breathe in as you say silently to yourself, "in, two, three"; (b) breathe out as you say silently to yourself, "out, two, three." **or** Each time you breathe out, say silently to yourself a word such as "peace" or "relax."
5. Do steps 1 through 4 only once or repeat steps 3 and 4 for up to 20 minutes.
6. End with a slow deep breath. As you breathe out say to yourself, "I feel alert and relaxed."

Exercise 2. *Simple Touch, Massage, or Warmth for Relaxation*

Touch and massage are age-old methods of helping others relax. Some examples are:

1. Brief touch or massage, e.g., handholding or briefly touching or rubbing a person's shoulder.
2. Warm foot soak in a basin of warm water, or wrap the feet in a warm, wet towel.
3. Massage (3 to 10 minutes) may consist of whole body or be restricted to back, feet, or hands. If the patient is modest or cannot move or turn easily in bed, consider massage of the hands and feet.
    - Use a warm lubricant, e.g., a small bowl of hand lotion may be warmed in the microwave oven, or a bottle of lotion may be warmed by placing it in a sink of hot water for about 10 minutes.

Relieving Cancer Pain without Medicines

- Massage for relaxation is usually done with smooth, long, slow strokes. (Rapid strokes, circular movements, and squeezing of tissues tend to stimulate circulation and increase arousal.) However, try several degrees of pressure along with different types of massage, e.g., kneading, stroking, and circling. Determine which is preferred.

Especially for the elderly person, a back rub that effectively produces relaxation may consist of no more than 3 minutes of slow, rhythmic stroking (about 60 strokes per minute) on both sides of the spinous process from the crown of the head to the lower back. Continuous hand contact is maintained by starting one hand down the back as the other hand stops at the lower back and is raised. Set aside a regular time for the massage. This gives the patient something to look forward to and depend on.

Exercise 3. Peaceful Past Experiences

Something may have happened to you a while ago that brought you peace and comfort. You may be able to draw on that past experience to bring you peace or comfort now. Think about these questions:

1. Can you remember any situation, even when you were a child, when you felt calm, peaceful, secure, hopeful, or comfortable?
2. Have you ever daydreamed about something peaceful? What were you thinking of?
3. Do you get a dreamy feeling when you listen to music? Do you have any favorite music?
4. Do you have any favorite poetry that you find uplifting or reassuring?
5. Have you ever been religiously active? Do you have favorite readings, hymns, or prayers? Even if you haven't heard or thought of them for many years, childhood religious experiences may still be very soothing.

Additional points: Very likely some of the things you think of in answer to these questions can be recorded for you, such as your favorite music or a prayer. Then, you can listen to the tape whenever you wish. Or, if your memory is strong, you may simply close your eyes and recall the events or words.

Exercise 4. Active Listening to Recorded Music

1. Obtain the following:
   - A cassette player or tape recorder. (Small, battery-operated ones are more convenient.)
   - Earphone or headset. (This is a more demanding stimulus than a speaker a few feet away, and it avoids disturbing others.)
   - Cassette of music you like. (Most people prefer fast, lively music, but some select relaxing music. Other options are comedy routines, sporting events, old radio shows, or stories.)
2. Mark time to the music, e.g., tap out the rhythm with your finger or nod your head. This helps you concentrate on the music rather than your discomfort.
3. Keep your eyes open and focus steadily on one stationary spot or object. If you wish to close your eyes, picture something about the music.
4. Listen to the music at a comfortable volume. If the discomfort increases, try increasing the volume; decrease the volume when the discomfort decreases.
5. If this is not effective enough, try adding or changing one or more of the following: massage your body in rhythm to the music; try other music; mark time to the music in more than one manner, e.g., tap your foot and finger at the same time.

Additional points: Many patients have found this technique to be helpful. It tends to be very popular, probably because the equipment is usually readily available and is a part of daily life. Other advantages are that it is easy to learn and is not physically or mentally demanding. If you are very tired, you may simply listen to the music and omit marking time or focusing on a spot.

Conclusion

We hope this chapter has helped you to understand treatments for pain and that it has given you useful information for dealing with pain. It is not intended to take the place of good communication between you and the health professionals who are caring for you. Remember that there are many ways to manage pain and that cancer pain can almost always be controlled.

Additional patient education materials (including information about diet and nutrition, chemotherapy, radiation therapy, emotional support, and the symptoms and treatment of many types of cancer) are available free of charge from both the American Cancer Society and the National Cancer Institute. Addresses and descriptions of the American Cancer Society and the National Cancer Institute are listed below.

Sources of Additional Information

American Cancer Society, Inc.
1599 Clifton Road, N.E.
Atlanta, GA 30329-4251
1-800-ACS-2345

The American Cancer Society (ACS) is a national nonprofit organization whose programs include research, education, and service. Local ACS Units offer service programs for cancer patients and their families. They provide information and guidance, referral to community health services and other resources, equipment loans for care of the homebound patient, transportation to and from treatment, and rehabilitation programs. Before contacting national headquarters, check your local telephone directory for an ACS Unit in your community.

Two mutual support programs, which began as grassroots efforts, have been designated as national programs of the American Cancer Society. Check to see if they are available in your community.

CanSurmount: CanSurmount brings together the patient, the family, the CanSurmount volunteer, and health professionals. On physician referral, a trained CanSurmount volunteer, who is also a cancer patient, meets with the patient and family in the hospital or home. The goal of the program is to improve mutual help and understanding through continuing education and support for volunteers, patients, families, health professionals, and the community.

I Can Cope: This program addresses the educational and psychological needs of people with cancer and their families. It is a series of classes covering information about cancer, types of treatments, communication with family, friends, and physicians and how to find additional resources. Through lectures, group discussions, and study assignments, the course helps people with cancer regain a sense of control over their lives.

For further information about CanSurmount and I Can Cope, contact your local Unit of the American Cancer Society.

National Cancer Institute
Office of Cancer Communications
Building 31, Room 10A24
Bethesda, MD 20892

The National Cancer Institute (NCI) is the US government's main agency for cancer research and information about cancer. Additional information about pain control and other cancer-related topics is available from the NCI-supported Cancer Information Service (CIS), a nationwide telephone service that answers questions from cancer patients and their families, health care professionals, and the public. Information specialists can provide information and publications on all aspects of cancer.

The toll-free number of the CIS is 1-800-4-CANCER.

You will reach a CIS office serving your area where a trained staff member can answer your questions and listen to your concerns. Spanish-speaking staff members are available.

Pain Organizations

American Academy of Pain Medicine
5700 Old Orchard Road
Skokie, IL 60077
(708) 966-9510

American Pain Society
5700 Old Orchard Road
Skokie, IL 60077
(708) 966-5595

American Society of Anesthesiologists
Pain Therapy Committee
515 Busse Highway
Park Ridge, IL 60068
(708) 825-5586

Commission on Accreditation of Rehabilitation Facilities
101 North Wilmot Road,
Suite 500
Tucson, AZ 85711
(602) 748-1212

Relieving Cancer Pain without Medicines

International Association for the Study of Pain
909 NE 43rd Street,
Suite 306
Seattle, WA 98105
(206) 547-6409

National Chronic Pain Outreach Association
7979 Old Georgetown Road,
Suite 100
Bethesda, MD 20814-2429
(301) 652-4948

Part Seven

Managing Pain

Chapter 39

Multidisciplinary Teams: The Integrated Approach to the Management of Pain

Introduction

We have come a long way in our social and professional attitudes toward the management of pain that have changed and developed during the last half century. A prior consensus statement, published in 1979, stressed the "caring" as well as the "curing" role in the management of pain associated with terminal disease and called for a more humanitarian approach. Since the time of that statement, further progress has been made in understanding and assessing the multidimensional character of pain, advancing the state of pharmacological techniques, and developing a variety of non-pharmacological approaches to the treatment of pain. In addition, recent years have witnessed the advent and growth of multi-disciplinary pain clinics employing a range of methods and styles for the treatment of pain. While no single model commands universal acceptance, this new commitment to utilizing multiple modes of treatment and employing the skills of a multi-disciplinary team of health professionals has come to be known as the "integrated approach to the management of pain."

Despite these recent scientific advances in the understanding and treatment of pain, it is important to recognize that there is no "magic bullet" or universally accepted treatment for the relief of pain and suffering. Contemporary science and clinical practice cannot assure

---

NIH Consensus Development Conference Statement Volume 6 Number 3. May 19-21, 1986.

the full relief of all pain. The data indicate that there remains a proportion of patients whose pain presents difficult, and so far unsolved, problems for successful management.

Yet over and above these limitations posed by current knowledge and technology, many informed observers, supported by some scientific data, perceive continuing deficiencies in the clinical management of pain. Concerns are focused on reported under-medication of individuals with acute pain and chronic pain associated with malignant diseases as well as reported over-medication of people with chronic pain not associated with malignant disease.

There is reason for concern that the education and training of many health care professionals for example, in schools of medicine, nursing, dentistry, and physical therapy, do not place adequate emphasis on contemporary methods of pain assessment and management. Furthermore, communications among physicians, dentists, nurses, other health care professionals, and patients regarding pain relief in clinical settings of both inpatient and outpatient types are less than adequate. These perceived deficiencies help to explain the attractiveness of collaborative approaches to pain management that stress joint efforts and enhanced communication among health care professionals. The multidimensional character of pain, the difficulty of assessment, and the multiplicity of possible interventions suggest the complexity of the task and reinforce the arguments favoring collaboration and shared responsibility among health care professionals in the management of pain. There is also an inherent role for the individual with pain, and often the family, in determining the course of treatment and participating in the process of pain management. Well-established ethical and legal principles require that individuals in-pain have a significant voice in treatment decisions. It is therefore important that they be informed sufficiently to understand, appreciate, and make intelligent decisions regarding the approach to pain management.

Estimation of the prevalence and incidence of pain as indicators of the magnitude of the problem addressed in this report is of great importance. Clearly, based on self-reports and clinical experience a large number of persons experience pain. However, reliable and valid estimates cannot be extrapolated from the data presented at this conference. Much of the information presented is based on reports from pain clinics that comprise only a small and non-representative sample of persons with pain. Yet epidemiological economic, and bio-statistical data delineating the magnitude of the problem of pain in this country—to individuals, communities, and health care facilities—are fragmented and inadequate.

Multidisciplinary Teams: The Integrated Approach

The term "integration" within the context of this consensus panel is used to describe an approach to the most effective use of pharmacological and non-pharmacological agents in the management of pain. In an effort to resolve some of the questions surrounding the integration of approaches to pain management, the Warren Grant Magnuson Clinical Center, the National Cancer Institute, the National Institute of Neurological and Communicative Disorders and Stroke, the National Institute of Dental Research, and the Office of Medical Applications of Research, NIH, jointly sponsored a Consensus Development Conference on the Integrated Approach to the Management of Pain. The conference brought together biomedical investigators, physicians, dentists, psychologists, nurses, other health care professionals, and representatives of the public on May 19-21, 1986.

Following a day-and-a-half of presentations by health care experts and discussion by the audience, a consensus panel, drawn from the health care and lay communities, considered the evidence and data presented and agreed on responses to the following questions:

- How should pain be assessed?
- How should pharmacological agents be used in an integrated approach to pain management?
- How should non-pharmacological interventions be used in an integrated approach to pain management?
- What is the role of the nurse in the integrated approach to pain management?
- What are the directions for future research in pain management?

How Should Pain Be Assessed?

Pain is a symptom that arises in response to a noxious stimulus or tissue injury. In some instances, pain may persist after the tissue damage has healed or in the absence of evident tissue damage. Clinicians have found it useful to classify pain into three major categories based on etiology: pain following acute injury, disease, or some types of surgery (acute pain); pain associated with cancer or other progressive disorders (chronic malignant pain), or pain in persons whose tissue injury is non-progressive or healed (chronic nonmalignant pain). An individual may have more than one type of pain.

Pain is a subjective experience that can be perceived directly only by the sufferer. It is a multi-dimensional phenomenon that can be described by pain location, intensity, temporal aspects, quality, impact, and meaning. Pain does not occur in isolation but in a specific human being in psychosocial, economic, and cultural contexts that influence the meaning, experience, and verbal and non-verbal expression of pain.

Verbal self-reporting and behavior measures have been developed to assess the characteristics of a person's pain. Self-reported pain assessments can range from a simple "yes" or "no" response to questions such as "Are you in pain?" to a complex battery of instruments that measure multiple factors. The McGill-Melzack Pain Questionnaire is a widely used tool that measures sensory, affective, and evaluative dimensions of pain. Other self-report tests consist of verbal descriptions that range from low to high amounts of the dimensions of pain to be measured and visual analog scales which may represent the entire continuum of a dimension of the pain experience. The degree of pain is reported by selecting a verbal descriptor or making a mark on the line to indicate the level of pain.

Pain behaviors can be measured by personal diaries kept by persons in pain to record such things as daily activities, self-reports of time of onset, pain severity, medication consumption, perceived effect of drugs, and reported response to pharmacological and non-pharmacological attempts at relief. In using direct observation, the clinician can document pain behaviors such as guarded movement, rubbing of painful areas, and sighing. Important to observe are the related practices of withdrawal and social isolation, drugs abused, over-utilization of the health care system, and inordinate pre-occupation with pain. Interpretation based on such observation warrants sensitivity to the patient's individuality, culture, and modes of pain expression.

The assessment of pain in children presents special problems and is a subject of current research interest. Clinical impressions suggest that children in pain may frequently be under-treated. The usual verbal testing techniques are not applicable for younger children, and measures of pain magnitude are imprecise in children at earlier stages of cognitive development. Since children of all ages can and do express their pain, innovations in assessment tools designed expressly for children must be developed. Assessment techniques that require magnitude estimates and cognition are also of limited applicability to special populations, for example, those who are cognitively impaired or faced with language, cultural, or educational barriers. More effective approaches to the assessment of pain in these persons with special needs deserve exploration.

The clinical assessment of the person with pain begins with diagnostic evaluation and clarification of the goals of therapy. These should be appropriate for the type of pain, its cause, and the characteristics of the individual affected. Also, when and how often pain assessments should be made varies. Expectations for improvement differ according to these factors. Repeated clinical measures of acute pain must be relatively short and should focus primarily on sensory description and comparative estimates of magnitude and intensity. At present, few valid and reliable acute pain measures exist. With chronic pain, assessment may be more productively focused on affective and evaluative aspects of the pain experience, as well as on its history and context. Many existing pain assessment measures are based on a chronic pain model. Recent research indicates that an attempt should be made to measure as many dimensions as feasible in all types of pain, although the relative importance of each dimension varies by pain type.

Acute Pain

The single most useful method for evaluating acute pain outside of the research environment is to ask the person how he or she feels. Assessment tools such as the visual analog scale may be adapted to the needs of the bedside and are easy to use. The McGill-Melzack Pain Questionnaire may be useful during the initial evaluation. However, it may not be practical on an ongoing basis in the clinical management of the individual experiencing pain. Further testing to establish reliability and validity of several different types of pain-specific self-report and visual analog scales in the clinical setting is indicated.

Chronic Pain Associated with Malignant Disease

Wide variations exist among persons with chronic pain associated with malignant disease. At such times, self-reports, the visual analog scale, and the McGill-Melzack Pain Questionnaire are useful when the person's condition permits. At other times, some individuals are quite ill and may be motionless and silent and only the simplest descriptions of discomfort can be elicited from them. Caregivers should review evidence of change in appetite, activity, social interaction, sleep patterns, and the impact of pain on the quality of life.

Chronic Pain Not Associated with Malignant Disease

The primary objective when evaluating individuals with this kind of pain should include the level of function as it may not be possible to achieve complete relief of pain. Both self-report measures and direct observation of motor activity are useful.

Measures of psychological function may be important in evaluating the individual's emotional state and coping mechanisms since depression can be an important factor for many persons. Outside the research environment practical measures such as an increase in physical activity or improvement in interpersonal relationships will reflect improvement.

Thus far, the evaluation of treatment effectiveness for pain has relied largely on clinical impressions of outcome. Clinical investigators are presently involved in the development of valid and reliable measures of appropriate short- and long-term outcomes. This includes measures that are useful for longitudinal study of change over time such as increase in physical activity, as well as measures of absolute endpoints. These include increased activities of daily living, improved patterns of socialization, and return to employment. Effective assessment has related economic effects as well since in part, it determines eligibility for benefits.

Should Pharmacological Agents Be Used in an Integrated Approach to Pain Management?

Individualization of Drug Therapy

There may be marked individual variation in intensity of effect for any dose of a drug. Variations in dose-response are due to variations in rates of drug absorption, metabolism, and excretion and to variations in cell or organ sensitivity to the drug, presence of disease and variations in age and body size. Attention should be given to these variations in dose-response in individualizing drug choice and drug dosage for patients with pain.

Acute Pain

Surveys of hospitalized people with acute pain have found that many continue to have moderate or severe pain because their treatment has been with doses of narcotic analgesics that have been too low or given at too long an interval between doses. Reasons for low doses or doses given infrequently include incorrect assessment, insufficient knowledge of the pharmacology of the prescribed drug, and personal attitudes of the caregivers and patients alike about narcotic analgesics. Concern about the problems of addiction and respiratory depression is greater than the actual risk. Approaches to addressing such problems include educating health care professionals about analgesic drugs and making them aware of how their attitudes may affect their use or nonuse of narcotic analgesics effectively. Public education with respect to these issues is also important.

One of the innovative ways that may provide effective individualized analgesia and comfort for these people has been the development of patient-controlled analgesia (PCA). This technique utilizes a device that permits intravenous self-administration of narcotic drugs within limits of dose and frequency established by the physician.

Chronic Malignant Pain

There are many parallels in the inadequate treatment of cancer pain with the inadequate treatment of acute pain. Surveys of people with metastatic cancer have revealed that the majority has moderate or severe pain. Research has shown that narcotic analgesics given on a scheduled basis in adequate doses is an improvement over the former p.r.n. (pro re nata or as occasion arises, according to circumstances, or as is necessary) method of physician-ordered narcotic use and nurse-or pharmacist-interpreted administration of drugs to address these pain problems.

An additional issue of concern in this patient population is the development of tolerance. There is an indication that when dosage requirement increases, the reason can be disease progression and not always increased tolerance. Physical dependence does occur but is not of clinical significance in advanced disease.

Some people with metastatic cancer cannot achieve pain control by systemic narcotics. In many situations, dose-limiting side effects are a problem. The addition of other drugs such as steroids or nonsteroidal anti-inflammatory drugs to the regimen may improve pain control without enhancing drug toxicity. In addition, other modalities of therapy such as nerve blocks, neuro-surgical procedures, radiation therapy, chemotherapy, and other appropriate interventions, while not considered in detail at this conference, should not be ignored in the care of the individual with cancer pain. An innovative approach to the treatment of cancer pain has been the exploration of new routes or methods of narcotic administration. These include continuous subcutaneous infusion, epidural and intrathecal routes, mucous membrane or transdermal absorption, oral formulations with slow release and absorption, and PCA.

One should be aware that many individuals with pain due to cancer early in the course of their illness can achieve pain control with non-narcotic analgesics. For this class of drugs as for the narcotics, individualization of dose and of drug is essential.

Chronic Nonmalignant Pain

People with chronic pain of non-malignant cause are a heterogeneous group with a variety of illnesses. They are treated with a wide variety of medications and other therapies, often with limited success. In an effort to alleviate the pain, drug dosage is often progressively raised to the point at which significant side effects appear. In addition to the established analgesics, tricyclic anti-depressants have been tried in some of these conditions with variable results. They are most effective when clinical depression accompanies pain. Phenothiazines may have been used in treating nausea or anxiety accompanying pain, but they are not effective as analgesics or as potentiators of analgesics. Special care should be taken to avoid over-treatment of these individuals, particularly with drugs that have a real risk of side effects or addiction.

Children and Infants

There are special problems in providing adequate analgesia for infants and children. These special problems are due to deficiencies in assessing pain and to the lack of sufficient knowledge about factors influencing drug action in this population. Special attention should be given to solving these problems.

Quality Assurance

We recommend that examination of the adequacy of pain relief for persons in the hospital or receiving services from other health care institutions and agencies should be made a part of existing quality assurance programs.

Should Non-pharmacological Interventions Be Used in an Integrated Approach to Pain Management?

This past decade has witnessed a dramatic increase in laboratory and clinical research on non-pharmacological approaches to pain management. Experienced clinicians report some success with a variety of non-pharmacological modalities, including acupuncture, biofeedback, transcutaneous electrical nerve stimulation (TENS), hypnosis, physical therapy, and behavioral approaches such as coping strategies, desensitization, modeling, operant conditioning, and relaxation. Diagnostic and therapeutic nerve blocks of many parts of the body may be useful in pain management and as predictors of the

Multidisciplinary Teams: The Integrated Approach

effect of neurosurgical intervention. Acupuncture and TENS are most commonly used for chronic musculo-skeletal disorders. Biofeedback is often used for the treatment of headaches and painful vascular conditions. Investigators agree that now is an appropriate time to evaluate the effectiveness of each of these modalities with specific patient populations through the use of controlled studies.

Behavioral therapies are used for some individuals with chronic pain. Practitioners believe that such therapies are indicated when excessive pain behavior is inconsistent with other clinical findings. They are also used when there is a progressive decline in activity, evidence of abuse in pain medications, or an inordinate dependence on spouse or family members.

Biofeedback involves giving individuals information about physiologic responses and ways to exercise voluntary control over these responses. It is useful in muscle tension headaches and migraine headaches. A variety of relaxation techniques can be used in reducing pain associated with stress or anxiety.

With regard to the non-pharmacological approaches to pain, there must be a willingness on the part of the patient to participate with the clinician in the decision about which modality to use. In addition, it is important that the family members be educated about the proposed modality and their role in its application. Persons uncomfortable with or unwilling to take potent drugs for the relief of pain may be more willing to consider non-pharmacological approaches.

The various modalities, singly or in combination, can be utilized in the management of acute or chronic pain. Some persons may require a simultaneous or sequential combination of multi-modal approaches incorporating pharmacological and non-pharmacological approaches in pain management.

What Is the Role of the Nurse in the Integrated Approach to Pain Management?

While the consensus panel was asked to investigate particularly the role of the nurse within this framework, it recognizes and supports the significant contributions made by all members of the health care team to the management of the person with pain. The expertise of the members of various specialties of the medical profession is critical to the management of pain.

However, the nurse may be the first health care provider to encounter the person experiencing pain as well as to identify the problem of uncontrolled pain. Thus, many opportunities exist for nurses to enhance the effectiveness of care delivery to individuals with pain. The nurse can be the key link in facilitating communication between the individual and the family and other members of the health care team. In so doing, nurses, along with other health care professionals, can make a significant contribution in facilitating effective patient participation in the decision making process.

The role of the nurse in the assessment and management of pain varies according to the type of patient population being served, the setting in which care is delivered, as well as the educational and professional experience of the individual nurse. In acute care settings, the nurse occupies a central position in assessing the individual with pain, in administering physician-selected therapeutic modalities, and in monitoring the condition of the person in pain.

For those individuals experiencing chronic pain who are being discharged from hospitals or other institutions, nurses are in a pivotal position to assess the congruence between the person's condition, need for care, and the community health, public health, or home health resources available for the management of the individual in the non-institutional setting.

For individuals managed at home, the nurse is frequently the professional who provides care, maintains ongoing communication with the individual and family, monitors the situation, and serves as the link with other care providers.

The role of the generalist nurse should not be underestimated. Nurses at this level have the most consistent interaction with the individual experiencing pain. Examples of the types of interventions that should be provided by the generalist nurse include:

- Preoperative patient education to lessen post-operative pain.
- Nursing care plans that reflect individual medication schedules based on individual preference and activity schedules.
- Implementation of non-pharmacological methods during acutely painful events such as childbirth, burn wound debridement, and diagnostic tests.

The nurse who specializes in the assessment and management of persons with pain may serve as part of an interdisciplinary team or may be individually identified as a resource within a particular setting. The nurse who specializes at this level must also possess increasingly sophisticated skills in the areas of pain assessment, pharmacology, choices of route and timing of drug administration, and participation in non-pharmacological interventions.

Multidisciplinary Teams: The Integrated Approach

Whether or not the nurse practices as a member of an interdisciplinary team, the nurse may be identified as the coordinator of patient care. In this role, the nurse must be able to communicate effectively not only with the person in pain but also with the entire family and health care team.

The role of the nurse with advanced preparation should include:

- Clinical management responsibilities such as titration of analgesics within a protocol according to the patient's level of analgesia, assessment, and participation in the use of both pharmacological and non-pharmacological modalities.

- Provision of consultation and educational services to other members of the nursing staff, other providers, and community groups.

- Active participation in research.

To fulfill these roles effectively, nursing curricula must include pain management content. Nurses practicing in nursing service, nursing education, and nursing research settings should be provided with fellowships for further study of pain management.

What Are the Directions for Future Research in Pain Management?

Future research should be directed to:

- Identify the factors that facilitate or hinder the dissemination and implementation of up-to-date information in clinical practice in the treatment of pain.

- Determine the appropriateness of using existing research measures in clinical settings and to evaluate their validity as adjuncts to clinical judgments in pain assessment. Investigators should consider the special issues related to children in pain, that have received less attention in the past.

- Identify the specific factors associated with outcome within treatment modalities.

- Assess more fully the potential value of each of the non-pharmacological approaches to pain in acute and chronic pain states through controlled studies in specific populations.

- Discover and develop more effective analgesic drugs with larger margins of safety. Precise knowledge about the pharmacology of known drugs is important, but the development of medicine with new intrinsic actions and new drug molecules is needed. The basic research needed to improve the pharmacological therapy of pain will have to be performed in humans and many species of animals and should utilize a wide variety of research disciplines and methodologies.

- Continue research on endorphins, enkephalins, and narcotic receptors that shows promise of producing better analgesic drugs. In addition, this research may contribute to a better understanding of the mechanisms of such non-pharmacological therapy as acupuncture and TENS.

- Develop and evaluate methods of drug delivery, including PCA, sustained release formulations, epidural administration, and transdermal absorption of narcotic drugs to improve pain management with presently available narcotic drugs.

- Conduct epidemiological studies of the incidence and prevalence of pain.

- Study the nature and meaning of pain in a variety of settings and within a broad range of populations as the basis of developing ethnoculturally and contextually appropriate assessment tools.

Conclusions

Pain is an important and complex phenomenon. Accurate pain assessment requires classification by type of pain and includes the establishment of treatment objectives. Different assessment tools are necessary to reflect the problems inherent in the various classifications of pain. Increasing numbers of assessment tools are available for use in research settings. Some of these tools are of clinical value when used with properly selected individuals.

Unfortunately, even when pain is reported and assessed, it may not necessarily be attended, monitored, treated, and satisfactorily managed. An integrated approach to the assessment and management of pain brings greater options to individuals seeking the alleviation of pain.

New methods are available to deliver drugs effectively with less toxicity. Pharmaco-therapy may be very effective in treating pain.

Multidisciplinary Teams: The Integrated Approach

However, personal attitudes may account for the undertreatment of persons in pain. Insight, education, attitude change, and accountability in the professional practice of health professionals will influence positively the implementation of adequate pain therapy. Non-pharmacological methods are playing an increasing role in the treatment of some types of pain.

Nurses have well-established pivotal roles in the assessment and management of pain that will increase in importance. All members of the multi-disciplinary health team urge effective teaching about the nature of pain and recommend that the integrated approach to pain management be included in both formal and continuing education of the various members of the pain team.

Throughout the conference, the theme emerged that no single treatment modality is appropriate for all or even for most individuals suffering from pain. The treatment, and the evaluation of that treatment, should vary with the constellation of factors surrounding that individual.

These considerations should guide future research.

Chapter 40

Guidelines to Help Select a Pain Unit

Many who suffer from chronic pain have been through a number of different treatments. They have tried physical therapy, biofeedback, surgery, medications, counseling, and other treatment modalities without much success. They find that the pain affects virtually every aspect of their everyday lives: work, home, school, and social activities are all controlled by the pain.

If you want to regain control of your life, it is important that you learn how to cope with chronic pain. Although your pain may never go away, it is possible to reduce pain levels and, more importantly, to improve the quality of your life. To do so, you may need a multidisciplinary approach to chronic pain. While many of you may have tried almost every available medical intervention without great success, sometimes these therapies are most effective when performed together in a controlled setting. To successfully regain control of your life, you must have all the necessary ingredients of pain management in the right quantity. It is possible to live with chronic pain.

A multidisciplinary pain program can provide you with the necessary skills, medical intervention, and direction to effectively cope with chronic pain. The following information will tell you how to go about locating a pain management program in your area, what to look for in a well-defined pain program, and what other issues to consider.

© American Chronic Pain Association. Reprinted with permission.

Multidisciplinary Pain Management Units

Make Sure You Locate a Legitimate Program

- Hospitals and rehabilitation centers are more likely to offer comprehensive treatment than are "stand alone" programs.

- Facilities that offer pain management should include several specific components, listed below.

- The Commission on Accreditation of Rehabilitation Facilities (CARF) [telephone: 1-(800)-444-8991] can provide you with a listing of accredited pain programs in your area (your health insurance may require that the unit be CARF accredited in order for you to receive reimbursement). You can also contact the American Pain Society, a group of health care providers, at (708) 966-5595 for additional information about pain units in your area.

Choose a Good Program That Is Convenient for You and Your Family

- Most pain management programs are part of a hospital or rehabilitation center. The program should be housed in a separate unit designed for pain management.

- Many pain management programs do not offer inpatient care. Choosing a program close to your home will enable you to commute to the program each day.

Learn Something about the People Who Run the Program

- Try to meet several of the staff members to get a sense of the people you will be dealing with while on the unit.

- The program should have a complete medical staff trained in pain management techniques including:
  - Physician (may be a neurologist, psychiatrist, physiatrist, or anesthesiologist but should have expertise in pain management)
  - Registered nurse
  - Physical therapist
  - Biofeedback therapist
  - Vocational counselor
  - Personnel trained in pain management intervention

Guidelines to Help Select a Pain Unit

- Psychiatrist or psychologist
- Occupational therapist
- Family counselor

Make Sure the Program Includes Most of the Following Features

- Biofeedback training
- Group therapy
- Counseling
- Occupational therapy
- Family counseling
- Assertiveness training
- TENS units
- Regional anesthesia (nerve blocks)
- Physical therapy (exercise and body mechanics training, not massage, whirlpool, etc.)
- Relaxation training and stress management
- Educational program covering medications and other aspects of pain and its management
- Aftercare (follow-up support once you have left the unit)

Be Sure Your Family Can Be Involved in Your Care

- Family members should be required to be involved in your treatment.

- The program should provide special educational sessions for family members.

- Joint counseling for you and your family should also be available.

Consider These Additional Factors

- What services will your insurance company reimburse, and what will you be expected to cover?

- What is the unit's physical set-up (is it in a patient care area or in an area by itself)?

- What is the program's length of stay?

- Is the program inpatient or outpatient (when going through medication detoxification, inpatient care is recommended)

- If you choose an out-of-town unit, can your family be involved in your care?
- Do you understand what will be required of you during your stay (length of time you will be on unit, responsibility to take care of personal needs, etc.)?
- Does the unit provide any type of job retraining?
- Make sure that, before accepting you, the unit reviews your previous medical records and give you a complete physical evaluation to be sure you can participate in the program.
- Your personal physician can refer you to the unit, but many programs also accept self-referral.
- Obtain copies of your recent medical records to prevent duplicate testing.
- Before you enter the unit, check with your insurance company to see what type of benefits it provides for pain management.
- Try to talk with both present and past program participants to get their feedback about their stay on the unit.

Pain management can make a significant difference in your life; however, you must realize that much of what you gain from your stay will be up to you. Treatment is designed to help you get out of the patient role and back to being a person. The program should help to restore your ability to function and to enjoy life. It will be up to you to become actively involved in the program if you expect to regain control of your life. Pain programs are difficult, but the benefits can improve your lifestyle!

If you need further information, please feel free to call the American Chronic Pain Association's national office at (916) 632-0922, or write to:

American Chronic Pain Association
P.O. Box 850
Rocklin, CA 95677
fax (916)632-3208

Chapter 41

The Challenge of Relieving Pain

The lucky among us have only an occasional headache. For others, pain is a constant, though unwelcome, companion.

Relieving pain is sometimes simple, sometimes impossible. It depends on the source of the pain and it may also depend on the person.

Everyday Aches and Pains

There are three main nonprescription choices for pain relief—aspirin, acetaminophen (Datril, Tylenol and others), and ibuprofen (Motrin IB, Advil, Nuprin, and others). All three block the production of chemicals called prostaglandins, which the body usually releases when cells are injured. Prostaglandins are believed to play an important role in the pain, heat, redness, and swelling that occur following tissue damage.

So what's the best choice for your headache, pulled muscle, or menstrual cramps?

When it comes to mild, nonspecific pain, headaches, or menstrual discomfort, "all three [nonprescription pain relievers] are quite useful," says Patricia Love, M.D., a rheumatologist with FDA's Center for Drug Evaluation and Research. "There are probably persons who are not able to detect a difference in the effectiveness of the OTC products."

It has been suggested, Love says, that aspirin or ibuprofen may be more effective than acetaminophen for pain caused by inflammation or

---

FDA Consumer, 09/01/1991.

mild menstrual discomfort because they have more prostaglandin-blocking effects. (For more information on menstrual cramps, see "Taming Menstrual Cramps" in the June 1991 *FDA Consumer*. and reprinted in this volume) "Our best advice at present is that, for mild pain, individuals may use what works best and is safe for them," says Love.

In other words, what doesn't cause them problems.

Because prostaglandins play a role in protecting the stomach lining from being attacked by the acid of digestive fluid, aspirin, ibuprofen, and, apparently to a lesser extent, according to Love, acetaminophen may cause stomach irritation, ulcers or bleeding. "If you have a history of stomach disorders, first talk to your doctor [before taking a nonprescription pain reliever]," says Love.

For some people who take aspirin, stomach irritation may be decreased by taking either enteric-coated aspirin, buffered aspirin, or other modified aspirin derivatives such as choline salicylate or magnesium salicylate. Buffered aspirin contains an ingredient that neutralizes some of the digestive system's acid and, therefore, may produce less irritation than plain aspirin.

Coated aspirin dissolves mainly in the intestine. (Uncoated aspirin dissolves in the stomach.) In theory, that difference may mean less stomach irritation says Love. But, she adds, it still depends on an individual's metabolism. For example, some people can't digest the coating, so while they don't get any stomach irritation, they don't get any benefit either. The aspirin passes out of the body undigested and unabsorbed.

People who can't take aspirin because of allergic reactions (e.g., rash, asthma, anaphylaxis) generally can't take ibuprofen either. For them, acetaminophen may be the only nonprescription choice.

"Persons with medication allergies should discuss the use of any nonprescription medication with their doctor," Love says.

She adds that all three drugs have the potential to cause liver damage, although liver toxicity is much less common than gastric ulcers or bleeding.

FDA is reviewing recent studies that suggest an association between use of all three nonprescription pain relievers and kidney disease. But the agency says that not enough is known yet about these possible associations to make any changes in current recommendations for use for healthy individuals.

"I think one of the important safety issues in choosing a medication is it's not just whether or not you have minor pain, but what is your medical history on top of the minor pain," says Love. "People who

The Challenge of Relieving Pain

have specific disorders—kidney disease, heart disease, bleeding problems, liver disorders, medication allergies—should talk to their physicians."

Acute Pain from Injury or Surgery

When the pain becomes too much to bear, or is the result of a serious injury or surgery, relief requires stronger medicine and a doctor's prescription. One class of frequently prescribed pain relievers is nonsteroidal anti-inflammatory drugs, often abbreviated NSAIDs. (The three nonprescription pain relievers are also NSAIDs, according to Love, although acetaminophen is not commonly referred to by that term.)

Prescription NSAIDs are given at higher doses than the nonprescription types, but the mechanism for pain relief is the same—blocking the production of prostaglandins. (For more information on NSAIDs, see "How to Take Your Medicine: Nonsteroidal Anti-Inflammatory Drugs" in the June 1990 *FDA Consumer* and reprinted in this volume.)

Opiate drugs are another class of pain-relieving prescription drugs. Commonly prescribed opiates include morphine, codeine, hydromorphone (Dilaudid), and meperidine (Demerol). (In some states, some forms of codeine are sold without a prescription in limited amounts.) Most of these drugs are derived from opium, the juice of the poppy flower.

Opiate drugs work by altering the transmission of pain messages in the brain and spinal cord, blocking pain messages or altering their character.

The pain-blocking action of the opiates can be enhanced by taking aspirin, ibuprofen or acetaminophen at the same time as the opiate. This hits pain with a "double-whammy." The NSAIDS block the pain at the site of injury, while the opiates suppress in the brain any remaining pain.

Unfortunately, the effect of opiates on the brain isn't limited to pain control. Opiates can cause drowsiness, nausea, constipation, and unpleasant mood changes in some people. However, sometimes simply trying a different opiate may be all that's needed to reduce these side effects.

Tolerance and Addiction

Because doctors are afraid patients may become dependent on opiate drugs, they sometimes hold back on the amount or number of doses, even if this means the patient doesn't get sufficient pain relief.

Ronald Dubner, D.D.S., chief of the Neurobiology and Anesthesiology Branch of the National Institute of Dental Research, says those fears are unfounded. But, he explains, "One needs to be very clear about making the distinction between tolerance and addiction." Tolerance occurs when the body no longer responds as well to the opiate's pain-relieving properties at the current dose. For example, some cancer patients with severe pain may need increasing amounts of morphine to maintain the same level of pain relief.

Addiction, on the other hand, is an overwhelming compulsion to continue use of the drug even when pain relief is no longer needed. While some of the addiction is physical, it is mainly considered a psychological dependence that has a detrimental effect not only on the individual, but also on society, because the addicted individual may have to obtain the drug illegally.

Addiction is "really a red herring in the field of pain control," says Dubner. The fear that giving patients opiates will turn them into addicts craving the drugs long after the pain has ended is unfounded, says Dubner.

"People who are truly seeking help for their pain and who are in good hands do not have addiction problems," he explains.

In any case, Dubner says, it is very rare for a patient to reach a point where no amount of an opiate will relieve pain and that should never be used as a reason for not increasing the drug's dose.

Anesthesiologist Francis Balestrieri agrees. "There's no reason to hold back the drug dose for people in acute pain," says Balestrieri, who is the director of the Woodburn Surgery Center at Fairfax Hospital in Falls Church, VA.

However, FDA's Curtis Wright, M.D., warns that the pain relief from higher doses of opiates must be weighed against the side effects these drugs can cause.

"It's a balancing act," says Wright, who is a medical review officer for the agency's center for drug evaluation and research. "The amount of pain relief must be weighed against the effects of adverse reactions such as agitation, nausea, confusion, and potentially lethal respiratory depression."

Patients in Control

Frequently, however, the doses of narcotics physicians prescribe are too low, not too high, and the time between doses is too long, according to a book by Barry Stimmel, M.D., *Pain, Analgesia, and Addiction: The Pharmacologic Treatment of Pain*. Stimmel writes that,

The Challenge of Relieving Pain

"Analgesic medications should be prescribed regularly around the clock in the presence of acute pain. The intervals between administration should be sufficiently close together to avoid swings in pain levels. Both laboratory and clinical studies have shown that the presence of anxiety will result in an increased need for narcotics, thus setting up a vicious cycle whereby escalating doses of analgesics are needed, without adequate pain relief being obtained."

The use of analgesics provides more benefits to the patient than just relieving pain.

"Evidence from laboratory experiments has begun to accumulate showing that pain can accelerate the growth of tumors and increase mortality after tumor challenge," writes John C. Liebeskind in an editorial in the January 1991 issue of *Pain*. "It appears that the dictum 'pain does not kill,' sometimes invoked to justify ignoring pain complaints, may be dangerously wrong."

Dubner agrees. "Pain is not a passive symptom. We consider pain, in many instances, an aggressive disease in itself. Therefore it becomes very, very critical to control pain as rapidly and as completely as possible." One solution to inadequate doses of pain relievers is patient-controlled intravenous analgesia (PCA), which is usually used in hospitals for acute pain following surgery. In PCA, the patient is connected to a machine called a PCA pump. When the patient pushes a control button, the machine delivers a dose of narcotic or other pain reliever intravenously. The doses are smaller than what would be given by injection, but because the drug goes directly into the bloodstream, relief can occur within seconds. A patient receiving traditional administration with an injection in the muscle or under the skin, may have to wait anywhere from 5 to 30 minutes for pain relief.

Although the pain relief with PCA's small doses may only last for 10 to 15 minutes, the patient can get another dose the second pain begins to return. Injections, on the other hand, may last up to two hours, but since the usual dosage schedule is three to four hours, the pain returns long before the nurse does.

"PCA matches the patients' relief to their pain," says Balestrieri. "It also relieves patients of the worry over their pain relief in the majority of cases."

It also helps patients deal with the side effects opiates can cause, says FDA's Wright.

"A substantial portion of patients don't want complete pain relief," says Wright. "They want as much pain relief as they can get without bad side effects."

Wright says that when the first studies were done on the effectiveness of PCA, "we thought that the pain scores [the patients gave] would be zero." (Patients generally rated pain on a four-point scale with four being the greatest amount of pain and zero, no pain.)

"What we found was that patients didn't titrate down to zero, but instead brought the pain down to one or two," he says.

The undesirable side effects of narcotics can be avoided completely with another form of continuous administration—epidural therapy. Epidurals, which inject the narcotics into the membrane surrounding the spinal cord, have been used for many years to block the pain of labor. Now this is being adapted to control pain after some major surgery, especially abdominal.

Drugs injected into the epidural space don't travel to the brain like other types of injections, explains Sherry Fisher, R.N., pain management coordinator at Fairfax Hospital. Therefore, complications such as nausea and respiratory depression don't occur.

With epidurals "patients can talk to me, take deep breaths, cough, and even be up and walking around, sometimes 24 hours after surgery," says Fisher. Normally, after the type of major surgery that requires the kind of pain control epidural therapy provides, "the patient would still be on a ventilator after 24 hours," she says.

However, epidurals aren't effective for every type of pain. Besides pain from abdominal surgeries, epidurals are best used for pain following major chest and urologic surgery, according to Fisher.

No matter what the form of administration, "I don't think people should be exposed to any more pain than they're willing to tolerate," says Dubner.

Implantable Pump Administers Morphine

A concentrated form of morphine specially developed for administration by implantable pump is now available to people in sever pain, such as terminal cancer patients.

The small pump provides a steady stream of the drug to nerves along the spine, giving more constant relief, without the "peaks and valleys" of pain sometimes associated with capsules, pills, and intravenous injections. FDA approved the drug in July 1991. It will be marketed under the trade name Influmorph.

The pumps, called microinfusion devices, can be implanted under the skin of the abdomen or worn outside the body. A specially concentrated morphine was needed because the pumps are so small (about 3 inches in diameter). At FDA's request, the drug was developed by

The Challenge of Relieving Pain

Elkins-Sinn Inc. of Cherry Hill, N.J., under the agency's orphan products program, which encourages the development of needed therapies for diseases or conditions affecting fewer than 200,000 people.

The pump is programmed with dosing information before being filled with concentrated morphine and is thus able to constantly administer fractional doses of the drug. If the pump is implanted, the dose can be changed by beaming information through skin and tissues.

Misjudgment in the starting dose can result in severe side effects, such as seizures and respiratory problems. Therefore, patients must be monitored in a fully equipped and staffed facility for at least 24 hours after the initial dose. After this first "test" dose, however, patients may go home and return periodically—sometimes only once a month—for the physician to refill the pump reservoir with the medication.

Chronic Pain

Unfortunately, "when it comes to chronic pain, there are situations where pain cannot be controlled as well with the approaches that are available to us today," says Dubner.

Opiate drugs are usually avoided in chronic pain management because of the potential for tolerance.

Some types of chronic pain that are difficult to control include:

- pain from nerve damage caused by diabetes or shingles
- lower back pain that continues long after the initial injury has healed
- arthritis
- migraine and other chronic headaches.

There is some hope though. Tricyclic antidepressants, especially amitriptyline, have been found to relieve pain in patients with nerve damage. These drugs aid the body's own defenses by trapping serotonin, a pain-blocking chemical, at its point of production in the nerve endings in the dorsal horn of the spinal cord (see Figure 41.1). An excess of serotonin builds up and suppresses pain signals longer than usual.

Although FDA has not approved tricyclic antidepressants for pain control, these drugs are gaining wide acceptance for this purpose. (The practice of medicine may include the prescribing of approved drugs for unapproved uses supported by research and not otherwise contraindicated.)

Treatment of chronic and migraine headache pain may include two drugs approved for heart problems—calcium channel blockers and beta blockers. Treatment for mild arthritis pain, on the other hand, often begins with aspirin. If the patient can't tolerate aspirin, ibuprofen is a reasonable substitute, says Love. She warns, however, that even though people can buy aspirin and ibuprofen without a prescription, the doses required to treat arthritis pain are too high to be taken without a physician's care.

"The treatment of chronic arthritis, regardless of severity, requires an adequate diagnosis and possible use of many different types of medications, physical therapy, or surgery," says Love.

TENS

Another potential source of relief for chronic pain is transcutaneous electrical nerve stimulation (TENS). Through the use of the TENS device—a battery-powered generator that could be mistaken for a Walkman portable radio or a beeper—electrical impulses are transmitted to the site of pain through electrodes placed on the skin.

With the most common course of treatment, the physician or physical therapist sets the TENS device to deliver 80 to 100 impulses a second for 45 minutes, three times a day.

But there are a wide variety of parameter ranges, and what works for one person may have no effect on another. Determining the most effective settings "is a real art," says Stephen M. Hinckley, a physiologist with FDA's Center for Devices and Radiological Health.

Pain can be very subjective, explains Hinckley. Two people whose pain is caused by the same problem may need very different settings to achieve relief.

If a patient doesn't require hospital care, the patient can use the TENS device, preset to the proper level, at home. The device does not interfere with most normal activities.

A study published in the *New England Journal of Medicine* in June 1990 questioned the effectiveness of TENS. The study concluded "that for patients with chronic low back pain, treatment with TENS is no more effective than treatment with a placebo, and TENS adds no apparent benefit to that of exercise alone."

But, because a number of previous studies support the use of TENS, FDA still considers TENS to be effective for pain relief for some people.

Though it isn't clear why TENS works, there are two plausible theories, according to the *Harvard Medical School Health Letter*. The first holds that nerves can easily carry only one message at a time.

The Challenge of Relieving Pain

The electrical pulses from TENS overload the nerves, and the pain message shuts down. A second theory hypothesizes that the electrical pulses stimulate the body to release its own painkilling molecules, called endorphins, into the fluid bathing the spinal cord.

Pain researchers are studying how to stimulate production of the brain's own opiates, such as endorphins, enkephalins and dynorphins, since they may act as natural painkillers, according to NIH's Dubner.

"There are clear indications that stimulation in certain parts of the brain can be helpful in some patients," he says.

Focus on Life

Sometimes, though, none of these therapies will completely relieve the pain for chronic sufferers. They don't have to give up hope, though. For many in chronic pain, behavior modification techniques such as biofeedback, meditation and relaxation training may offer some relief. These treatment approaches are designed to alter a patient's reactions and behavior in response to pain.

"They learn that they can deal with their pain effectively if they focus on improving their quality of life instead of focusing on their pain," says Dubner.

Seymour Rubin, 67, who has suffered with chronic back pain for 40 years, agrees. "If I focus on the pain, it just gets worse," he says. Instead, Rubin keeps busy with walking, reading, and running errands with his wife.

"Singing helps, talking helps," adds Rubin. "And I've just learned to accept the fact that I have pain."

How You Know That You Stubbed Your Toe

1. Nociceptors are specialized nerve endings in the skin and other peripheral tissues that respond exclusively to tissue-damaging stimuli. Prostaglandins sensitize these nerve endings, and the pain message starts on its way to the brain. Aspirin and ibuprofen and, to a lesser extent, acetaminophen can block prostaglandin production at this point.

2. Pain travels along special nerve fibers to the part of the spinal cord called the dorsal horn.

3. Tricyclic antidepressants work here by enhancing the effects of the body's own natural painkillers.

Pain Sourcebook

How You Know That You Stubbed Your Toe

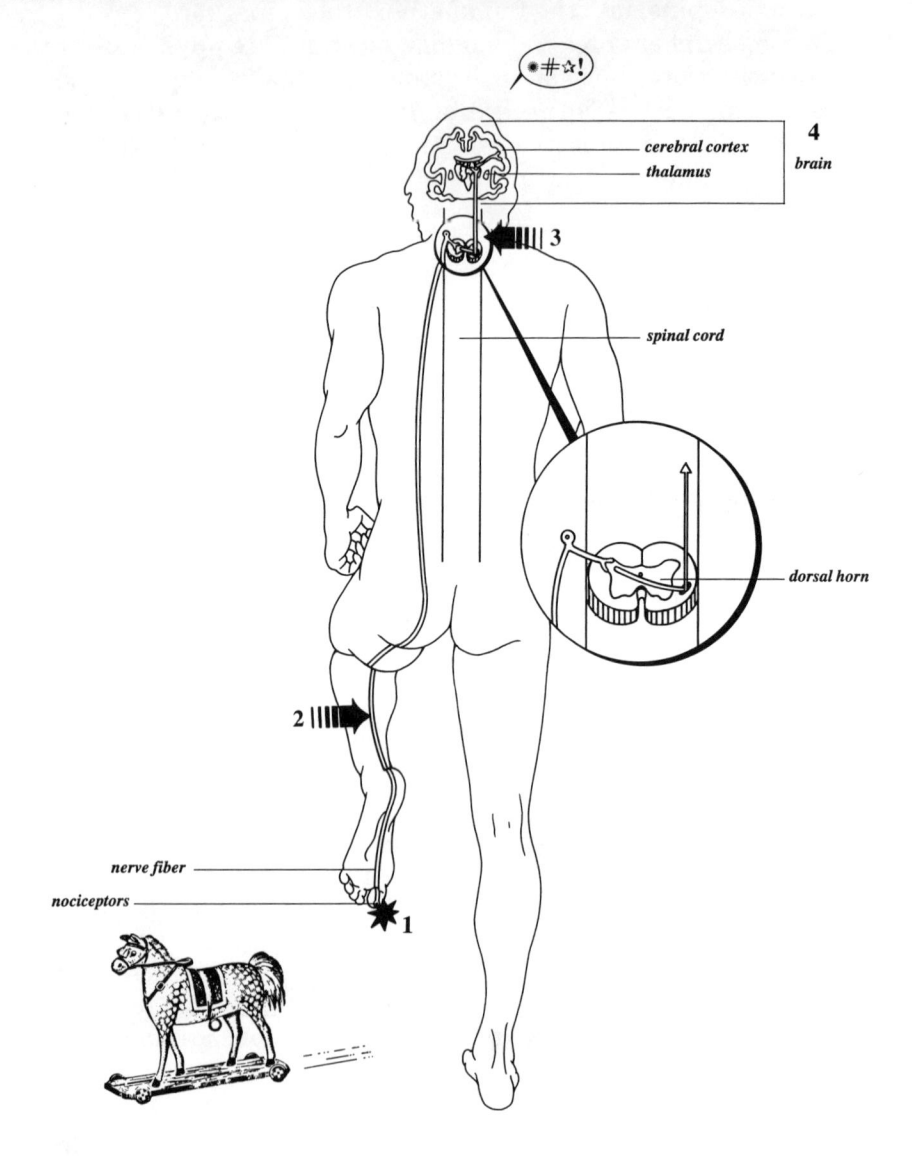

Figure 41.1.

The Challenge of Relieving Pain

4. From the dorsal horn, the pain ascends to the thalamus and then to the cerebral cortex. Opiates cause the brain to suppress pain messages before they leave the dorsal horn.

Clinical Studies

The Pain Research Clinic at the National Institutes of Health has ongoing studies in the following areas:

- wisdom tooth extraction
- painful diabetic neuropathies
- causalgic-type pains, including reflex sympathetic dystrophy
- oral-facial pain, including temporomandibular disorders.

To find out how to become a patient in these studies, write:

Jean Itkin
National Institute of Dental Research
National Institutes of Health
Building 10, Room 3C407
Bethesda, MD. 20892
Telephone: (301) 496-0394

—by Dori Stehlin

Dori Stehlin is a staff writer for *FDA Consumer*.

Chapter 42

Pain, Pain, Go Away: An FDA Guide to Nonprescription Pain Relievers (OTC)

Used to be, aspirin and other salicylates were the only medications available for nonprescription relief of minor ailments—from headaches and fever to muscle strain and minor arthritis. Today, consumers looking for temporary relief from such garden-variety ills have their pick of what can be a bewildering array of "regular," "extra-strength," and "maximum pain relief" tablets, caplets and gel caps on the drugstore shelf.

Though this cornucopia can seem confusing, the products' pain-relieving ingredients fall into just four categories: aspirin (and other salicylates), acetaminophen, ibuprofen, and naproxen sodium. For the most part, these over-the-counter (OTC) analgesic ingredients are equally effective. However, some may be more effective for certain types of ailments, and some people may prefer one type to another because of their varying side effects.

"Knowing the pros and cons of each type of pain reliever will allow you to choose among them," says William T. Beaver, M.D., professor of pharmacology and anesthesia at Georgetown University School of Medicine in Washington, D.C.

Old Faithful

Americans have been reaching for aspirin for almost 100 years as an all-purpose pain reliever (see "Aspirin: A New Look at an Old Drug" in the January-February 1994 *FDA Consumer* and reprinted in this

---

FDA Consumer, January/February 1995.

volume). Aspirin (or acetylsalicylic acid) works in part by suppressing the production of prostaglandins, hormone-like substances that have wide-ranging roles throughout the body, such as stimulating uterine contractions, regulating body temperature and blood vessel constriction, and helping blood clotting. "Regular" strength aspirin contains 325 milligrams (mg) per tablet; "extra" or "maximum" strength, 500 mg per tablet. The usual adult (defined as 12 years and older) dosage is one to two 325-mg aspirin tablets every four hours.

Some manufacturers add caffeine to aspirin.

"There is no evidence that caffeine relieves pain, but it can enhance the effects of aspirin, possibly by lifting a person's mood," says Michael Weintraub, M.D., director of FDA's Office of OTC Drug Evaluation.

Since a two-tablet dose provides roughly the same amount of caffeine as a cup of coffee, you can get the same effect by taking two plain aspirin with coffee. To minimize the stomach irritation aspirin can cause, some brands are "buffered" with calcium carbonate, magnesium oxide, and other antacids or coated so the pills don't dissolve until they reach the small intestine. Buffered formulas may offset aspirin's directly irritating effects on the stomach lining. They may be useful for people who get heartburn or stomach pain when they take aspirin, as well as for those with arthritis, who need to take as much as 4,000 mg every day.

Aspirin also causes gastrointestinal (GI) upset indirectly (by inhibiting production of a prostaglandin that protects the stomach lining by stimulating mucus production); buffering does nothing to offset this effect.

The downside of coated aspirin products is that they may take up to twice as long to provide pain relief as plain aspirin, according to Weintraub. In September, 1994, an FDA advisory panel recommended that labels on products containing aspirin warn that heavy drinkers are especially vulnerable to developing GI bleeding.

Aspirin should not be taken by people who have:

- ulcers, because it can worsen symptoms

- asthma, because it can trigger an attack in some asthmatics

- uncontrolled high blood pressure, because of an increased risk of one type of stroke

- liver or kidney disease, because it may worsen these conditions

- bleeding disorders or who are taking anticoagulant medication, because it may cause bleeding.

Continual high dosages of aspirin can cause hearing loss or tinnitus—a persistent ringing in the ears. FDA requires products containing aspirin and other salicylates to carry a label warning that children and teenagers should not use the medicine for chickenpox or flu symptoms because of its association with Reye syndrome, a rare disorder that may cause seizures, brain damage, and death.

The label also alerts pregnant women that use of aspirin in the last trimester may increase the risk of stillbirth and of maternal and fetal bleeding during delivery.

One Aspirin Alternative

Twenty years ago, FDA approved acetaminophen (Tylenol, and other brands and generics) in dosages of 325 mg and 500 mg for OTC use. "Nobody knows exactly how acetaminophen works, but one theory is that it acts on nerve endings to suppress pain," says Weintraub. Acetaminophen is as effective as aspirin in relieving mild-to-moderate pain and in reducing fever, but less so when it comes to soft tissue injuries, such as muscle strains and sprains, he adds. The usual adult dosage is two 325-mg tablets every four hours. Acetaminophen-based products to ease menstrual cramps often contain other ingredients, such as pamabrom (a diuretic) or pyrilamine maleate (an antihistamine used for its sedative effects).

"While these ingredients are safe, they have not been proven effective against uterine cramps, although they may relieve other symptoms associated with menstrual pain," says Weintraub.

Though acetaminophen is no better or faster at pain relief than aspirin, the drug is gentler on the stomach and reduces fever without the risk of Reye syndrome. However, even at moderate doses, acetaminophen can cause liver damage in heavy drinkers. At press time, FDA was planning to require a warning about this on the labels of OTC products containing the drug.

From Rx to OTC

Like aspirin, ibuprofen and naproxen sodium inhibit prostaglandin production. However, they are more potent pain relievers, especially for menstrual cramps, toothaches, minor arthritis, and injuries accompanied by inflammation, such as tendinitis. FDA approved ibuprofen for OTC marketing in 1984 at a dosage level of 200 mg every 4 to 6 hours, and naproxen sodium in 1994 at a dosage level of 200 mg every 8 to 12 hours.

Table 42.1. Over-the-Counter pain relief primer

Type/Dosage	Common Brands	What It Does	Possible Side Effects
aspirin 325 mg 500 mg	Anacin[1] Ascriptin[2] Bayer Bayer Plus[2] Bufferin[2] Ecotrin[3]	Relieves mild to moderate pain from headaches, sore muscles, menstrual cramps, and arthritis; reduces fever.	Prolonged use may cause gastrointestinal bleeding, especially in heavy drinkers; may increase the risk of maternal and fetal bleeding and cause complications during delivery if taken in the last trimester; can cause Reye syndrome if given to children and teenagers who have the flu or chickenpox.
acetaminophen 325 mg 500 mg	Anacin-3 Excedrin[1] Pamprin[4] Midol[4] Tylenol	Relieves mild to moderate pain from headaches and sore muscles; reduces fever.	May cause liver damage in drinkers and those taking excessive amounts (more than 4,000 mg daily) for several weeks.
ibuprofen 200 mg	Advil Motrin-IB Nuprin Pamprin-IB	Relieves mild to moderate pain from headaches, backaches, and sore muscles; relieves minor pain of arthritis; provides good relief of menstrual cramps and toothaches; reduces fever.	Gastrointestinal bleeding, especially in heavy drinkers; stomach ulcers; kidney damage in the elderly, people who have cirrhosis of the liver, and those taking diuretics.
naproxen sodium 200 mg	Aleve	Relieves mild to moderate pain from headaches, backaches, and sore muscles; relieves minor pain of arthritis; provides good relief of menstrual cramps and toothaches; reduces fever.	Gastrointestinal bleeding; stomach ulcers; kidney damage in the elderly, people who have cirrhosis of the liver, and those taking diuretics.

1. *Contains caffeine.*
2. *Contains buffers.*
3. *Enteric coated.*
4. *Contains ingredients other than analgesics.*

"Ibuprofen and naproxen sodium were converted to OTC status after their manufacturers did the necessary studies to show that these pain relievers were effective at OTC dosages, which are lower than prescription dosages," explains Weintraub. The lowest dosage strength for prescription-strength ibuprofen (Motrin and others) is 300 mg per tablet, and 275 mg per tablet for the prescription version of naproxen sodium (Anaprox, for example).

"In addition, the pharmaceutical companies had to show that these drugs were safe for use by a larger, more varied group of people [than would have received them by prescription only] and that the drugs were safe to use without medical supervision, as is the case with all nonprescription drugs."

Taken at the recommended adult dosage, OTC ibuprofen (Advil and others) and naproxen sodium (Aleve) are somewhat gentler on the stomach than aspirin. However, people who have ulcers or who get GI upset when taking aspirin should avoid both. In addition, asthmatics and people who are allergic to aspirin should avoid ibuprofen and naproxen sodium. An FDA advisory panel has recommended labeling on ibuprofen products like that recommended for aspirin, warning heavy drinkers about increased risk of gastric bleeding and impaired liver function (products with naproxen sodium labels already include this information). Although ibuprofen and naproxen sodium interfere with blood clotting much less than aspirin does, they should not be used by people who have bleeding disorders or who are taking anticoagulants.

Children under 12 should not be given either drug, except under a doctor's supervision, and people over 65 are advised to take no more than one naproxen sodium tablet every 12 hours.

Choosing an OTC pain reliever involves balancing effectiveness for a particular ailment with side effects. Often this is a very individual choice, based in part on your health history and how the drug affects you. Regardless of which type of OTC pain reliever you choose, remember that it is intended to be used on a short-term basis, unless directed by a doctor, cautions Weintraub.

The warning labels on these products include limitations on duration of use to ensure that chronic or serious illnesses are not masked. Typically, labels advise against taking the product for more than 10 days to relieve pain (for children, the upper limit is five days), or more than three days to reduce fever. If symptoms worsen, pain persists, or there is redness or swelling, medical attention should be sought.

—by Ruth Papazian

Ruth Papazian is a writer in New York City.

Chapter 43

Taking Nonsteroidal Anti-Inflammatory Drugs (NSAIDs)

How you take a drug makes a big difference in how well it will work and how safe it will be for you. Timing, what you eat and when you eat, proper dose, and many other factors can mean the difference between feeling better, staying the same, or even feeling worse. This drug-information chapter is about nonsteroidal anti-inflammatory drugs, often abbreviated NSAIDs. It is intended to help you make your treatment work as well as possible. However, this is only a guideline. You should talk to your doctor or pharmacist about how and when to take any prescribed drugs.

Conditions These Drugs Treat

- symptoms such as redness, warmth, swelling, stiffness, and joint pain caused by rheumatoid arthritis, osteoarthritis, and other rheumatic conditions.

- menstrual cramps.

- pain, especially that associated with dental problems, gout, episiotomy (an incision made in a woman's perineum and vagina during childbirth to prevent tearing), tendinitis, bursitis, and injuries such as sprains and strains.

FDA Consumer, June, 1990.

NSAIDs are not a cure for arthritis or any other disease. These drugs temporarily relieve pain by blocking the body's production of chemicals known as prostaglandins, which are believed to be associated with the pain and inflammation of injuries and immune reactions.

How to Take

Indomethacin and phenylbutazone should always be taken with food. The food helps prevent an upset stomach, which NSAIDS can cause. Meclofenamate may be taken with meals. For other NSAIDs, however, your doctor may tell you to take the first several doses 30 minutes before or two hours after eating. This will help the medicine relieve the symptoms more quickly.

Like food, antacids may prevent an upset stomach when you're taking NSAIDs. However, both food and some over-the-counter antacids may interfere with an NSAID's effectiveness. Ask your doctor for the best approach for a particular NSAID.

NSAID tablets and capsules should be washed down with eight ounces of water to help prevent the drugs from irritating the delicate lining of the esophagus and stomach. In addition, to let gravity help move the pills along—don't lie down for at least 15 to 30 minutes after each dose.

Be sure to take the right number of tablets or capsules for each dose. Liquid doses are best measured in special spoons available from your pharmacist. Teaspoons or tablespoons from the kitchen drawer are rarely the right dosage size.

Missed Doses

Ask your doctor what to do if you forget to take a dose. Some NSAIDs have a longer-lasting effect in the body than others, so you'll need your doctor's guidance on whether to make up a missed dose of the specific NSAID you are taking, or just wait until it's time for the next dose.

But never take a double dose.

Be sure to refill your prescriptions soon enough to avoid missing any doses.

Relief of Symptoms

Most NSAIDs start to relieve pain symptoms in about an hour. However, for long-term inflammation and for severe or continuing arthritis, relief may not come for a week to several weeks.

Taking Nonsteroidal Anti-Inflammatory Drugs (NSAIDs)

How long you will need to take the medicine depends on the condition being treated. Make sure you understand your doctor's instructions.

Side Effects and Risks

Common side effects include nausea, cramps, indigestion, and diarrhea or constipation. Other side effects can include increased sensitivity to sunlight, nervousness, confusion, headache, drowsiness, or dizziness. If you have any of these side effects, notify your doctor, but don't stop taking your medication on your own.

Occasionally, NSAIDs can cause ulcers or bleeding in the stomach or small intestine. Warning signs include severe cramps, pain, or burning in the stomach or abdomen; diarrhea or black tarry stools; severe, continuing nausea, heartburn, or indigestion; or vomiting of blood or material that looks like coffee grounds. If any of these side effects occurs, stop taking the medicine and call your doctor immediately.

Other serious but rare reactions are:

- **Anaphylaxis**. Signs of this severe allergic reaction are very fast or difficult breathing, difficulty in swallowing, swollen tongue, gasping for breath, wheezing, dizziness, or fainting. A hive-like rash, puffy eyelids, change in face color, or very fast but irregular heartbeat or pulse may also occur. If any of these occurs, get emergency help at once.

- **Sore throat or fever.** With phenylbutazone, sore throat or fever can be early signs that the drug has impaired the bone marrow's ability to produce blood cells. Call your doctor immediately. Because of the seriousness of this side effect, phenylbutazone is usually prescribed as a last resort and then for short periods only.

- **Swelling.** Unusual swelling of the fingers, hands or feet, weight gain, or decreased or painful urination can indicate worsening of an underlying heart or kidney condition. If any of these symptoms occurs, call your doctor.

Precautions and Warnings

- NSAIDs should not usually be taken during pregnancy or while breast-feeding.

- People 65 and older are more likely to experience the side effects of NSAIDs and get sicker with those effects than younger adults.

- Alcoholic beverages should be avoided, as they increase the potential for stomach problems while taking NSAIDs.

- Don't take acetaminophen or aspirin or other salicylates with NSAIDs unless directed by your doctor. Taking these drugs along with NSAIDs may increase the risk of side effects.

- Tell your physician if you are taking any other medication—prescription or nonprescription.

- Before any surgery or dental work, tell the physician or dentist that you are taking NSAIDs.

- Don't drive or operate machines if the medicine makes you confused, drowsy, dizzy, or lightheaded. Learn how the medicine affects you first.

- NSAIDs can increase sensitivity to sunlight in some people. To avoid the risk of a serious sunburn, stay out of direct sunlight, especially between 10 a.m. and 3 p.m.; wear protective clothing; and apply a sunblock with a skin protection factor of 15.

Generic Names

diclofenac	ketoprofen	phenylbutazone
diflunisal	ketoralac	piroxicam
fenoprofen	meclofenamate	sulindac
ibuprofen	mefenamic acid	tolmetin
indomethacin	naproxen	

Don't store drugs in the bathroom medicine cabinet. Heat and humidity may cause the medicine to lose its effectiveness.

Keep all medicines, even those with child-resistant caps, out of the reach of children. Remember, the caps are child-resistant, not child-proof.

Discard medicines that have reached the expiration date shown on the label.

— by Dori Stehlin

Chapter 44

Aspirin: Potent Pain Relief, but Misuse Can Be Dangerous

Chapter Contents

Section 44.1—A New Look at an Old Drug 488
Section 44.2—Reye Syndrome: The Decline of a Disease 493

Section 44.1

A New Look at an Old Drug

FDA *Consumer*, January/February 1994, *FDA Consumer*, October 1990.

In purses and backpacks, in briefcases and medicine chests the world over, millions of people keep close at hand a drug that has both a long past and a fascinating future. Its past reaches at least to the fifth century BC, when Hippocrates used a bitter powder obtained from willow bark to ease aches and pains and reduce fever. Its future is being shaped today in laboratories and clinics where scientists are exploring some intriguing new uses for an interesting old drug.

The substance in willow bark that made ancient Greeks feel better, salicin, is the pharmacological ancestor of a family of drugs called salicylates, the best known of which is the world's most widely used drug—aspirin.

Americans consume an estimated 80 billion aspirin tablets a year. The Physicians' Desk Reference lists more than 50 over-the-counter drugs in which aspirin is the principal active ingredient. Yet, despite aspirin's having been in routine use for nearly a century, both scientific journals and the popular media are full of reports and speculation about new uses for this old remedy. The National Library of Medicine's main computerized catalog includes more than 2,700 scientific articles about aspirin. And those are only the English language publications that have appeared in the last five years.

Yet aspirin's beginnings were rather unspectacular. Nearly 100 years ago, a German industrial chemist, Felix Hoffmann, set about to find a drug to ease his father's arthritis without causing the severe stomach irritation associated with sodium salicylate, the standard anti-arthritis drug of the time. In the forms then available, the large doses of salicylates used to treat arthritis—6 to 8 grams a day—commonly irritated the stomach lining, and many patients, like Hoffmann's father, simply could not tolerate them.

Figuring that acidity made salicylates hard on the stomach, Hoffmann started looking for a less acidic formulation. His search led

Aspirin: Potent Pain Relief, but Misuse Can Be Dangerous

him to synthesize acetylsalicylic acid (ASA), a compound that appeared to share the therapeutic properties of other salicylates and might cause less stomach irritation. ASA reduced fever, relieved moderate pain, and, at substantially higher doses, alleviated rheumatic and arthritic conditions. Hoffmann was confident that ASA would prove more effective than salicylates then in use.

His superiors, however, did not share his enthusiasm. They doubted that ASA would ever become a valuable, commercially successful drug because at large doses salicylates commonly produced shortness of breath and an alarmingly rapid heart rate. It was taken for granted—incorrectly as it turns out—that ASA would weaken the heart and that physicians would be reluctant to prescribe it in preference to sodium salicylate, a drug they at least knew. Hoffmann's employer, Friedreich Bayer & Company, gave ASA the now-familiar name aspirin, but in 1897 Bayer didn't think aspirin had much of a future. It could not have foreseen that almost a century after its development aspirin would be the focus of extensive laboratory research and some of the largest clinical trials ever carried out in conditions ranging from cardiovascular disease and cancer to migraine headache and high blood pressure in pregnancy.

How Does it Work?

The mushrooming interest in aspirin has come about largely because of fairly recent advances in understanding how it works. What is it about this drug that, at small doses, interferes with blood clotting, at somewhat higher doses reduces fever and eases minor aches and pains, and at comparatively large doses combats pain and inflammation in rheumatoid arthritis and several other related diseases?

The answer is not yet fully known, but most authorities agree that aspirin achieves some of its effects by inhibiting the production of prostaglandins. Prostaglandins are hormone-like substances that influence the elasticity of blood vessels, control uterine contractions, direct the functioning of blood platelets that help stop bleeding, and regulate numerous other activities in the body.

In the 1970s, a British pharmacologist, John Vane, Ph.D., noted that many forms of tissue injury were followed by the release of prostaglandins. In laboratory studies, he found that two groups of prostaglandins caused redness and fever, common signs of inflammation. Vane and his co-workers also showed that, by blocking the synthesis of prostaglandins, aspirin prevented blood platelets from aggregating, one of the initial steps in the formation of blood clots.

This explanation of how aspirin and other nonsteroidal anti-inflammatory drugs (NSAIDs) produce their intriguing array of effects prompted laboratory and clinical scientists to form and test new ideas about aspirin's possible value in treating or preventing conditions in which prostaglandins play a role. Interest quickly focused on learning whether aspirin might prevent the blood clots responsible for heart attacks.

A heart attack or myocardial infarction (MI) results from the blockage of blood flow not through the heart, but to heart muscle. Without an adequate blood supply, the affected area of muscle dies and the heart's pumping action is either impaired or stopped altogether.

The most common sequence of events leading to an MI begins with the gradual build-up of plaque (atherosclerosis) in the coronary arteries. Circulation through these narrowed arteries is restricted, often causing the chest pain known as angina pectoris.

An acute heart attack is believed to happen when a tear in plaque inside a narrowed coronary artery causes platelets to aggregate, forming a clot that blocks the flow of blood. About 1,250,000 persons suffer heart attacks each year in the United States, and some 500,000 of them die. Those who survive a first heart attack are at greatly increased risk of having another.

Could Aspirin Help?

To learn whether aspirin could be helpful in preventing or treating cardiovascular disease, scientists have carried out numerous large randomized controlled clinical trials. In these studies, similar groups of hundreds or thousands of people are randomly assigned to receive either aspirin or a placebo, an inactive, look-alike tablet. The participants—and in double-blind trials the investigators, as well—do not know who is taking aspirin and who is swallowing a placebo.

Over the last two decades, aspirin studies have been conducted in three kinds of individuals: persons with a history of coronary artery or cerebral vascular disease, patients in the immediate, acute phases of a heart attack, and healthy men with no indication of current or previous cardiovascular illness.

The results of studies of people with a history of coronary artery disease and those in the immediate phases of a heart attack have proven to be of tremendous importance in the prevention and treatment of cardiovascular disease. The studies showed that aspirin substantially reduces the risk of death and/or non-fatal heart attacks in

Aspirin: Potent Pain Relief, but Misuse Can Be Dangerous

patients with a previous MI or unstable angina pectoris, which often occurs before a heart attack.

On the basis of such studies, these uses for aspirin (unstable angina, acute MI, and survivors of an MI) are described in the professional labeling of aspirin products, information provided to physicians and other health professionals. Aspirin labeling intended for the general public does not discuss its use in arthritis or cardiovascular disease because treatment of these serious conditions—even with a common over-the-counter drug—has to be medically supervised. The consumer labeling contains a general warning about excessive or inappropriate use of aspirin, and specifically warns against using aspirin to treat children and teenagers who have chickenpox or the flu because of the risk of Reye syndrome, a rare but sometimes fatal condition.

Aspirin for Healthy People?

Once aspirin's benefits for patients with cardiovascular disease were established, scientists sought to learn whether regular aspirin use would prevent a first heart attack in healthy individuals. The findings regarding that critical question have thus far been equivocal. The major American study designed to find out if aspirin can prevent cardiovascular deaths in healthy individuals was a randomized, placebo-controlled trial involving just over 22,000 male physicians between 40 and 84 with no prior history of heart disease. Half took one 325-milligram aspirin tablet every other day, and half took a placebo.

The trial was halted early, after about four-and-a-half years, and the findings quickly made public in 1988 when investigators found that the group taking aspirin had a substantial reduction in the rate of fatal and non-fatal heart attacks compared with the placebo group. There was, however, no significant difference between the aspirin and placebo groups in number of strokes (aspirin-treated patients did slightly worse) or in overall deaths from cardiovascular disease.

A similar study in British male physicians with no previous heart disease found no significant effect nor even a favorable trend for aspirin on cardiovascular disease rates. The British study of 5,100 physicians, while considerably smaller than the American study, reported three-quarters as many vascular "events." FDA scientists believe the results of the two studies are inconsistent.

The U.S. Preventive Services Task Force, a panel of medical-scientific authorities in health promotion and disease prevention, is one of many groups looking at new information on the role of aspirin in cardiovascular disease. In its *Guide to Clinical Preventive Services*, issued in 1989, the task force recommended that low-dose aspirin therapy "should be considered for men aged 40 and over who are at significantly increased risk for myocardial infarction and who lack contraindications" to aspirin use. A revised Guide, scheduled for publication in the fall of 1994, is expected to include a slightly revised recommendation concerning aspirin and cardiovascular disease but no major change in advice to physicians about aspirin's possible role in preventing heart attacks.

Better understanding of aspirin's myriad effects in the body has led to clinical trials and other studies to assess a variety of possible uses: preventing the severity of migraine headaches, improving circulation to the gums thereby arresting periodontal disease, preventing certain types of cataracts, lowering the risk of recurrence of colorectal cancer, and controlling the dangerously high blood pressure (preeclampsia) that occurs in 5 to 15 percent of pregnancies.

None of these uses for aspirin has been shown conclusively to be safe and effective, and there is concern that people may be misusing aspirin on the basis of unproven notions about its effectiveness. Last October, FDA proposed a new labeling statement for aspirin products advising consumers to consult a doctor before taking aspirin for new and long-term uses. The proposed statement would read, "IMPORTANT: See your doctor before taking this product for your heart or for other new uses of aspirin because serious side effects could occur with self treatment."

The Other Side of the Coin

While examining new possibilities for aspirin in disease treatment and prevention, scientists do not lose sight of the fact that even at low doses aspirin is not harmless. A small subset of the population is hypersensitive to aspirin and cannot tolerate even small amounts of the drug. Gastrointestinal distress—nausea, heartburn, pain—is a well-recognized adverse effect and is related to dosage. Persons being treated for rheumatoid arthritis who take large daily doses of aspirin are especially likely to experience gastrointestinal side effects.

Aspirin's antiplatelet activity apparently accounts for hemorrhagic strokes, caused by bleeding into the brain, in a small but significant percentage of persons who use the drug regularly. For the great majority of occasional aspirin users, internal bleeding is not a problem. But aspirin may be unsuitable for people with uncontrolled high blood pressure, liver or kidney disease, peptic ulcer, or other conditions that might increase the risk of cerebral hemorrhage or other internal bleeding.

Aspirin: Potent Pain Relief, but Misuse Can Be Dangerous

New understanding of how aspirin works and what it can do leaves no doubt that the drug has a far broader range of uses than Felix Hoffmann and his colleagues imagined. The jury is still out, however, on a number of key questions about the best and safest ways to use aspirin. And until some critical verdicts are handed down, consumers are well-advised to regard aspirin with appropriate caution.

— by Ken Flieger

Ken Flieger is a writer in Washington, D.C.

Section 44.2

Reye Syndrome: The Decline of a Disease

FDA Consumer, October 1990.

Each year between March 1951 and March 1962, the Royal Alexandra Hospital for Children in New South Wales, Australia, admitted one or two children in such a critical state that most of them could not be saved, despite the most advanced medical care.

The cases had a number of unusual features in common. When admitted, all but two of the 21 children were in a coma or stupor, although their illness had started out a few days or weeks earlier with only common childhood upper respiratory symptoms—usually cough, sore throat, runny nose, or earache. Some children had even appeared to be recovering before the more serious phase of the illness began, with fever, relentless vomiting, convulsions, wild delirium, screaming, intense irritability, and violent movements.

Seventeen of the children died within an average of 27 hours after admission. At autopsy, all were found to have brain swelling, a slightly enlarged, firm and uniformly bright yellow liver, and a change in the appearance of the kidneys. Douglas Reye, M.D., the hospital's director of pathology, and his colleagues believed this set of symptoms represented a distinct disease, which they called fatty degeneration of the viscera (internal organs) of unknown cause. Though they suspected that ingestion of drugs or poisons may have been responsible for the condition, an investigation into the children's homes revealed they had no access to these substances.

In 1963, George Johnson, M.D., and his co-workers reported an epidemic of 16 fatal cases of an encephalitis-like disease occurring within a four-month period during an outbreak of influenza B in a small North Carolina community. Although children in this group were older than those studied by Reye, and their preceding illness was flu, it was subsequently theorized from Johnson's description of the symptoms and post-mortem findings that several of the children who died may have also had the syndrome described by Reye. It became known as Reye-Johnson syndrome, though it's usually referred to as Reye (pronounced rye) syndrome.

After the Reye-Johnson reports were published, numerous reports came in from the United States and other parts of the world showing that the syndrome was both more widespread and more common than was thought. Though this was not a new disease—it had been reported as early as 1929—for the first time it had been identified and characterized as a distinct entity.

During the 1960s and 70s, when regional and then national surveillance of Reye syndrome was established by the Atlanta-based Centers for Disease Control, scientists observed that the syndrome occurred in association with outbreaks of the flu, especially influenza B. They also noted that it followed chicken pox, with children aged 5 to 15 most often affected. Less often it was associated with other viruses and acute respiratory and diarrheal illnesses.

When Is it Reye?

Many toxic substances (such as carbon tetrachloride, phosphorus and alcohol) and other diseases (such as acute hepatitis and viral encephalitis) can produce symptoms like Reye syndrome. Since most physicians were completely unfamiliar with the syndrome at the time, they needed to know what constituted a positive diagnosis.

CDC established case definitions for regional surveillance and outbreak investigations in the late 1960s. Criteria for a case included mental status changes, such as delirium or coma, and a liver biopsy (tissue sample) showing fat accumulation in the liver (or high levels of liver enzymes and ammonia in the blood). There also needed to be no other more reasonable explanation for the brain or liver abnormalities.

Aspirin: Potent Pain Relief, but Misuse Can Be Dangerous

Records show that Reye syndrome has affected an infant as young as 4 days old and has occurred in a 59-year-old man; however, more than 90 percent of reported cases are in children under 15. About 2 percent are in adults over 20.

How the Illness Progresses

The course of the illness is variable. Reye syndrome can be mild and self-limiting, or it can progress rapidly, causing death within hours of onset, usually from brain swelling. But the progression may also stop at any stage, with complete recovery in 5 to 10 days and the quick return of normal liver function.

Doctors classify stages of Reye syndrome based on the level of the patient's consciousness and corresponding physical signs: Stages 0 to 2 are pre-comatose, with lethargy or delirium, and sometimes combativeness, but with the child still responding to stimuli. Coma progressively deepens in stages 3 to 5; the child is unresponsive to stimuli, and heart and lung function begin to shut down.

The earlier the diagnosis and treatment, the better the chance for survival. Intense supportive care in a hospital experienced in dealing with Reye syndrome also improves odds. Children who survive but experience the most severe stages of the illness—especially infants—are sometimes left with neurological abnormalities, often mental retardation or disorders of voice and speech.

Fatality rates when national surveillance began on a regular basis in 1976 were as high as 40 percent, declined to between 20 and 30 percent from 1978 to 1987, but rose in 1988 and 1989. CDC experts speculate that this higher death rate may reflect decreasing interest in the syndrome—because of its rarity—resulting in the reporting of only the most serious cases.

The Aspirin Connection

Just as Reye suspected that a drug or poison may have triggered the disease's development, investigators in the United States looked for some common factor among children who developed the syndrome. They found it in aspirin taken during flu or chicken pox.

In 1980, results of studies conducted in Ohio, Michigan and Arizona demonstrated an association between Reye syndrome and aspirin use during a preceding respiratory tract or chicken pox infection.

"It was those initial studies that we reviewed in 1980 that first led CDC to report in its Morbidity and Mortality Weekly Report [MMWR] that there was an association," states Lawrence B. Schonberger, M.D., an epidemiologist with the agency. In 1981, CDC reported in MMWR results of a fourth study that revealed the same association. In 1982, the Surgeon General of the U.S. Public Health Service issued a warning against giving aspirin to children with flu or chicken pox.

The public was quick to pick up on the association. "A kind of natural study was occurring, because once people heard about the results [of the studies], they started to lower the use of aspirin in their children," says Schonberger. "If aspirin had nothing to do with it [Reye syndrome], then one might anticipate that there would be no clear decrease in the incidence of Reye syndrome."

That's not what happened. Aspirin use in children under 10 declined by at least 50 percent from 1981 to 1988, and the number of Reye syndrome cases went down correspondingly. In the opinion of Peter C. Rowe, M.D., assistant professor of pediatrics, Children's Hospital of Eastern Canada, Ottawa, Ontario, the declining use of aspirin and the decreasing incidence of Reye syndrome represent a "natural ecological experiment."

Other Government Actions

The federal government made other moves. To confirm the preliminary findings of the state studies, in 1985-1986 the government sponsored the "Public Health Service Study of Reye's Syndrome and Medications." Twenty-seven children who developed Reye syndrome after a preceding respiratory illness or chicken pox were matched with 140 children who had had the same illnesses at the same time, but did not develop Reye syndrome. More than 96 percent of the Reye syndrome cases, compared with 38 percent of the controls (the children who did not develop Reye syndrome), had received aspirin (or other salicylates) to treat the preceding illness. The study was prematurely ended because not enough Reye syndrome children who had not been exposed to aspirin could be found to justify the expense of continuing the investigation, in itself an indication of a public health triumph.

In 1986, FDA adopted a preliminary rule requiring aspirin manufacturers to add warnings to product labels about the possible association between aspirin use and the development of Reye syndrome. The permanent rule became final in 1988, and the labeling reads: Children and teenagers should not use this medicine for chicken pox or flu symptoms before a doctor is consulted about Reye syndrome, a rare but serious illness reported to be associated with aspirin.

Aspirin: Potent Pain Relief, but Misuse Can Be Dangerous

The number of Reye syndrome cases, which reached a high in 1980 with 555 cases, has steadily decreased, compared with years in which there has been similar types of influenza activity. The decline has been most dramatic among children from 5 to 10 years of age. In 1989, a heavy influenza B year, 27 cases of Reye syndrome were reported to CDC, almost half of them fatal. According to CDC, since 1985, 40 to 65 percent of reported Reye syndrome patients have been older than 10. Because this age group often self-medicates, recent educational efforts have been geared to reach them.

Other Factors

Some questions about the relationship between aspirin and Reye syndrome still remain. Although figures show that 90 to 95 percent of Reye syndrome patients in the United States have taken aspirin during a preceding viral illness, it is estimated that less than 0.1 percent of children having a viral infection and treated with aspirin develop the syndrome.

Are Other Factors Involved?

Apparently so. Reye syndrome has always been a puzzling disease. Research on possible causes has been hampered because no one can come up with a simple specific diagnostic test for the syndrome. The waters are further muddied by the existence of at least 19 viruses, including the chicken pox and flu viruses, which cause infectious illnesses that can precede Reye syndrome development. Some experts have proposed that Reye syndrome develops from the interaction of a viral illness, genetic susceptibility to the disease, and exposure to chemicals, such as salicylates, pesticides and aflatoxin. Others speculate that unidentified viruses or other infectious agents are involved.

That some children may be more susceptible to Reye syndrome than others has been shown by cases appearing among children in the same family and by recurrent episodes of the illness in the same child. It is possible that more than one type of Reye syndrome exists, or that some of these cases may not be Reye syndrome at all.

Reye-like Disorders

In the light of what we know now, it is even questionable whether all pathologist Reye's cases were true Reye syndrome. Recent research indicates that some children diagnosed in the past with Reye syndrome, particularly those under 5, may have had underlying metabolic abnormalities that produce similar symptoms.

"There may well be certain cases that come in even today—in the very young—that five years from now we'll find are really some other abnormal congenital problem—where they have a metabolic defect and it expresses itself in a form that looks very much like Reye syndrome," says CDC's Schonberger. Because these children require different treatment, proper diagnosis can be a matter of life or death. In children 5 or older, the diagnosis of Reye syndrome is more conclusive—especially when symptoms occur during flu and chicken pox epidemics—since few other diseases in this age group mimic common Reye syndrome symptoms.

It's possible that metabolic disorders will prove some day to be the chief cause of Reye syndrome. However, until then, it's important to remember that aspirin use during flu or chicken pox is asking for trouble.

In Schonberger's words: "The association between aspirin and Reye syndrome is so strong that it has now become literally foolhardy to act as if no etiologic [cause-and-effect] relationship exists."

Reye Syndrome Symptoms

In most cases, children seem to be recovering from a viral illness when lowing symptoms occur:

- nausea
- vomiting, usually very severe
- fever
- lethargy
- stupor or coma, sometimes followed by convulsions
- wild delirium and unusual restlessness noted in about half of patients

—by Evelyn Zamula

Evelyn Zamula is a freelance writer in Potomac, MD.

Chapter 45

A Burning Question: When Do You Need an Antacid?

You can't believe you ate the whole thing. But you did. All seven courses. Then you had two helpings of dessert. Then, to be social, you had a couple of drinks. Or maybe three or four.

And now you're paying for it. You've got a "burning sensation" in your stomach or your chest, or maybe you feel all knotted up inside.

Your first reaction may be to reach for your favorite antacid to make the hurting go away. And if you do, you won't be alone.

Americans are currently spending close to $1 billion per year on these popular, over-the-counter drugs. Used according to directions and in moderation, they can quickly relieve the symptoms associated with occasional heartburn and indigestion. But these useful products may not always be necessary, and they have their dark side if used improperly.

"Improperly" means taking too much of an antacid over a short period, or using antacids frequently over a long period (weeks, months or years). Frequent and prolonged use of these products can cause irreparable harm to your heart, kidneys or bones.

Even if used occasionally and in moderation, antacids can mean bad news for people with special medical conditions.

Hugo Gallo-Torres, M.D., a medical officer with FDA's Center for Drug Evaluation and Research, said it's a good idea to consult your doctor before using antacids if you:

- are on any kind of medication
- are pregnant or breast-feeding

FDA Consumer, 06/02/1991.

- have kidney problems
- have chronic constipation, diarrhea or colitis
- have stomach or intestinal bleeding
- have an irregular heartbeat
- have any kind of chronic illness
- have symptoms that may indicate appendicitis.

Though they cause problems for some, most people can take antacids without worrying. Consumers who use them only once in a while, and as directed, are unlikely to experience significant side effects.

But, like most everything else in life, moderation is the key.

"Antacids are useful drugs—they serve a purpose," said Gallo-Torres.

"Ideally, though, it's always better to try dealing with heartburn and indigestion—at least initially—without taking any medications at all, or by avoiding trouble in the first place."

Gallo-Torres said there are some simple steps you can take that may help prevent heartburn or indigestion.

- Don't eat big meals. Your stomach has to work long and hard to process them, which means it has to produce a lot of acid. It helps to eat more frequent—but smaller—meals.

- Eat more slowly. Downing a lot of food in a hurry can overwhelm your stomach, which responds by producing extra digestive acids.

- After you eat, don't lie down right away. If you do, you're more likely to have heartburn, because gravity is now preventing food from going speedily to the intestines. It's also a good idea to eat your last big meal at least three hours before bedtime. When you go to sleep, everything slows down, including your digestive system, so food you've eaten right before bedtime will stay in your stomach longer. It won't feel good.

- Don't wear tight-fitting garments. They can literally compress your stomach, making it more likely that the stomach's acid contents will enter your esophagus and cause a burning sensation.

- Cut down on caffeine; it makes your stomach produce more acid. Caffeine-heavy items include coffee, tea, chocolate, and some sodas.

A Burning Question: When Do You Need an Antacid?

- Avoid foods that contain a lot of acid, such as citrus fruits and tomatoes, and any other food that gives you problems.

- Cut back on alcohol and smoking. Both irritate the lining of your stomach and both tend to lower esophageal sphincter pressure. When this happens, it's easier for the contents of your stomach to shoot back up into your esophagus.

- Sleep with your head and shoulders propped up six to eight inches, so that your body is at a slight angle. This gets gravity working for you and not against you, and the digestive juices in your stomach are more likely to head south, for your intestine, instead of back up into your esophagus.

"If you do take an antacid, remember that what you're taking is a drug," Gallo-Torres said. "It is a drug that, in the vast majority of cases, should be used only for occasional relief of mild heartburn or indigestion. Antacids are fast-acting. They should bring relief within minutes. If you're taking antacids and there's no relief, then something else may be going on, something that requires a physician's evaluation."

Igor Cerny, a pharmacist with FDA's Center for Drug Evaluation and Research, agreed. "If you find yourself taking antacids frequently," he said, "you need to say to yourself: 'Wait a minute.... I wasn't doing this before, so why am I doing it now? Something might be wrong with me.'"

"If your symptoms last more than two weeks, go see your doctor," he recommended. "Two weeks is the general rule of thumb. Beyond that, taking antacids can actually mask a more serious medical problem."

Cerny said it's a good idea to see your doctor even sooner—preferably right away—if you're experiencing any symptoms severe enough to interfere with your lifestyle, symptoms such as continuous vomiting or diarrhea, extreme discomfort or pain in your gastrointestinal (GI) tract, vomiting of blood or material that looks like coffee grounds (but which is actually digested blood), or any of these accompanied by fever.

"Using antacids to alleviate serious symptoms like these is like trying to put out a building fire with a hand-held extinguisher," Cerny said. "Serious symptoms require professional evaluation and treatment."

A Quick Look Inside

Your entire digestive system is called the alimentary canal, or GI tract. About 30 feet from beginning to end, it includes your mouth (where digestion actually begins), esophagus, stomach, small intestine, and colon (also called the large intestine). Antacids do most of their work in the stomach.

The stomach serves as a kind of "holding tank" for food before it moves on to the intestines, where the major part of digestion takes place. But the stomach does more than just hold food. It helps with digestion, too. It secretes pepsin and hydrochloric acid, which work together to break down proteins into simpler compounds.

Under normal conditions, the digestive process rolls along quietly and efficiently, unnoticed. But every once in a while something happens down there that catches your attention: a burning sensation, a cramped or bloated feeling, or other unpleasant phenomena that tell you something is not quite right.

The pH Factor

Antacids make you feel better by increasing the pH balance in your stomach. The pH system is a scale for measuring the acidity or alkalinity of a given environment (in this case, your stomach). The scale goes from zero to 14.

Seven is neutral. Below seven is acid. Above seven is alkaline.

Normally, the acid level in your stomach is about 2 or 3. Trouble may start when your pH drops below those numbers.

To make you feel better, an antacid need not bring the pH level all the way up to 7 (neutral), which would be a highly unnatural state for your stomach anyway. In order to work, all the antacid has to do is get you to 3 or 4. It does this by neutralizing some of the excess acid.

So What's Wrong with Me Anyway?

The world of gastrointestinal disorders is a complex and sometimes baffling one. If you're feeling pain or discomfort in your GI tract, it could be something as unworrisome as simple indigestion, or maybe a stress ulcer.

Or it could be cancer.

In between these extremes are a billion other possibilities (a slight exaggeration, but you get the idea).

A Burning Question: When Do You Need an Antacid?

For example, your doctor may say you're suffering from non-ulcer dyspepsia. According to the *Handbook of Nonprescription Drugs* (ninth edition), non-ulcer dyspepsia "refers to intermittent [on and off] upper abdominal discomfort, the cause of which is not clearly defined."

In other words, when you get right down to it, non-ulcer dyspepsia is a catch-all term used for all sorts of stomach upset problems. Some symptoms include upper abdominal pain, nausea, vomiting, bloating, and indigestion.

Indigestion is another fuzzy word. Some people like to call it sour stomach, or acid indigestion, or upset stomach, or acid stomach.

It could mean that you have a touch of gastritis (when your stomach lining becomes inflamed by too much acid secretion). Or it could mean you've simply eaten too much at once, and all that food is sitting heavy in your stomach, like a bowling ball, trying to get digested (as in the case of the massive overindulgence described at the beginning of this article).

Then there's heartburn, which is another matter.

Heartburn happens when the stomach's contents, along with all its corrosive digestive juices, goes into reverse and shoots back up into the esophagus (the tube that extends from the pharynx, or throat, into the stomach). Normally, the pressure in your stomach is lower than the pressure in your esophagus, which helps prevent food from reentering the esophagus. But once in a while the delicate pressure system can break down.

This unsettling event, called gastroesophageal reflux (heartburn), may sometimes announce itself with an embarrassing belch.

But whether you make a noise or not, you feel the burning. The lining of your stomach is fairly accustomed to an acid environment, but your esophagus definitely isn't, so even a little acid in there will sometimes be enough to get your attention.

If gastroesophageal reflux is happening to you all the time, then you may have something called gastroesophageal reflux disease. It could be that your esophageal sphincter (the "door" between your esophagus and your stomach) is weak, chronically allowing the stomach's contents to push back out into the esophagus, burning it.

If the burning sensation is a little lower, and stays around for more than a few days, you could have another problem altogether: a peptic ulcer. An ulcer is simply a sore in your stomach that keeps getting irritated by all the acid swirling around down there.

Antacids can be used to treat all these GI problems. But most people who experience occasional discomfort somewhere along the GI tract, are likely not dealing with an ulcer, or stomach cancer, or anything else major. Chances are it's run-of-the-mill heartburn or indigestion.

You don't need to see a doctor for occasional heartburn or indigestion. The hurting will disappear on its own. If you want some relief in the meantime, antacids will fit the bill nicely.

Again, it should be emphasized that if you experience unpleasant GI symptoms for more than two weeks, or if your symptoms are severe, it may be more than something run-of-the-mill.

Get it Checked out.

Recipe for Relief

FDA requires that every antacid on the market be safe (which means the antacid won't cause serious side effects, provided you take it in the proper dosage over the recommended period of time) and effective (which means the antacid will do what it's supposed to do).

Drug manufacturers must make and label their antacids according to specific guidelines in FDA's monograph on antacids. If manufacturers don't follow this federal antacids "recipe," they are not allowed to market their products.

According to FDA's monograph, an antacid is safe and effective if it meets the following conditions:

- It must contain at least one of the antacid active ingredients (acid neutralizers) approved by the agency. (All the approved ingredients are listed in the antacid monograph.)

- It must contain a sufficient amount of the active ingredients. Specifically, each active ingredient included in the antacid product must contribute at least 25 percent to the product's total neutralizing capacity.

- In a laboratory test, the antacid must neutralize a specific amount of acid and keep it neutralized for at least 10 minutes.

- The label on the antacid must state that the product is good only for relieving the symptoms of "heartburn," "sour stomach," "acid indigestion," and "upset stomach associated with these symptoms." The label can't make any other medical claims.

A Burning Question: When Do You Need an Antacid?

- The label must contain certain warnings concerning proper dosage, side effects (such as constipation or diarrhea), and how much sodium the product contains.

- The label must warn about the product's possible interactions with other drugs. Antacids can increase or decrease the speed at which some medications are eliminated from the body. For example, antacids can block the body's absorption of tetracycline, an antibiotic.

- The label must give directions for using the product, and it must carry a warning not to use the product for more than two weeks except under the advice and supervision of a physician.

What's in an Antacid?

The opposite of an acid is a base, and that's exactly what antacids are.

But a base all by itself can't neutralize the acid inside you. For reasons that are best explained on a blackboard in chemistry class, a base needs some chemical "helpers," or ingredients, to accompany it on its neutralizing mission into your stomach.

All antacids contain at least one of the four primary "helpers" or ingredients: sodium, calcium, magnesium, and aluminum.

Here's a brief rundown of the composition and some potential side effects of various antacids:

Sodium (Alka-Seltzer, Bromo Seltzer, and others)

Sodium bicarbonate or baking soda, perhaps the best known of the sodium-containing antacids, is potent and fast-acting. As its name suggests, it's heavy in sodium. If you're on a salt-restricted diet, and especially if the diet is intended to treat high blood pressure, take a sodium-containing antacid only under a doctor's orders.

Calcium (Tums, Alka-2, Titralac, and others)

Antacids in the form of calcium carbonate or calcium phosphate are potent and fast-acting.

Regular or heavy doses of calcium (more than five or six times per week) can cause constipation. Heavy and extended use of this product may clog your kidneys and cut down the amount of blood they can process, and can also cause kidney stones.

Magnesium (Maalox, Mylanta, Camalox, Riopan, Gelusil, and others)

Magnesium salts come in many forms—carbonate, glycinate, hydroxide, oxide, trisilicate, and aluminosilicates. Magnesium has a mild laxative effect; it can cause diarrhea. For this reason, magnesium salts are rarely used as the only active ingredients in an antacid, but are combined with aluminum, which counteracts the laxative effect. (The brand names listed above all contain magnesium-aluminum combinations.)

Like calcium, magnesium may cause kidney stones if taken for a very prolonged period, especially if the kidneys are functioning improperly to begin with. A serious magnesium overload in the bloodstream (hypermagnesemia) can also cause blood pressure to drop, leading to respiratory or cardiac depression—a potentially dangerous decrease in lung or heart function.

Aluminum (Rolaids, AlternaGEL, Amphogel, and others)

Salts of aluminum (hydroxide, carbonate gel, or phosphate gel) can also cause constipation. For these reasons, aluminum is usually used in combination with the other three primary ingredients.

Used heavily over an extended period, antacids containing aluminum can weaken bones—especially in people who have kidney problems. Aluminum can cause dietary phosphates, calcium and fluoride to leave the body, eventually causing bone problems such as osteomalacia or osteoporosis.

It should be emphasized that aluminum-containing antacids present virtually no danger to people with normal kidney function who use these products only occasionally and as directed.

Simethicone

Some antacids contain an ingredient called simethicone, a gastric defoaming agent that breaks up gas bubbles, making them easier to eliminate from your body.

FDA says simethicone is safe and effective in combination with antacids for relief of gas associated with heartburn. But not all antacids contain this ingredient.

If you're looking for relief of symptoms associated with gas, read the antacid's label carefully to make sure it contains simethicone.

—by Tom Cramer

Tom Cramer is a staff writer for *FDA Consumer*.

Chapter 46

Taking Beta Blocker Drugs

How you take a drug can be very important to both its effectiveness and safety. Sometimes it can be almost as important as what you take. Timing, what you eat and when you eat, proper dose, and many other factors can mean the difference between feeling better, staying the same, or even feeling worse. This drug-information chapter is intended to help you make your treatment work as effectively as possible. It is important to note, however, that this is only a guideline. You should talk to your doctor about how and when to take any prescribed drugs.

Conditions These Drugs Treat

All beta blockers are used to treat high blood pressure. Many are also used to prevent the heart-related chest pain or pressure associated with *angina pectoris* (a condition often occurring during exertion where too little blood reaches the heart). Atenolol, metoprolol, timolol, and propranolol are used to improve survival after a heart attack. Propranolol is used to treat heart rhythm problems, other specific heart conditions, migraine headaches, and tremors. Beta blockers can be used for other conditions as determined by your doctor.

Beta blockers cannot cure these conditions. However, by blocking certain receptors in the body, beta blockers lower and regulate the heartbeat and lessen the heart's workload.

FDA Consumer, 12/03/1990.

While taking beta blockers, it is important that you continue any diet and exercise program prescribed by your doctor, as these are often important parts of the therapy for the conditions being treated.

How to Take

Beta blockers can be taken either with food or on an empty stomach.

If you are taking an extended-release product such as Inderal LAR (propranolol), swallow it whole. Don't chew it or crush it in any way.

If you are taking the concentrated solution of propranolol, always use the dropper provided. You can mix the solution with water or any other beverage (or, if you prefer, pudding or applesauce). After taking a dose, rinse the glass with some liquid and drink that liquid as well to be sure that the entire dose is taken.

Be sure to take the right number of tablets or capsules for each dose.

Taking your medicine at the same time each day will help you remember to take it regularly.

Missed Doses

Do not suddenly stop taking a beta blocker without first talking to your doctor. Your condition could worsen if you stop taking this medicine or miss many doses.

If you miss a dose, take it as soon as you remember. If you take the beta blocker once a day, you can take it up to eight hours before the next scheduled dose. If you take the medication more often than once a day, you can take it up to four hours before the next scheduled dose. Ask your doctor or pharmacist if you have questions.

Never take two doses at the same time.

Always have enough of your beta blocker medicine to last over weekends, holiday periods, and when you travel.

Relief of Symptoms

For conditions such as high blood pressure, angina, heart rhythm disturbances, or tremors, some effects can be seen immediately and usually peak within a week. If treating migraine headaches, it may take up to six weeks before the full effects occur. For any of these conditions, the dosage of the beta blocker may need to be adjusted by your doctor when you first begin taking it. Also, the appropriate dosage can vary greatly among people, depending on individual response.

Since many of the conditions that beta blockers treat are chronic, you may have to take this medicine for the rest of your life.

Side Effects and Risks

Common side effects include slowed heartbeat, tiredness, nausea, diarrhea, constipation, and decreased sexual ability. Other mild side effects can include difficulty sleeping or nightmares, headache, drowsiness, and numbness or tingling of the fingers, toes or scalp. Also, if you have diabetes, beta blockers can obscure some of the signs of low blood sugar, such as tremors or rapid heartbeat. Check with your doctor if any of these side effects seems troublesome or if you have any questions.

More serious reactions can sometimes occur with beta blockers. These include the following:

- the beginning or worsening of heart failure. Symptoms of this include shortness of breath (especially on exertion), coughing, weakness, weight gain, and swelling of feet, ankles, or lower legs.

- severe wheezing or difficulty breathing, especially in people who have or have had asthma, chronic bronchitis, emphysema, or other breathing conditions. Because beta blockers can trigger or worsen these conditions, make sure your doctor knows about them.

- an extremely slow heartbeat (less than 50 beats per minute)

- cold hands and feet or blue fingernails, which could mean reduced circulation to these areas

- confusion, hallucinations or depression. If any of these or other serious reactions occur, call your doctor immediately.

Precautions and Warnings

If you suddenly stop taking a beta blocker, you could worsen your condition and experience potentially dangerous side effects, such as chest pain, fast or irregular heartbeat, high blood pressure, and headaches. Always check with your doctor before discontinuing a beta blocker.

Consult with your doctor if you think you could become pregnant or plan to breast-feed while on a beta blocker.

Learn how the medicine affects you. Don't drive or operate machines if this medicine makes you drowsy, dizzy or lightheaded. If you are taking labetalol, dizziness or light-headedness can occur when getting up from sitting or lying down. If this happens, sit up slowly, placing your legs over the side of the bed or couch, and stay there for a few minutes before trying to stand.

Before any surgery or dental work, tell the physician or dentist that you are taking beta blockers. Tell your physician if you are taking or considering taking any other prescription or nonprescription medication.

Drinking alcohol while on beta blockers can sometimes increase the chance of side effects such as dizziness or tiredness.

Generic Names

- acebutolol
- atenolol
- betaxolol
- carteolol
- labetalol
- metoprolol
- nadolol
- penbutolol
- pindolol
- propranolol
- timolol

Drug Tips

- Don't store drugs in the bathroom medicine cabinet. Heat and humidity may cause the medicine to lose its effectiveness.

- Keep all medicines, even those with child-resistant caps, out of the reach of children. Remember, the caps are child-resistant, not child-proof.

- Discard medicines that have reached the expiration date.

— by Igor Cerney

Igor Cerney is on the staff of FDA's Drug Labeling, Education and Research Branch.

Chapter 47

Patches, Pumps, and Timed Release: New Ways to Deliver Drugs

If, 25 years ago, someone tried to sell you an adhesive patch, telling you to stick it behind your ear and it would keep you from getting sick on the high seas, you could make a safe bet that you were being sold up the river by a modern-day snake oil salesman.

Today, however, a similar patch can be legitimately prescribed by your doctor. Technological advances over the last 20 to 30 years have enabled scientists to develop new forms of delivering drugs to our bodies, including a transdermal patch containing the drug scopolamine to prevent motion sickness.

Drug dosage forms are keeping pace with the high-tech times. Indeed, the ubiquitous tablet of 1990 may one day become obsolete, going the way of the spirits, powders and tinctures of a century ago.

What might replace the tablet? How about pills that are pumps and implanted drug-filled devices with or without tiny computers to regulate the time and amount of drug dispensed? These and other unconventional dosage forms already exist, heralding advances in drug delivery that promise even safer and more effective treatments.

One of the most active areas of research and development in drug delivery involves "controlled-release" products. Rather than develop new drug entities at great cost, some drug therapies already on the market can be improved simply by controlling the rate at which they enter the bloodstream.

"Virtually all the delivery systems marketed are initially in what we would call 'immediate-release preparations'—things that disintegrate

FDA Consumer, June 1991.

and dissolve in 5 or 10 minutes," says FDA visiting scientist Gordon Amidon, Ph.D. "For some drugs, dissolution may take longer because of drug or dosage form properties, but the controlled release is not designed in."

Timing Is Everything

"Drugs that are released rapidly produce a relatively rapid and high concentration in the body, followed by a sharp decline—a peak and valley effect," says Amidon. "We know that at too low a blood level the drug is not effective, at optimum level it's effective, and at too high a level undesirable effects are produced. The objective is to try to maintain the range in between."

Controlled-release systems deliver a drug at a slower rate for a longer period. The dosage form contains more drug than a conventional tablet or injection, for example, but delivers the medication far more slowly—over a period of hours, days, or even years, rather than seconds or minutes.

Depending on the mechanism, the delivery system may simply release the drug at a variable, but slower, rate, or release it at a constant rate over the period of release. Sometimes, by decreasing the variability of blood levels, it may reduce side effects.

The Ways to Delay

Milo Gibaldi, Ph.D., dean of the University of Washington's School of Pharmacy in Seattle, writes in *Biopharmaceutics and Clinical Pharmacokinetics*: "The early history of the prolonged-release oral dosage form is probably best forgotten. Products were developed empirically, often with little rationale, and ... problems were common. Today, the situation has improved; many of the available products are well-designed drug delivery systems and have a defined therapeutic goal. In some cases, the prolonged-release dosage form is the most important and most frequently used form of the drug."

Prolonged-release preparations usually require less frequent dosing. Being able to take a pill once a day instead of four times or more, for example, can help improve patient compliance. That is, it's often easier and less bothersome for patients to remember to take fewer doses of medications.

There are a number of ways of controlling the rate of delivery of oral medicines. One system uses the principle of osmosis to release the drug. The drug and an osmotic agent are surrounded by a semipermeable

Patches, Pumps, and Timed Release

membrane pierced by one or more small, laser-drilled holes. As water from the digestive tract is drawn through the membrane, the osmotic layer expands, pushing the drug through the holes.

In other systems, the drug simply diffuses through a polymer coating of the pill. The drug may be contained in a reservoir surrounded by a polymer film, or it may be uniformly distributed through the polymeric material.

"Most of the polymers used in human pharmaceuticals are derivatives of natural products such as gelatin and cellulose, or the synthetic polymer silicone," says Amidon. "When designing a drug delivery system, you select the polymer best suited for that particular system based on the properties of the specific polymer."

An erosion-controlled release system uses a polymer that is relatively water-soluble with the drug incorporated in it. As the polymer dissolves, it releases the drug. The formulation of *Contac*'s "tiny time pill" capsules is based on an erosion system. It consists of coated and uncoated granules that erode at various rates, thus releasing the drug at varying rates and providing relief for an extended period.

Skin Patches

Some drugs that have the right properties to penetrate the skin and are potent enough to be effective at low doses can be delivered transdermally (through the skin). The first transdermal patch was approved by FDA in 1979. It contained the drug scopolamine, used to treat motion sickness.

Scopolamine can cause dry mouth, drowsiness, blurred vision and other eye problems, and sometimes more serious side effects, including dizziness and confusion, hallucinations, difficulty urinating, and rashes. Delivered through the skin at a slow rate in small amounts over three days, however, the drug can protect against motion sickness with fewer or less severe side effects.

One patch design consists of four layers of thin, flexible membranes: an impermeable backing, a drug reservoir, a rate-controlling membrane, and an adhesive. When the patch is applied, the drug begins flowing through the skin into the bloodstream at a rate regulated by the membrane, pre-programmed to keep the drug at levels that provide effectiveness with acceptable adverse effects.

Another transdermal preparation is a nitroglycerin patch for patients with angina pectoris (chest pain). Unlike nitroglycerin tablets placed under the tongue at the onset of an attack to relieve pain, the patch is applied once a day (usually to the chest) to help prevent angina attacks.

As with scopolamine, a goal of delivering a steady concentration of nitroglycerin was to provide the lowest effective blood level of the drug while minimizing adverse effects, such as headaches in the case of nitroglycerin.

With the nitroglycerin patch, however, it was discovered that maintaining constant blood levels is not advantageous. Studies showed that when patches are worn continuously, drug tolerance develops within 24 hours and the medication is no longer effective. Revised labeling recently approved by FDA recommends a dosing schedule alternating a daily patch-on period of 12 to 14 hours a day with a patch-off period of 10 to 12 hours.

Another extended-release preparation that did not prove as successful as originally expected is *Ocusert*, a reservoir system in a wafer-like disk, designed to treat glaucoma. Glaucoma is characterized by increased pressure in the eye that can cause blindness. At the time Ocusert was developed, the standard treatment for glaucoma was application four times a day of eye drops containing the pressure-lowering drug pilocarpine. The drops often caused side effects, however, and patients sometimes did not take them as prescribed. *Ocusert*, on the other hand, placed in the lower eyelid, where it floats in the tear film, delivers low-dose pilocarpine continuously for one week.

Although it was seen as having the potential to solve patient compliance problems, Ocusert was never widely used, in part because older patients were reluctant to place the object in their eyes. Also, *Ocusert* costs the patient approximately five times more than the pilocarpine drops. A new drug, timolol, has since been developed, which, although not a controlled-release preparation, requires only two applications of drops a day instead of the four needed with pilocarpine.

Implants and Intrauterine Devices

Devices implanted under the skin are also being developed to deliver drugs at a controlled rate. FDA approved one such device for contraception in December 1990. The Norplant system is implanted under the skin and protects against pregnancy for five years, unless removed sooner. It consists of six flexible silicone tubes filled with a five-year supply of the hormone levonorgestrel. It is implanted in the upper arm, and small amounts of the hormone continuously seep through the permeable tubes into the bloodstream, providing contraception. (For more on this device, see "Norplant: Birth Control at Arm's Reach" in the May 1991 *FDA Consumer*.)

Similarly, an intrauterine device called *Progestasert* releases the hormone progesterone directly into the uterus for one year to prevent pregnancy. An advantage of these controlled-release contraceptives over contraceptive pills is convenience; their effectiveness does not depend on remembering to take a daily pill.

The Mechanical Pump

Although the advantages of a steady rate of drug release are evident, some drugs are more effective given in intervals. Infusion pumps can be programmed to deliver drugs at very precise dosages and delivery rates. These pumps may have a feedback device that controls drug delivery according to need.

"I think we're going to see more complex dosing patterns that are going to be more difficult to regulate orally," says Amidon. "With further development of electronics and miniaturization of pumps and sensors, we'll be able to monitor various vital signs, and that will lead to feedback systems." Such a feedback system could monitor blood glucose levels and deliver insulin when needed.

Amidon explains that the size of the pump depends on the amount of drug and the intended length of treatment. Some pumps are portable, some wearable. For miniaturized, implantable pumps, methods will have to be devised to refill the device externally, perhaps once a month or once a year, through a catheter.

"I would say that 50 years from now we're going to have implantable pumps with multiple drugs that we can externally program once a month and, rather than going to the doctor for checkups, we will plug ourselves into a telephone monitoring device," Amidon predicts. "To solve problems like drug tolerance, we're going to have to develop drug delivery programs that are not constant, but programmed with time or circadian doses. We're going to see more complicated therapy in order to be able to reduce the amount of drug exposure and increase its efficacy."

If Amidon's vision is to become reality, several technological roadblocks will have to be solved first. Donald Marlowe, director of FDA's division of mechanics and material science, points out just one, as an example. Before feedback technology can be applied in humans, problems with the pump's sensor mechanism must be overcome, Marlowe says. "For example," he explains, "contact with body proteins causes reduced sensitivity of the sensors, compromising [feedback] reliability."

One implanted pump, approved by FDA in 1982, allows chronic infusion of the liver cancer drug FUDR directly into the artery leading to that organ, thereby delivering a high concentration of the drug to the target organ.

William Ensminger, M.D., Ph.D., Professor of Internal Medicine and Pharmacy at the University of Michigan Medical School in Ann Arbor, says that people live and function with implanted pumps quite well. One of his patients had a pump for eight years, which was refilled every couple of weeks. "We've had other people who have had them in for four years and a few people who have had them taken out when the liver tumor was eradicated."

Last July, FDA approved a concentrated form of morphine specially developed for microinfusion pumps that can be implanted under the skin of the abdomen or worn outside the body. Given this way, the drug can provide more constant relief to people in severe pain, such as terminal cancer patients. Programmed with dosing information before it is filled with the concentrated morphine, the pump constantly delivers fractional doses of the drug. The dose can be changed by beaming information through skin and tissues to the implanted pump.

Concentrated morphine can have severe side effects, such as seizures and respiratory depression if the starting dose is misjudged. Therefore, patients must be monitored in a fully equipped and staffed facility for at least 24 hours after the initial "test" dose. Patients may then go home and return periodically—sometimes as seldom as once a month—for a physician to refill the reservoir in the pump.

It's clear that we're witnessing an evolution—or revolution—in drug delivery, with many innovations in administering drugs to improve safety and effectiveness. The process continues, using techniques as varied as advanced electronics and genetic engineering.

—by Marian Segal

Marian Segal is a member of FDA's public affairs staff.

Chapter 48

Treating Chronic Pain with Implantable Therapies

A Patient's Guide to Spinal Cord Stimulation and Intraspinal Drug Infusion

Introduction

Chronic pain is constant or recurring pain that lasts longer than six months. It can affect a person's relationships, job, and quality of life. This chapter discusses two implantable therapies (spinal cord stimulation and intraspinal drug infusion) which may be appropriate when conservative treatments fail. For carefully selected patients, these two implantable therapies have been proven effective in reducing pain and improving quality of life.

How Is Pain Felt?

Although pain seems to be felt at the point of injury, the sensation is actually registered in the brain. Pain messages are sent from muscles, organs, and other tissues, through the spinal cord to the brain. Blocking those pain messages from reaching the brain can prevent pain. Spinal cord stimulation (SCS) blocks the pain messages with electrical impulses to the spinal cord. Intraspinal drug infusion therapy blocks pain signals with low doses of morphine delivered to the spinal cord.

©1993 Medtronic Neurological. Reprinted with permission.

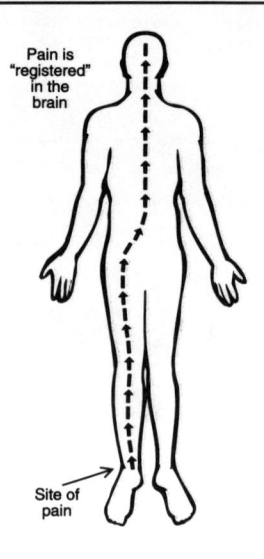

Pain Sourcebook

Figure 48.1. Pain receptors in the leg send pain messages to the brain through the spinal cord.

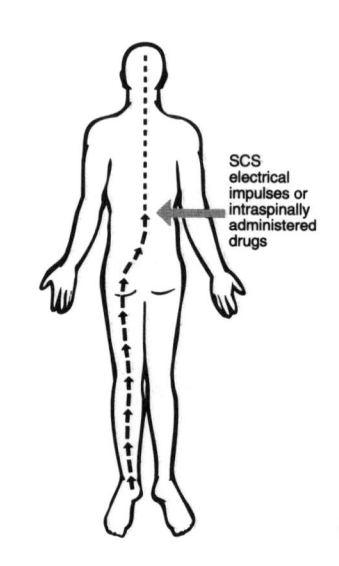

Figure 48.2. Spinal cord stimulation blocks pain signals to the brain using electrical impulses. Intraspinal drug infusion therapy blocks pain signals to the brain with morphine.

What Is Spinal Cord Stimulation (SCS)?

Spinal cord stimulation (SCS) is a procedure for the control of chronic pain that has helped thousands of patients worldwide since the early 1970s. SCS stimulates the spinal cord with tiny electrical signals to interfere with the transmission of pain signals to the brain, thus reducing the sensation of pain. The affected area of the patient's body feels a gentle tingling. SCS is a reversible procedure that does not damage the spinal cord or nerves.

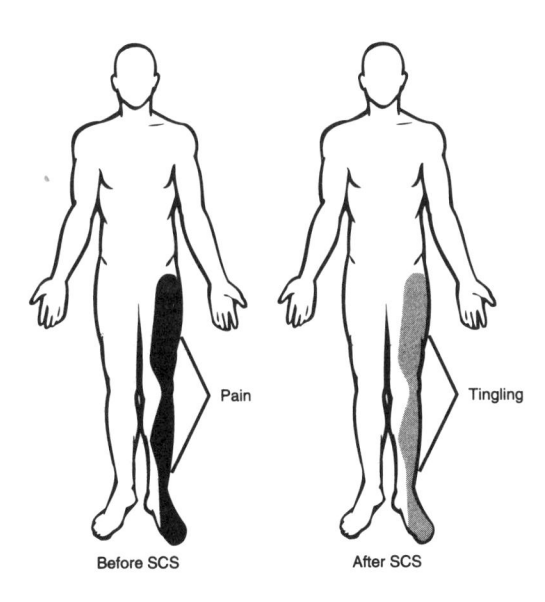

Figure 48.3. This is one example of successful spinal cord stimulation.

Who Is a Candidate for SCS Therapy?

The best candidates for SCS therapy have severe, chronic pain in the arms or legs. Patients with leg pain primarily and some pain in the lower back may also benefit from SCS therapy. Most patients have tried other methods of pain control (such as behavior modification, oral narcotics, nerve blocks, or surgery), but have not experienced sufficient pain relief.

What Is an SCS System?

There are two types of SCS systems: fully implanted systems and systems with an external power source. For fully implanted systems, a battery in the implanted pulse generator provides the power. The pulse generator, which looks like a pacemaker, also contains circuitry that allows it to be programmed for each individual patient.

For patients who require a permanent external power source, a receiver is implanted. The power for external units is provided by a transmitter which is worn externally. Both types of systems are connected to a lead (pronounced "leed").

The lead is a flexible insulated wire which carries electrical impulses from the pulse generator or receiver. The tip of the lead has tiny electrodes that stimulate the spinal chord.

Figure 48.4. A totally implantable SCS system has no external components.

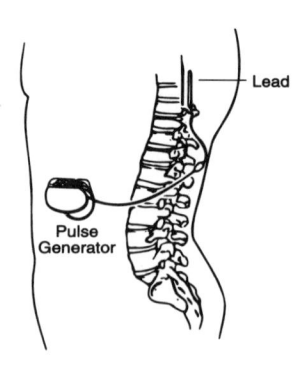

Figure 48.5. An "external" SCS system has both implanted and external components.

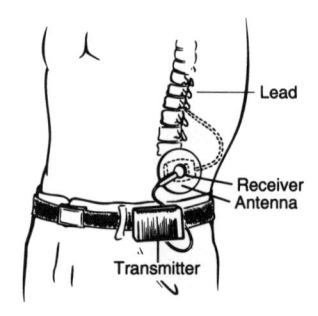

How Will the Doctor Know Whether SCS Will Work?

Patients undergo a trial of stimulation to determine whether SCS will be effective for them. The patient remains awake during the trial (under local anesthesia) and there is little discomfort involved. The physician inserts the lead along the spinal cord so that tingling is felt in the area where the patient normally feels the pain. During the procedure, the patient tells the physician where he or she feels the tingling, and when the tingling completely covers the painful area. During this trial period, which may last from a few hours to several days, the effectiveness of stimulation is tested using an external power source. Some patients are observed on an outpatient basis; others are admitted to the hospital. Patients who experience significant pain relief (at least 50 percent reduction) during the trial may have the SCS system implanted.

If the patient does not experience significant pain relief during the trial, the lead is removed, and the patient may be evaluated for intraspinal drug infusion therapy or other alternatives.

How Is an SCS System Implanted?

The lead is implanted during the stimulation trial. If the patient continues to experience significant pain relief during the SCS trial, the physician will surgically implant either a permanent pulse generator or receiver under the skin, in the abdomen or upper buttock area. The lead is then connected to the implanted pulse generator or receiver, and stimulation patterns are again tested and adjusted.

What Can Be Expected from SCS Therapy?

Patients using SCS therapy can expect 50 to 75 percent pain relief, which is considered a good to excellent result. Occasional adjustments to the stimulation output will be required. Most adjustments can be made in the physician's office using a computer which "communicates" to the implanted pulse generator via radio waves. Adjustments to external units are made via the transmitter. Some models allow patients to adjust the stimulation themselves using a handheld programmer.

SCS has reduced pain for thousands of people worldwide. However, because SCS does not eliminate the source of pain, the extent of its effectiveness may vary. When SCS therapy is successful, the patient may have a more active lifestyle because pain is reduced.

What Is Intraspinal Drug Infusion Therapy?

Intraspinal drug infusion is an implantable therapy which blocks pain by administering small doses of morphine directly to the spinal cord. Intraspinal drug infusion requires much smaller doses of morphine for pain relief than with oral (pills) or intravenous methods. Patients may have fewer side effects and greater pain relief.

Who Is a Candidate for Drug Infusion Therapy?

Patients with severe, chronic pain in broad areas of the body, either from cancer or other causes, may benefit from intraspinal drug infusion therapy. Most patients have unsuccessfully tried other pain control methods. While their pain may respond to oral drug therapy, they either do not achieve adequate pain relief or cannot tolerate the side effects of the pain drug at effective doses. Some patients may have had an unsuccessful SCS trial as well.

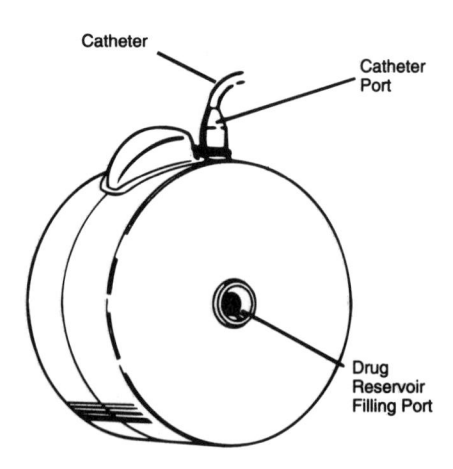

Figure 48.6. *An intraspinal drug infusion system consists of a pump and spinal catheter implanted under the skin.*

Treating Chronic Pain with Implantable Therapies

What Is an Intraspinal Drug Infusion System?

An intraspinal drug infusion system consists of a pump and catheter. The pump is a round metal disk about one inch thick and three inches in diameter. It weighs about six ounces. The pump stores and releases prescribed amounts of morphine into the spinal canal. The pump can be refilled by inserting a needle through the patient's skin into a filling port in the center of the pump. The catheter is a flexible tube that delivers the morphine from the pump to the spinal canal.

How Does the Doctor Know If a Drug Infusion System Will Work?

Selected candidates for this therapy undergo a trial of intraspinal drug therapy. During this trial, the physician injects a small dose of morphine into the spinal canal to determine whether the pain can be diminished with this treatment. This procedure is not uncomfortable for the patient. Patients who experience significant pain relief during the trial may have a drug infusion pump and catheter implanted.

Where and How Is the Pump Implanted?

The drug pump is surgically placed just underneath the skin usually in the lower abdominal area. The spinal catheter is inserted through a needle into the spinal canal. The other end of the catheter is placed under the skin and connected to the pump. The pump is filled with the morphine prescribed by the physician.

How Is the Medication Dispensed?

Some drug infusion systems dispense at a steady rate, with the dosage determined by the concentration of the medication injected into the pump reservoir. Medication changes in steady-rate systems are accomplished by withdrawing the old strength of medication and re-infusing the new strength drug. With a programmable pump, a tiny motor moves the medication from the pump reservoir through the catheter. Adjustments in the dose, rate, and timing of the medication can be made using an external programmer. This allows greater flexibility for matching the dosage of pain relief medication with patient needs.

What Can Be Expected from Intraspinal Drug Infusion Therapy?

Patients can expect good to excellent pain relief if they had a successful trial. Patients will need to return to their physician's office for pump refills and adjustments to their medication (approximately every four to 12 weeks). Compared with intravenous (I.V.) drug infusion or oral medications, intraspinal drug infusion usually controls pain with much smaller dosages because the drug is delivered directly into the intraspinal space. With this delivery method, therapeutic benefits are maximized and side effects are minimized. Benefits of intraspinal drug infusion therapy may include a more active lifestyle, better sleep, and reduced need for oral pain medications.

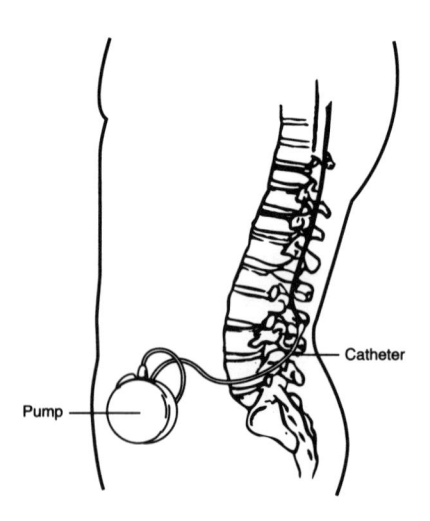

Figure 48.7. An implanted drug pump delivers very small doses of morphine through the catheter to the spinal cord. With intraspinal drug infusion therapy, pain relief can be achieved with much smaller doses of morphine than would be required with oral or intravenous methods.

Is Addiction a Concern with Intraspinal Drug Infusion Therapy?

This is a very rare, unlikely outcome. Research has shown that fewer than one in 1,000 patients becomes "addicted" to morphine with intraspinal drug infusion therapy because the dose required for pain control is so small. Addiction refers to compulsive drug-seeking behavior and using pain medication for emotional gratification. Patients in pain rarely get addicted because they use morphine to control pain, not for emotional gratification.

Ask Your Doctor

Patients whose chronic pain has not responded to more conventional treatment may be considered by their physician for spinal cord stimulation or intraspinal drug infusion therapy. If you have questions regarding these treatments, feel free to discuss them with your physician.

Chapter 49

Integration of Behavioral and Relaxation Techniques for the Treatment of Chronic Pain and Insomnia

What behavioral and relaxation approaches are used for conditions such as chronic pain and insomnia?

Pain

Pain is defined by the International Association for the Study of Pain as an unpleasant sensory experience associated with actual or potential tissue damage or described in terms of such damage. It is a complex, subjective, perceptual phenomenon with a number of contributing factors that are uniquely experienced by each individual. Pain is typically classified as acute, cancer-related, and chronic nonmalignant. Acute pain is associated with a noxious event. Its severity is generally proportional to the degree of tissue injury and is expected to diminish with healing and time. Chronic non-malignant pain frequently develops following an injury but persists long after a reasonable period of healing. Its underlying causes are often not readily discernible, and the pain is disproportionate to demonstrable tissue damage. It is frequently accompanied by alteration of sleep, mood, sexual, vocational, and avocational function.

Insomnia

Insomnia may be defined as a disturbance or perceived disturbance of the usual sleep pattern of the individual that has troublesome

National Institutes of Health Technology Assessment Conference Statement. October 1995.

consequences. These consequences may include daytime fatigue and drowsiness, irritability, anxiety, depression, and somatic complaints. Categories of disturbed sleep are:

1. inability to fall asleep,
2. inability to maintain sleep, and
3. early awakening.

Selection Criteria

A large variety of behavioral and relaxation approaches are used for conditions such as chronic pain and insomnia. The specific approaches that were addressed in this technology assessment conference represent three important selection criteria. First, somatically directed therapies with behavioral components (e.g., physical therapy, occupational therapy, acupuncture) were not considered. Second, the approaches were drawn from those reported in the scientific literature. Many commonly used behavioral approaches are not specifically incorporated into conventional medical care. For example, religious and spiritual approaches, which are the most commonly used health-related actions by the U.S. population, were not considered in this conference. Third, the approaches are a subset of those discussed in the literature and represent those selected by the conference organizers as most commonly used in clinical settings in the United States. Certain commonly used clinical interventions such as music, dance, recreational, and art therapies also were not addressed.

Relaxation Techniques

Relaxation techniques are a group of behavioral therapeutic approaches that differ widely in their philosophical bases as well as in their methodologies and techniques. Their primary objective is the achievement of non-directed relaxation (rather than direct achievement of a specific therapeutic goal). They all share two basic components: (1) repetitive focus on a word, sound, prayer, phrase, body sensation, or muscular activity and(2) the adoption of a passive attitude toward intruding thoughts and a return to the focus. These techniques induce a common set of physiologic changes that result in decreased metabolic activity. Relaxation techniques may also be used in stress management (as self-regulatory techniques) and have been divided into deep and brief methods.

Integration of Behavioral and Relaxation Techniques

Deep Methods

Deep methods include autogenic training, meditation, and progressive muscle relaxation (PMR). Autogenic training consists of imagining a peaceful environment and comforting bodily sensations. Six basic focusing techniques are used: heaviness in the limbs, warmth in the limbs, cardiac regulation, centering on breathing, warmth in the upper abdomen, and coolness in the forehead. Meditation is a self-directed practice for relaxing the body and calming the mind. A large variety of meditation techniques are commonly used; each has its own proponents. Meditation generally does not involve suggestion, autosuggestion, or trance. The goal of mindfulness meditation is development of a non-judgmental awareness of bodily sensations and mental activities occurring in the present moment. Concentration meditation trains the person to passively attend to a bodily process, word, and/or a stimulus. Transcendental meditation focuses on a "suitable" sound or thought (the mantra) without attempting to actually concentrate on the sound or thought. There are also many movement meditations, such as yoga and walking meditation in Zen Buddhism. PMR focuses on reducing muscle tone in major muscle groups. Each of the 15 major muscle groups is tensed and then relaxed in sequence.

Brief Methods

The brief methods, which include self-control relaxation, paced respiration, and deep breathing, generally require less time to acquire or practice and often represent abbreviated forms of a corresponding deep method. For example, self-control relaxation is an abbreviated form of PMR. Autogenic training may be abbreviated and converted to a self-control format. Paced respiration teaches patients to maintain slow breathing when anxiety threatens. Deep breathing involves taking several deep breaths, holding them for five seconds, and then exhaling slowly.

Hypnotic Techniques

Hypnotic techniques induce states of selective attention focusing or diffusion combined with enhanced imagery. They are often used to induce relaxation and also may be a part of cognitive-behavioral techniques (CBT). The techniques have pre- and post-suggestion components. The pre-suggestion component involves attention focusing through the use of imagery, distraction, and/or relaxation. Subjects focus on relaxation and passively disregard intrusive thoughts. The pre-suggestion component of hypnosis has features that are similar to other relaxation techniques. The suggestion phase is characterized by introduction of specific goals, for example, analgesia may be specifically suggested. The post-suggestion component involves continued use of the new behavior following termination of hypnosis. Individuals vary widely in their hypnotic susceptibility and suggestibility, although the reasons for these differences are incompletely understood.

Biofeedback Techniques

Biofeedback techniques are treatment methods that use monitoring instruments of varying degrees of sophistication to provide patients with physiologic information that allows them to reliably influence psycho-physiological responses of two kinds:

1. responses not ordinarily under voluntary control and
2. responses that ordinarily are easily regulated, but for which regulation has broken down.

Technologies that are commonly used include electromyography (EMG-BF), electroencephalography (EEG-BF), thermometers (thermal-BF), and galvanometry (electrodermal-BF). Biofeedback techniques often induce physiological responses similar to those of other relaxation techniques.

Cognitive-behavioral Techniques

Cognitive-Behavioral techniques (CBT) attempt to alter patterns of negative thoughts and dysfunctional attitudes in order to foster more healthy and adaptive thoughts, emotions, and actions. These interventions share four basic components: education, skills acquisition, cognitive and behavioral rehearsal, and generalization and maintenance. Relaxation techniques are frequently included as a behavioral component in CBT programs. The specific programs used to implement the four components can vary considerably. Each of the aforementioned therapeutic modalities may be practiced individually, or they may be combined as part of multimodal approaches to management of chronic pain or insomnia.

Relaxation and Behavioral Techniques for Insomnia

Relaxation and behavioral techniques corresponding to those used for chronic pain may be employed for specific types of insomnia. Cognitive

Integration of Behavioral and Relaxation Techniques

relaxation, various forms of biofeedback, and PMR may all be used in the treatment of insomnia. In addition, the following behavioral approaches are generally used in the management of insomnia.

- **Sleep hygiene**, which involves educating patients about behaviors that may interfere with the sleep process, with the hope that education about maladaptive behaviors will lead to behavioral modification.

- **Stimulus control therapy**, which seeks to create and protect conditioned association between the bedroom and sleep. Activities in the bedroom are restricted to sleep and sex.

- **Sleep restriction therapy**, in which patients provide a sleep log and are then asked to stay in bed only as long as they think they are currently sleeping. This usually leads to sleep deprivation and consolidation followed by a gradual increase in the length of time in bed.

- **Paradoxical intention** in which the patient is instructed not to fall asleep, with the expectation that efforts to avoid sleep will in fact induce it.

How Successful Are These Approaches?

Pain

A plethora of studies using a range of behavioral and relaxation approaches to treat chronic pain is reported in the literature. The measures of success reported in these studies depend on the rigor of the research design, the population studied, the length of follow-up, and the outcome measures identified. As the number of well-designed studies using a variety of behavioral and relaxation techniques grows, the use of meta-analysis as a means of demonstrating overall effectiveness increases.

One carefully analyzed review of studies on chronic pain, including cancer pain, was prepared under the auspices of the U.S. Agency for Health Care Policy and Research (AHCPR) in 1990. A great strength of the report was the careful categorization of the evidential basis of each intervention. The categorization was based on design of the studies and consistency of findings among the studies. These properties led to the development of a four-point scale that ranked the evidence as strong, moderate, fair, and weak; that scale is used in this panel report in evaluating both the AHCPR studies and additional data.

Evaluation of behavioral and relaxation interventions for chronic pain reduction in adults found the following:

Relaxation. The evidence is strong for the effectiveness of this class of techniques in reducing chronic pain in a variety of medical conditions.

Hypnosis. The evidence supporting the effectiveness of hypnosis in alleviating chronic pain associated with cancer is strong. In addition, the panel was presented with other data suggesting the effectiveness of hypnosis in other chronic pain conditions such as irritable bowel syndrome, oral mucositis, temporomandibular disorders, and tension headaches.

Cognitive-Behavioral Techniques. The evidence was moderate for the usefulness of cognitive-behavioral techniques (CBT) in chronic pain. In addition, a series of eight well-designed studies found CBT superior to placebo and to routine care for alleviating low back pain and rheumatoid arthritis and osteoarthritis, but inferior to hypnosis for oral mucositis, and, as mentioned, to EMG biofeedback for tension headache.

Biofeedback. The evidence is moderate for the effectiveness of biofeedback in relieving many types of chronic pain. Data were also reviewed showing EMG-BF to be more effective than psychological placebo for tension headache but equivalent in results to relaxation. For migraine headache biofeedback is equivalent to relaxation therapy and better than no treatment, but the superiority to psychological placebo is less clear.

Multimodal Treatment. Several meta-analyses address the effectiveness of pain clinic multimodal treatments. These studies indicate a consistent positive effect of the program of these centers on several categories of regional pain. Back and neck pain, dental or facial pain, joint pain, and migraine headaches have all shown a significant benefit.

Although there is relatively good evidence for the effectiveness of several behavioral and relaxation interventions in the treatment of

Integration of Behavioral and Relaxation Techniques

chronic pain, there is insufficient data to conclude that one technique is more effective than another for a given condition. For any given individual patient, however, one approach may indeed be more appropriate than another.

Insomnia

Behavioral treatments produce improvements in some aspects of sleep, the most pronounced of which are for sleep latency and time awake after sleep onset. Relaxation and biofeedback were both found to be effective in alleviating insomnia. Cognitive forms of relaxation such as meditation were slightly better than somatic forms of relaxation such as PMR. Sleep restriction, stimulus control, and multimodal treatment were the three most effective treatments in reducing insomnia. No data were presented or reviewed on the effectiveness of CBT or hypnosis. Improvements seen at treatment completion were maintained at follow-ups averaging six months in duration. Although these effects are statistically significant, it is questionable whether the magnitude of the improvements in sleep onset and total sleep time are clinically meaningful.

To adequately evaluate the relative success of different treatment modalities for insomnia a number of major issues need to be addressed.

First, valid objective measures of insomnia are needed. Some investigators rely on self-reports by patients, while others believe that insomnia must be documented electro-physiologically.

Second, what constitutes a therapeutic outcome should be determined. Some investigators use time until sleep onset, number of awakenings, and total sleep time as outcome measures, whereas others believe that impairment in daytime functioning is another important outcome measure. Both of these issues require resolution for research in the field to move forward.

Critique

Although this literature offers substantial promise, the state of the art of the methodology in this field of behavioral and relaxation interventions indicates a need for thoughtful interpretation of these findings and prompt translation into programs of health care delivery. It should be noted that similar criticisms can be made of many conventional medical procedures.

Several cautions must be considered threats to the internal and external validity of the study results. The following problems exist regarding internal validity:

1. The full and adequate comparability among treatment contrast groups may be absent;

2. The sample sizes are sometimes small, lessening the ability to detect differences in efficacy;

3. Complete blinding, which would be ideal, is compromised by patient and clinician awareness of the treatment;

4. The treatments may not be well described and adequate procedures for standardization such as therapy manuals, therapist training, and reliable competency and integrity assessments have not always been carried out; and

5. A potential publication bias in favor of authors dropping studies with small effects and negative results is a concern in a field characterized by studies with small numbers of patients.

With regard to the ability to generalize the findings of these investigations, the following considerations are important:

- The patients participating in these studies are usually not cognitively impaired. They must be capable not only of participating in the study treatments, but also of fulfilling all the requirements of participating in the study protocol.

- The therapists must be adequately trained to conduct the therapy competently.

- The cultural context in which the treatment is conducted may alter its acceptability and effectiveness.

In summary, this literature offers substantial promise and suggests a need for prompt translation into programs of health care delivery. At the same time, the state of the art of the methodology in the field of behavioral and relaxation interventions indicates a need for thoughtful interpretation of these findings. It should be noted that similar criticisms can be made of many conventional medical procedures.

Integration of Behavioral and Relaxation Techniques

How do these approaches work?

The mechanism of action of behavioral and relaxation approaches can be considered at two levels:

1. Determining how the procedure works to reduce cognitive and physiological arousal and to promote the most appropriate behavioral response and,

2. Identifying effects at more basic levels of functional anatomy, neuro-transmitter and other biochemical activity, and circadian rhythms. The exact biological actions are often unknown.

Pain

There appear to be two pain transmission circuits. Some data suggest that a spinal cord-thalamic-frontal cortex-anterior cingulate pathway plays a role in the subjective psychological and physiological responses to pain, whereas a spinal cord-thalamic-somatosensory cortex pathway plays a role in pain sensation. A descending pathway involving the periaquaductal gray region modulates pain signals. This system can augment or inhibit pain transmission at the level of the dorsal spinal cord. Endogenous opioids are particularly concentrated in this pathway.

At the level of the spinal cord, serotonin and norepinephrine appear to play important roles. Relaxation techniques as a group generally alter sympathetic activity as indicated by decreases in oxygen consumption, respiratory and heart rate, and blood pressure. Increased slow wave activity on electroencephalography has also been reported. Although the mechanism for the decrease in sympathetic activity is unclear, one may infer decreased arousal (due to alterations in catecholamines or other neurochemical systems) plays a key role.

Hypnosis, in part because of its capacity for evoking intense relaxation, has been reported to reduce nausea associated with chemotherapy and has been shown to be helpful in reducing several types of pain, e.g., lower back and burn pain. Hypnosis does not appear to influence endorphin production, and its role in the production of catecholomines is not known. Hypnosis has been hypothesized to block pain from entering consciousness by activating the thalamic-frontal cortex-anterior cingulate pathway to inhibit impulse transmission from thalamic to cortical structures. Similarly, other CBTs may decrease transmission through this pathway. Moreover, the overlap in brain regions involved in pain modulation and anxiety suggest a possible role for CBT approaches affecting this area of function, although data are still evolving.

CBT also appears to exert a number of other effects that could alter pain intensity. Depression and anxiety increase subjective complaints of pain, and cognitive-behavioral approaches are well-documented for decreasing these affective states. In addition, these types of techniques may alter expectation, which also plays a key role in subjective experiences of pain intensity. They also may augment analgesic responses through behavioral conditioning. Finally, these techniques help patients feel empowered or less helpless and better able to deal with pain sensations.

Insomnia

A cognitive-behavioral model for insomnia (see Figure 49.1) elucidates the interaction of insomnia with emotional, cognitive, and physiologic arousal: dysfunctional conditions, such as worry over sleep; and maladaptive habits (e.g., excessive time in bed and daytime napping) and the consequences of insomnia (e.g., fatigue and performance in impairment of activities).

In the treatment of insomnia, relaxation techniques have been used to reduce cognitive and physiological arousal and thus assist the induction of sleep as well as decrease awakenings during sleep.

Relaxation is also likely to influence decreased activity in the entire sympathetic system, permitting a more rapid and effective

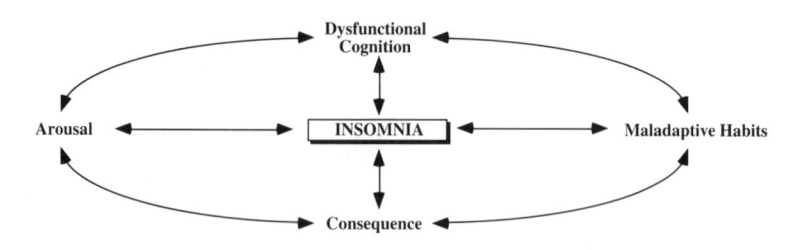

Figure 49.1 MORIN CM (1993) Insomnia—The Guilford Press Adapted From Presentation by D. J. Buysse, M.D. at NIH Technology Conference 10-17-95.

"deafferentation" at sleep onset at the level of the thalamus. Relaxation may also enhance para-sympathetic activity in turn further decreasing autonomic tone. In addition, it has been suggested that alterations in cytokine activity (immune system) may play a role in insomnia or in response to treatment.

Cognitive approaches may decrease arousal and dysfunctional beliefs and thus improve sleep. Behavioral techniques including sleep restriction and stimulus control can be helpful in reducing physiologic arousal, reversing poor sleep habits, and shifting circadian rhythms. These effects appear to involve both cortical structures and deep nuclei (e.g., *locus ceruleus* and *suprachiasmatic nucleus*).

Knowing the mechanisms of action would reinforce and expand use of behavioral and relaxation techniques, but incorporation of these approaches into the treatment of chronic pain and insomnia can proceed on the basis of clinical efficacy, as has occurred with the discovery of other practices and products before their mode of action was completely delineated.

Are there barriers to the appropriate integration of these approaches into health care?

One barrier to the integration of behavioral and relaxation techniques in standard medical care has been the emphasis on the biomedical model as the basis of medical education. The biomedical model defines disease in anatomic and patho-physiologic terms. Expansion to a bio-psychosocial model would increase emphasis on a patient's experience of disease and balance the anatomic/physiologic needs of patients with their psychosocial needs.

For example, of six factors identified to correlate with treatment failures of low back pain, all are psycho-social factors. The integration of behavioral and relaxation therapies with conventional medical procedures is necessary for the successful treatment of such conditions. Similarly, the importance of a comprehensive evaluation of a patient is emphasized in the field of insomnia where failure to identify a condition such as sleep apnea will result in inappropriate application of a behavioral therapy. Therapy should be matched to the illness and to the patient.

The integration of psycho-social issues with conventional medical approaches will necessitate the application of new methodologies to assess the success or failure of interventions. Therefore, additional barriers to integration include lack of standardization of outcome measures, lack of standardization or agreement on what constitutes successful outcome, and consensus on what constitutes appropriate follow-up. Methodologies appropriate for the evaluation of drugs may not be adequate for the evaluation of some psycho-social interventions, especially those involving patient experience and quality of life. Psycho-social research studies must maintain the high quality of those methods that have been painstakingly developed over the last few decades. Agreement needs to be reached for standards governing the demonstration of efficacy for psycho-social interventions.

Psychosocial interventions are often time intensive, creating potential blocks to provider and patient acceptance and compliance. Participation in biofeedback training typically includes up to 10 to 12 sessions of approximately 45 minutes to 1 hour each. Additionally home practice of these techniques is usually required. Thus, patient compliance and willingness to participate in these therapies will have to be addressed. Physicians will have to be educated on the efficacy of these techniques. They must also be willing to educate their patients about the importance and potential benefits of these interventions and to provide encouragement for the patient through the training processes.

Insurance companies provide a financial incentive or barrier to access of care depending upon their willingness to provide reimbursement. Traditionally, insurance companies have been reluctant to reimburse for some psycho-social interventions and reimburse others at rates below those for standard medical care. Psycho-social interventions should be reimbursed as part of comprehensive medical services at rates comparable to those for other medical care particularly in view of data supporting their effectiveness and data detailing the costs of failed medical and surgical interventions.

The evidence suggests that sleep disorders are significantly underdiagnosed. The prevalence and possible consequences of insomnia have begun to be documented. There are substantial disparities between patient reports of insomnia and the number of insomnia diagnoses, as well as between the number of prescriptions written for sleep medications and the number of recorded diagnoses of insomnia. Data indicate that insomnia is widespread, but the morbidity and mortality of this condition are not well understood. Without this information, it remains difficult for physicians to gauge how aggressive their intervention should be in the treatment of this disorder. Additionally, the efficacy of the behavioral approaches for treating this condition has not been adequately disseminated to the medical community.

Finally, who should be administering these therapies? Problems with credentialing and training have yet to be completely addressed in the field. Although the initial studies have been done by qualified and highly trained practitioners in each of these fields, the question remains as to how this will best translate into delivery of care in the community. Decisions will have to be made about which practitioners are best qualified and most cost-effective to provide these psycho-social interventions.

What are the significant issues for future research and applications?

Research efforts on these therapies should include additional efficacy and effectiveness studies, cost-effectiveness studies, and efforts to replicate existing studies. Several specific issues should be addressed:

Outcomes

- Outcome measures should be reliable, valid, and standardized for behavioral and relaxation interventions research in each area (chronic pain, insomnia) so that studies can be compared and combined.

- Qualitative research is needed to help determine patients' experiences with both insomnia and chronic pain and the impact of treatments.

- Future research should include examination of consequences/outcomes of untreated chronic pain and insomnia; chronic pain and insomnia treated pharmacologically versus treated with behavioral and relaxation therapies; and combinations of pharmacologic and psycho-social treatments for chronic pain and insomnia.

Mechanism(s) of Action

- Advances in the neuro-biological sciences and psycho-neuro-immunology are providing an improved scientific base for understanding mechanisms of action of behavioral and relaxation techniques, and need to be further investigated.

Covariates

- Chronic pain and insomnia, as well as behavioral and relaxation therapies, involve factors such as values, beliefs, expectations, and behaviors, all of which are strongly culturally shaped.

Research is needed to assess cross-cultural applicability, efficacy, and modifications of psycho-social therapeutic modalities.

- Research studies that examine the effectiveness of behavioral and relaxation approaches to insomnia and chronic pain should consider the influence of age, race, gender, religious belief, and socio-economic status on treatment effectiveness.

Health Services

- The most effective timing of the introduction of behavioral interventions into the course of treatment should be studied.

- Research is needed to optimize the match between specific behavioral and relaxation techniques and specific patient groups and treatment settings.

Integration into Clinical Care and Medical Education

- New and innovative methods of introducing psycho-social treatments into health care curricula and practice should be implemented.

Conclusions

A number of well-defined behavioral and relaxation interventions are now available, some of which are commonly used to treat chronic pain and insomnia. Available data support the effectiveness of these interventions in relieving chronic pain and in achieving some reduction in insomnia. Data are currently insufficient to conclude with confidence that one technique is more effective than another for a given condition. For any given individual patient, however, one approach may indeed be more appropriate than another.

Behavioral and relaxation interventions clearly reduce arousal and hypnosis reduces pain perception. However, the exact biological underpinnings of these effects require further study, as is often the case with medical therapies. Although the literature demonstrates treatment effectiveness, the state of the art of the methodologies in this field indicates a need for thoughtful interpretation of the findings as well as an urgency to translate them into programs of health care delivery.

Although specific structural, bureaucratic, financial, and attitudinal barriers exist to the integration of these techniques, all are potentially

Integration of Behavioral and Relaxation Techniques

surmountable with education and additional research, as patients shift from being passive participants in their treatment to becoming responsible, active partners in their rehabilitation.

The conference was co-sponsored by the National Institute of Mental Health, National Institute of Dental Research. National Heart, Lung, and Blood Institute, National Institute on Aging, National Cancer Institute, National Institute of Nursing Research, National Institute of Neurological Disorders and Stroke, and the National Institute of Arthritis and Musculoskeletal and Skin Diseases.

More Information

This statement and the full text of other NIH statements are also available online through an electronic bulletin board system and through the Internet:

NIH Information Center BBS
1-800-NIH-BBS1 (644-2271)

Gopher
gopher://gopher.nih.gov/Health and Clinical Information

World Wide Web
http://text.nlm.nih.gov

ftp
ftp://public.nlm.nih.gov/hstat

Publications Ordering Information

NIH Consensus Statements, NIH Technology Statements, and related materials are available be writing to the NIH Consensus Program Information Center, P.O. Box 2577, Kensington, Maryland 20891; by calling toll-free 1-888-NIH-CONSENSUS (1-888-644-2667); or by visiting the NIH consensus Development Program home page on the World Wide Web at http://consensus.nih.gov.

Chapter 50

What Can Be Done When the Pain Won't Go Away?

"Ouch!"

Smash a finger while hammering and your body responds with a jolt of pain that overpowers your other senses and commands: "Stop, you've injured your finger!"

Reacting to the sudden pain and the soreness that follows the blow, you immobilize and favor the hurt finger and thereby promote healing.

For the fact is, pain plays a vital biological function. Its importance is dramatically illustrated by people who are unable to feel pain because of disease or injury. Lacking this important warning system, they suffer cuts, burns, broken bones, and other injuries that a sense of pain helps most of us either avoid or react to quickly, preventing worse injury.

But not all pain is useful. Chronic pain that persists long after its cause has been diagnosed serves only to torment the patient. Produced by conditions like a nerve or back injury or cancer, chronic pain has been compared to a burglar alarm that can't be switched off.

The more research scientists learn about the nature and physiology of pain, the more complex it seems to be. Only recently have medical scientists begun to understand the mechanism of pain. Armed with greater knowledge, they hope to mobilize new resources to control pain.

Moreover, interdisciplinary medical teams focusing on pain at hospitals and pain treatment centers are developing new strategies to

---

FDA Consumer, July-August, 1989.

treat pain more effectively with traditional painkilling medicines and techniques.

Blocking the Pain Pathway

Pain impulses are sent from the site of the damage to the spinal cord and then on to the brain. The pain from that misdirected hammer blow, for example, is flashed to the nervous system from nociceptors, pain receptors in peripheral tissues—in this case, your thumb. Damaged cells release substances that raise the sensitivity of nociceptors, causing them to send out strong pain pulses.

Prostaglandins are a group of sensitizing substances produced by injured cells. Aspirin and aspirin-like compounds kill pain by inhibiting prostaglandin production by cells of the peripheral nervous system.

Pain can be stopped further up the line—in the spinal cord. Pain impulses originating in peripheral nerves—in your smashed thumb, for instance—travel along special nerve fibers to cells in a part of the spinal cord known as the dorsal horn. In the microscopic spaces—called synapses—between dorsal horn cells, chemical neurotransmitters enable pain messages to move from one cell to the next on their way to the brain. The dorsal horn cells, however, release a neurotransmitter called serotonin that blocks the passage of pain impulses between cells. Antidepressant drugs such as amitriptyline are thought to prevent nerve cells from pulling serotonin out of the synapses between dorsal horn cells, which may explain why these drugs can relieve pain.

Clinicians are now trying amitriptyline and newer tricyclic antidepressant drugs such as desipramine in patients suffering pain caused by shingles and to treat the severe burning foot pain sometimes associated with diabetes.

Moreover, they are looking for the substances involved in pain transmission from the peripheral nerve cells to the dorsal horn so they can suppress pain even earlier along this route.

Pain impulses ascend from the spinal cord to the thalamus in the midbrain and then to the cerebral cortex. Morphine, codeine, and other drugs derived from the opium poppy have long been used to control severe pain by causing the brain to suppress pain messages received from the dorsal horn. Synthetic opiates include methadone, hydromorphone and meperidine.

While both natural and synthetic opiate drugs are very effective in handling severe pain, they can have bothersome side effects, including nausea, drowsiness, constipation, and mood changes.

What Can Be Done When the Pain Won't Go Away?

One of the most important breakthroughs in pain research in the past decade was the discovery that the body makes its own opiates—endorphins, enkephalins and dynorphins. After finding these natural painkillers in the brain and spinal cord, scientists discovered that injecting opiates directly into the spinal fluid would relieve pain.

They found that very small dosages of opiates injected at sites in the spinal cord where pain is inhibited not only relieved pain, but also prevented some of the side effects associated with large dosages.

Research scientists are also investigating newer opiate-like drugs that they hope will have less troublesome side effects than those caused by currently available drugs.

Problem of Drug Tolerance

Patients with chronic pain who take opiates for extended periods tend to build up a tolerance to the drugs and need ever larger doses to control their pain. But new findings point to an approach that may enable doctors to circumvent the problem of tolerance.

Researchers have learned that morphine and enkephalins attach themselves to different places on the surface of nerve cells that transmit pain impulses. They speculate that, if enkephalin-like drugs could be developed, patients tolerant to morphine might get effective pain relief by being switched to drugs that mimic the enkephalins.

Pain experts say that many doctors are overly concerned about the risks of opiate dependence in their patients treated for severe pain, such as that caused by cancer. The specialists say these concerns are largely unfounded, basing their assurance on a study of 11,000 hospitalized patients who had been given opiates. Only four patients had any difficulty giving up painkilling medication once it was no longer needed.

Pain experts are now recommending that severe acute pain, like that following major surgery, or the severe chronic pain of cancer be treated more aggressively by simultaneously administering two or more drugs that act at different pain control sites. To dampen the pain signals generated at the peripheral nervous system, doctors can prescribe aspirin-like drugs. To suppress the pain messages going to the spinal cord and brain, they can use opiates.

The experts say that pain medication works better if adequate doses are begun early and maintained on a regular schedule, before the pain becomes severe. Furthermore, since patients vary greatly in their need for pain relief, they also advise adjusting the dose according to individual need.

Doctors can stop pain cold by blocking the pain at the peripheral nerve level with local anesthetics. Unfortunately, these nerve blocks also shut down other sensations, such as hot and cold, as well as the nerve impulses that control muscles. Another disadvantage: The effects of the anesthetics wear off, and the pain blockage is only temporary.

Control Without Drugs

Severe, intractable pain that cannot be successfully controlled by drugs may be relieved surgically by cutting the bundles of nerve fibers in the spinal cord that carry the pain messages from damaged nerve tissues. Called a "cordotomy," the operation blocks pain on the entire side of the body fed by the nerve fibers. But in time the pain tends to return. Other surgical attempts to control pain by severing nerve pathways or destroying nerve tissue also fail to bring enduring relief in many if not all cases. Somehow the body succeeds in establishing other nerve pathways to circumvent the surgically disrupted channel.

Another intriguing approach to pain relief involves the use of electricity. The idea that electrical stimulation can be used to treat pain is hardly new. Some scholars trace it back to ancient Egypt, and we know from historic records that it was used by the Romans. The ancients had to rely on electric eels and torpedo fish as sources of electricity. But in the 19th century, when man-made electricity became first available and then commonplace, electrotherapy was viewed as a panacea. The fact that it turned out not to be gave it a bad name.

In the 1960s, however, two investigators, Ronald Melzack and Patrick D. Wall, proposed a new "gate-control" theory, which provides a scientific rationale for electrical stimulation in the control of pain. They postulated a neural "gate" in the dorsal horn of the spinal cord shared by the large nerve fibers, which carry sensory and motor control signals, and the small ones, which transmit pain impulses. By stimulating large nerve fibers with weak currents of electricity, the gate is closed and pain transmission along the small fibers is shut down, according to the theory.

The work of Melzack and Wall revived the interest of respected research scientists in electrical stimulation therapy. In an experiment at the University of California at San Francisco, neuroscientists are studying the safety and effectiveness of a device that is intended to control pain by direct electrical stimulation of the thalamus. A small

What Can Be Done When the Pain Won't Go Away?

battery-powered device worn at the patient's waist sends a radio frequency signal to a receiver implanted just under the skin of the abdomen. Wires under the skin lead from the receiver to one or more pairs of electrodes implanted in the thalamus. By varying the amplitude (strength) of the radio signal, doctors—and, with experience, patients themselves—may be able to control intractable pain that does not yield to other measures. Researchers now believe that the electrical stimulation relieves pain because it causes the brainstem and the spinal cord to release endorphins.

While clinical investigators are reporting some success with the use of electrical implants, this technique is yet to be validated by comprehensive clinical studies. In addition, as with most other methods of pain relief, the effects of electrical stimulation appear to weaken over time.

Investigators hope that as equipment and techniques improve and as physicians learn to identify the patients who are most likely to benefit, electrical stimulation will prove to be a useful tool for pain management.

TENS, or transcutaneous electrical nerve stimulation, is a noninvasive form of electrical pain control. Electrodes are placed directly on the skin over the painful area or at selected points along the pain nerve pathway. A small battery-powered generator about the size of a pack of playing cards sends pulses of current to the electrodes.

Early experience with TENS convinced some investigators and their patients that it was a promising technique of pain control. However, according to a summary of clinical literature published by the Department of Health and Human Services, after 20 years of experience with TENS, its effectiveness remains uncertain. The department's survey revealed broad variability in pain relief from patient to patient and from one type of pain to another.

Fortunately, to treat the average headache or other minor, short-term ache or pain, most people don't need to seek out a doctor. Instead, they take aspirin, acetaminophen, or some other over-the-counter analgesic until the pain goes away.

But persistent pain often signals an underlying health problem. Headaches can sometimes be a symptom of disorders of the brain, heart and circulatory system, the ear, and the eye. Severe, intermittent headaches may be caused by a brain tumor.

So besides simply looking for relief from pain, when pain persists or recurs, it's good common sense to see a doctor to diagnose and treat its cause.

Use of Analgesics

Most people can safely self-medicate with nonprescription analgesics (pain relievers) as long as they stay within the dosage limits given on the label. Overdosing with aspirin or similar drugs may cause symptoms such as gastric irritation or ringing in the ears. Reye syndrome, a rare but life-threatening malady affecting children and young adults, has focused attention on the safe use of over-the-counter pain relievers that contain aspirin. Overdoses of acetaminophen can also be toxic. Extended self-medication with analgesic drugs at recommended dosages may not cause symptoms. But prolonged use without medical supervision may mask a serious illness. To use over-the-counter analgesics safely:

- Always read the label and follow instructions, cautions and warnings.

- Do not exceed the maximum dosages on the product's label.

- Adults should not take pain relievers for more than 10 days unless directed by a doctor. (For fever, the limit is three days.)

- Children and teenagers should limit use to five days for pain and three days for fever.

- Because of the danger of Reye syndrome (a rare but sometimes fatal illness), children and young adults (2 to 20 years of age) should not take aspirin for chicken pox, flu, or flu-like symptoms. When in doubt, consult a doctor.

- Those allergic to aspirin should not take any medicine containing aspirin-like ingredients, such as carbaspirin calcium, choline salicylate, magnesium salicylate, and sodium salicylate.

- Pregnant women should not take aspirin in the last three months of pregnancy unless instructed by a doctor. Aspirin taken near time of delivery can cause bleeding in both mother and child.

—by Egon Weck

Chapter 51

Living with Chronic Pain: A How-to-Manage Manual for Families of Chronic Pain Patients

This chapter reprints a manual developed for use in Patient/Family Education at the Tampa General Rehabilitation Center by Dana S. DeBoskey, Ph.D., Fred L. Alberts Jr., Ph.D., Stuart J. Greif, PSV.D., Karen Morin, M.S.W. and Dennis Todd, Ph.D. This manual and the others in the series were written and produced by the staff of the Tampa General Rehabilitation Center, Tampa General Hospital, Tampa, Florida.

Dedication

To the unrecognized sufferers of chronic pain—the families and loved ones.

Preface

Chronic pain is not just the experience of one person suffering. Pain changes everyone associated with it. It imposes enormous physical and mental hardships on the patient and burdens the entire family with frustration, stress, and a host of social, emotional and economic consequences.

©1989 Tampa General Rehabilitation Center, Tampa General Hospital, Tampa, Florida. HDI Publishers, 10131 Alfred Lane Houston, Texas 77041. Extracted from *Living with Chronic Pain: A How-to-Manage Manual for Families of Chronic Pain Patients*. Reprinted with permission.

For the patient, recent advances in multi-disciplinary treatment approaches offer the promise of relief and a return to a more normal and active life.

For the family, little has been done to help them deal with the many problems that result from living with a person in chronic pain. Ironically, it is the family members who often silently suffer the brunt of the chronic pain patient's problems. It is the family who listens to the complaints and pleas for help. It is the family who frequently can be found calling the physicians or running to the drug store in the middle of the night. It is also the family members who are deprived of a normal life. Living with a chronic pain sufferer can place stress on the family's entire lifestyle such that emotional reactions become commonplace and relationships are strained to the breaking point. Everything that was normal about the family's daily activities becomes lost in the many changes that occur because of the existence of chronic pain.

Essentially, this chapter is intended to be a source and a new beginning for the all too often neglected sufferer of chronic pain—the family.

Introduction

"How can this be happening to us? My family isn't even a family anymore! We walk on eggs around the house and still it does not seem to help reduce the pain or angry outbursts. I'm tired and confused. Why can't the doctors do anything? Why can't they just cut the nerves or prescribe some medication before it drives us all crazy! I want to help but everything I do is not enough. It makes me feel mad and guilty and I can't take it much longer." Sound familiar? These comments are just a few of the common concerns expressed by families. Most family members become quite distressed when their loved one has pain that doesn't go away. At first you try to help by showing kindness and providing as much comfort as possible. Later, when the pain persists, even after doctors have tried everything. You may become frustrated and exhausted. You might even express angry feelings and then feel guilty afterwards.

These are all normal reactions to chronic pain. It is normal to feel a whole range of emotions and it is good for you to talk about these feelings with other family members. You will be surprised at how similar your feelings are to those experienced by others. You may need help in expressing your feelings, and if so, take that step first. Ask around for a chronic pain support group in your area. Find a friend, counselor, or social worker and take this manual with you and begin sharing your feelings by discussing the various topics you find important to your situation. The more you talk and share experiences and use this chapter as a guide, the better your life situation will be. Not only will you benefit, but so will your loved one who has chronic pain.

It is important for you to keep in mind that you can help the one you love by first helping yourself. When you have a good basic understanding and use of the techniques in this chapter, you will have a tremendous positive effect in helping to reduce the stress, tension and pain of the sufferer and the entire family. Keep the chapter handy and share it with all family members, including the children. They also need information about chronic pain so that they can help as well.

Finally, a word of encouragement. This chapter was written for you. We believe in the power of the family in helping chronic pain sufferers overcome their disability. We believe in you. No matter how hopeless or discouraging your life may seem at this point, you can make a difference if you try. Although we are quite aware that not all pain patients are male, for the sake of simplicity we have used the pronoun he to represent all chronic pain patients and hope this will not be offensive to any of our readers.

Begin now by reading. Continue later by doing. You have nothing to lose and everything to gain. We wish you the best in all your efforts and we are confident you will make a difference.

Soft-cover versions of this chapter are available from HDI Publishers. Call 1-800-321-7037 for ordering information.

Medical Aspects

Chronic pain is one of the most frustrating problems a physician has to contend with. Physicians are used to thinking about a symptom as the presentation of a specific disease process which can be diagnosed by a specific test and which can be treated by a specific treatment method. Chronic pain defies many of these rules.

In most cases there is no single specific cause to explain the chronic pain. Even the most sophisticated tests which have become available to physicians recently are unable to pinpoint a specific cause in the majority of these patients. Many additional factors, normally not taken into account by many physicians, like family interactions, stress, anxiety, social situations, etc., play a significant role in the causation and persistence of chronic pain. More and more physicians are recognizing that chronic pain should be treated by a group of professionals in an interdisciplinary cooperative set up than by individual physicians. This chapter is the result of such a collaborative effort, by many medical professionals from different specialties. It attempts to simplify many of the complex issues involved into simple, practical easy to follow instructions.

This chapter can be used by those who themselves suffer from chronic pain, but is intended for those who are closely related to a pain patient.

It also can be used by medical and health professionals as an adjunct to their treatment.

Lack of a Specific Cause

It is very frustrating for the patients and their families not to know exactly what is causing their pain. Multiple visits to many doctors only add to their confusion, because of the different and, at times, conflicting opinions they hear. This is because in the majority of patients with chronic pain, the pain is not caused by a single source or cause. Many factors, such as scarring, muscle spasms, entrapped nerves, irritated nerves, changes in blood vessels, soft tissue injury, etc. help initiate or maintain the pain. Unfortunately, many of these factors are not detected by the tests available at this time. Because of this fact, many patients undergo repeated testing in the hope of "nailing down" a cause for the pain. Such repeated testing is unnecessary in many patients, rarely ever gives more information and, more importantly, can be harmful.

Another important factor which contributes to pain is the fear of reinjury or fear of hurting oneself. This fear results in the patient's perceived need for further testing to correct "a specific cause" which might "further injure him."

Examples of Lack of a Specific Cause:

1. Patient goes from doctor to doctor hoping that the next doctor will be able to "diagnose correctly" the cause of pain.

2. Patient undergoes a myelogram every six months to a year— which can result in a debilitating condition called Arachnoiditis.

3. Patient refuses to take part in treatment programs because of the concern that he may hurt himself when one is not sure of the "exact diagnosis."

Resolutions for Lack of a Specific Cause:

1. Consult a physician who has enough experience with chronic pain and one in whom you and the patient have confidence.

2. Even though a second opinion in many cases is valuable and necessary, multiple consultations with physicians of the same specialty are counterproductive.

3. When you do obtain a second opinion, have that physician review all of the tests already undergone rather than repeat them unnecessarily.

4. Accept the fact that in the majority of cases, a specific cause for the pain cannot be identified.

5. Discuss with the medical doctor any treatment concerns that you have.

Role of Medications

Even though there are many excellent pain medications, none of them are intended for long term use. Narcotic medications are powerful pain killers, but even they are not effective in controlling pain generated by muscle spasms, scarring, etc., which are the common sources of pain in many patients. These medications are commonly used only because of the perceived lack of alternatives. In fact, many patients on large doses of narcotics do not notice any difference in pain levels even after they are taken off their narcotic medications. The side effects of these medications can be serious.

On the other hand, there are some medications not known as "pain medications" which can be very helpful and necessary. Some of these medicines like Elavil are used by psychiatrists and, hence, are not well accepted by pain patients. Certain anti-inflammatory medicines and muscle relaxants do not appear to have any effect at all after administration of each dose, but in the long run are very beneficial.

Examples of Role of Medication:

1. A patient required increasing doses of narcotics for pain control and ultimately was on 160mg/hour of morphine given in an intravenous drip, but still had severe pain. The patient was

able to come off all narcotics without any increase in pain. Pain was controlled by other techniques better than it ever was on the large dose of narcotics.

2. A patient was on 8-10 Dilaudid tablets and 3-5 Valium tablets per day for 7-10 years. He still had uncontrolled pain and spent most of the time in bed. After he was taken off the medications, it was evident that not only the medicines were not helping his pain, but were part of the problem. He was able to carry on daily activities because he was not drowsy from the medications, and not constipated, and now could think clearly.

3. Elavil used in small doses decreases pain, helps sleep, increases appetite and increases the endorphin levels of the body. It is used in pain patients for these reasons and not psychiatric reasons.

Resolutions for Role of Medication:

1. Consult a physician associated with a pain clinic that can help control medication and provide freedom from drug dependence.

2. Try to avoid the temptation of thinking that "medication" will be the answer to all problems. This is dangerous and can lead to drug abuse and dependence.

Role of Surgical Procedures

Surgical procedures like a laminectomy, spinal infusion, etc. and destructive procedures such as nerve blocks, rhizotomies, etc. do not have an important role in pain control and only apply in a limited number of specially selected patients.

However, in the majority of chronic pain patients, these procedures are of no value and in many patients can aggravate the problem. Repeated back surgeries lead to excessive scarring of tissue, arachnoiditis and nerve injury. Nerve blocks can lead to loss of function of extremities, loss of sensation and occasionally painful numb areas.

Examples of Role of Surgical Procedures:

1. A patient had severe foot pain which was not controlled by medication. He persuaded a surgeon to amputate his foot in the hope of getting rid of the painful area. Not only did the

Living with Chronic Pain: A How-to-Manage Manual

original pain persist after the amputation, but the patient developed phantom limb pain in addition to his original pain.

2. A patient had a benign tumor in the chest area. He underwent a nerve block which relieved his pain, but developed numbness in the area which was more difficult to live with than his original pain.

Resolutions for Role of Surgical Procedures:

1. Consult a physician who has experience in dealing with chronic pain about various treatment options.

2. Ask questions about all side effects of the procedures.

3. Never undergo a surgical procedure without obtaining a second opinion.

4. Accept the fact that there are no surgical treatments available for many of the chronic pain problems.

Extent of Testing Necessary

Modern medicine has many armaments in store to diagnose medical problems. Technological breakthroughs like CT Scans, MRI Scans and special imaging techniques have vastly improved the chances of fast and accurate diagnosis.

These techniques can positively rule out serious diseases as a cause of pain, even though the exact cause of pain cannot be determined in many cases. Some of these tests need to be repeated frequently, e.g., a cardiogram needs to be done every time there is severe chest pain, urine examination needs to be repeated every time you have burning while urinating. However, there are other tests which do not give any additional information by repeating them, e.g., EMG exams each time a muscle hurts. There are some other tests which can actually be harmful each time they are repeated, e.g., myelogram.

Learn to trust your doctor once you have selected one. After the patient has undergone a thorough testing, repeating those tests is useless, expense and, in many cases, harmful.

What Results to Expect

Chronic pain is a very difficult problem to deal with. In many cases it is caused by scarring, nerve injury, nerve irritations, etc.

which cannot be cured. Do not expect the patient to be "cured." Do not expect him to be completely pain free.

What you can expect is to have him able to cope and manage the pain at a tolerable level, to be able to have a decent, meaningful life, in spite of some pain and be able to go back to productive life without the help of pain medications. The results that can be obtained, however, entirely depend on the motivation, cooperation and efforts of everyone involved; the family as well as the patient.

Once relief is obtained, be sure to follow the recommendations of the physician and treatment team regarding what to do at home to continue enjoying reduced levels of pain. It will require a change in lifestyle in order to avoid backsliding and having the pain return as before. A few simple exercises and relaxation techniques practiced faithfully every day can produce long lasting results and end the cycle of stress, frustration and pain.

Patient Behaviors

Although individuals suffering chronic pain are quite different, there are many common experiences that they tend to share that sheds light on the reasons why particular behaviors are adopted by many pain patients.

For a moment, consider the typical pain experiences most of us have had. Usually the pain lasts for relatively short periods of time. Most likely, we were able to comprehend the underlying cause of this pain experience and we were well aware of what was necessary to reverse the discomfort. With these occurrences where discomfort was intense and irreversible at that moment, we began to experience considerable concern and perhaps fear, thinking that perhaps our formulation of the problem was wrong and that this is more serious than we thought. However, a visit to the family physician provided an understanding and solution, and a decrease in anxiety followed.

With chronic pain, however, all previous behaviors that served to reverse discomfort are no longer effective. Anxiety increases. There is no way to relieve it. Confusion may follow regarding the reason for this painful experience. Many may feel they are being punished or may feel bitter that they have been the one chosen to suffer. Mostly, however, there is the feeling of despair. Feelings of helplessness, hopelessness tend to follow. Sleep is disrupted and the suffering becomes a lonely ordeal.

Worries may begin to increase. There may be concerns about the pain getting worse or that the pain will interfere with their work.

Living with Chronic Pain: A How-to-Manage Manual

Sleepless nights turn into nightmares of improbable fears. Without sleep, exhaustion and irritability follow. Other similar feelings and attitudes follow from experiences with "doctor shopping." The pattern may initially begin with a visit to the family physician who, after unsuccessful attempts to relieve discomfort, refers to a specialist or neurologist. After several hospitalizations, numerous diagnostic procedures and perhaps a number of drastic measures, the pain gradually returns, perhaps to the same intensity. Medication is ineffective and, oftentimes, addiction occurs. Following detoxification, either another round of consultants are called and the cycle begins again or a psychiatrist is called. Considerable resentment for the medical community emerges. The patient is drained emotionally, physically and financially. Reexamining past experiences, the patient may begin to feel that something has been missed. As such, the patient may overfocus on feelings that previously were never attended to, in hopes of providing information that will help doctors find the missing link. Feeling more desperate, the individual may seek new treatment or techniques. Typically, however, the pain returns to the same intensity. Perhaps surgical relief is sought. Again, the pain returns.

The subjective experiences of the person in chronic pain are intense. We hope that our descriptions of these behaviors will assist the family in both understanding the reasons for these reactions as well as providing suggestions for dealing with them.

Anger and Irritability

Anger and irritability are common chronic pain patient behaviors. The patient experiencing pain may possess many angry feelings and may often be irritable and express a lower tolerance to annoyances and changes in day-to-day events. Patients express anger at the family, employer, institutions, and even themselves. Sometimes the anger is expressed directly at the actual cause of the angry feelings, while at other times it is expressed indirectly or even displaced. Displaced anger is that anger which results from intense angry feelings at one individual or event and is "displaced" upon another individual or event. That is, the patient may be angry at his physician, but may express feelings of anger at a spouse or family member. Passive expression of anger is as problematic as angry outbursts and chronic irritability. In these cases, the patient may have difficulty expressing feelings, particularly those of anger, and respond "passively." For example, a patient who harbors

Pain Sourcebook

many angry feelings may not outwardly express those feelings, but may slam doors, become very irritable, set up situations in which others suffer, etc.

Examples of Anger/Irritability:

1. The patient refuses to comply with treatment.

2. The patient threatens health care workers, family and friends.

3. The patient is angry at his employer because the employer will not let him work.

4. The patient shows irritability to mild disruption in routine day-to-day events, such as any change of plans, having to wait to see a physician, the weather, etc.

5. The patient refuses to attend a family picnic.

6. The patient blames others for his pain and/or his current negative situation with statements such as "If you only knew what I am going through, you would treat me differently!" or "You don't understand-you will never understand!"

7. The patient becomes moody and unpredictable. One minute things are fine; the next minute all hell breaks loose.

8. The anger behavior is directed at the patient himself and he tends to stop taking care of himself, such as forgetting to shave, change clothes or clean up in general.

9. Angry and resentful, the patient begins to withdraw to himself by the excessive use and abuse of alcohol, cigarettes, Junk food and drugs.

Resolutions for Anger/Irritability:

1. Do not react to the angry outbursts or actions personally.

2. Remove yourself from potentially "explosive" situations.

3. Allow the patient to vent his feelings, but do not engage with the anger by arguing or trying to reason. A straightforward

Living with Chronic Pain: A How-to-Manage Manual

"I'll talk with you later, when you're feeling better," or similar comment will do. Don't expect the pain patient to understand or agree with your actions. He is angry and likely will not be happy with anything you do.

4. Help develop structure to assist the patient in dealing with angry episodes and feelings. Let him know that when he gets angry, you will try to understand but may not always agree, or talk about it until he calms down.

5. Encourage patient to write down the angry feelings. Even if no one reads it but him this is a good way to release anger.

6. If the patient has been through a multidisciplinary pain management program or has learned through some other means to reduce pain with specific relaxation techniques, encourage the use of it. These techniques are very powerful in reducing anger, stress and pain, all at the same time!

7. Don't deny your own feelings. You are human and will get angry yourself at times. When you do, you might "blow your top" at the patient. Although you should remember that your anger is usually a result of your frustration with living with someone in pain, you must realize that if you're normal, you will occasionally have a bad day yourself. You're entitled to "let off steam" once in awhile.

8. Keep in mind that the patient's anger and irritability is likely a result of the pain, but may not always be. He can be angry for other reasons that have nothing to do with pain. You will find it difficult to know which is which. Don't worry. You don't have to always know the difference when anger is expressed. Later, when things have calmed down and you both talk about it, you will begin to learn which is which. Your behavior should still be the same no matter what is causing the pain.

9. Redirect the anger toward the pain. Let him know that "pain" is most likely responsible for his upsettedness. This will help focus the emotions where they belong and not at irrelevant people, places or events.

Dependency

In addition to the presence of depression, distress, frustration, apprehension, tension and perhaps fear, chronic pain patients develop a considerable degree of dependency that becomes quite burdensome to family members. This often occurs as a result of feeling overwhelmed by present life circumstances and feeling immobilized. They feel, perhaps, that they are unable to accomplish things previously handled without any effort. A point is reached where a major impact on their self-confidence and self-esteem is experienced. Support and encouragement from others are no longer effective. Out of concern, perhaps, family members begin to resume responsibilities previously handled by the patient. However, to remove these responsibilities often results in negative ends, i.e., lowered self-esteem and further withdrawal from responsibility demands. Perhaps considerable guilt is experienced. The experience of inner conflict may result for many who have placed such a heavy weight on functioning throughout their life independently, and now are crippled by their difficulties and dependency on others. For these people, the distress is significantly intensified. For others, many seek nurturing behaviors from family members. Once family members have given their all, the patient may seek nurturing from others. They begin to arrange their lives to ensure a constant supply of nurturing and reinforcement from their environment. Certain characteristic attitudes may be noted. The most apparent is the pervasive feeling that they are helpless—the "poor me" attitude. A striking lack of initiative and general avoidance of independent functioning or responsibilities often is noted. By displaying physical helplessness, by acting weak, by expressing self-doubt, and by communicating a need for assurance, they are likely to obtain the nurturing and protection they seek. By adopting this inferior role, they provide others with a feeling of being sympathetic, useful, stronger and quite competent. These strategies succeed well in achieving the nurturing that they desire.

Examples of Dependency: Example patient statements are as follows:

1. "Please make me independent again!"

2. "God, the pain is unbearable! Please tie my shoes... take out the garbage... turn on the T.V....before going to work."

3. "Look at me! There's no way I'll ever be able to do that again. Could you do that for me?"

4. "I really hate to ask you again, but..."

5. "Can't you see I'm in pain? Why won't you do it for me?"

6. "I'd really like to eat... take a bath... put on some nice clothes... clean up around here... it's just that this pain is so bad today."

7. "Could you call the doctor again for me? He'll listen to you better than me."

Resolutions for Dependency:

1. Have a reasonable understanding of what the true physical limitations are by consulting with the patient's physician.

2. Set reasonable expectations.

3. The family will need to avoid doing things that the physician feels the patient is capable of doing.

4. Do not mistake love for assuming their responsibilities.

5. Do not assume guilt.

6. Remember that assisting them to relinquish their dependency behaviors will prove a slow process. Do not get discouraged.

7. Step-by-step, rebuild an image of competence and self esteem by carefully and slowly disengaging that habit of having others doing things for them.

8. Be consistent.

9. You may need to make changes in the patient's environment in order to maximize independent functioning.

10. Do not allow yourself to be available to the patient on a continual basis.

Egocentricity

After an individual has experienced chronic pain, he can become completely self-centered, displaying behavior that is characteristic of a three- or four-year-old. Initially, following the injury or incident, the patient finds that everything has been focused on him, his pain, and resolving the pain. Many families find it very difficult or impossible to readjust the center of focus to other family members and/or issues.

The chronic pain patient often believes that "until his pain is taken care of" the entire family should be readily available to assist him with his problem. This belief is reinforced by such statements as "My problems are the worst" or "No one knows the pain I feel." At times when the family may try to attend to other members, the patient (thinking and/or fearing that he will be forgotten) may say such things as "If you really understood the pain I am in you would not treat me like this."

This generalized "everybody for me" attitude can be very wearing for the family, especially if it becomes expected at all costs. We are all willing to go the extra mile for someone who realizes and appreciates our efforts. However, we are trained to be unresponsive to selfish behavior, and this is often how the patient is viewed. As a result, families either unknowingly or sometimes knowingly pull away from the self-centered behavior, and this in turn often results in the individual becoming even more egocentric. There is a fine line between offering enough attention and actually fostering continued self-centered orientation.

Examples of Egocentricity:

1. The patient wonders why the family member is not able to get off work and spend every lunch hour at the hospital while he is in the Pain Management Program.

2. The patient wonders why he can only spend four hours at home on an LOA (leave of absence). He does not understand that his spouse needs to get some sleep before she works the midnight shift.

3. The patient screams, "Why can't you find me the right doctor?"

4. The patient wonders why the spouse is playing golf on Sunday instead of keeping him company at home.

5. The patient accuses the spouse of being on the doctor's side instead of his.

6. The patient is astounded that the family would want to go out to eat when he is in pain.

Resolutions for Egocentricity:

1. Do not relinquish everything to the pain patient's needs.

2. Do not allow the patient to get to the point of expecting that all his demands will be met.

3. Be aware that his egocentricity may interfere with your desire to assist with his rehabilitation.

4. Do not expect the patient to respect your rights—you may have to do some demanding of your own.

5. Redirect his focus when he continues to center verbalizations around his thoughts and desires.

6. Do not allow the patient's desires to immobilize the family.

7. Sign up for an assertiveness training class.

8. Praise the patient when he allows the family to attend to another family member's problems.

9. Offer noticeable recognition if the patient himself focuses his concerns on another family member.

10. Consider family therapy if the patient's problems consume your entire life. Even if the patient refuses to attend himself, it's important that the rest of the family receive some professional supportive counseling.

Manipulation

Manipulation is a common characteristic of pain patients. It is not a pastime engaged in for fun. More often than not, the patient is not even aware of what he is doing. For many, compensation, addiction, the confounding of doctors, or the sick role itself may be the major motivating factor. An accident or illness markedly alters a person's way of living. It is not unusual following painful illness or injury that unmet emotional needs become a significant concern. Reinforcement of pain behavior by family/involved others partially serves to meet these needs. A new lifestyle develops. Pain can serve as an excuse to get out of responsibilities without disgrace. A family member would have to be cruel to make the patient perform responsibilities given the amount of pain frequently displayed. The word "can't" can often be looked at as "I don't want to."

Getting others to do things for them that they are capable of doing themselves is also accomplished through expression of pain. Others feel sympathetic for the patient. As noted in the previous chapter, by adopting this illness role, they provide others a feeling of being useful, stronger and competent. This is quite powerful in acquiring the nurturing that they are seeking. The patient gains tremendous sympathy, attention and care. The difficulties that follow are many. For example, to invest himself in improving and giving up the illness role would mean giving up the tremendous amount of attention, sympathy, etc., not to mention that he would have to reassume previous responsibilities. Additionally, difficulties become quite intense for the spouse who oftentimes has to assume the role of sole supporter as well as the role of parent to a helpless childlike patient.

How does the patient wield such power? By expressing pain, the patient can elicit guilt feelings in both spouse and children. The patient can control family members' behavior, avoid responsibilities and get a variety of payoffs while lying around feeling sorry for himself.

All of this can be done without the patient himself and the family ever being aware that manipulation is occurring! In fact, everyone would most likely deny the suggestion that it exists at all.

Examples of Manipulation: Example patient statements are as follows:

1. "The doctor said that you need to do this for me."

2. "Dear, you know how unbearable this is. You know I can't return to work."

3. "That doctor doesn't realize how badly I hurt, he won't give me any pain medication. Let's find another doctor who will understand."

Living with Chronic Pain: A How-to-Manage Manual

4. "I need the insurance company to buy this for my pain."

5. "Please stay with me, you can always go out another time."

6. "You're the only one who really understands my pain. You know the doctors are wrong when they want me to get off this medication and exercise."

7. "That Pain Management Program is crazy! They expect me to get better by doing all those silly activities. You'll talk to them won't you?"

8. "How could you leave me here alone in pain while you were having fun?"

Resolutions for Manipulation:

1. The family should participate in the patient's medical evaluations and within the patient's pain program regime. A clear understanding of true limitations can be acquired, and information obtained will then be accurate.

2. Constructive family discussions should be held for the patient to learn what effect he has on immobilizing the family.

3. The family should not feel guilty and should not tolerate being immobilized.

4. The family can help by reinforcing constructive behaviors rather than feeding into the sick role.

5. Avoid triangulations—do not allow the patient to work one family member against another. Often someone in the family will serve as the patient's advocate, validating their pain and freeing them from responsibilities.

6. Triangulations will also occur between patient, family member and doctor or health professional. If you find yourself upset with the medical staff because they refuse to be manipulated by the patient's sick role, alert yourself to the possibility of falling victim to triangulation and discuss it with a counselor or social worker. Your advocacy may or may not be appropriate to

the situation, and talking about it with others will help shed light on the matter.

Denial

The behavior that works at complete odds with pain rehabilitation efforts is that of denial. If the patient is not willing to admit that non-medical issues are affecting the presence of pain, he will see no reason for therapies (physical therapy, occupational therapy, work hardening, biofeedback, etc.) and will eventually sabotage all therapeutic efforts.

Denial is a method of preserving one's self-image. The patient often feels that if he admits that anything other than organic factors are leading to pain, that people will believe that all his pain is "psychological." Therapists and family members must help the patient to feel comfortable with recognizing and admitting that various factors impinge upon the pain experience; otherwise, therapies will have little impact.

It is important for everyone involved to recognize that the various non-medical factors that contribute to and maintain chronic pain are stress, inactivity, emotional vulnerability, drug dependency, physical-occupational-recreational debilitation, depression, low tolerances and coping levels, and a gradual withdrawal into complete focus on self and bodily concerns. Ironically, while most of these factors are the result of having chronic pain, they are additionally responsible for maintaining and increasing the pain condition. Therefore, chronic pain no longer needs a physical problem to carry on its existence! It can survive quite persistently with some combination of the non-medical factors mentioned above. In addition, psychological problems result from chronic pain—not the other way around. Denial is a psychological condition—chronic pain is not.

Examples of Denial: The following statements are often representative of the presence of denial:

1. "My marriage is fine—we have a great relationship."

2. "I am not under any stress."

3. "There is no particular time when my pain worsens—it's always random."

4. "My head has nothing to do with my pain."

5. "There is no way I can work with this pain."

6. "I know the doctors have missed something. Maybe another x-ray will show them where my problem is."

7. "No, I won't talk to a psychologist. I'm not crazy!"

8. "My problem is physical, stress and those other things have nothing to do with my problem."

Resolutions for Denial:

1. Do not feed into the denial statements

2. Do not challenge the denial statements.

3. Let the patient know that you believe his pain is real.

4. Help the patient to recognize that stress does have an impact on pain.

5. Eliminate references to psychological issues.

6. Recommend stress management for the patient and the family.

7. Be supportive of non-medical alternatives such as biofeedback, relaxation, and counseling.

8. Realize that denial is not something that the patient can be made aware of by you. The best you can do to help is to make the patient aware of how non-medical factors are also involved. Professional help by a therapist familiar with the treatment of chronic pain is necessary.

Overfocus on Physical Concerns

The chronic pain patient has been faced with pain that has been debilitating. For some, and certainly not all, the focus on health and body illness is a behavior that the patient relies on for avoiding responsibility, engaging in conversations with others, and meeting their dependency needs. Some patients, for example, are simply confused about the relationship between their emotional health and their physical health. Certainly, some pain that chronic pain patients experience has a known medical origin. However, some pain reports are complaints resulting from lower tolerances to pain experienced by the patient. The patient's focus on physical concerns is of considerable frustration to both the patient and the family.

Examples of Overfocus on Physical Concerns:

1. A patient with low back pain may get a headache to avoid a potentially stressful or unwanted interaction with others.

2. A patient may develop stomach problems in order to avoid going out to dinner.

3. The patient may focus on additional and/or new pain in order to maintain status as a pain patient.

4. New pain locations or problems may demonstrate to family and friends that the condition is worse than doctors first thought.

Resolutions for Overfocus on Physical Concerns:

1. Reinforce the patient for efforts that he makes at managing the pain.

2. Limit that patient's opportunity to talk about pain by structuring the day or by literally insisting that pain is discussed only between, for example, 6:00 and 6:30 p.m.

3. Monitor the patient's health, but avoid reinforcing the patient's discovery and discussion of pain.

4. Talk with the patient's physician about his pain so that the family is aware of the degree of the pain, any medical limitations, and side effects that may complicate the family situation.

5. Reinforce and use non-medical alternatives to pain management, such as relaxation techniques, counseling, biofeedback, etc.

6. Discourage "doctor shopping" by reinforcing the physician's recommendations.

Depression

Most people experience some degree of depression at one time or another in their lifetime. The frequency and intensity varies with this very common emotional difficulty. "Depression" can range from sad feelings to immobilization and suicidal thoughts and plans. The chronic pain patient is at risk for some degree of depression, as a result of significant life stress (e.g., hospitalization, inability to work). Depressive symptoms include sadness, loss of interest in activities, unusual sleeping and eating habits (either too much or too little), difficulty concentrating, tearfulness, poor self-concept, feelings of helplessness and hopelessness, and suicidal thoughts. Mood swings are also a symptom of a fairly significant depression. Chronic pain and depression usually go hand in hand and tend to reinforce each other in a kind of mutually deteriorating pattern.

Examples of Depression:

1. The patient may refuse to attend social functions such as a dinner party or family get-together.

2. The patient verbalizes statements such as, "Life is over and will never be the same again," or "I got a raw deal from life."

3. The patient may be suicidal and express more alarming evidence of depression by verbalizing a suicidal thought, intent, or plan.

4. The patient may be overly involved with alcohol and/or drugs to "mask" a depression.

5. The patient may appear to lack energy and/or be tearful much of the time.

6. The patient's mood swings from good too bad at the drop of a hat.

7. Unpredictable angry outbursts occur followed by long periods of silence.

8. The patient loses interest in sex and casual displays of affection.

9. The patient loses interest in getting better.

Resolutions for Depression:

1. The family must sympathize with the depression that the patient experiences. Being a "good listener" is helpful.

2. Be alert to suicidal threats and take them seriously. People who express suicidal thoughts are asking for help. Direct the patient to a qualified mental health specialist when suicidal issues are present.

3. Discourage use of medication and/or alcohol to alleviate the depression.

4. Encourage the patient to seek counseling to explore the relationship between depression and pain and the confusions between the two that is often present.

6. Encourage the patient to mobilize as much as medically advisable. Exercise, within medically prescribed limits, is beneficial.

6. Discourage the patient from staying in bed and avoiding family and friends.

7. Avoid comments such as "cheer up!" Usually this only backfires and worsens the condition.

8. If no concern for suicide exists, try to carry on routinely without providing undue attention to the patient. This is not to suggest that the depression be ignored, but simply means avoid making it the focus of the family attention.

Anxiety and Fears

The pain patient is usually full of anxiety-provoking questions such as, "What if there is something wrong with me that the doctors cannot discover?" "What if I'm really dying?" or "What if I really am crazy?" Although there is an unending list of fears that could be enumerated, there are three main fears upon which we will focus.

The first is the patient's fear that doctors, friends, employers, etc., think he is crazy. As time goes on, this is expanded to a fear that he, in fact, may actually become crazy if a solution to the pain is not found.

Secondly, there is the fear of reinjury. This fear is a true detriment to rehabilitation as it significantly interferes with the patient participating in therapeutic activities. It becomes a vicious cycle whereby the individual stays immobile for fear of hurting himself again and, while inactive, has increased time on his hands to ruminate regarding all other concerns.

Last, there is the fear of discovery of wellness. Most family members believe that the patient's pain is continuous; however, chronic pain usually is episodic or intermittent. There are times when the patient feels better and can actually engage in productive tasks. What sometimes occurs is that families inadvertently feel or overtly express the view that the person must be better if he was able to accomplish a specific job. Such comments might include "If you could wash the car this morning, then you are well enough to help me bring in the groceries" or "You can't be that sick if you were able to help Ron fix his car yesterday." When families draw these types of conclusions based on "good times," they scare the person off from engaging in productive activity when their pain has decreased intensity. Thus, the patient becomes anxious when he is not maintaining the sick role.

We are not, of course, saying that a chronic pain patient's fears or anxieties are unfounded. The individual has many legitimate fears and the family can best assist by understanding the basis of the emotions and providing a supportive stance for increased activity and decreased rumination.

Examples of Anxiety and Fears:

1. The patient is fearful that he will no longer be able to provide financially for his family.

2. The patient is afraid to go to a psychiatrist.

3. The patient fears that others think the pain is only in his head.

4. The patient fears that the pain could be related to cancer that has not been identified by the doctors.

5. The patient "doctor shops" and continues to search for a documented medical cause in order to avoid confronting various psychological factors.

6. The patient is afraid that activity will lead to reinjury so he refuses to go to physical therapy.

7. As anxiety and fear increase, so does the pain. In addition, anxiety reduces the patient's ability to use reason and good judgement.

Resolutions for Anxiety and Fears:

1. Identify anxiety-provoking situations and work on alleviating the patient's stress.

2. Do not share your own fears and anxieties with the patient.

3. Do not reinforce these emotions by belaboring a discussion of the patient's fears.

4. Encourage the patient to utilize stress management and/or relaxation techniques.

5. Avoid "walking on eggs" around the house. It is not effective and may serve to increase everyone's tension.

6. When anxiety is expressed by the patient over physical or psychological issues, encourage him to discuss it with the doctor.

Low Self-Esteem

One of the most attitudinal changes which the pain patient experiences is the loss of self-esteem. Considerable frustration initially occurs with the experience of being incapable of accomplishing everyday things that previously required little to no effort. A vicious cycle emerges that involves frustration, apprehension, tension and perhaps the fear that circumstances will deteriorate even further. Feelings of helplessness, hopelessness, and inadequacy translate into lowered self-esteem.

Financially, the burden of medical bills mounts. Typically, the pain patient will find himself relinquishing the role of financial supporter/contributor, which further intensifies family difficulties. Feelings of guilt and inadequacy are experienced. This lowered self-esteem often leads to a display of depressive behaviors which were discussed earlier.

Living with Chronic Pain: A How-to-Manage Manual

Examples of Low Self-Esteem:

1. "I can't do this now and I'll never be able to do it again."

2. "My wife has got to work full-time now! God, what has become of me?"

3. "I'm never going to get better."

4. "I can't even make love anymore. My wife will probably leave me for sure."

5. "I must be being punished for something!"

6. "If I can't learn what I did before, then what's the use?"

Resolutions for Low Self-Esteem:

1. The family should make attempts at reinforcing all efforts made toward change.

2. Family should engage in regular discussions where it can be made clear to the patient that respect and selfworth are not contingent upon pre-morbid or pre-pain condition.

3. The family should encourage the patient to participate in all family activities.

4. The family can rebuild self-esteem in a step-by-step program of decreasing the patient's habit of leaning on others and learning new independent skills.

5. Remind the patient that although he may be down, it does not mean that he is out! He can contribute by following the recommended treatment routine of exercise and therapeutic relaxation.

6. Human beings are better off (no matter what the extent of their handicap) when they can accomplish and do for themselves. Remind the patient of the truth of this assertion and encourage him to think about returning to some form of employment. Earning one's own income is eminently important to one's self-esteem.

Social Isolation

Social isolation is a double-edged problem. On the one hand, the chronic pain patient often pulls away from social contacts; and, on the other hand, he may drive people away by focusing continually on his physical problems. Each of these facets is detrimental to both the patient and family.

Through the process of attempting to solve a chronic pain problem, the patient has found security in primarily one setting—the home. This secure feeling is tied to the fact that he has become comfortable with an environment where he controls whom he sees and when he sees them. Either inadvertently or at times on purpose, the patient has been able to manipulate all facets of the home setting. It should not be surprising that an individual would enjoy this control since he feels he has very little control over any other aspect of his life; thus, he resists socializing outside the home.

Moreover, for some people, leaving the bed or the house can be associated with wellness, and we explained that anxious behaviors and fears are associated with people assuming that the patient is now "normal." Along with this comes concerns that the patient is not so different and that they must be better off than they are indicating. Again, we have the vicious circle of avoiding activities or socializing for fear that he will be expected to do all the other things "normal" people are capable of doing. Thus, it is safer and less threatening to stay home.

Examples of Social Isolation:

1. Extended family members quit stopping by on Sunday afternoons.

2. The patient's closest friends from his former job no longer call him to go on their regular Friday night outings.

3. The patient refuses to go to his son's ball games, even though he previously attended them on a regular basis.

4. The patient finds that in a large group setting people actively avoid engaging him in a conversation.

5. The patient, by his negative attitude, discourages others from being around him.

Living with Chronic Pain: A How-to-Manage Manual

Resolutions for Social Isolation:

1. Each family member must let the individual know that they believe the person is in pain, but they do not want to continuously hear about his physical ailments.

2. The family should remind the individual that friends are easily scared off by social interactions that focus primarily on "sickness."

3. Tell your friends not to ask, "How are you feeling today?"

4. Select family activities that are structured rather than open for complaining sessions.

5. Plan family activities away from the home.

6. Open up communication within the family so that other members will feel free to openly discuss their reactions and concerns with the patient.

Stress

"Stressed out" is a term used to describe the impact of life stress on an individual in which anxiety, tension, high blood pressure, depression, anger, distractibility, and physical problems may result. Not all stress is "bad stress," since manageable stress gives one the energy to do productive and creative work. Thus, stress should not necessarily be eliminated, but "managed." The pain patient experiences life stress in almost all areas. There are physical stress (the pain), social stress (feeling left out and cheated), and work stress (unable to work or uncomfortable at work), and certainly family stress (feeling the need to "return to normal"). Heightened levels and combinations of stress result in the immediate symptoms noted above, and ultimately result in decreased quality of life. Dealing with the patient's stress as well as managing their own stress is important for families of chronic pain patients.

Examples of Stress:

1. Because of loss of income and/or medical bills, the patient may blurt out, "If one more bill collector calls, I'm going to scream!"

2. The patient may exhibit increased levels of agitation, tension, and even depression.

3. The patient may be very irritable and overreact to the noise of children or to not being able to locate something they have misplaced.

4. The patient may become very irritable or depressed, following job interviews, due to stress.

5. The patient becomes quiet and reserved one minute and "lashes out" the next.

6. New pain problems develop or other physical complaints increase.

Resolutions for Stress:

1. As a family project, enroll in a stress management class offered at the local community mental health center or school.

2. For high levels of stress resulting in increased physical symptoms (e.g., high blood pressure, headaches, anxiety attacks), be sure to have the patient see a physician.

3. A psychologist would be helpful in assisting the patient and family in learning relaxation training and stress management techniques.

4. Biofeedback training and other techniques have proven effective in treating moderately high levels of stress. A referral to a psychologist may be appropriate.

5. Stress management books and relaxation training tapes are available at most bookstores and would be a good adjunct to the patient's rehabilitation.

Decreased Sexual Contact

Chronic pain almost always results in a general and gradual reduction in physical and emotional contact between pain patient and partner. There are many reasons for this and our experience leads us to believe that the least likely reason is a loss of love. In fact, we find that persons with chronic pain are extremely frustrated with their reduction of affection and sexual contact. They state that they are humiliated or ashamed of their withdrawal of affection and would dearly like to have a normal relationship, but do not know how.

In our pain management program we have noticed a common pattern that occurs to contribute to this problem. First, pain causes disruption of sexual activity which then causes fewer attempts which, in turn, causes a reduction in affectionate behavior. This triggers emotions such as depression, frustration, suspicion, anger, mistrust, and alienation. With emotions now increased, the inclination to communicate verbally and sexually are hindered. The cycle continues until there exists an unspoken agreement: "We don't do that anymore." One of our patient's spouses regretfully admitted to obtaining sexual gratification elsewhere because of the lack of it at home. Interestingly, both pain patient and spouse knew of this independently, but never discussed it with each other.

Examples of Decreased Sexual Contact:

Sexual problems do not exist in a vacuum. They exist in conjunction with many other problems surrounding communication.

1. The person with chronic pain seems uncomfortable with touching or any displays of affection. This behavior reflects the fear by the person that touching will lead to kissing and kissing will require sex. And, if sex is attempted, it will be a failure or cause an increase in pain. Therefore, these persons come to believe that to avoid pain and failure it is best to avoid sex. This happens to be true, but the logic misses the point that some failure and some pain are always a part of life, and to avoid these things means withdrawal from almost every human activity.

2. Discussion or frank talk about the lack of sexual contact are nonexistent, or when the subject is raised so are tempers. In many situations between normal couples, candid talk about sex and need for affection does not exist. With chronic pain as an added problem, the likelihood that discussion will take place gets even smaller. The person in pain soon learns to avoid any attempts by the partner to discuss the problem by withdrawing or complaining of the unreasonable pressure to perform that is implied when such discussions take place. One

of our patient's spouses displayed her anger when she blurted out, "He not only won't let me touch him, but he won't even let me talk with him about why he won't let me touch him. I feel rejected and frustrated!"

Resolutions for Decreased Sexual Contact:

1. Begin by not requiring discussion of sex or affection by your partner. This will reduce the anxiety and feeling that discussion is mandatory. Forced discussion is not possible. Inform your partner that you wish to discuss the matter, but only when he feels ready.

2. Display unconditional affection. That is, give quick hugs or a kiss on the cheek or a squeeze of the arm and do not wait for a return display. Go on about your business as if you do not expect to receive affection just because you offered it. This will help reduce the pressure your partner may feel to "perform."

3. Use humor in your contacts. Nothing releases pent up energy more quickly and efficiently than humor. Laughing at life's frustrations is not easy to do, but is very effective when done.

4. Should you not be able or inclined to improve communication with your partner for any reason, please seek professional help.

Nonproductive Behaviors

Pain, because of its very nature and our experience, is most often recognized by everyone as a warning signal. Humans have long histories of experiencing pain followed by the normal reaction of increased anxiety and the orientation to obtain relief. Very simply, pain seems to produce a reflex reaction of behaviors that are geared toward reducing the pain. Touching a hot stove produces the reflex behavior of quickly withdrawing the hand. Stubbing the toe on a hard object produces the reflexive behavior of withdrawing the foot and perhaps avoidance of its use until the pain goes away.

With chronic pain, however, there also exists the tendency to reflexively respond to it as a warning signal. But now the behavioral habit of withdrawing or avoiding physical movement serves to hinder instead of help. Lack of movement is not good because physical activity is not likely to cause further damage. In fact, the opposite is more often true.

Living with Chronic Pain: A How-to-Manage Manual

Physical activity over time reduces pain. Lack of physical activity increases pain by reducing muscle tone and contributing to poor posture and overall body weakness.

What does the normal tendency to be inactive because of pain have to do with productivity? Everything! We are creatures of habit and, as such, we have many features which allow us to go about our daily lives with relative ease. We drive a car and shift gears and avoid other cars without giving much thought to the complexity of the task. We arise in the morning and perform a ritual of getting ourselves ready for work without a thought to the matter. We simply and easily perform many difficult behaviors throughout the day and we owe this to our ability to learn and develop habits. Inactivity is a learned habit response to pain. With chronic pain, inactivity is nonproductive.

Problems develop, though, when we develop habits that are nonproductive or are not in our best interest. Cigarette smoking is nonproductive for healthy lungs. Staying in bed when it is time to go to work may not be a problem if it happens only once. But, what if it happens again and again? A nonproductive habit is being formed. Now our ability to function well because we learn to develop habits serves us poorly. We have learned to respond to the alarm clock with a nonproductive behavior instead of a productive one.

The normal nonproductive habit response to pain is to be inactive. Once a habit like this is learned, it is hard to break. If pain is reduced or avoided by lack of movement, then continuing to not move or only moving very carefully should avoid or reduce all forms of pain, right? Wrong! Continuing to be inactive with chronic pain is a normal learned habit response, but it is the wrong response. Inactivity is the enemy of chronic pain!

First and foremost is to understand that as a family member you are not in control of the behaviors of another family member. You have some influence, but make no mistake about it, each family member is ultimately in control of only their own behavior. This means you must not take responsibility for the behavior of the person in chronic pain. Your responsibility is to gear your behavior such that your influence contributes to producing the best conditions for the person with chronic pain to change his own behavior. In this way, you can help.

Examples of Nonproductive Behavior:

1. Lying in bed beyond sleep time.

2. Not dressing or wearing only pajamas or underwear.

3. Avoiding even small tasks like helping out around the house or picking up after oneself.

4. Avoiding work of any kind.

5. Personal hygiene and grooming habits are replaced with sloppiness and neglect of self-care.

6. Avoidance of attention to family and economic needs.

7. Avoidance of making plans for the future or dealing with necessary issues.

Resolutions for Nonproductive Behavior:

1. Encourage activity. The patient may resist, but you must be just as persistent. Take opportunities to make it difficult for him to be inactive.

2. Do not do for the person in pain what he can do for himself.

3. You must realize that your helping behavior helps the person in pain to stay in pain. We thrive when we produce and wither when we do not.

4. Encourage and allow productive behaviors by structuring the family environment to help the person in chronic pain feel and be productive.

Drug/Alcohol Abuse

Pain relief is the natural consequence of altering our consciousness through the use of drugs and alcohol. Both physical and emotional pain can be dulled by the use of narcotics or a few drinks. The relief, unfortunately, is short lived and when the physical pain returns, the emotional pain can be made much worse. In addition, the repeated cycle of this behavior can add more problems, such as addiction, kidney and liver damage, and other physical and mental complications.

Narcotics, when used for acute pain, work quite well because they buy the body pain-relieving time for it to heal. When the body heals and the pain leaves, there is no need for further medication. This is good because all pain medication has short-term effects. That is, they

Living with Chronic Pain: A How-to-Manage Manual

work for a short time, then, because of the body's ability to build tolerance for drugs, they lose their effect.

Alcohol is a general depressant and will dull the awareness of pain, but brings with it the danger of requiring more and more for the same effect. In addition, alcohol is often used in conjunction with narcotics. This places the user at great risk because the effect of mixing the two often results in toxic levels for the body. The body's ability to withstand nonprescribed combinations is limited.

For the user, the pain may or may not subside. In fact, the increased use of drugs and alcohol only serves to produce "zombie-like" effects, and often the person is left with pain plus confusion.

Remember, drugs and alcohol are poor ways to control pain. Certain drugs may be of value, but you must be careful by making sure that the drugs are intended for chronic pain—not acute pain. If you are not sure, it is wise to check with a chronic pain program in your area.

Examples of Drug/Alcohol Abuse:

1. The person will become upset without cause or justification. Flying off the handle at unpredictable times and situations can be a regular occurrence.

2. Often persons suffering from drug and alcohol effects will perceive things differently than those around them. The distortion to them is not a distortion and they often become frustrated with why others do not see things the way they do. Most drug and alcohol abusers do not want to believe that their perception is distorted.

3. Mood changes are evident. One minute happy, one minute sad is typical of these individuals.

4. The patient will assign all his problems to pain rather than to drug or alcohol misuse or abuse. "It's the pain that causes me to do this."

Resolutions for Drug/Alcohol Abuse:

1. The number one priority, if you suspect drug and/or alcohol abuse, is to get help. If you observe the behaviors given in the examples and confront the person, you may only aggravate the situation.

2. Detoxification, or obtaining help to rid the person of dependence on drugs/alcohol, is part of many pain management programs' regular treatment. It cannot be done easily by you or the person in pain alone without serious side effects and potential complications for your relationship.

3. Avoid encouraging the use of medication for pain relief. It is tempting for you to provide a pill in your effort to help your loved one obtain relief. Fight the temptation and, instead, encourage them to use distraction or relaxation techniques.

4. Find a pain management support group by checking with hospitals and physicians or social workers. The group can be beneficial for you as well as your loved one.

5. Try to administer the medication on a regular basis, rather than when the person asks for it. This procedure can be only used if your loved one agrees for you to "manage" the medication. Before you attempt this, talk about it with your loved one and discuss the advantages and disadvantages of using this procedure. We have listed some here for you. Perhaps you can think of others.

    Advantages:

    - Less worry about medication mistakes or excesses.

    - Person in pain does not have to "display" pain behavior to obtain medication.

    - Anxiety about not receiving enough medication is reduced. "Enough" is what the physician has prescribed as safe to take in one day.

    Disadvantages:

    - Takes responsibility for pain relief control out of hands of person in pain.

    - Person may feel dependent upon caretaker of medication and resent him.

    - "Enough" medication may not be enough since, as we stated before, medication breeds the need for more with less and less effect on pain.

6. Avoid nagging about excessive drinking. This usually only increases the behavior.

7. Avoid making drinking as a means of solving your own problems. If you demonstrate that when you are frustrated you "need" a drink, then it becomes unfair to expect that your loved one in pain should not have the same option.

Relief at All Costs

Pain causes people to seek relief. When relief does not come, anxiety and stress are increased and, thus, the experience of pain is made worse. Patients then will go to extreme limits to obtain relief.

"Just cut my foot off and I'll be happy." This was a quote from one of our patients whose pain was so intense and persistent that he felt he would rather not have a foot than put up with the pain. The problem here was that removal of the foot would not have reduced the nerve pain that this man was experiencing. The fact is that even with his foot removed he might still "feel" his foot and the pain. Amputees are well aware of how one can feel a limb that is not there or feel pain in a limb that has long since been removed. In desperation, pain patients will do many things no matter how bizarre or self-destructive. This is quite understandable, but it still remains a problem. That is, most of the time these extreme attempts to obtain relief do not work. This cruel reality becomes known to the dejected patient only after the attempt.

Examples of Relief at All Costs:

1. The patient overdoses on pain medication thinking more pills will alleviate his suffering.

2. The patient reads about new medical developments and travels all over the country in an attempt to obtain a miracle cure.

3. A patient buys street drugs and doubles his effects with alcohol.

4. The patient pushes the physician to do surgery even though the tests do not always support the idea. In response to the pressure, exploratory surgery may be considered and perhaps a fusion or laminectomy. If the result is negative, the patient can become quite depressed and discouraged. Soon the patient stops doing anything and becomes dependent and withdrawn.

5. The patient seeks out several different physicians asking each one for medication and then three times what each doctor independently has prescribed. Worry follows that this deception may be discovered and then he will be a "cut off."

Resolutions for Relief at All Costs:

1. Find a physician who specializes in the treatment of chronic (not acute) pain. Avoid the temptation to "doctor shop."

2. Avoid being the patient's spokesperson. Most patients are quite able to speak for themselves and do better when they are allowed to engage in negotiations about their treatment. If you become the spokesperson, you may find yourself quickly in the uncomfortable position of having to provide explanations for why your negotiation with the medical staff has not produced relief Leave it up to the medical staff to perform the job they are paid to do.

3. Finally, realize that there are going to be times when nothing can be done to stop the pain, but much can be done to reduce the experience of pain. Finding a physician with experience and involvement in a chronic pain program is your first step.

Gender Differences in Pain

The effects of chronic pain do not occur in the same way for males and females. Their responses can be different to the experience of pain. Their interpretations and feelings about what pain has done to them can be different. This does not mean that all males or females respond in a uniform manner. There are tendencies, however, which can produce unique behavior because of the conditioning and experience differences of one sex or the other. The importance here is for female spouses to be aware of possible male tendencies in chronic pain, and male spouses to be aware of tendencies for female sufferers of chronic pain.

Notice how male comments tend to involve being brave or acting tough, while females tend to be a bit more direct and open with their feelings. Males also tend to display anger, while females find it easier to relate a wider range of emotions, such as depression and the need for understanding. Of course, there are elements of male and female traits in all of the comments listed below. The point here is that there are tendencies which may explain certain persistent behavior of the chronic pain patient.

Living with Chronic Pain: A How-to-Manage Manual

Examples of Gender Differences in Pain:

- **Male Issues**

    1. "I should be tough and not let others know that I hurt, but I'm afraid."

    2. "I can't do hard labor I'm not a man anymore. I feel worthless."

    3. "I don't care what anybody says, I'm going to do what I want, when I want!"

    4. "Sure, I'm angry. Wouldn't you be?"

    5. "Just cut my leg off and let me go home. Do anything, but do something!"

- **Female Issues**

    1. "I want to be strong, but I feel better when I let others know about how I hurt."

    2. "How will I support myself? Who would want to share a life with me anymore?"

    3. "I'm tired of being this way. No one seems to understand or care anymore. I feel worthless!"

    4. "Of course, I'm depressed. Wouldn't you be?"

    5. "I can't seem to stand it much longer you must help me. Can't you see I'm suffering?"

Resolutions for Gender Differences in Pain:

1. It is not appropriate to view males and females in a stereotyped manner. We are not encouraging or suggesting that you do. We are asking for you to be sensitive to the tendencies for males to behave differently than females with chronic pain. From our experience, neither males nor females have an advantage in being able to deal with their chronic pain. We have seen males fall apart while females remained strong and vice versa.

2. Pain is a unique and subjective experience. It is important to recognize that the person in pain still has values, ideals, habits, and viewpoints which contribute to their interpretation of what the effects of chronic pain means to them. As a result, there will always tend to be differences in behavior. One difference which may seem obvious is gender. Recognize the possibility of these differences and it will help you understand to a small extent why your loved one persists in certain behaviors related to pain. With understanding comes tolerance, and with tolerance comes the opportunity to respond to your loved one with support and encouragement when they must face the difficult notion that they may no longer "feel" like a strong male or attractive female.

Family/Significant Other Behaviors

All too often, the primary focus of professionals is on the pain patient. In so doing, there is a disregard for the family who suffers considerably as a result of the changes in their life circumstances. Feelings of despair occur with the family as well and are not limited to the pain patient. Among the many disturbances experienced by pain patients' families, a few of the most pronounced, often shared, center around the intense changes in family interactions, actual alterations in family roles and ineffectual attempts using old methods that were successful in the past when dealing with the pain patient's difficulties. These are but a few of the reasons underlying the extremely intense feelings of frustration, anger, despair, guilt and apprehension that are continually experienced by family members.

For example, at previous times, compassion, concern and care were appropriate in relieving the patient of his distress. However, this approach may actually undermine the patient's efforts to acquire new ways to deal with problem areas. The family is often unaware of the new behaviors it must acquire, yet they are quite uncomfortable with the occurrence of new intense family interactions. As such, the family unconsciously contributes to the maintenance of the patient's self-defeating behaviors.

It is the purpose of this section of our manual to provide a more productive route that will provide a more positive outcome. Many behaviors which families of pain patients experience will be presented in these next sections. Suggestions will be made in an attempt to provide an awareness, understanding and approach that might prove to be beneficial. However, it is important to note that these are just suggestions. In no way is this manual a substitution for professional help. Many families may find themselves at a point where there are no other alternatives, and professional help should be sought.

Fostering Dependency—The Mistake of Love

The most persistent behaviors of family members toward the chronic pain sufferer involve those of providing "help." Why not? Shouldn't we help others when they are ill? Would not helping be unkind and cruel? These are tough issues, but you must come to grips with them if you want your behavior to really be helpful. First of all, doing something for the sufferer will most likely be received with much enthusiasm and gratitude. Sometimes help is refused at first, then later it may be asked for, or even demanded. The problem is not whether we help or do not, but rather when and how much help we give. The key to successful helping, then, is knowing the right time to offer help and the right amount of help to provide.

Before you can be of real help to someone, two conditions must be met. First, the person you help must actually need the help. Otherwise your help, at best, would be a showing of affection and, at worst, perhaps contributing to the problem. Helping a little old lady across the street may seem like a kind and helpful thing to do, but as the old joke goes, if she didn't want to go across the street in the first place, you're not doing her a favor by helping her. The second condition requires that the help you give must be somehow related to the need. It does no one any good to give the wrong kind of help. For example, helping a person fix her stalled vehicle by changing her tire is not likely to get the car moving.

With chronic pain, the first condition is usually always met. That is, we know the person is in need of help. The second condition is where we begin to have trouble. What kind of help should we give? Once we know this, then we can deal with when and how much. Attend a chronic pain family group and discuss with other family members ways to help that are effective.

The "mistake of love" simply means doing for others what they need to be doing for themselves if they are to get better. Persons with chronic pain usually are quite inactive and become physically unfit, which will tend to complicate and increase pain. Most sufferers need to be active, not inactive. Yet, many family members find themselves running themselves ragged trying to keep their loved one from experiencing pain by doing everything for him. This behavior not only may not prevent the pain, but will tend to cause the sufferer to require more and more help, thus, fostering dependency.

Make no mistake about it, love does not mean doing for others when it is not good for them. Many of us need to ask ourselves whom we are really doing this for. Could we be doing or helping because we feel we must do something?

Examples of Fostering Dependency—The Mistake of Love: You may feel you already know the answer to the "when and how much" question. Here are some answers we have received from family members.

1. "I feel I should always help!"

2. "I know when to help—she tells me!"

3. "I started out helping a little. Now I feel I am doing too much—he doesn't want to do anything for himself anymore!"

4. "Everything I do just doesn't seem to be enough."

Resolutions for Fostering Dependency—The Mistake of Love: We would like to ask you to direct your motivations toward the types of family behaviors that do not foster dependency. You can begin by considering and trying some of the following behavioral suggestions.

1. Make a list of all the household things that need to be done and discuss with everyone including the chronic pain sufferer who should do what. This will allow for a routine to be established so that everyone's chores will be clear. The pain sufferer should have responsible chores as well. Make sure you check with the physician or chronic pain management staff on what chores the pain sufferer could reasonably be expected to perform.

2. As a rule of thumb, avoid doing for the pain sufferer what he can do for himself. This does not mean you must stop doing favors or acts of kindness, but does require you to carefully consider whether you are really helping the sufferer stay inactive by your help.

3. If the pain sufferer is already overly dependent, it will be difficult for you to stop fostering the dependency. One way is to

have an open and honest discussion with the sufferer about the need for you to help by sometimes not helping.

4. Establish clearly what you and others will do and what the sufferer will do for himself and then stick to it.

5. Avoid making excuses to yourself for why you need to do for the sufferer. Remember, the best reason to do for others is when they really need your help. If your help prevents them from learning to help themselves, your help is not help at all.

6. Show your appreciation whenever they do something for themselves.

7. Remember—you can help, but the manner in which you help makes a difference. Sometimes not helping is the best form of help you can provide.

Frustration

Frustration is usually the result of unachieved expectations and often goes hand in hand with anxiety and anger. If you are a person who is used to being in control of your life and the lives of family members, the presence of chronic pain in your loved one will be one of the most frustrating times of your life. It seems there is no relief from the multitude of problems that mount up. You may wish you could say things to the patient that would at least help you let off steam, but you become acutely aware that this only leads to added problems later.

The egocentricity displayed by the patient is often the greatest source of frustration. Again, we can become very easily annoyed with the person who focuses primarily on his own needs. As more and more goals and wishes of other family members are blocked, the cumulative frustration within an entire family can make the home environment a powder keg.

Examples of Frustration: The following statements exemplify frustration.

1. "Everything I do is not enough."

2. "We do not have a life of our own anymore."

3. "This is as bad as raising another child."

4. "The insurance company doesn't return my calls."

5. "What about me... don't I count?"

Resolutions for Frustration:

1. Recognize that the patient's behavior is essentially outside your control and do not attempt to change him drastically. There are some things you just cannot change.

2. Begin addressing other family members' needs.

3. Give yourself some time away so that you can be refreshed and effectively deal with the issues when you are at home.

4. Develop alternative methods of reaching your goals if you find that certain avenues are blocked.

6. Seek professional help if you are at your wit's end.

Anger

The family of a chronic pain patient soon realizes that it is not just the patient who has a problem. Although the family may not have physical pain, there is no question that living with a chronic pain patient stirs a variety of emotions. Some family members, like the chronic pain patient, harbor many angry feelings. The family may express anger at the patient, other family members, the patient's employer, hospitals, and even themselves. Recognize that anger and irritability may be present when the family's goals are temporarily blocked. Attempt to rechannel these emotions and energy in a positive direction.

Examples of Anger:

1. A husband becomes irate with hospital staff because they are not feeding the patient properly.

2. The family blames the patient's employer for the patient's inability to work, claiming that the work place is unsafe.

Living with Chronic Pain: A How-to-Manage Manual

3. A wife blames the hospital for a patient's lack of progress.

4. A family member becomes sarcastic with the patient or other family members.

Resolutions for Anger:

1. Recognize that the family has been affected by the current situation and recognize the legitimacy of your anger.

2. Attempt to identify what provokes your anger and learn to deal with it or avoid it if possible (e.g., a particular friend of the patient, a specific health care worker, etc.).

3. Substitute a vigorous and/or productive activity for anger (e.g., physical exercise, housecleaning, yard work).

4. Do not allow the anger to eat away at you and affect your own health.

5. Attend family support groups of chronic pain patients, or, if necessary, seek individual or family (including couple) counseling to deal effectively with your anger.

Guilt

If you have been a "guilt accumulator" in the past, you will be easily trapped into taking on even greater volumes of guilt during the "doctor shopping" process. If you previously stayed free of guilt, you will now have some difficulty avoiding it. The circumstances surrounding living with a chronic pain patient provide a multitude of possibilities for thinking or feeling that you have not done the best thing in a given situation. Guilt will arise from at least four main sources: 1) you; 2) the patient; 3) other family members; 4) concerned others.

Examples of Guilt:

1. You may feel guilty every time you go out of the house without your loved one.

2. You may feel guilty that you have not done more to help alleviate the patient's pain.

3. You may feel guilty that you have ignored and/or avoided your friends.

4. You may feel guilty that at times you fantasize about a three-week vacation alone.

5. You may feel guilty that you have not been able to help the patient find a doctor with whom he is perfectly satisfied.

Resolutions for Guilt:

1. Accept guilt as a normal human feeling over which you have minimal control.

2. Substitute some engrossing activity to get your mind off the guilt—gardening, exercising, biking, etc.

3. Schedule your guilt time—only feel guilty on Wednesdays.

Escape/Avoidance

After we have been involved in a problem situation for six months or more, it is only human nature to experience the desire to escape. On the contrary, there would actually be something wrong if you enjoyed living day after day with the conflicts presented by a pain patient. It is best to accept the fact that absolute escape is not feasible, but intermittent, short, scheduled escapes are perfectly appropriate and, in fact, necessary to maintain your sanity and health.

Examples of Escape/Avoidance:

1. The spouse finds that he spends longer and longer hours at the office.

2. Being alone has increased appeal.

3. Travel posters look inviting.

4. You enjoy it when the patient sleeps in late and you have the morning to yourself.

Resolutions for Escape /Avoidance:

1. You should not avoid thoughts of escape—schedule your escapes within reason.

2. Make sure that you have time to yourself each day.

3. Do not cancel your vacation plans.

4. Admit that you are avoiding the patient and make attempts to change the behaviors that are involved in this avoidance. If changes are not forthcoming, spare yourself the guilt of wanting to escape at times.

Fatigue

There is probably no other time in your life when you have been this fatigued for such an extended period. You have been involved in a problem that often consumes and interferes with your sleeping hours. On top of this actual reduction in rest, the demand for your waking hours has been tremendous. The responsibility of caring for an individual in pain and searching for a cure is often a 24-hour job and analogous to the care of a new baby. Moreover, all tension resulting from anxiety, anger, and frustration are very tiring and add to the overall debilitating effect of fatigue.

Examples of Fatigue:

1. Hours and days are spent searching for the answer from the right doctor.

2. The family members become physically drained from waiting on the loved one in pain.

3. Much energy is expended just keeping life going from day to day.

4. The patient makes a great commotion and wakes everybody up when he goes to listen to his relaxation tape so that he can get back to sleep.

5. Attempts to nap are often fruitless due to racing thoughts regarding unsolved problems.

6. You experience a reoccurring back problem which interferes with your night's rest.

Resolutions for Fatigue:

1. Utilize relaxation techniques for insomnia. If you are unfamiliar with these, consult a psychologist.

2. Put off until tomorrow what is not absolutely necessary.

3. Delegate responsibilities. Others should pitch in and help, including the patient.

4. Do not feel you have to constantly be by the patient's side. Ignore accusations that you are not always available.

5. Structure time away by yourself.

Stress

The chronic pain patient experiences stress because of major life stress, such as not being able to work, living with pain, etc. The family is also faced with significant life stress. The impact of life stress on an individual is often exhibited by increased anxiety, tension, blood pressure, anger, distractibility, depression, and physical problems. As discussed earlier, not all stress is "bad stress" (distress), and it is often proposed that stress not be eliminated, but managed. Heightened levels and combinations of life stress result in the various symptoms noted above, and ultimately result in decreased quality of life. The recognition of the impact of stress on individuals has become an important issue in wellness and preventive health programs.

Examples of Stress:

1. Family members may show increased levels of agitation, tension, and even depression.

2. A family member may be very irritable and overreact to minor nuisances (e.g., noise, a particular television show selected by others, misplacing the newspaper).

3. A spouse may become overwhelmed by the financial stress (e.g., overly worrying about mounting medical costs) or with the complications of the spouse's condition (e.g., limited socializing, decreased sexual contact).

Living with Chronic Pain: A How-to-Manage Manual

Resolutions for Stress:

1. As a family project, enroll in a stress management class offered at the local community mental health center or school.

2. Whenever high levels of stress result in physical symptoms (e.g., high blood pressure, headaches, anxiety attacks), be sure to see a physician.

3. Psychologists are helpful in assisting families in learning relaxation training and stress management.

4. Stress management books and relaxation training tapes are available at most bookstores and would be helpful in learning to manage stress.

5. Recognize that your stress is a consequence of living and dealing with chronic pain.

Depression

As discussed earlier, most individuals experience some degree of depression at one time or other in their lifetime. Families witness depression in chronic pain patients, but often hide or do not admit their own depression. Some pain clinics have reported that spouses of chronic pain patients report being up to four times more depressed than the patients! This is not so surprising when you consider the intensity of life situations many chronic pain families must endure. The family is at risk for some degree of depression, as a result of significant life stress (e.g., financial stress, change in family goals). Symptoms of depression include sadness, loss of interest in activities, unusual sleeping and eating habits (either too much or too little), difficulty concentrating, tearfulness, poor self-concept, feelings of helplessness and hopelessness, and suicidal thoughts.

Examples of Depression:

1. A family member refuses to attend a graduation or other special function.

2. A family member may verbalize such things as, "It's hopeless. I don't know what keeps me going."

3. Sometimes individuals attempt to hide a depression by being overly involved with alcohol and/or drugs.

4. A family member may be suicidal and express more alarming evidence of depression by verbalizing a suicidal thought, intent, or plan.

Resolutions for Depression:

1. Increase physical exercise within medically prescribed limits.

2. Encourage the family members to continue to be involved in activities.

3. Take suicidal threats seriously. People who express suicidal thoughts are asking for help. Direct the individual to a qualified mental health specialist when suicidal issues are present.

4. Consider individual and/or family (couple) counseling.

5. Attend family support groups.

6. If depression doesn't subside, see a physician, psychologist or a psychiatrist. There are antidepressant medications and therapy which can help.

Social Isolation

As is often the case when a "pained" loved one is at home, the family reduces its contact with the outside world to allow the patient to have a quiet environment and to provide emotional support. The danger here is that this pattern will become a habit that will be hard to break. Studies have shown that the support of family and friends is more important than the assistance of hospital personnel, doctors, or the clergy. Thus, it is a mistake to isolate yourself from your old contacts.

Even though you may make every effort to foster old friendships, you may find that many will gradually drift away due to a variety of reasons:

1. they are not able to understand the patient's obsession with his physical condition;

Living with Chronic Pain: A How-to-Manage Manual

2. they are not able to accept the patient as he presents himself in a group setting;

3. they find that they are uncomfortable in the patient's presence because they no longer share common interests and goals. If you find this occurring with a large portion of your former friends, make every effort to form new acquaintances.

Examples of Social Isolation:

1. A retired woman takes on the responsibility of her daughter who is in chronic pain and her three children, and does not make arrangements to see her friends on a social basis.

2. A wife quits her job and gives up outside contacts to attempt to meet all the needs of her husband.

3. The family refuses to go out until the patient can go to social engagements with them.

Resolutions for Social Isolation:

1. Do not set up an early pattern of decreased social contacts.

2. Do not quit your job unless absolutely necessary.

3. When friends call, talk about things other than the patient and how or what he is doing.

4. Schedule outings for social activities and then follow through.

5. Do not convince yourself that you are the only one who can care for the patient.

Sexual Frustration

No area is more difficult to understand than sexual effects of chronic pain on family members. One reason for this is often family members do not openly discuss such sensitive issues. Nevertheless, we offer some ideas on the subject based upon our experiences working with families.

"We don't touch or do anything anymore!" was a comment from a wife of one of our patients. It was not an uncommon statement. How does this happen and why does it continue? Usually, when chronic pain occurs, inactivity leads to dependence and this leads to depression. This results in a loss of desire for sex as well as a fear of increased pain or poor performance. Thus, anxiety increases, which starts the cycle of avoiding sex all over again. You may begin to wonder if you have lost your desirability or attractiveness. Do not worry, this is not usually the case. What seems to be the case is a sort of pain-imposed impotence that is placed upon the patient.

Examples of Sexual Frustration:

1. Little or no romance exists. You become frustrated.

2. Every attempt by your to achieve tenderness and closeness is rebuffed or avoided by the patient.

3. Thoughts of infidelity occur.

4. You begin questioning your "desirability."

Resolutions for Sexual Frustration:

1. Find a counselor or certified sex therapist and go yourself until the patient agrees to go later. Most patients will not agree to marital counseling in the beginning, but will after a while.

2. Do not make overt attempts to touch or kiss the patient. Use quick, but tender touches, hugs or kisses and then leave the room or go about your business right away. This will take the pressure off the patient to "perform" and may encourage him to even want more.

3. Finally, realize that the problem is not unresolvable. With counseling and proper treatment, you can enjoy a good sexual relationship again.

Communication Problems

Communication is the everyday exchange of information between and among individuals. Communication can be formal, informal, direct, indirect, written, oral, and even in the form of "body language" (i.e., a particular facial response or body movement that "communicates" to others). Often the complaint is, "We don't communicate anymore." This is generally not the case. The communication may be indirect and not clear, but some form of communication takes place. "Communication problems" become the "catch-all" term for many interpersonal, family, or marital problems. Communication "gaps" and deficiencies can be corrected.

Examples of Communication Problems:

1. A spouse complains, "We never discuss anything anymore."

2. A husband may feel that he has communicated his feelings to his wife, but the communication may have been inadequate and not direct.

3. "Chit-chat" and superficial issues are discussed with ease, but when an emotional issue is discussed, there is an overreaction or avoidance of the topic.

Resolutions for Communication Problems:

1. Be direct with your communication. Say what you mean. That is not to say to be rude or to hurt someone, but simply say what you are trying to communicate in a simple and direct manner.

2. Avoid indirect communication, such as grimaces, slamming doors, sarcasm, "beating around the bush," etc.

3. Practice expressing emotional feelings with someone you trust. Try to translate that experience to other loved ones.

4. Consider a brief community education course on "Enhancing Communication Skills," as available through community mental health centers.

5. Consider family and/or marital counseling to enhance communication in interpersonal relationships.

Problems with the Health Care System

Typically, chronic pain becomes an intense and draining focus with not only the pain patient, but the family member becoming its victim. The pain patient's constant agony and complaints begin to affect everyone. Medications, physicians' bills, and hospitalizations reach the point until they break the family's financial security. Role reversals, the demands for attention, and increased irritable interactions turn to resentment. In turn, the patient begins to resent the family feeling it is "unfair" the way he is being treated. Chronic pain can not only destroy the patient, but can destroy the family as well. It is only normal to see families turning to physicians seeking solutions. The family only experiences further anger and resentment following expensive physician visits, further hospitalizations and numerous diagnostic procedures. The results only leave them further financially strapped and the problems still remain.

It is not surprising that families become unusually intolerant of professionals involved in the process. Emotional clashes increase to great proportions. Family members find themselves affected at their place of employment and often find themselves attempting to salvage home life and business life. Anger, guilt, tension, and apprehension only build. It is not unusual to see families on the verge of divorce.

Despair shifts the course of events to move from visits with physicians to focusing on insurance companies. "How can we pay these bills?" "Doesn't the insurance company pay for things like this?" "Doesn't the insurance company owe us?" These are typical and understandable stages of thinking experienced by now desperate families. However, the families perceive insurance companies as uncooperative. They lose sight of many facts. For just a moment, try to understand that insurance companies focus on attempting to keep people out of hospitals. By this nature, an adversarial situation appears to arise where they are forced to take a position. Additionally, consider for one moment that the monies available to insurance companies must serve a large number of people. The insurance carriers are obligated to protect the rights of many, but for those who should receive it. Everyone cannot receive these services nor can one receive services for prolonged periods of time.

Examples of Problems with the Health Care System: The following statements are often heard

1. "Why won't you pay for a pain management program?"

2. "What do you mean she is not disabled?"

3. "It's too worker's compensation related!"

4. "We have paid our premiums on time and now they won't pay our bills!"

Resolutions for Problems with the Health Care System:

1. Families must understand the insurance carriers and businesses. To make a profit, they must limit the number of hospitalizations, diagnostic procedures, etc.

2. If finances are strained, families might seek the support provided professionally at a community mental health center.

3. Examine carefully your insurance plan. Determine precisely for what you can and cannot be reimbursed.

Loss of Financial Security

The most universal form of stress encountered by pain patients is the tremendous impact on their financial security. It has been estimated that there are 50 million sufferers of arthritis, 25 million migraine sufferers, and seven million Americans who suffer low back pain. Approximately $900 million is spent on over-the-counter analgesic pills, with $100 million spent on aspirin. For individual pain patients, one study at the University of Washington found that as many as 20 to 25 surgical operations were experienced, with many spending more than $25,000 in health services per year. The pain patient and his family become victimized by chronic pain. Medications, hospitalizations, and physicians' bills mount and reach the point of breaking the family's financial security. The pain patient often finds himself unable to contribute to the family any longer, resulting only in leaving the family in further financial despair. Anger, guilt, tension, and apprehension build to intense levels for all family members. Considerable intolerance for any frustrations are experienced. In addition to attempting to salvage family security, family members frequently find themselves attempting to salvage their employment security.

Examples of Loss of Financial Security:

1. The family is irate because the pain patient has been sitting in front of the TV several days per week.

2. The family panics when accumulating hospital bills arrive, especially in relation to lost income.

3. The insurance company refuses to fund the pain patient's hospital expenses.

Resolutions for Loss of Financial Security:

1. Discuss financial arrangements with your insurance carrier and determine the coverage to which you are entitled.

2. Inquire from your local board regarding Medicare and Medicaid benefits.

3. Discuss financial arrangements with a well recognized pain management program. These people have experience with many different insurance carriers and may be able to make arrangements not previously considered.

Gender Differences in Response to Family Member's Pain

Like the gender differences in response to pain by the patients themselves, there are also gender differences in the family member's response to the pain patient. Female family members may tend to expect a male with pain to not complain or be tough. Male family members may tend to expect the female with pain to always complain since they are used to females being better at expressing emotions. The result of these expectations can be a decrease in communication and an increase in misunderstanding and family discord.

Examples of Gender Differences in Response to Family Member's Pain: Not much is known about what specifically goes on as a result of the gender differences because much of the effect is subtle. Interestingly, though, two examples from our experience may shed some light on the form of the problem.

1. A male family member in counseling revealed that he had had it with all his wife's complaints about pain. We were quite surprised because our observations of his wife had not resulted in us viewing her as a complainer. In fact, she was what we term a pain diminisher, meaning that she had more pain than she would talk about. How, then, was the husband's views so different? After several sessions, we discovered that he "inflated" the number of complaints she expressed. He could offer no reason for this exaggeration on his part. Further sessions revealed that he expected her to complain because she was a female and this expectation affected what the actual experience was.

2. In another case, a man who had chronic pain was "trapped" at home while his wife worked. The traditional roles were now reversed and the relationship between them became confused. He was not able to view himself as a man while she was uncomfortable with being in a more dominant position.

Resolutions for Gender Differences in Response to Family Member's Pain:

1. Realize that cultural expectations are learned and are normal in everyone's lives. You will tend to expect the opposite sex to behave a certain way when they may, in fact, behave differently. Chronic pain places a great strain on behavior so it is likely that behavior may not be typical.

2. Open lines of communication so that you do not have to guess at what to expect from each other. Men can cry and express emotions, but usually only when they feel their manhood is not in question. Women can take charge and dominate, but usually only when they are not at risk of losing their female traits.

3. Finally, remember that sex roles can easily be reversed in chronic pain conditions. Do not be afraid when this happens. Seek counseling to understand and deal with it.

4. It might be important to realize that while recommended prescription items may not be paid for, your prescription bill will be considerably reduced if not eliminated following successful completion of a pain management program.

5. Discuss financial arrangements with pain clinic staff. These people have experience with many different insurance carriers and may be able to help you understand your benefits.

6. Inquire from your local board regarding Medicare and Medicaid benefits.

Conclusions

We hope that we have provided you with informative and useable information. In describing these behaviors and offering suggestions for management, we were well aware that some readers might misinterpret and take offense, especially if they are the chronic pain patient. There are always two sides to every story, so we are in the process of developing a manual that is specifically for the patient. If changes are to be made and problem issues resolved, all involved must adapt to the presence of chronic pain. We hope that here we have assisted family members with the present publication. Please remember, however, that you may need a professional to help you modify these procedures to your life or to provide support for you to be consistent in your actions. You can make a difference! You're certainly not alone. Thousands of families like yours have used the concepts presented in this manual and enhanced the quality of their lives with a lot of patience, a little humor, and courage—you will be successful.

Chapter 52

Aggressive Pain Management as an Alternative to Euthanasia for the Terminally Ill Patient

One of the nagging ironies of modern medicine is that while it has enormously extended life spans, it has also stretched out the dying process. In his 1908 book *Science and Immortality* the physician William Osler reported on his study of 486 deaths at Johns Hopkins Hospital in Baltimore. He found that only about one in five of the deceased seemed to be suffering in their final days. For "the great majority," he stated, "death was a sleep and a forgetting."

Of the 2.5 million people who now die in the U.S. annually, roughly two-thirds succumb after protracted struggle with chronic illnesses such as heart disease and cancer. The dying are also increasingly "sequestered" from the rest of society says David Rothman of Columbia University, who is writing a book on the history of death in America. The percentage of deaths occurring in hospitals, nursing homes or other institutions has risen steadily since the 1930s to nearly 80 percent today. And recent research has found that most of those who are conscious while dying feel distress.

Given this situation, it is hardly surprising that euthanasia is winning so many adherents. Polls show that a majority of Americans support the right of patients to receive a lethal overdose from their doctors. Last year a Michigan jury acquitted Jack Kevorkian, alias "Doctor Death," of charges related to his having helped two women kill themselves. Meanwhile, appellate courts in California and New

---

Reprinted with Permission ©1997 by Scientific American, Inc. All rights reserved. From May 1997 issue of Scientific American.

York struck down state prohibitions against physician-assisted suicide. The U.S. Supreme Court is expected to rule this summer (1997) on the constitutionality of such prohibitions.

The issue has riven the health care community. The American Medical Association (AMA), the American Nursing Association, the National Hospice Organization and dozens of other groups have filed briefs with the Supreme Court opposing physician-assisted suicide. Supporters of legalization include the American Medical Student Association, the Coalition of Hospice Professionals, and Marcia Angell, editor of the *New England Journal of Medicine.*

Nevertheless, this dispute masks a deep consensus among health care experts that much can and should be done to improve the care of the dying.

While the media have focused on euthanasia, a diverse collection of physicians groups, foundations, hospitals and other organizations has quietly begun seeking alternative solutions. The avenues being explored include treating physical and psychological distress more aggressively, relaxing restrictions on the use of opioids, educating health care workers and the public about the needs of the terminally ill, and expanding the use of hospices, which emphasize comfort rather than cure.

Some observers draw an analogy between euthanasia and abortion: the ideal situation in each case would be to reduce the need for such drastic solutions. "Even though people disagree on physician-assisted suicide," says Rosemary Gibson of the Robert Wood Johnson Foundation a major supporter of programs addressing the needs of the dying, "they are working together on this."

The Lessons of SUPPORT

The largest investigation to date of the problems posed by end-of-life care is the Study to Understand Prognoses and Preferences for Outcomes and Risks of Treatments. Called SUPPORT, it followed more than 9,000 severely ill patients admitted to five teaching hospitals during the early 1990s. This past January the SUPPORT team published data on 3,357 deceased patients whose final days had been observed by their relatives.

According to the reports of the family members, 40 percent of those patients who were conscious experienced severe pain "most of the time," and more than 25 percent were anxious or depressed. Overall almost two-thirds of the patients "had difficulty tolerating" their condition, the researchers wrote in the *Annals of Internal Medicine.*

Aggressive Pain Management as an Alternative to Euthanasia

On the other hand, the study contradicted the widespread belief that tyrannical physicians are keeping many patients alive against their will. Nine out of 10 patients approved of their medical treatment, even invasive procedures that seemed contrary to desires indicated in living wills and other "advanced directives."

None of the patients requested or received lethal overdoses of drugs, at least to the knowledge of the researchers. "It is very rare for people this sick to be looking to die faster than they have to," says Joanne Lynn, the lead author of the paper and head of the Center to Improve Care of the Dying at George Washington University.

The tendency of even extremely ill patients to cling to life makes sense, Lynn adds, given the intractable uncertainties of medical prognoses. In a recent paper in the *Duquesne Law Review,* the SUPPORT group notes that of those subjects with congestive heart failure, the second most common cause of death (after cancer) in the U.S., 28 percent who were expected to live less than six months survived for at least another year.

Although predictions for cancer patients were more accurate, 13 percent of the lung cancer patients with prognoses of less than six months survived a year or more. Conversely, after examining prognoses calculated by a statistical model from the day before patients actually died, the researchers found that 17 percent were expected to live for at least two more months and 7 percent for six months.

Expanding Hospice Care

Lynn thinks it is inappropriate to legalize assisted suicide when so little effort has been expended on exploring alternatives. "Having been involved with some wonderful hospices and nursing homes," she says, "I'm very impressed with what can be achieved with relatively modest investments." Indeed, many experts consider the most successful model for the delivery of palliative care to be hospices, which are often termed "the gold standard in care of the dying." Only a few decades old, the hospice concept involves providing comfort—including medical, psychological, social and even spiritual services—for those beyond cure and approaching death.

Since 1985, two years after the federal Medicare program began covering hospice care for people expected by physicians to live less than six months, the number of hospice providers in the U.S. has surged from 500 to more than 2,500. Some 400,000 patients—about one sixth of all those dying—now receive some hospice care every year in the U.S., according to the National Hospice Organization, based in

Arlington, VA. More than 80 percent must be served in their homes, under the terms of the Medicare legislation; the rest are in hospitals, nursing homes, or facilities dedicated to hospice care.

Studies have estimated the median duration of hospice care at just over one month. Medicare provides hospice coverage for indefinite periods, but payments lasting much more than six months are reviewed; Medicare officials can retroactively deny payment or require co-payment for patients whose prognoses are deemed to have been too positive.

Most hospice patients are dying of cancer, though all increasing number are afflicted with AIDS. John J. Mahoney, president of the National Hospice Organization, says many more people should be eligible for hospice treatment, and they should be admitted at earlier stages in their disease.

Hospice care is also economical, according to Mahoney. A 1995 study sponsored by the hospice organization examined records of all Medicare beneficiaries who died of cancer in 1992. The investigation—which was not controlled for independent variables—found that Medicare spent almost 50 percent less on hospice patients during their last month of life than on those receiving standard care. Medicare currently spends well over $1 trillion annually on hospice reimbursements, and the average daily cost for individual patients is about $100, roughly the same as for nursing home care.

The effort to expand the hospice population has run into a roadblock recently as a result of an investigation by the U.S. Department of Health and Human Services, which oversees Medicare. Last year department inspectors charged hospices in Puerto Rico, Florida and elsewhere with admitting patients who were not terminally ill and thus not eligible for Medicare funding; some patients had allegedly remained at hospices for three or four years. Mahoney fears that the accusations, which have been disputed, will make doctors and hospices even more conservative in deciding when patients should he enrolled in hospice care.

Combating Pain

One possible solution to this problem—proposed by Lynn of the Center to Improve Care of the Dying—is a program called MediCaring. It is intended to extend hospice-like services to patients who have incurable diseases but do not qualify for hospice care because they have unpredictable conditions or are expected to live longer than Medicare guidelines allow. Unlike hospice patients, participants in MediCaring would in some cases be eligible for aggressive, expensive treatments such as

Aggressive Pain Management as an Alternative to Euthanasia

chemotherapy, bone marrow transplants and surgery, although access to such treatments would be restricted. Pilot projects employing MediCaring approaches are now under way in four states and the District of Columbia.

All patients, not just those in hospices, should be able to receive expert palliative care, according to Kathleen M. Foley of the Memorial Sloan-Kettering Cancer Center in New York City. An authority on the treatment of pain, Foley is also director of the Project on Death in America. Created by the investor and philanthropist George Soros in 1994, the New York-based project has already dispensed more than $15 million for programs on death and dying. They range from studies of how different ethnic groups view death to an initiative of the United Hospital Fund to improve end-of-life care at 12 New York hospitals.

Foley opposes legalizing physician-assisted suicide, which she denigrates as "treating suffering by eliminating the sufferer." In the course of her career, she says, she has repeatedly encountered patients who asked to be put out of their misery. In almost every case, she says, the requests abated after the patients had received supportive care, including analgesics, antidepressants or counseling.

There have been enormous advances in the management of pain, Foley asserts. Drugs can be delivered through skin patches, topical creams and implanted pumps as well as intravenously. New automated delivery systems, which measure levels of medication in the blood, can stop pain before it starts while minimizing side effects such as nausea, grogginess and constipation. Too few health care professionals, Foley adds, are integrating these advances into practice—in large part because they have not been trained to view end-of-life care as an important part of medicine. Searching the medical literature for articles on "death," she notes, will yield more articles on cell death than on human death.

Foley advocates making pain a "vital sign" that is monitored along with other important parameters of health by nurses and physicians. Pain should also be treated as early as possible in the trajectory of a disease, according to Neil MacDonald, an oncologist at the Clinical Research Institute of Montreal. "Preventing a problem is preferable to reacting to it," he states. Recent animal studies, he says, reveal that chronic pain can alter the central nervous system, making the discomfort more severe and intractable through a "kindling effect."

Clinical observations, MacDonald notes, suggest that the seriously ill may also become trapped in a vicious cycle of intensifying distress. Chronic pain often becomes more severe over time, he explains, leading to psychological distress that in turn makes the physical pain harder to endure. In the same way, shortness of breath, which is common among the dying, may trigger panic that exacerbates the breathing problem.

Major obstacles to proper treatment of pain, MacDonald points out, are the laws and social attitudes that hinder prescriptions of analgesics—and opioids such as morphine in particular. This problem is being addressed by the Pain and Policy Studies Group at the University of Wisconsin. In 1991 the researchers surveyed state medical boards—which monitor prescriptions of drugs and discipline physicians deemed to be overprescribing—on their attitudes about painkillers. The survey determined that board members had too little appreciation of the importance of pain management and excessive anxiety about the dangers of addiction. Many members wrongly equated addiction with physical dependency on a drug, says David E. Joranson, head of the study group. In fact, Joranson explains, addiction is a psychological condition characterized by obsessive craving. Many patients become physically dependent on opioids—requiring increased doses to bring about the same effect and displaying withdrawal symptoms when medication ceases—but psychological addiction is rare.

The researchers have held six workshops to educate medical board members in different states about the importance of pain treatment and the true risks of opioids. They plan to conduct a second survey of state medical boards in 1999 to determine how much the boards' attitudes and practices have changed. The Wisconsin investigators are also working with the World Health Organization and other groups to reform international regulations hampering the prescription of opioids for pain treatment.

Physicians, Educate Yourselves

This summer the American Medical Association plans to launch a program to educate physicians about palliative care.

Spearheading the program is Linda L. Emanuel, director of the AMA's Institute for Ethics. Emanuel was the primary author of the brief opposing physician-assisted suicide that the AMA submitted to the Supreme Court. In her past 12 years as an internist, she says, only two patients have asked her to kill them; both changed their minds after she made it clear that they had other options for treating their distress.

Nevertheless, "the need to improve things is enormous," Emanuel says. The AMA educational project, she explains, will encourage physicians to discuss patients' attitudes toward dying in advance of terminal illness

Aggressive Pain Management as an Alternative to Euthanasia

and to learn how to treat common afflictions of the severely ill, including pain, bedsores, incontinence, depression and psychosis.

During the program's first phase, panels of experts will discuss palliative care and other issues with health care leaders from many states at a few large, regional conferences; those meetings will be followed by many smaller assemblages for separate states and communities. "We hope to directly train about half of all physicians" in the U.S. "and indirectly reach all the others," Emanuel says. The goal, she adds, is to "change the culture of medicine."

The Faculty Scholars Program could be another instrument of change. Funded by the Project on Death in America, it provides fellowships of up to $70,000 a year to "outstanding clinicians and academic leaders who want to make a career-level commitment to care of the dying," says Susan Block of Harvard Medical School, director of the program. Twenty-six scholars have already been chosen, and 10 more selections are pending.

Scholars are pursuing a variety of projects. These include revamping curricula for medical schools and residency programs and developing new models of service delivery, such as one in which teams of clinicians provide hospice-like care for terminally ill patients in hospitals. Such units have already been established at Massachusetts General Hospital, Sloan-Kettering and elsewhere.

Unlike Emanuel, Foley and others who oppose physician-assisted suicide, Block believes that for a very small number of people it may be the best way to die "on their own terms." Block nonetheless agonizes over whether such acts should be legalized. "I can't find a stance that feels right," she remarks. "I can't say it's always wrong, but I am afraid of what might happen with legalization." Moreover, she adds, "the vast majority of patients who want physician-assisted suicide have problems like depression that we can help them with."

But changing the practice of medicine is not enough, according to Ira Byock, a veteran hospice physician based in Missoula, Mont., and president of the American Academy of Hospice and Palliative Medicine. Several years ago, Byock created the Missoula Demonstration Project to identify new solutions to end of-life care. Although dying patients must receive competent medical care, Byock says, "this is too important to be left to the medical experts. We are exploring nonmedical ways to support patients and their families."

One goal of the project—which is supported by the Robert Wood Johnson Foundation, the Pioneer on Death in America and other foundations—is to create what Byock calls a "very detailed, high-definition snapshot" of death and dying in Missoula. The study will compile information on all the deaths occurring within Missoula, including medical histories of the deceased and surveys of the attitudes of surviving family members. The project will also sponsor discussions in churches, schools and workplaces with the goal of finding innovative ways to make death less agonizing.

Premortem Eulogies

Possibilities under consideration are training volunteers to spend time with terminally ill people; allowing dying patients to express themselves through art or by recording their life histories for a permanent archive; combining child care facilities with hospices so that the very young and very old can mingle; using pets to raise patients' spirits; having choirs of neighbors sing songs outside the homes of the dying; having friends and relatives give eulogies to a dying person before death.

Researchers will then track how attitudes and behaviors change over time. Comparison of Missoula to a control population in Pocatello, Idaho, will help determine if any of the interventions is working. Byock hopes the project will become a model for similar one across the country. Eventually, the project may do for end-of-life care what the more famous Framingham Heart Study—which for almost half a century has tracked the habits and cardiac histories of the residents of Framingham, Mass.—has done for the treatment of heart disease.

The problems posed by caring for those near death will surely become more pressing as society ages. The percentage of the U.S. population age 85 or older is expected to grow from just over 1 percent, its current level, to 5 percent by the middle of the next century, according to the Alliance for Aging Research, a nonprofit group in Washington, D.C. Several studies nearing completion should inject more data into the discussion of end-of-life care. The Institute of Medicine, a branch of the National Academy of Sciences, has been examining the issue for more than three years and is expected to publish a major report on the subject this summer.

A group led by Diane E. Meier of the Mount Sinai Medical Center is just about to make public the largest survey to date of physicians' attitudes toward assisted suicide and related issues. The preliminary data suggests that doctors with the most experience prescribing lethal doses of drugs to patients tend to be more comfortable with their decisions. Meier finds that tentative result disturbing. Ideally, she says, physicians committing such acts would never "get over their fear and trembling."

Aggressive Pain Management as an Alternative to Euthanasia

Many health care workers have already privately admitted to having helped patients die. According to a report in the May 23, 1996, issue of the *New England Journal of Medicine,* 20 percent of a group of 850 nurses working in intensive care units acknowledged having deliberately hastened the death of a patient. A survey of 118 San Francisco-based doctors, published in the *New England Journal of Medicine* this past February, found that half had prescribed lethal doses of drugs to patients suffering from AIDS.

Such acts are likely to become still more common if the Supreme Court rules in favor of physician-assisted suicide this summer. Sloan-Kettering's Foley contends that, given its lack of knowledge about palliative care, the medical profession is simply not prepared for such a responsibility. "Doctors don't know enough to kill," she declares.

—by John Horgan, staff writer.

Part Seven

Pain Resources

Chapter 53

Finding Help

Helpful Sources of Information on General Pain:

Organizations

American Academy of Pain Medicine
4700 West Lake Avenue
Glenview IL 60025-1485
(847) 375-4731, fax (847) 375-4777
e-mail aapm@dial.cic.net

American Pain Society
4700 West Lake Avenue
Glenview, IL 60025-1485
(847) 375-4715, fax (847) 375-4777

American Chronic Pain Association
National Office
P.O. Box 850
Rocklin, CA 95677
(916) 632-0922, fax: (916)632-3208

HDI Publishers
PO Box 131401
Houston, TX 77219
(800) 32-7037, fax (713) 956-2288

International Association for the Study of Pain
909 NE 43rd Street,
Suite 306
Seattle, WA 98105
(206) 547-6409

Mayday Pain Resource Center
City of Hope National Medical Center
1500 East Duarte Road
Duarte, CA 91010
Phone (818) 359-8111 Ext 3829, fax (818) 301-8941

National Chronic Pain Outreach Association
7979 Old Georgetown Road,
Suite 100
Bethesda, MD 20814-2429
(301) 652-4948, fax (301) 907-0745

Pain Clinics

While there is no official certifying agency accrediting pain clinics throughout the country, there are many excellent clinics, often affiliated with university-associated medical centers. Your family doctor or university medical center may be able to refer you to reputable clinics nearby. If not, physicians can request a worldwide pain clinic directory published by:

American Society of Anesthesiologists
515 Busse Highway
Park Ridge, IL 60068

To find an accredited pain treatment center nearby, you may write:

The Commission on Accreditation of Rehabilitation Facilities,
101 N. Wilmot Rd., Suite 500,
Tucson, AZ 85711

Selected Publications

Living with Chronic Pain: Personal Experiences of Pain Sufferers, by Laura S. Hitchcock, Ph.D., National Chronic Pain Outreach Association.

Finding Help

Pain: Making Life Liveable, by Dana S. DeBoskey, Ph. D., HDI Publishers.

Principles of Analgesic Use in the Treatment of Acute Pain and Cancer Pain, American Pain Society.

Helpful Sources of Information on Back Pain

Organizations

Agency for Health Care Policy and Research
Publications Clearinghouse
P.O. Box 8547
Silver Spring, MD 20907
800-358-9265

American Osteopathic Association
142 E Ontario St.
Chicago, IL 60611
(800) 621-1773

American Congress of Rehabilitation Medicine
5700 Old Orchard Rd.
1st floor.
Skokie, IL 60077-1057
(708)966-0095

American Red Cross
430 17th St. N.W
Washington, DC 20005
(202) 789-5600, fax (202) 639-3711

American College of Occupational and Environmental Medicine
55 W. Seegers Rd.
Arlington Heights, IL 60005-3919
(708) 228-6850

American Academy of Orthopaedic Surgeons
6300 N. River Rd.
Rosemont, IL 60018-4262
(708) 823-7186

American Academy of Physical Medicine and Rehabilitation (AAPMR)
IBM Plaza, Suite 2500
Chicago, IL 60611-3604
(312) 464-9700

Physiatric Association of Spine, Sports and Occupational Rehabilitation (PASSOR).
IBM Plaza, Suite 2500
Chicago, IL 60611-3604
(312) 464-9700

Selected Publications

Acute Low Back Problems in Adults: Assessment and Treatment
Department of Health and Human Services AHCPR Publications
Clearinghouse Box 8547
Silver Spring, MD 20907-8547
(800) 358-9295 (voice mail, 24 hours a day)
This and all other AHCPR Clinical Practice Guidelines are also available online through the National Library of Medicine (Health Services/Technology Assessment Text).

American Medical Association Pocket Guide to Back Pain
This 80-page minibook discusses the anatomy of the back, offers tips on preventing injury, and describes back problems ranging from muscle aches and pains to trauma, infections, and other disorders. $4.99. For information on bulk discounts, write to Special Markets, Random House, Inc., 201 E 50th St.. New York. NY 10022.

Back in Action: A Guide to Understanding Your Low-Back Pain and Learning What You Can Do About It
A brochure published by the Group Health Cooperative of Puget Sound, University of Washington Schools of Medicine and Public Health, and Seattle Veterans Affairs Medical Center. It can be ordered through the AHCPR Clearinghouse.

Good News for Bad Backs
Robert L. Swezey, MD, and Annette M. Swezey. Published in 1993 by Cequal Publishing Co., 1328 Sixteenth St., Santa Monica, CA 90404. A video by Dr. Swezey titled "No More Back Pain" is also available.

Finding Help

Helpful Sources of Information on Headache:

Organizations

American Council on Headache Education (ACHE)
875 Kings Highway
Suite 200
Woodbury, NJ 08096-3172
(609) 384-8760, fax (609) 384-5811
toll free 1-800-255-ACHE

American Association for the Study of Headache (AASH)
875 Kings Highway
Suite 200
Woodbury, NJ 08096-3172
(609) 384-384-5811

National Headache Foundation (NHF)
5252 N. Western Ave.
Chicago, IL 60625
Telephone (1-800) 843-2256
NHF offers a list of headache clinics and a state list of National Headache Foundation physician members interested in treating headache.

Neurology Institute
P.O. Box 5801
Bethesda, MD 20824
Telephone (1-800) 352-9424

Selected Publications

Headache and Diet: Tyramine-free Recipes, by Seymour Diamond, M.D., National Headache Foundation:
A 172-page spiral-bound book, this resource contains recipes for soups, salads, appetizers, entrees, beverages, and desserts. Additional information about headache causes and treatments is also included.

Migraine: The Complete Guide, by Lynne M. Constantine and Suzanne Scott, the American Council on Headache Education. A 1994 Dell Trade Paperback:
Based on the best information available including medical research, clinical experience of leading experts, and personal stories from those afflicted with migraines.

No More Headaches, National Headache Foundation:
Developed to educate consumers on causes and triggers of headache as well as effective diagnostic procedures, this 37 minute video tape provides solutions to for relief of pain and nausea, discusses new treatments and offers suggestions on how to change daily habits to prevent or abort headaches.

Relief from Migraine, video by Drs. J. Keith Campbell, Neil Raskin, and Joel Saper, American Association for the Study of Headache:
This video offers a fresh and innovative look at current theory on migraine, insights from patients, and the role of new and existing treatment therapies. Aired originally on American Medical Television.

Stretch and Relax Tape, National Headache Foundation:
This audio tape is based on a series of progressive relaxation techniques which involve the tightening and relaxing of specific muscle groups. It also contains guided visualization and imagery in two exercises: a thirty-minute program and a fifteen-minute session.

The Relaxation Tape, National Headache Foundation:
This audio tape contains techniques to assist the listener in experiencing greater self control and relaxation. The tape is narrated by a physical therapist, and is broken down into two exercises: a thirty-minute program and a fifteen-minute "Bus Stop" exercise.

Helpful Information on Nerve and Muscle Pain:

American Chronic Pain Association
P.O. Box 850
Rocklin, CA 95677
(916) 632-0922

Bell's Palsy Research Foundation
9121 E. Tanque Verde, Suite 105-286
Tucson, AZ 85749
(520) 749-4614

National Chronic Pain Outreach Association
7979 Old Georgetown Road
Suite 100
Bethesda, MD 20814-2429
(301) 652-4948

Finding Help

National Rehabilitation Information Center (NARIC)
Macro Systems-Suite 935
8455 Colesville Road
Silver Spring, MD 20910-3319
(301) 588-9284
(800) 346-2742
TTY (301) 495-5626
FAX (301) 587-1967
http://www.naric.com/naric

Office of Scientific and Health Reports
National Institute of Neurological Disorders and Stroke
Building 31, Room 8A06
National Institutes of Health
9000 Rockville Pike
Bethesda, MD 20892
(301) 496-5751

Trigeminal Neuralgia Association.
PO Box 340
Baranegat Light, NJ 08006
(609) 361-1014, fax (609) 361-0982

Massachusetts General Hospital
Neurosurgical Service
Fruit Street
Boston, MA 02114
617-726-2000 (main switchboard)

REPETITIVE STRESS DISORDERS

Arthritis Foundation
1330 Peachtree St.
Atlanta, GA 30309
(404) 872-7100, fax (512) 872-0457
WWW: http://www.arthritis.org
Arthritis Foundation's 24-hour National Hotline at (800) 283-7800.

Carpal Tunnel Syndrome/RSI Association
PO Box 514
Santa Rosa, CA 95402
(707) 571-0397

National Institute of Occupational Safety and Health
Mail Stop C13
4676 Columbia Parkway
Cincinnati, OH 45226-1998
(513) 533-8287
(800) 356-4674.

Occupational Safety and Health Administration
U.S. Department of Labor
200 Constitution Avenue, N.W.
Washington, DC 20210
(202) 219-4667 (Publications Office)

Safety and Health Assessment and Research for Prevention
Washington State Department of Labor and Industries
PO Box 44330
Olympia WA 98504-4330
(206) 956-5669

Helpful Sources of Information on Cancer Pain

Organizations

American Cancer Society, Inc.
1599 Clifton Road, N.E.
Atlanta, GA 30329-4251
1-800-ACS-2345

The American Cancer Society (ACS) is a national nonprofit organization whose programs include research, education, and service. Local ACS Units offer service programs for cancer patients and their families. They provide information and guidance, referral to community health services and other resources, equipment loans for care of the homebound patient, transportation to and from treatment, and rehabilitation programs. Before contacting national headquarters, check your local telephone directory for an ACS Unit in your community.
Two mutual support programs, which began as grassroots efforts, have been designated as national programs of the American Cancer Society. Check to see if they are available in your community.

CanSurmount: CanSurmount brings together the patient, the family, the CanSurmount volunteer, and health professionals. On physician

Finding Help

referral, a trained CanSurmount volunteer, who is also a cancer patient, meets with the patient and family in the hospital or home. The goal of the program is to improve mutual help and understanding through continuing education and support for volunteers, patients, families, health professionals, and the community.

I Can Cope: This program addresses the educational and psychological needs of people with cancer and their families. It is a series of classes covering information about cancer, types of treatments, communication with family, friends, and physicians and how to find additional resources. Through lectures, group discussions, and study assignments, the course helps people with cancer regain a sense of control over their lives.

For further information about CanSurmount and I Can Cope, contact your local Unit of the American Cancer Society.

National Cancer Institute
Office of Cancer Communications
Building 31, Room 10A24
Bethesda, MD 20892

The National Cancer Institute (NCI) is the US government's main agency for cancer research and information about cancer. Additional information about pain control and other cancer-related topics is available from the NCI-supported Cancer Information Service (CIS), a nationwide telephone service that answers questions from cancer patients and their families, health care professionals, and the public. Information specialists can provide information and publications on all aspects of cancer.
The toll-free number of the CIS is 1-800-4-CANCER.
You will reach a CIS office serving your area where a trained staff member can answer your questions and listen to your concerns. Spanish-speaking staff members are available.

If you have difficulty locating a pain program or specialist, contact a cancer center, a hospice, or the oncology department at your local hospital or a medical center. The following sources can provide names of pain specialists, pain clinics, or programs in your area:

The Cancer Information Service (CIS). Supported by the National Cancer Institute, is a nationwide telephone service that answers questions from cancer patients and their families, health care professionals, and the public. At the CIS, health information specialists provide information and publications on all aspects of cancer, including pain control. They can give you information about clinical trials (research studies) that are open to patients and that test new and promising treatments for cancer and cancer pain. They also may know about cancer-related services in local areas. By dialing 1-800-4-CANCER (1-800-422-6237), you will reach a CIS office serving your area. A trained staff member will answer your questions and listen to your concerns. Spanish-speaking staff members are available.

Selected Publications

Management of Cancer Pain: Adult Patient's Guide; National Cancer Institute (NCI) 800-4-CANCER.

You Don't Have to Suffer (Oxford University Press, 1994). by Susan S. Lang and Richard Patt, M.D.

Additional patient education materials (including information about diet and nutrition, chemotherapy, radiation therapy, emotional support, and the symptoms and treatment of many types of cancer) are available free of charge from both the American Cancer Society and the National Cancer Institute.

Helpful Sources of Information on Surgical Pain

American Academy of Orthopaedic Surgeons
6300 N River Rd
Rosemont, IL 60018
(847) 823-7186, fax (847) 823-8125
e-mail custserv@aaos.org

American Orthotic and Prosthetic Association
Orthotics & Prosthetics National Office
1650 King Street, Suite 500
Alexandria, Virginia 22314
(703) 836-7114/6/8 fax (703) 836-0838

Finding Help

American Society of Anesthesiologists
Pain Therapy Committee
515 Busse Highway
Park Ridge, IL 60068
(708) 825-5586

Commission on Accreditation of Rehabilitation Facilities
101 North Wilmot Road,
Suite 500
Tucson, AZ 85711
(602) 748-1212

Duke University Medical Center
Department of Prosthetics and Orthotics
MO4 Davison Building
PO Box 3885
Durham, NC 27710
(919) 684-2474 fax (919) 681-8496

Selected Publications

Pain Control after Surgery: Patient's Guide, AHCPR, 800 358-9295.

For the New Amputee, Duke University Medical Center

Selected Resources on the Internet

American Academy of Neurology
http://www.aan.com

American Academy of Orthopaedic Surgeons
http://www.aaos.org

American Association of Suicidology
http://www.cyberpsych.org/aas.htm

American Cancer Society
http://www.cancer.org

American Chiropractic OnLine (ACA OnLine).
http://www.cais.net/aca/

American College of Sports Medicine
http://www.acsm.org/sportsmed

American Dental Association
http://www.ada.org

American Red Cross
http://crossnet.org

Arthritis Foundation
http://www.arthritis.org

Centers for Disease Control and Prevention
http://www.cdc.gov

City of Hope National Medical Center
http://www.cityofhope.org

Duke University Medical Center
http://www.mc.duke.edu

International Association for the Study of Pain
http://weber.u.washington.edu/~crc/IASP.html

IVI Publishing's OnHealth
http://www.healthnet.ivi.com/onhealth/common/htm/index.htm

Mayo Clinic
http://www.mayo.edu

National Headache Foundation
http://webcrawler.com/select/genmed.20.html

National Health Information Center
http://nhic-nt.health.org

National Institutes of Health
http://www.nih.gov/home.html
http://consensus.nih.gov

National Library of Medicine
http://www.nlm.nih.gov

National Organization for Rare Disorders, Inc.
http://www.stepstn.com/nord/rdb_sum

University of Massachusetts Medical Center
http://www.ummed.edu

U.S. Department of Health and Human Services
http://www.os.dhs.gov

Index

Index

Page numbers in *italics* refer to figures; the letter n after a page number denotes a note.

A

Abbott, F. V. 269, 283, 296, 300, 350, 360
abdominal aortic aneurysm, low back pain and 158
abdominal pain, medical emergency and 14
Abrass, I. B. 320, 322, 351
Absi, E. G. 280, 356
acebutolol 510
acetaminophen 10, 86–97
  for acute low back pain 167
  for cancer pain 410–11, 413
  for dental surgery 292
  for everyday aches and pains 465–66
  for headaches 91, 121
  for infants 318
  for menstrual cramps 258
  for postoperative pain 280
  safe dosages of 413
  see also Tylenol
acid indigestion 503
acid stomach 503
Acta Anaesthiologica Scandinavica 345, 348, 349, 351, 357
Acta Chiurgica Scandinavica 359, 360
Acta Obstetrica Gynecologica Scandinavica 347
Acta Orthopaedica Belgica 353
acupuncture 454–55
  for arthritis pain 51
  and cancer pain 436
  defined 362
  low back pain problems and 178
  pain relief and 11
  as pain therapy 37–38
acupuncture points *38*
acute low back pain 165, 167–68
  see also back pain; low back pain
Acute Low Back Pain in Adults: Assessment and Treatment 620
acute low back problems 173–82
  see also back pain; low back pain
Acute Low Back Problems in Adults: Assessment and Treatment 169
acute pain
  assessment and measurement of 55–65, 450, 451
  cancer and 398
  control of 9, 471–72

acute pain, continued
  described 6, 31
  integrated approach to 452–53
  management of 263–381
    responsibility for 335–37
  treatment therapies for 16–17
Acute Pain Management: Operative or Medical Procedures and Trauma Guidelines Report 369, 371
Acute Pain Management Guideline Panel (1992) 55–56, 57, 64, 65, 337
Adams, J. 305, 339
Adams, S. 307, 347
addictions 467–68
  to morphine 21, 525
    misconceptions about 26
  to narcotics 417
  to pain 7–9
  terminal illnesses and 610
adjuvant, described 117
adolescents 548
  back pain and 158–59
  menstrual pain and 253–54
  postoperative pain management and 300
adrenaline 34
  see also epinephrine
Advil 83, 219, 258, 410, 481
  see also ibuprofen; nonsteroidal anti-inflammatory drugs
aerobic exercise
  acute low back pain and 167
  endorphin stimulation and 5
  for fibromyalgia 210
  pain relief and 13
age factor
  degenerative conditions and 142
  low back pain and 156
  plantar fasciitis and 242
  spinal stenosis and 235
  tic douloureux and 195
Agency for Health Care Policy and Research (AHCPR) 56, 366, 531–32
  Clinical Practice Guideline for Acute Pain Management 264
  Clinical Practice Guidelines 150, 152, 159–60, 161, 162, 163, 167, 169, 182

Agency for Health Care Policy and Research (AHCPR), continued
  guidelines 185
  panels 159
  publications 65, 66, 171, 173n, 347, 369, 371, 397n, 407n, 425n
  publications clearinghouse 619
AHCPR *see* Agency for Health Care Policy and Research (AHCPR)
alarm clock headache *see* cluster headaches
Alberts, Fred L., PhD 549
alcohol use 580–83
  antacids and 501
  aspirin and 412
  cancer pain and 435
  nonsteroidal anti-inflammatory drugs and 486
Aleve 481
  see also naproxen sodium; nonsteroidal anti-inflammatory drugs
Alexander, J. I. 283, 339
Alexander, L. L. 313, 356
Alka-2 505
Alka-Seltzer 505
Alksne, John, MD 201–2
Allen, D. A. 301, 357
Alliance for Aging Research 612
Alloza, J. L. 267, 359
AlternaGEL 505
Altimier, L. 56, 66
Altman, A. 306, 309, 311, 361
Ambien 112–13
Ambrosio, F. 290, 345
American Academy of Hospice and Palliative Medicine 611, 612
American Academy of Orthopaedic Surgeons 170, 619, 626
American Academy of Pain Medicine 405, 442, 617
American Academy of Pediatrics 310, 339, 361
American Academy of Physical Medicine and Rehabilitation 170, 620
American Association for the Study of Headache (AASH) 101–2, 103, 108–9, 621
American Association of Anesthesiologists 54

Index

American Cancer Society 402, 405, 441, 624, 625
  publications 397n, 407n, 425n
American Chiropractic Association 185
American Chiropractic OnLine 183n
American Chronic Pain Association 53, 215, 451n, 464, 617, 622
American College of Occupational and Environmental Medicine 170, 619
American College of Rheumatology 209, 210
American Congress of Rehabilitation Medicine 170, 619
American Council for Headache Education (ACHE) 96, 101, 102, 108–9, 621
  publications 93n, 115n
    Headache 75n, 95n, 101n, 131n
American Family Physician 135
American Journal of Chinese Medicine 345
American Journal of Clinical Hypnosis 344
American Journal of Nursing 359
American Journal of Ophthalmology 350
American Journal of Orthopsychiatry 345
American Journal of Pediatric Hematology and Oncology 355
American Journal of Sports Medicine 343, 350, 358
The American Journal of Surgery 343, 352, 359
American Medical Association (AMA) 606
American Medical Association Institute of Ethics 610
American Medical Association Pocket Guide to Back Pain 170, 186, 620
American Medical Student Association 606
American Nurses Association 268, 340
American Nursing Association 606
American Orthotic and Prosthetic Association 626

American Osteopathic Association 171, 619
American Pain Society 29, 33, 268, 269–70, 274, 278, 335, 340, 405, 442, 462, 617
American Physical Therapy Association 24
American Red Cross 171, 619
American Society of Anesthesiologists 386, 405, 442, 618, 627
Amidon, Gordon, PhD 512, 513
Amidrin 86
Amiel-Tison, C. 304, 341
amitriptyline (Elavil) 10, 113, 544
Amphogel 505
amputation
  for leg cramps 232
  phantom pain and 7, 51
  postoperative pain and 383
Anacin 410
  see also aspirin; nonsteroidal anti-inflammatory drugs
Anaesthesia 340, 342, 344, 349, 351, 355, 356
Anaesthesia and Intensive Care 342, 352, 356
analgesics 10, 548
  described 407
  forms of 279
  for menstrual pain 255
  for migraine headaches 83
  see also over-the-counter drugs; patient-controlled analgesia; prescription medications
Anand, K. 310, 340
Anand, K. J. 269, 310, 313, 340
Andersen, K. H. 312, 340
Anderson, J. E. 301, 314–15, 345
Andolsek, K. 311, 340
anesthesia
  safety factors and 385–87
  during surgery 279
Anesthesia and Analgesia 341, 342, 343, 344, 351, 352, 354
Anesthesiology 344, 348, 352, 353, 354, 356, 358, 359, 360
Anesthesiology Clinics of North America 355

Ang, M. 281, 354
Angel, A. 290, 345
Angell, Marcia 606
angina pectoris 507, 513
 see also chest pain
angioplasty, for leg cramps 232–33
animal studies
 nociceptin and 70–71
 thermal angioplasty and 233
Annals of Internal Medicine 171, 353, 359, 606
Annals of Neurology 350
Annals of the Royal College of Surgeons of England 343
Annals of Thoracic Surgery 356, 359, 360
Anscombe, A. R. 267, 341
antacid medication 499–506
anti-anxiety medications 424
anti-convulsant medications
 for cancer pain 424
 as chronic nerve pain relieving medication 10
 tic douloureux and 196
anti-depressant medications 10, 24, 544
 for cancer pain 424
 for fibromyalgia 210
 for pain 43
 serotonin and 75
 for tension-type headaches 91
anti-epileptic medications 43–44
anti-migraine medications 83
anxiety 570–72
 cancer pain and 402
 dental surgery and 291
 postoperative pain and 286–87
 tension-type headaches and 80, 85, 89
 see also emotions
anxiolysis, defined 362
aortic bypass 297
APLD *see* aspiration percutaneous lumbar diskectomy (APLD)
Applied Neurophysiology 347
Applied Nursing Research 343
Aradine, C. R. 303, 341
Archives of Internal Medicine 344

Archives of Pediatric and Adolescent Medicine 171
Archives of Surgery 358
arm pain 14–15, 213
Armstrong, P. J. 329, 341
Arneson, S. W. 311, 359
Aro, X. 171
Arora, M. K. 298, 343
arteriosclerosis, leg cramps and 231
arteritis, leg cramps and 231
arthritis
 back pain and 142
 hand problems and 219–21
 low back pain and 151
 treatment for
  omega-3 fatty acids 219
"Arthritis: Modern Treatment for that Old Pain in the Joints" 219
Arthritis and Rheumatism 345
Arthritis Foundation 221, 623
arthritis pain
 chronic pain and 32
 medication for 11
 treatment for 9–10, 50–51
Arthritis Sourcebook 219
artificial sweeteners, headaches and 116–17
Ascriptin 410
Ashley, L. C. 301, 342
as needed doses of medication
 versus around-the-clock (atc) doses 27, 278, 283
 described 8
aspiration percutaneous lumbar diskectomy (APLD) 146
aspirin 10, 477–79, 488–98
 for arthritis 50, 219
 for cancer pain 410–14
 for dental surgery 292
 for everyday aches and pains 465–66
 for headaches 91, 121
 for knee pain 240
 for low back pain 151, 167
 for migraine headaches 83
 for pain relief 42, 77
 for repetitive strain injuries 223
 safe dosages of 413

Index

"Aspirin: A New Look at an Old
　Drug" 477
*Association of Operating Room
　Nurses Journal* 350
asthenopia (tired eyes) 98
Atarax 424
Atchison, N. E. 330, 331, 341
atenolol 507, 510
atherosclerosis, eye pain and 99
athletes
　back pain and 158–59
　reports of little pain from 77
　see also sports injuries
Ativan 112, 424
Atkinson, J. H. 64, 66
atrophied muscles, chronic pain and 24
Attia, J. 304, 341
audiotapes
　The Relaxation Tape 622
　Stretch and Relax 622
aura *see* migraine aura; migraine headaches
autogenic training 529
autonomic nervous system
　biofeedback and 12
　described 34
　pain signals and 5
　sympathetic nerves of
　surgical treatment of 47
Aynsley-Green, A. 269, 310, 313, 340

B

Bach, S. 269, 299, 341
Back and Neck Disorders Sourcebook 186
Back in Action 182
Back in Action: A Guide to Understanding Your Low-Back Pain and Learning What You Can Do About It 169, 620
back muscles *174*
back pain
　causes of 135–37
　information sources for 619–20
　see also low back pain
back supports, for spinal stenosis 237

back surgery 298–99
　see also surgery
baclofen 194, 196
Bagge, L. 300, 354
Bains, M. 289, 356
Balduc, Howard, DC 185
Balestrieri, Francis, MD 468
balloon angioplasty, for leg cramps 232
Banning, A. 294, 358
barbiturates 309
Barcus, C. S. 302, 348
Barlow, W. 171
Barrier, G. 304, 341
Bartlett, M. K. 270, 286, 344
Bartlett, R. H. 269, 342
Bartoszek, D. M. 214
Battit, G. E. 270, 286, 344
Bauchner, H. 307, 341
Bayer *see* aspirin; nonsteroidal anti-inflammatory drugs
Bayer, A. J. 321, 341
Bayer, Jay D., DO 113
Bayer (Friedrich) and Company 489
Beaver, William T., MD 477
Beck, A. 307, 357
Bedford, Robert, MD 391
bed rest
　acute low back pain and 167
　back pain and 143
　low back pain and 149, 150, 160–61
　low back problems and 179
　misconceptions about 25
Beebe, A. 57, 66, 288, 353, 381, 425n, 438
Beecher, H. K. 330.341
behavioral indicators
　chronic pain and 7
　of families and significant others 586–99
　of patients 556–86
　for presence of pain 61
　see also emotions
Behavioral Research and Therapy 345, 350
behavioral therapy 455
　for chronic pain 527–40
　for insomnia 527–40
　for pain relief 45–46

635

Behavior Therapy 358
Bell, Sir Charles 205
Bell's palsy 205–8
Bell's Palsy Research Foundation 622
Bellville, W. J. 322, 341
Benadryl 230
Bender, J. S. 321, 341
Benedetti, C. 268, 348, 356
benzodiazepines 112, 308–9
Berde, C. B. 61, 66, 315, 318, 341, 342
Berde, C. V. 275, 342
Bergstrom, I. 300, 301, 304, 349
Bernstein, B. A. 307, 357
Bernstein, N. 312, 342
Berrisford, R. G. 280, 295, 356–57
Bersten, A. 329, 341
best evidence synthesis 361
beta blockers 507–10
  for migraine headaches 83
betaxolol 510
Bevan, J. C. 313, 350
Beyer, J. E. 61, 66, 275, 301, 303, 341, 342
Bianchi, M. 329, 360
Bibby, S. R. 280, 295, 356–57
Bickford-Smith, P. J. 280, 295, 356–57
Bigler, D. 296, 357
Bigos, Stanley J., MD 159, 171
biofeedback 454–55, 473
  for cancer pain 429
  headaches and 119–20
  low back pain problems and 178
  for pain relief 12, 45, 530
  for postoperative pain 288
  tension-type headaches and 91, 92
Biopharmaceutics and Clinical Pharmacokinetics 512
Black, R. E. 315, 316, 348
bladder dysfunction 153
Block, Susan 611
blood clots
  aspirin and 489–90
  pain associated with 14–15
Bloom, S. R. 313, 340
Blyth, A. 280, 349
Bollish, S. J. 269, 342
bone scans
  evaluation of pain and 8
  low back pain and 160

Bonica, J. J. 214, 359
Borg, T. 300, 354
Boston Collaborative Drug Study 323
Bourson, A. 72
Bowyer, O. 171
braces, for spinal stenosis 237
brachial plexus 213
Bradley, J. W. 295, 358
bradykinin 77
Braen, G. 171
brain
  endorphin production and 5
  main regions of 76
  message-routing section in 4–5
  pain messages and 517, *518*, 544
  parts of 75, 76, 544
  sense of pain of 75
  see also central nervous system; spinal cord; *individual brain parts*
Brain Research 71, 342, 355
brain stem
  described 77
  headaches and 94
Brandt, M. R. 267, 351
Branthwaite, M. A. 267, 349
Bray, R. J. 315, 342
Brebner, J. 295, 358
Bresler, David 429
Brigham and Women's Hospital, Boston 210
British Journal of Anaesthesia 339, 349, 351, 353, 354, 356, 357
British Journal of Clinical Pharmacology 348
British Journal of Haematology 358
British Journal of Surgery 356–57
British Medical Journal 341, 357
Brody, Jane E. 208
Bromage, P. R. 328, 342
Bromo Seltzer 505
Brown, B. W., Jr. 322, 341
Brown, M. J. 313, 340
Browne, G. 320, 343
Brundage, D. 317, 318, 352
Buckley, J. 317, 318, 352
Bufferin 410
  see also aspirin; nonsteroidal anti-inflammatory drugs

Index

Bulletin of the Hospital for Joint Disease Orthopaedic Institute 358
Bullit, E. 268, 342
bupivacaine 292
buprenorphine (Buprenex) 16
Burnett, M. L. 269, 322, 344
burns
 children and 312–13
 pain management and 329–31
Burns, J. 280, 349
bursitis 483
Burt, R. A. 280, 344
Bush, J. P. 310, 342
butorphanol tartrate 281
Butt, W. 317, 352
Buxton, R. J. 267, 341
Buysse, D. J., MD *536*
Byock, Ira 611, 612
bypass surgery, for leg cramps 232

C

Cabanela, D. J. 300, 354
Cafergot 83, 85, 86
Cafermine 86
caffeine 414
 headaches and 117
 as headache treatment 86
 tension-type headaches and 91
Caldwell, S. 301, 350
Calimlim, J. 275, 358
Camalox 505
Campbell, D. T. 364
Campbell, N. N. 301, 342
Campoersi, E. 328, 342
Campos, R. G. 310–11, 314, 342
Canadian Anaesthetists' Society Journal 347
Canadian Journal of Anaesthesia 360
Cancer Information Service 442, 625–26
cancer pain 397–441
 causes of 398
 chronic pain and 32
 describing 400–401
 in elderly patients 436
 information sources for 624–26

cancer pain, continued
 medications for 10, 408–24
 deciding about 416–17
 treatment for 22–23, 50, 398–99, 403
 without medication 425–41
cancer pain diary 401
Cancer Pain Management Guideline Panel (1994) 56, 66
Caplan, R. 268, 356
Capogna, G. 295, 298, 342
capsaicin 11, 197
carbamazepine 10, 43, 196–97
 see also Tegretol
CARF *see* Commission on Accreditation of Rehabilitation Facilities (CARF)
carpal tunnel syndrome 217–22
 described 218
Carpal Tunnel Syndrome/RSI Association 623
Carr, D. B. 330, 331, 341
Carrieri, V. K. 61, 66
Carroll, D. 269, 354
carteolol 510
Caruso, F. S. 281, 351
case study design, described 361
Cassuto, J. 331, 350
catheters, pain relief delivery and 279, *522*
CAT scans *see* computerized axial tomography (CAT scans)
Caty, S. 311, 345
cauda equina 137, 141
cauda equina syndrome 152
Causon, R. C. 313, 340
Ceccherelli, F. 290, 345
Ceccio, C. M. 269, 343
Celleno, D. 295, 298, 342
Centers for Disease Control and Prevention (CDC) 494, 496
 publications 495
central nervous system
 chronic pain care costs and 33
 kappa opioid receptors and 281
 mu opioid receptors and 281–82
 pain messages and 34
 surgery on
  pain management and 293–94
 see also brain; spinal cord

cerebellum, described 77
cerebral cortex 544
cerebral cortex, pain signals in 4–5
Cerny, Igor 501, 510
Cervero, F. 353
cervical spine disorders
  described 187
  neck pain and 187–90
cesarean section 298
Chada, J. S. 321, 341
Chadwick, H. S. 268, 356
Champagne, M. T. 344, 346, 348, 356
Chanarin, I. 331, 358
Chang, W. D. 171
Chapman, C. 348
Chapman, C. R. 274, 343
Chapman, J. 304, 353
Chawla, R. 298, 343
Cheigh, J. 282, 359
chemicals
  neurotransmitters as 4, 75, 544
  released by injured tissues 77
Cherkin, D. 171
Chestnut, D. 328, 342
chest pain, medical emergency and 14
Child Development 342
Child Health Care 345
children
  anesthesia for 389–94
  colic and 81
  integrated approach to pain for 454
  lollipop pain relief medication for 16
  over-the-counter drugs for 481, 548
  pain assessment in 450
  postoperative pain management and 300–316, 318–20
Children's Health Care 345
Children's Hospital, Boston 158
Children's Hospital of Eastern Canada, Ottawa 496
Children's Memorial Hospital, Chicago 390
Chinyanga, H. 317, 352
chiropractic manipulation
  back pain and 143
  for chronic pain relief 23
  low back pain treatment and 183–85

chloral hydrate 112
Chlorpromazine 309
Chmela, Jan 219–20
Choiniere, M. 331, 343
cholecystectomy 297
choline magnesium trisalicylate 280
Chou, C. S. 171
Christofides, N. D. 313, 340
chronic headaches 79
chronic pain
  cancer and 398
  causes of 551–53
  common misconceptions about 25–26
  described 7
  how-to manual for families 549–604
  hypersensitivity and 43
  implants for 517
  malignant disease and 450, 451
    integrated approach to 453–54
  nonmalignant disease and 450, 451–52
    integrated approach to 454
  pain unit selection and 461–64
  research into 31–54
  treatment for 23–25, 527–40
Church, J. J. 292, 360
Chymodiactin 169
chymopapain 145–46, 163
  for low back pain 169
cigarette smoking
  antacids and 501
  leg cramps and 231
  migraine headaches and 83
cingulotomy 48
circumcision pain 312
City of Hope National Medical Center 618
Clark, W. E. 330, 358
Cleeland, Charles S., PhD 22, 61, 67
Clinical Neurology 214
Clinical Pediatrics 354
Clinical Pharmacology and Therapeutics 350, 353, 354, 358, 360
Clinical Pharmacy 342
Clinical Practice Guideline 57
Clinical Practice Guideline: Acute Low Back Problems in Adults 182

Index

Clinical Practice Guideline for Acute Pain Management 264, 265, 266–367
Clinical Practice Guideline for Acute Pain Management: Operative or Medical Procedures and Trauma **374**
Clinical Research Institute of Montreal 609
Clinics in Geriatric Medicine 344
Clinics in Sport Medicine 214
clochicine 168
clonazepam 197
Clotz, M. 309, 354
Clum, G. A. 288, 355
cluster headaches 84–85
  described 80
  hypothalamus and 76
  medication for 11
Coalition of Hospice Professionals 606
Cockrell, J. L. 310, 342
codeine 10, 43, 83, 281, 416
cognitive-behavioral treatment 285–90, 529, 530
  see also behavioral therapy
Cohen, D. 306, 309, 311, 361
Cohn, B. T. 289, 343
Cohn, Jeffrey E. 232
cold treatment
  for acute low back pain 168
  for back pain 143
  for cancer pain 432–33
  for hemorrhoids 247
  for knee pain 240
  for low back pain 161
  for low back problems 177
  pain relief and 12, 48
  for postoperative pain 279, 289
collars, for cervical spine disorders 189
College of Anesthetists 356
Collins, C. 313, 317, 343
Collins, C. L. 269, 342
Columbia University 390, 605
Commission on Accreditation of Rehabilitation Facilities (CARF) 29, 406, 442, 462, 618, 627

computerized axial tomography (CAT scans) 144
computerized tomography (CT)
  cervical spine disorders and 188
  evaluation of pain and 8
  low back pain and 160
  low back problems and 180
computer users, carpal tunnel syndrome and 222
Conn, I. G. 290, 343
Conn, R. R. 289, 350
Consensus Development Conference on the Integrated Approach to the Management of Pain 449
Constantine, Lynn M. 131n
continuous subcutaneous infusion 423
controlled-release systems 511–12
Cook, T. D. 364
Cooperman, A. M. 289, 343
coping strategies 454
Copp, L. A. 344, 346, 348, 356
cordotomy 46–47, 546
Cornell University 29
coronary artery diseases 33
Corry, J. 311, 345
corsets
  low back pain problems and 178
  for spinal stenosis 237
cortex
  described 77
  migraine headaches and 93
corticosteroids 10, 237
  acute low back pain and 168
  for low back pain 162
  for plantar fasciitis 243
Costley, E. C. 317, 360
Cote, Charles, MD 390
counterirritant, defined 362
Cousins, M. J. 268, 282, 323, 355, 360
Covington, E. C. 328, 343
Covino, B. G. 269, 345
Cowley, R. A. 330, 358
Craig, K. D. 305, 347
Cramer, Tom 506
cramps *see* leg cramps; menstrual pain
Crean, P. 313, 317, 343

Critical Care Medicine 352
Crook, J. 320, 343
Crozer-Chester Medical Center, Chester, PA 246
Crul, J. F. 295, 348
cryotherapy
  defined 362
  for postoperative pain 289
  see also cold therapy
Cuetter, A. C. 214
cultural factors
  emotional response to pain and 6
  pain assessment and 450
Currie, K. O. 328, 343

D

Daake, D. R. 287, 288, 343
Dalessio, Donald J., MD 197
Dalmane 112
Daly, J. C. 290, 343
Daly, Tom 185
Danesh, B. J. 280, 343
Daniels, L. K. 288, 344
Dartmouth Medical School, Hanover, NH 392
Darvon 51
  see also propoxyphene (Darvon)
Datril 258, 410, 465
Daut, R. L. 61, 67
Davie, I. T. 280, 344
Davies, J. R. 289, 344
Davis, M. A. 320, 344
Day, W. C. 267, 352
D'Bras, B. E. 295, 298, 356
DeBoskey, Dana S., PhD 549
Debrovner, Charles H., MD 256, 257, 258
Decadron 424
DeConno, F. 329, 360
DeGood, D. E. 301, 342
DeMeester, T. R. 280, 285, 359
Demerol 257, 282, 309
  see also meperidine (Demerol)
demon headache *see* cluster headaches
dental surgery 483
  pain management and 291–92

Depakene 197
Depakote 197
Department of Health and Human Services (DHHS) 264, 547, 608
  Agency for Health Care Policy and Research (AHCPR) 65, 183
  guidelines 184, 185
  publications 169, 182
depression 569–70
  cancer pain and 402
  family response to pain and 595–96
  low back problems and 180
  serotonin and 43
  tension-type headaches and 80
  see also spreading depression
descriptive study, described 361
desensitization 454
desipramine 544
Desyrel *see* trazodone (Desyrel)
de Veber, L. L. 303, 353
Developmental Medicine and Child Neurology 346
Dewan, D. M. 269, 296, 344
Dexadrine 424
Dextroamphetamine 424
D.H.E. 45 *see* digyhdroergotamine mesylate (D.H.E. 45)
DHHS *see* Department of Health and Human Services (DHHS)
diabetes
  chronic pain and 7
  eye pain and 99
  leg cramps and 227, 233
diabetic neuropathy 11
Diamond, Seymour, MD 84
The Diamond Headache Clinic 84
diaries
  for cancer pain 401
  for headaches 117, 127, *129*
  for pain assessment 450
  for sleep 112–13
diazepam 309
dichloralphenazone 86–87
Dick, Margaret Jorgensen, RN, PhD 56, 66, 67
Dickinson, Emily 31
Dickman, M. 267, 352
diclofenac 486

Index

diet and nutrition
  antacids and 500
  beta blockers and 508
  headaches and 116–17
  hemorrhoids and 246, 249
  potassium and 229
diflunisal 486
digydroergotamine mesylate (D.H.E. 45) 83, 86
Dilantin 10, 196–97
  see also phenytoin (Dilantin)
Dilaudid 416, 423
Dillon, P. 267, 344
Dimensions in Critical Care Nursing 349
Dinarello, C. 267, 344
Dionne, R. A. 267, 348
disabilities
  headaches and 103–4
  low back pain and 150
diskectomy 169
diskography 188
disk syndrome 151
distraction therapy, for cancer pain 430–31
diuretic drugs, leg cramps and 229, 233
doctors
  back pain and 143–44
  consultations with
    for migraine headaches 106
  consultation with
    for repetitive strain injuries 224
  how to find
    for headache treatment 131–32
  pain questionnaires and 8
  as specialists in pain treatment 52
  see also physicians
Dolphine 416
Donovan, M. 267, 344
Donovan, M. I. 56, 57, 67
Doral 112
Doriden 112
Dormon, F. 301, 317, 355
Doucette, E. J. 280, 344
DPT mixture 309
Drabman, R. S. 312, 351
Draeger, R. I. 289, 343

Dripps, R. D. 331, 344
drugs *see* over-the-counter drugs; prescription medications
drug therapy 452
  see also over-the-counter drugs; prescription medications
drug tolerance 417, 545–46
  versus addiction 467–68
  described 417–18
  drug abuse and 580–83
Dubner, R. 353
Dubner, Ronald, DDS 468, 469, 470, 471, 473
Duke University Medical Center, Department of Prosthetics and Orthotics 383n, 627
Dunn, J. 304, 353
Duquesne Law Review 607
Duragesic 390, 393
dysmenorrhea 252–59
  explanation of 253–54
  types of 256–57
  see also menstrual pain
dyspesia 503

E

Eason, A. L. 289, 352
Eckenhoff, J. E. 331, 344
Ecotrin 410
Edgar, L. 300, 350
education
  low back pain and 165
  migraine awareness and 107–9
  for patients, defined 362
  postoperative pain control 278, 285–86
Educational Researcher 367
EEG *see* electroencephalogram (EEG)
Egan, T. M. 280, 344
Egbert, A. M. 269, 322, 344
Egbert, L. D. 270, 286, 344
Egdahl, G. 267, 344
Eisenach, J. C. 269, 296, 344
Ekblom, A. 290, 347
Eland, J. M. 301, 311, 314–15, 344, 345
Elavil 10, 113, 424, 553–54

electrical stimulation
  for Bell's palsy 207
  of brain 39, *39, 40,* 546–47
  for neurogenic pain 51
  pain relief and 11, 38–39
  see also transcutaneous electrical nerve stimulation (TENS)
electroencephalogram (EEG) 93
electrolyte balance 229
electromyogram (EMG) 144
electrostimulator *39, 40*
Elkind, Arthur, MD 92
Elkind Headache Center 92
Elkins-Sinn Inc. 471
Ellerton, M. 311, 345
Elliott, C. 311, 350
Elliott, C. H. 301, 312, 345, 350
Emanuel, Linda L. 610–11
EMG *see* electromyogram (EMG)
emotions
  anger and irritability 557–59, 590–91
  anxiety and fears 570–72
  avoidance 592–93
  chronic pain and 7, 13, 452
  communication problems 598–99
  denial 566–67
  dependency 560–61, 587–89
  depression 569–70, 595–96
  egocentricity 562–63, 589
  escape 592–93
  fatigue 593–94
  frustration 589–90
  guilt 591–92
  headaches and 115, 118
  low back problems and 180
  low self-esteem 572–74
  manipulation 563–66
  nonproductive behaviors 578–80
  overfocus on physical concerns 567–69
  pain signals and 6
  produced in limbic system 5
  sexuality issues 576–78, 597–98
  social isolation 574–75, 596–97
  stress 575–76, 594–95
  see also behavioral indicators
endometriosis 256–57

endorphins
  acupuncture and 11
  decrease of pain with 5
  and gate theory of pain 37
  headaches and 124
  pain reduction and 76
  research into role of 41
  transcutaneous electrical nerve stimulation and 11
Endress, M. P. 306, 350
Endress, P. 287, 350
Eng, J. 280, 295, 356–57
Engberg, G. 280, 285, 345
English, M. J. 269, 283, 296, 360
enkephalins, described 5, 37
Ensminger, William, MD, PhD 516
epidural
  analgesia
    for children 316
  corticosteroids 162
    for acute low back pain 168
  described 363
  opioids 278
Epilim 197
epinephrine (adrenaline) 34
episiotomy 298
episiotomy pain 64, 483
equianalgesic, defined 363
Ercaf 86
Ercata 86
Ergo-Caff 86
Ergomar 83, 86
Ergostat 83, 86
ergotamines 83
ergotamine tartrate 86
Eriksson, S. 327, 348
Estes, D. 280, 345
estrogens 253
European Journal of Obstetrics, Gynecology, and Reproductive Biology 345
eutectic mixture of local anesthetics (EMLA) 308, 363
euthanasia, alternatives to 605–13
Evan, G. 268, 349
Evron, S. 290, 345
exercise
  acute low back pain and 167
  beta blockers and 508
  for fibromyalgia 210

Index

exercise, continued
  headaches and 120
  low back pain and 150, 161
  low back problems and 180
  menstrual cramps and 259
  for pain relief 13
  for postoperative pain 289
exercises
  endorphin stimulation and 5
  for knee pain 240
  in warm water
    for arthritis pain 51
experimental study, described 361
eye pain 14, *97,* 514
  cluster headaches and 84
  headaches and 97–99

F

Facco, E. 290, 345
facet syndrome 151
facial pain
  Bell's palsy and 205
  tic douloureux and 33, 43, 194
Facts About Dysmenorrhea and Premenstrual Syndrome 252n
Faculty Scholars Program 611
Fairfax Hospital, Falls Church, VA
  Woodburn Surgery Center 468, 470
family issues
  chronic pain and 549–604
  headaches and 104, 118
  low back problems and 179
  multidisciplinary pain units and 462, 463
  pain relief therapy and 13
Farag, R. R. 321, 341
Farley, Dixie 88
Fassler, D. 311, 345
fatigue
  cancer pain and 402
  family response to pain and 593–94
FDA Consumer 79n, 88, 135n, 217n, 219, 227n, 229, 245n, 249, 256n, 389n, 465n, 466, 467, 477, 477n, 483n, 488n, 493, 499n, 507n, 511n, 514, 543n
Feldman, H. R. 287, 288, 354

fenoprofen 486
fentanyl 15–16, 281, 390, 393
Ferguson, B. F. 313, 345
Fermin, P. 296, 353
Fernald, C. 311, 345
Ferrante, F. M. 269, 345
Ferrell, B. A. 320, 321, 322, 323, 345
Ferrell, B. R. 320, 321, 323, 345
fibromyalgia 151, 209–11
  causes of 209–10
  diagnosis of 210
  research on 210–11
  treatment for 210
Field, M. D. 364, 366
Field, T. 311, 314, 346
Fields, H. L. 353
financial issues 601–2
Fisher, D. 317, 348
Fisher, D. M. 309, 361
Fisher, Sherry, RN 470
Fitzgerald, M. 268, 301, 346
Fitzpatrick, J. J. 287, 346, 349
Flaherty, G. G. 287, 346, 349
Flexeril 230
Flieger, Ken 493
fluoxetine (Prozac) 24
Foldes, F. F. 281, 354
Foley, K. M. 282, 294, 320, 321, 329, 346, 350, 353
Foley, Kathleen M. 609, 611, 613
food allergies 116
Food and Drug Administration (FDA) 259, 366, 491
  advisory committee on anesthetic and life support drugs 390
  advisory panels 478, 481
  approvals 83, 145, 230, 232, 247, 280, 295, 389, 410, 470, 471, 479, 506, 513, 514, 515, 516
  center for devices and radiological health 472
  center for drug evaluation and research 465, 468, 499, 501
  center for food safety and applied nutrition 246
  division of cardio-renal drugs 228
  division of mechanics and material science 515

643

Food and Drug Administration (FDA), continued
  division of metabolism and endocrine drug products 257
  division of neuro-pharmacological drugs 80
  division of nutrition 219
  division of oncology 228
  division of over-the-counter drug evaluation 247
  drug labeling, education and research branch 510
  labeling 492, 504–5
  office of OTC drug evaluation 478
  pilot drug evaluation program 391, 392, 393
  reviews 466
  spontaneous reporting system 391
  warnings 496
foot pain 241–44
  stubbed toe and 473–75, *474*
  see also heel pain
Fordyce, W. E. 321, 346
Forrest, W. H. 322, 341
Forster, Jeff 171
Fortin, F. 270, 286, 346
Foster, R. 300, 304, 305, 348–49
Foster, R. L. 301, 303, 346, 348
Foundation for Chiropractic Education and Research 186
Fowler-Kerry, S. 301, 307, 311, 346, 347
Fox Chase Cancer Center Pain Management Center, Philadelphia 22
Fradet, C. 307, 347
Framingham Heart Study 612
Franck, L. S. 301, 347
Frank, Barbara, MD 246, 247
Frank, H. 289, 360
Friedman, Arnold 90
Fritz, D. J. 275, 347
Fuller, S. 287, 350
Funk, S. G. 344, 346, 348

G

Gallagher, E. G. 280, 285, 295, 351
Gallo-Torres, Hugo, MD 499–501
Gallup Organization polls 101, 102, 184
Gamma Knife 199–200
gastritis 503
gastrointestinal bleeding 100
gate control theory of pain 4, 35–36, 546
Gauntlett, I. 317, 348
Gauvain-Piquard, A. 304, 347
Gedaly-Duff, V. 314, 347
Gelfand, M. M. 289, 358
Gelusil 505
gender factor
  headaches and 95–96
  lower back pain and 142–43
  migraine headaches and 80
  response to pain and 584–86, 602–3
  tension-type headaches and 91
generic drugs 486
  versus name brand drugs 410–11
genetic factors
  back pain and 143
  Bell's palsy and 206
  headaches and 96
  migraine headaches and 49
Georgetown University Hospital, Washington D. C.
  department of neurology 137, 145
Georgetown University School of Medicine 477
George Washington Hospital, Center to Improve Care of the Dying 607, 608
George Washington University Medical Center, Washington, D. C.
  division of colon and rectal surgery 245
geriatric pain management 320–23
Geriatrics 346
Gibaldi, Milo, PhD 510
Gibbons, P. 305, 357
Gibbs, J. M. 288, 354
Gibson, Rosemary 606
Gielen, M. 295, 348
Gilbertson, William E. 247
Giron, G. P. 290, 345
glaucoma 97–99, 514
glycerol rhizotomy 198, 203
Gode, G. R. 298, 343

Index

Goldiner, P. 289, 356
Goldson, E. 311, 314, 346
Gonsalves-Ebrahim, L. 328, 343
Good Housekeeping 19n
Goodman, J. T. 304, 353
Good News for Bad Backs 170, 620
Gotamine 86
Goulding, G. 295, 298, 356
gout 483
Grabinski, P. Y. 282, 294, 322, 350, 351, 353
Gracely, R. H. 275, 347
Granat, M. 290, 345
Grant, I. S. 298, 356
Greif, Stuart J., PSV.D 549
Grey-Donald, K. 300, 350
Grice, S. C. 269, 296, 344
Group Health Cooperative of Puget Sound 169
Grunau, R. V. E. 305, 347
Gueldner, S. H. 287, 288, 343
Guide to Clinical Preventive Services 491, 492
Gunn, M. L. 267, 352
Guralnick, M. S. 289, 358

H

Haarmann, I. 268, 355
Haddox, J. D. 326, 360
Haig, M. J. 313, 350
Hakkinen, U. 171
Hale, Ellen 259
Hall, B. 289, 343
Hand, C. W. 327, 357
Handbook of Nonprescription Drugs 503
Hand Clinics 214
hand pain 213
hand problems 219–21
Hanley, M. R. 268, 347
Hannallah, R. S. 313, 347
Hanson, A. L. 269, 298, 347
Hanson, B. 298, 331, 350
Hanson,B. 269, 347
Hansson, P. 290, 347
Hardy, R. 289, 343
Hargreaves, A. 289, 290, 348

Hargreaves, K. M. 267, 292, 348, 349
Harkins, S. W. 321, 348
Harris Organization polls 184
Hart, L. 307, 357
Harvard Medical School, 48, 611
Harvard Medical School Health Letter 472–73
Harvard University, Boston 365
Hasenbos, M. 295, 348
Haug, C. 214
Hazelrigg, G. 289, 350
HDI Publishers 549n, 551, 617
Headache and Diet: Tyramine-free Recipes 621
headache diary 117, 127
  form for *129*
headache management 115–29
headaches
  causes of 115
  chronic pain and 32
  diagnosis of 80
  information sources for 621–22
  treatment for 49, 79–87, 128, 547
  see also migraine headaches
head pain, medical emergency and 14
Health Care for Women International 67
health care providers
  low back problems and 175
  system problems 599–601
  see also doctors; nurses; physicians; specialists
health maintenance organizations
  lack of second opinions and 225
Health Psychology 350
Health Tips 239n
Hearn, M. T. 303, 353
Heart and Lung 351
heart attack, aspirin and 490–91
heartburn 499–504
heat treatment
  for acute low back pain 168
  for back pain 143
  for cancer pain 432–33
  for fibromyalgia 210
  for low back problems 177
  pain relief and 12, 48
  for plantar fasciitis 243

heat treatment, continued
  for postoperative pain 279, 289
  thermocoagulation as
    for neurogenic pain 51
heel pain, plantar fasciitis and 241–44
Hegland, M. 317, 318, 352
Hehenberger, D. 289, 358
Heidrich, G. 282, 350
Heimbach, D. M. 301, 357
hemorrhoids 245–49
  surgery for 298
  treatment for 246–48
  types of 245
Hendrickson, M. 315, 316, 348
Hendrix, B. E. 289, 352
heredity *see* genetic factors
Herman, S. J. 280, 344
hernia repair 298
herniated discs 188
  diagnosis of 156
  surgical treatment for 164, 169
  treatment for 145
heroin, cancer pain and 423–24
herpes simplex, Bell's palsy and 206
  see also shingles
Hertzka, R. 317, 348
Herz, A. 268, 355
Hester, N. K. O. 303, 348–49
Hester, N. O. 300, 301, 302, 303, 304, 305, 307, 314, 346, 348, 349
Hewett, J. E. 289, 350
Hewlett, A. M. 267, 331, 349, 358
Hickey, P. 313, 340
high blood pressure medication 11, 83
Hinckley, Stephen M. 472
Hinkle, Allen, J., MD 392, 393
Hinnant, D. 287, 352
Hinshaw, J. R. 255, 280
histamines, released by injured tissues 77
Hodsman, N. B. 280, 349
Hoffmann, Felix 488–89, 493
Holditch-Davis, D. 56, 66
Hollt, V. 268, 355
Holmbeck, G. N. 310, 342
Holzemer, W. L. 63, 67, 303, 304, 357, 359
Hopodarsky, J. 287, 351
Horan, J. J. 287, 288, 349

hormones
  changes in
    headaches and 116
  implants for 514–15
  menstrual cycle and 252–53
  prostaglandins
    speed-up of pain messages and 5
  see also individual hormones
Horowitz, B. F. 287, 349
hospice care 607–8
Hospodarsky, J. 288
hotlines
  Arthritis Foundation 221
  Cancer Information Service 402, 405, 442
  National Cancer Institute 625
Houde, R. 282, 359
Houde, R. W. 275, 322, 349, 351
"How to Take Your Medicine: Nonsteroidal Anti-Inflammatory Drugs" 467
Hsueh Tsa Chih 171
Hunt, S. P. 268, 349
hurt *versus* pain 63
Huskisson, E. C. 275, 357
Hutchins, R. C. 289, 358
hydrocodone 281
hydromorphine 416
hydromorphone 281
Hyman, R. B. 287, 352
hyperalgesia, described 43
hypnosis 454
  for cancer pain 436
  for pain relief 42, 45, 529–30
  for postoperative pain 288
hypnotic medications 112
hypothalamus 75, 78
hysterectomy 298

I

ibuprofen 479, 481, 486
  for arthritis 219
  arthritis pain and 50
  for cancer pain 410, 411, 413
  for dental surgery 292
  for everyday aches and pains 465
  for headaches 121

Index

ibuprofen, continued
  for menstrual cramps 258
  as nonsteroidal anti-inflammatory drug 10
  for repetitive strain injuries 223
  safe dosages of 413
  for tension-type headaches 91
I.D.A. 86
Ignelzi, R. J. 64, 66
Image 353
imagery *see* visualization therapy
imaging tests
  for low back pain *159,* 159–60
imaging tests, for low back pain 150
imipramine (Tofranil) 10
Imitrex 11, 87
implants for pain management 514–15, 517–25
inactivity, low back pain and 150
Inderal 83
Inderal LAR 508
Indian Journal of Medical Research 343
indigestion 499–500
indomethacin 50, 484, 486
infants
  integrated approach to pain for 454
  postoperative pain management and 302–20
infrared photocoagulation 248
injuries 77
  acute pain and 467, 527
  back pain and 135–36
  chronic pain and 7, 527
  see also repetitive strain injuries; sports injuries
insomnia
  headaches and 111–13
  treatment for 527–40
  see also sleep
Institute of Medicine 366
insurance coverage 463–64
  insomnia treatment and 538
integration, defined 449
intensity scale, for pain assessment 63
Intensive Care Medicine 341
intermittent claudication 231, 233

International Anesthesiology Clinics 356
International Association for the Study of Pain 33, 57, 66, 267, 268, 349, 364, 406, 443, 527, 618
International Headache Society 79, 90, 103
International Intradiscal Therapy Society 163
International Journal of Nursing Studies 346, 354
internet addresses 541, 627–28
  Agency for Health Care Policy and Research 263n, 270
  American Chiropractic OnLine 183n, 185
  National Institute of Neurological Disorders and Stroke 213n
  National Institutes of Health 213n
  National Rehabilitation Information Center 214, 623
interpleural, defined 363
intraocular inflammation *see* uveitis (intraocular inflammation)
intraspinal drug infusion therapy 517–25
Inturrisi, C. E. 282, 294, 329, 346, 350, 353, 359
Iso-Acetazone 86
Isocom 83, 86
isometheptene 83, 86–87
Issues in Comprehensive Pediatric Nursing 356
Itoh, M. 289, 352

J

Jackson, D. 269, 296, 349
Jackson, D. L. 290, 349
Jackson, D. W. 289, 343
Jacox, A. K. 268, 345, 349
Jaffer, M. 290, 343
Jain, S. 289, 356
Jarvie, G. J. 312, 351
jaw pain 194
Jay, S. M. 301, 309, 311, 350, 361
Jeans, M. E. 269, 283, 289, 296, 300, 350, 358, 360

Jensen, J. E. 289, 350
Jick, H. 281, 323, 355
John, M. E., Jr. 288, 350
Johns Hopkins Hospital, Baltimore 605
Johns Hopkins University, Baltimore 365
Johns Hopkins University Hospital, Baltimore 36
Johnson, D. G. 315, 316, 348
Johnson, G. 304, 353
Johnson, George, MD 494
Johnson, J. 287, 350
Johnson, J. E. 306, 350
Johnston, C. C. 300, 313, 350
Jonsson, A. 331, 350
Joranson, David E. 610
Journal of Advanced Nursing 352
Journal of American Association of Nurse Anesthetists 355
Journal of American Osteopathic Association 351
Journal of Applied Behavioral Analysis 351
Journal of Burn Care and Rehabilitation 356, 357
Journal of Child Psychology and Psychiatry 342
Journal of Clinical Psychology 356
Journal of Consulting and Clinical Psychology 351, 352, 355, 358
Journal of Developmental and Behavioral Pediatrics 357
Journal of Family Practice 340
Journal of Foot Surgery 352
Journal of Intravenous Nursing 349
Journal of Neurophysiology 71
Journal of Obstetric, Gynecologic, and Neonatal Nursing 347
Journal of Obstetric, Gynecologic and Neonatal Nursing 55n
Journal of Occupational Medicine 184
Journal of Pain and Symptom Management 66, 342, 343, 347, 354
Journal of Parenteral and Enteral Nutrition 351
Journal of Pediatric Nursing 66, 341, 360
Journal of Pediatric Psychology 342, 357
Journal of Pediatrics 342, 352, 361
Journal of Pediatric Surgery 340, 348
Journal of the American Academy of Child Psychology 351
Journal of the American Dental Association 349
Journal of the American Geriatric Society 341, 345
Journal of the American Medical Association 341, 347, 359
Journal of the Formosan Medical Association 352
Journal of the New York State Nurses Association 354
Joynt, R. J. 214

K

Kaiko, R. F. 282, 294, 322, 350, 351, 353
Kallos, T. 281, 351
Kane, R. L. 320, 322, 351
Kaplan, J. A. 280, 285, 295, 351
Kaplan, K. 280, 345
Karamanian, A. 281, 354
Karas, S. E. 214
Karlstrom. G. 300, 354
Karusaitis, Vincent, MD 228, 229, 230, 231
Katz, E. R. 305, 351
Katz, Russell, MD 79–80, 83, 85
Kavanagh, C. 312, 351
Kay, J. 307, 347
Kehlet, H. 258, 267, 296, 298, 351, 357
Kellerman, J. 305, 351
Kelley, M. L. 312, 351
Kelvie, W. 267, 275, 358, 359
Kenny, G. N. 280, 349
ketoprofen 10, 486
ketoralac 486
ketorolac 280, 292
Kevorkian, Jack, MD 605
Kieckhefer, G. M. 63, 66
Kiefer, R. C. 287, 288, 351
Kirchoff, K. 306, 350

Index

Kirking, D. M. 269, 342
Kirnon, V. 313, 350
Kirouac, S. 270, 286, 346
Klein, J. 313, 317, 343
Klonopin 197, 424
knee pain 239–40
Koehntop, D. 317, 318, 352
Koerner, S. 281, 354
Kondziolka, Douglas, MD 200
Konikoff, Fred 231
Koren, G. 313, 317, 343, 352
Korpela, R. 308, 353
Krane, E. G. 346, 349, 350
Kremer, E. 64, 66
Kriegler, Jennifer, MD 24, 25
Kristensen, K. 300, 301, 303, 304, 348–49, 353
Krogg, E. 309, 354
Kwentus, J. 321, 348

L

labetalol 510
labor pains, similarity to menstrual cramps 254
Lamb, M. 331, 358
laminectomy 145, 190, 238
Lanatrate 86
Lancet 340, 346, 350, 360
Lander, J. 289, 290, 348
Lander, J. R. 311, 347
Lang, Susan S. 19n, 29
language of pain, described 13
Langvod, J. 355
Lanham, R. H., Jr. 289, 352
Lanzafame, R. J. 255, 280
Lasagna, L. 267, 275, 358, 359
laser coagulation 248
Laska, E. M. 341, 348
Latimer, R. J. 267, 352
Lawless, S. 56, 66
Lawlis, G. F. 287, 352
Laws, Edward R., Jr., MD 145
laxatives 247
Laying, F. C. 287, 288, 349
LeBaron, S. 305, 306, 309, 311, 352, 361
Lee, K. A. 63, 66

Lee, M. 289, 352
leg cramps 227–33
  causes of 227–29
  treatment for 230–31, 232–33
leg pain 14–15
  spinal stenosis and 225–38
Lehn, B. M. 315, 342
Lemerle, J. 304, 347
LeNeel, J. C. 316, 354
Lenox Hill Hospital, New York
  Pain Treatment Program at 19
Lertakyamanee, J. 312, 359
Levin, R. F. 287, 288, 352, 354
Levo-Dromoran 416
levorphanol 281, 416
Levy, Michael, MD, PhD 22–23
Lewis, J. D. 331, 358
Lewith, G. T. 290, 360
Li, C. H. 294, 353
Liao, W. S. 289, 352
Liberman, H. 295, 298, 356
Liebeskind, John C. 469
Lien, I. N. 289, 352
lifestyles
  physical activity and
    low back problems and 178
  sedentary
    low back pain and 136
  see also inactivity
light sensitivity, migraine headaches and 105
limbic system
  described 78
  emotions produced in 5
Lindeman, C. 270, 359
Lindsey, A. M. 61, 66
Lioresar 196
Lipicky, Raymond 228
Lipton, Richard B., MD 101, 109
Liu, Y. C. 289, 352
liver disorders
  hemorrhoids and 245
  leg cramps and 231
Living with Chronic Pain: Personal Experiences of Pain Sufferers 618
local anesthetics 308, 363, *370*, 387
  see also epidural
Locsin, R. G. 287, 352

Loffreda-Mancinelli, C. 295, 298, 342
Lohr, K. N. 364, 366
lollipop medication 15–16
Long, D. 289, 358
Love, Patricia, MD 465, 466, 467, 472
lovonorgestrel 514
low back pain 135
  chronic pain and 32
  new treatment of 149–69
  possible causes of 157
  treatment for 49–50, 160–63
  see also back pain
low back problems
  causes of 174–75
  things to do about 175–76
  treatment for 176–78
Lowe, G. D. 280, 343
Lowe, N. K. 63, 67
Lowe, N. R. 63, 66
Lowinson, J. H. 355
Luke, B. 307, 347
lumbar strain 151
Lynn, A. M. 315, 317, 352
Lynn, Joanne 607, 608

M

M. D. Anderson Cancer Center, Houston 21
Maalox 505
MacDonald, Neil 609–10
Machin, D. 290, 360
MacIntosh, N. 301, 346
MacKenzie, N. 298, 356
Mackie, J. 300, 301, 353
MacLeod, S. M. 313, 317, 343
Macrae, W. A. 298, 356
Madden, C. 287, 288, 352
magnetic resonance imaging (MRI)
  cervical spine disorders and 188
  evaluation of pain and 8
  low back pain and 159
  low back problems and 180
  tic douloureux and 196
Magora, F. 290, 345
Mahoney, John J. 608
Majid, M. R. 280, 295, 356–57

"Making a Stand Against Leg Cramps" 229
malignant pain 56
Malloy, G. B. 287, 352
Malovany, R. 281, 354
Malrnivaara, A. 171
managed care, low back pain and 149
Management of Cancer Pain: Adult Patient's Guide 28, 626
The Management of Pain 214
Management of Severe Pain 354
Manani, G. 290, 345
Manipulation for My Back Problem? 185
manipulative therapy
  for acute low back pain 168
  for back pain 143
  for low back pain 50, 151, 162, 163
  see also chiropractic manipulation
Marcus, Norman J., MD 19
marijuana, and cancer pain 436
Maripuu, E. 300, 354
Marks, R. M. 267, 282, 353
Marlowe, Donald 515
Marshall, A. H. 290, 343
Marshall, B. E. 267, 353
Martens, M. 353
Martini, N. 289, 356
Marvin, J. A. 301, 357
Massachusetts General Hospital, Boston 365, 611
Massachusetts General Hospital, Neurological Service 623
massage therapy
  for cancer pain 432, 438–39
  for fibromyalgia 210
  headaches and 120–21
  for low back pain 50
  low back pain problems and 178
  pain relief and 12
  for postoperative pain 279, 289
mastectomy pain 11
Mather, L. 300, 301, 353
Matlak, M. E. 315, 316, 348
Matousek, M. 269, 298, 347
Maunuksela, E. L. 306, 308, 309, 311, 353, 361
Max, M. B. 294, 341, 348, 353

Index

Maxwell, L. 312, 353
Mayer, M. N. 304, 341
Mayo Clinic 15, 243, 256
Mayo Clinic Health Letter 3n, 217n, 222n, 235n, 241n, 385n
Mayo Foundation for Medical Education and Research 3n, 217n, 222n, 235n, 241n, 385n
Mayor's Commission for Disabilities, Richmond, VA 221
McArdle, C. S. 280, 349
McCaffery, M. 57, 66, 288, 353, 381, 425n, 438
McCormack, P. 289, 356
McCoy, C. E. 287, 352
McGill-Melzach Pain Questionnaire 450, 451
McGill Pain Questionnaire 61
McGlothlin, James, PhD 217, 220
McGrath, D. 296, 353
McGrath, K. 289, 359
McGrath, M. M. 313, 353
McGrath, P. A. 303, 353
McGrath, P. J. 61, 66, 275, 303, 304, 307, 342, 347, 353, 354
McGuire, L. 267, 344
Mcleod, R. S. 280, 344
McNeer, M. F. 312, 351
McQuay, H. 269, 354
McQuay, H. J. 327, 357
Mearns, A. J. 280, 295, 356–57
meclofenamate 484, 486
Medical Clinics of North America 341, 346, 351
Medical College of Virginia, Division of Rheumatology, Allergy and Immunology 221
medical examinations *see* physical examinations
medical history
  leg cramps and 228
  low back pain and 151–56
  low back problems and 175–76
  trigeminal neuralgia and 195
MediCaring program 608–9
medication delivery systems
  described 15–16
  new methods for 511–16
  see also patient-controlled analgesia

medications *see* over-the-counter drugs; prescription medications
meditation therapy 12, 44–45, 473, 529
Medtronic Neurological 517n
mefenamic acid 258, 486
Meharry Medical College, Nashville, TN 69, 70
Mehta, G. 275, 358
Meier, Diane E. 612
Meignier, M. 316, 354
Melzack, R. 57, 63, 66, 67, 331, 343
Melzack, Ronald 546
Memorial Sloan-Kettering Cancer Center, New York 609, 611, 613
menstrual pain 252–59, 483
  causes of 256–57
  medications for 465–66
  research and 254
  treatment for 254–55
menthol preparations, for cancer pain 433–34
meperidine (Demerol) 10, 43, 282, 309
Merskey, H. 267, 354
meta-analysis 361
methadone 10, 281, 416
methysergide maleate 86
methysergide (Sansert) 83
metoprolol 507, 510
Meunier, J. C. 72
Micheli, L. J. 171
microdiskectomy 169
microiontophoresis 70
microvascular decompression (MVD) 201–3
midazolam 309, 392
Middlebrook, J. L. 312, 351
Midol 258
Midrin 83, 86
Migergot 86
Migraine: The Complete Guide 131n, 621
migraine aura 81, 82, 84, 93–94
  study of 105
  see also migraine headaches
migraine headaches
  chronic pain and 32
  described 80
  medication for 11

651

migraine headaches, continued
  origin of 82–83
  sleep and 111–13
  study of 101–9
  treatment for 49
  types of
    classic migraine 81, 90
    migraine with aura 81, 89
  see also headaches
migraineurs, defined 81
migraineurs, study of 103–4
Migratine 86
Migrazone 86
Migrex 86
Mikalacki, K. 289, 343
Millard, C. 301, 346
Miller, E. 322, 341
Miller, E. D., Jr. 280, 285, 295, 351
Miller, Edward D., Jr. MD 390, 392, 393, 394
Milman, R. 355
Missoula Demonstration Project 611, 612
Mitride 86
mixed opioid agonist-antagonist, described 363
modeling 454
Modig, J. 300, 354
Moffat, Marilyn, PT, PhD 24
Mogan, J. 288, 354
Mogensen, T. 296, 357
Mokha, Sukhbir S. 69–71
Mollereau, C. 72
monosodium glutamate (MSG) 116
Montefiore Hospital 90
Montefiore Medical Center, New York, Headache Unit 94
Moon, M. H. 288, 354
moonface, described 50
Moore, P. A. 292, 349
Moore, R. A. 269, 327, 354, 357
Morbidity and Mortality Weekly Report 495–96
Moricca, G. 348
Morin, C. M. *536*
Morin, Karen, M.S.W. 549
morphine 10, 43
  cancer pain and 416, 423
  for chronic pain relief 23–24

morphine, continued
  implantable pump for 470–71, 515–16, 517, *524*
  as pain reliever 5
  for postoperative pain 283–84
morphine receptors 5
Motrin 258, 410, 416, 424
Motrin IB 83, 219, 258
  see also ibuprofen; nonsteroidal anti-inflammatory drugs
Mount Sinai Hospital, New York 232
Mount Sinai Medical Center 612
Mount Sinai Medical Center, Cleveland
  Neuro-Ophthalmology Section 99
Mullen, B. V. 255, 280
Mullooly, V. M. 287, 288, 354
multiple sclerosis (MS) 195, 199
Muscle and Nerve 214
muscle contractions 85
  see also tension-type headaches
muscle cramps 228
  see also leg cramps
muscle pain, information sources for 622–23
muscle relaxants 91, 167, 230
muscle strains, low back pain and 136, 151, 553
myelogram
  for back pain 144
  for low back pain 49
myelography, cervical spine disorders and 188
myelopathy 188
Mylanta 505
Myre, L. 315, 316, 348
myths
  regarding headaches 95–96
  regarding pain 2627

N

Nachemson, Alf 143
Nadeau, Stephen, MD 19
nadolol 510
Nagashima, H. 281, 354
Nahata, M. 309, 354
nalbuphine hydrochloride 281

Index

Nalfon 416
Naprosyn 258, 416
naproxen 258, 486
naproxen sodium 479, 481
  as nonsteroidal anti-inflammatory drug 10
  for repetitive strain injuries 223
  for tension-type headaches 91
narcotics 391
  for cancer pain 417–20
  for headaches 124
  as mimics of endorphins 77
  pain management and 8–9, 553–54
  as pain relievers 5, 10
  withdrawal from 422–23
  see also prescription medications; synthetic narcotics (opioids)
NARIC *see* National Rehabilitation Information Center (NARIC)
National Academy of Sciences 366
  Institute of Medicine 612
National Cancer Institute 33, 442, 449, 541, 625
  publications 397n, 407n, 425n
National Center for Research Resources 69, 71
National Chronic Pain Outreach Association 29, 53, 215, 406, 443, 618, 622
National Headache Foundation 53, 79, 81, 84, 87, 89n, 97n, 621
  publications 111n
National Health and Medical Research Council (Australia) 268, 354
National Heart, Lung, and Blood Institute 541
National Hospice Organization 606, 607–8
National Institute for Occupational Safety and Health 217, 220, 221
National Institute of Arthritis and Musculoskeletal and Skin Diseases (NIAMS) 210, 211, 541
  Multipurpose Arthritis and Musculoskeletal Diseases Centers 211
  office of scientific and health communications 209n
  publications 187n

National Institute of Dental Research (NIDR) 33, 40, 71, 449, 468, 541
National Institute of Mental Health (NIMH) 33, 541
National Institute of Neurological and Communicative Disorders and Stroke 449
National Institute of Neurological Disorders and Stroke (NINDS) 33, 39, 40, 87, 541, 623
  office of scientific and health reports 54
  research programs 213
National Institute of Nursing Research 541
National Institute of Occupational Safety and Health 624
National Institute on Aging 541
National Institutes of Health (NIH) 211, 245, 274, 275, 320, 335, 347, 354
  conferences 143
  Consensus Development Conference Statement 447n
  information center electronic bulletin board 541
  office of medical applications of research 449
  pain research clinic 475
  publications 31n, 252n, 263n, 541
  reports 145
National Institutes of Health (NIH) Technology Conference 536
National Institutes of Health Technology Assessment Statement 527n
National Library of Medicine 169, 365, 488
National Rehabilitation Information Center (NARIC) 214, 623
National Science Foundation (NSF) 71
Nature 72, 349
Nayman, J. 287, 288, 352
NCRR Reporter 69n
NCRR Research Centers in Minority Institutions 69
Neary, J. 289, 355
neck pain, causes of 187–88

653

nerve blocks
 cancer pain and 403, 435
 local, defined 363
nerve conduction test 218
nerve fibers 48
 surgical severing of 46–47, 47
nerve impulses, nociceptors and 4
nerve pain, information sources for 622–23
nerve roots
 slipped discs and 137
 surgical treatment and 164
nerve spasms 218
neural blocks 278
neuralgias, health care costs of 33
neurogenic pain, treatment for 51
neurologists 52
 Bell's palsy and 205
The Neurology Center, Alexandria, Headache Program 80
The Neurology Institute 87, 621
Neuron 347
neurons
 and gate theory of pain 36
 source of pain and 69
neuropathic pain, defined 362
Neuroscience Letters 360
neurosurgeons 52
 back pain treatment by 146
 tic douloureux and 196
neurotransmitters 4–5, 544
 described 75
 and gate theory of pain 36
 serotonin 43, 544
New England Journal of Medicine 171, 340, 344, 346, 355, 472, 606, 613
Newman, Lawrence 101
New York Medical College, Valhalla 211
The New York Times 205n
New York University School of Medicine, New York City 256
New Zealand Medical Journal 354
NIAMS *see* National Institute of Arthritis and Musculoskeletal and Skin Diseases (NIAMS)
Niebyl, J. 312, 353

Nikolarakis, K. 268, 355
NINDS *see* National Institute of Neurological Disorders and Stroke (NINDS)
nitrites, headaches and 116
nitroglycerin patches 513–14
NMDA receptors, described 70
nociception, defined 362
nociceptors 11, 473
 described 4, 34
nocideptin, as pain inhibitor 70
No More Back Pain 170
No More Headache 622
nonpharmacologic management
 integrated approach to pain 454–4555
 of postoperative pain 285–90, 287
nonsteroidal anti-inflammatory drugs (NSAID) 9–10, 368
 acute low back pain and 167
 for arthritis 219
 for arthritis pain 50
 for dental surgery 292
 described 363
 dosages for 372–73, 413, 483–86
 for knee pain 240
 for low back pain 151, 161
 for menstrual cramps 257–58
 for postoperative pain 278
 for repetitive strain injuries 223
 for spinal stenosis 237
 see also *individual drugs*
Noreng, M. F. 269, 299, 341
norepinephrine 5
Normand, S. L. 280, 344
normeperidine 282
Norplant 514
"Norplant: Birth Control at Arm's Reach" 514
Northwestern University Medical School 390
Norwood, S. 56, 66
Nothacker, H. P. 72
Novik, B. 311, 340
NSAID *see* nonsteroidal anti-inflammatory drugs
Nubain 281
Numorphan 416

Index

Nunn, J. F. 331, 358
Nuprin 83, 219, 258, 410
   see also ibuprofen; nonsteroidal anti-inflammatory drugs
nurses
   pain assessments and 56
   role of, in integrated approach to pain management 455–57
Nursing Research 67, 346, 348, 350, 357, 359, 360

O

obesity, hemorrhoids and 245
Obstetrics and Gynecology 353
Occupational Safety and Health Administration (OSHA) 624
occupational therapy, for pain relief 12
occupations
   assembly line workers tension-type headaches and 85
   carpal tunnel syndrome and 222
   cervical spine disorders and 188
   low back pain and 136
   repetitive strain injuries and 218
ocular ischemic syndrome 97, 99
Ocusert 514
Oden, R. 267, 268, 355, 356
Olness, K. 311, 355
Olshwang, D. 290, 345
Olson, R. 311, 350
Olson, R. A. 312, 345
Omnigraphics 219
Oncology Nursing Forum 347
Ontario (Canada) Ministry of Health 184
operant conditioning 454
   see also behavioral therapy
Opheim, K. E. 315, 352
opiates see opium (opiates)
opioids 308, *368–69*
   acute low back pain and 167
   agonist, described 363
   for dental surgery 292
   discovery of 69
   dosages for *374–75*
   myths about 25
   partial agonist, described 363

opioids, continued
   postoperative pain and 263, 280–85
   terminal illnesses and 610
   see also synthetic narcotics (opioids)
opium (opiates)
   as pain reliever 5
   source for *42,* 545
oral contraceptives, menstrual cramps and 259
Oralet 390, 392–93
oral transmucosal fentanyl citrate (OTFC) 16
Orap 197
ordinary headache see tension-type headaches
Oregon Health Sciences University, Portland 70
orphanin FQ 70
Orthopedic Nursing 343
Orthopedic Review 355
orthopedists 52, 146
orthotic devices, for plantar fasciitis 243
Orudis KT see ketoprofen; nonsteroidal anti-inflammatory drugs
Osgood, P. F. 330, 331, 341
OSHA see Occupational Safety and Health Administration (OSHA)
Osler, William 605
osteoarthritis 142, 219
   spinal stenosis and 235
osteopaths, back pain and 143
osteoporosis 142
Osterweil, D. 320, 323, 345
Ostheimer, G. W. 269, 345
OTC see over-the-counter drugs
OTFC see oral transmucosal fentanyl citrate (OTFC)
Ouslander, J. G. 320, 322, 351
over-the-counter drugs
   antacids as 499–506
   for arthritis 219
   for cancer pain 407, 410–15
   guide to *20,* 477–81, *481*
   for headaches 85, 91, 121
   for hemorrhoids 247–48
   for leg cramps 230
   for menstrual cramps 258

over-the-counter drugs, continued
  for migraine headaches 83, 105
  for pain relief 9
  see also prescription medications
overuse strain injury 222–25
oxcarbazepine 197
oxycodone 10, 281, 284, 416
oxygen, as treatment for cluster
  headaches 85
oxymorphone 416
Ozolins, M. 301, 311, 350

P

Paice, Judith, RN, PhD 21
pain
  categories of 449
    acute pain 449, 451
    chronic malignant pain 449, 451
    chronic nonmalignant pain 449,
      451–52
  classifications of 56
  defined 57–58, 362, 397–98, 449, 527
  types and characteristics of 6–7
  types of 398
Pain 66, 67, 341, 342, 343, 344, 346,
  347, 348, 349, 353, 354, 355, 357,
  358, 360, 364, 469
*Pain, Analgesia, and Addiction: The
  Pharmacologic Treatment of Pain*
  468–69
*Pain: Clinical Manual for Nursing
  Practice* 66, 288
*Pain: Clinical manual for nursing
  practice* 381
Pain: Making Life Liveable 619
pain assessments
  distress scales for 377
  forms for 62, 378–79
  instruments used for 62–64
  integrated approach to 449–52
  intensity scales for 63, 376
  terms used in 363
  verbal descriptor scales for 63–64
  visual analog scales for 63–64
pain behavior
  described 7
  see also emotions

Pain Center, Mount Sinai Medical
  Center, Cleveland 24, 25
pain clinics 52–53, 54, 618
*Pain Control After Surgery: Patient's
  Guide* 28
pain distress scales 377
pain intensity scales 376
pain management
  challenge of relieving pain 465–75
  evaluation of 65
  future research into 457–58
  integrated approach to 447–59
  methods for 12–13
  multidisciplinary units for 461–64
  new concepts of 3
  new trends in 27–28
  terminal illnesses and 610
Pain Management 85
Pain Management: Nursing Perspective 67
Pain Management and Evaluation,
  Greencastle, PA 113
Pain Management Center, Beth Israel Hospital, Boston 23
Pain Measurement and Assessment
  66
pain measurement standards 58–59
pain patterns, determination of 188
pain plans, described 9
pain threshold 398
  defined 362
pamabrom 258
Pamelor 113
Pamprin 258
Panerai, A. E. 329, 360
Papazian, Ruth 481
Pape, K. 317, 352
Papillon, J. 331, 343
parathyroid glands, leg cramps and
  231
Parikh, R. K. 283, 339
Parks, L. H. 269, 322, 344
Parrino, J. P. 288, 350
PASSOR *see* Psychiatric Association
  of Spine, Sports and Occupational
  Rehabilitation (PASSOR)
Patel, J. M. 255, 280
patellofemoral pain 239–40

Index

Pathophysiological Phenomena in Nursing: Human Responses to Illness 66
pathways for pain 34, 47, 77, 544–45
  see also nerve fibers; central nervous system
Pathy, M. S. 321, 341
Patient Care 149n
patient-controlled analgesia (PCA) 469–70
  children and 315
  described 363
  integrated approach to 453
  for postoperative pain 278, 284–85, 383
  see also self-controlled medication
patient history *see* medical history
Patt, Richard, MD 21, 23, 25, 29
Paul, S. M. 63, 67, 304, 359
Payne, R. 324, 355
Pazzuconi, F. 329, 360
PCA *see* patient-controlled analgesia (PCA)
Peck, C. 287, 288, 352
Pediatric Clinics of North America 257, 341, 361
Pediatric Nursing 359
Pediatrics 339, 341, 345, 346, 357, 360, 361
Pediatrics: Nursing Update 348
Peebles, R. J. 267, 355
peer review 361
pelvic inflammatory disease 256–57
pelvic pain, medical emergency and 14
penbutolol 510
peptides (amino acids) 69
Perceptual and Motor Skills 349
Percodan 416
percutaneous procedures, trigeminal neuralgia and 198–200
peridural, described 363
perineural, defined 363
Perioperative Nursing Quarterly 359
peripheral nervous system 4, 544
Perkins, G. 301, 342
permanent pain *see* chronic pain
Persson, A. 327, 348

Peterson, L. 311, 358
Pettine, K. A. 300, 354
phantom pain
  described 402–3
  introduced 7
  treatment for 51, 383–84
  see also amputation
pharmacologic management
  integrated approach to pain 452–54
  of postoperative pain 280–85
Phenergan 309
phenylbutazone 484, 486
phenytoin (Dilantin) 10, 196–97
Phillips, G. D. 268, 355
physical examinations
  back pain and 143–44
  for low back pain 153, 156–64
  low back problems and 176
  prior to vigorous exercise 5–6
physical therapy
  Bell's palsy and 207
  for chronic pain relief 23–24
  for fibromyalgia 210
  headaches and 120
  for pain relief 12, 13
  for repetitive strain injuries 224
  for spinal stenosis 237
physicians
  headaches and 87
  pain management and 4
  suicide assistance and 609, 610, 612–13
  see also doctors
Physicians' Desk Reference 488
Physiotherapy Practice 360
Pickett, C. 288, 355
pilot review 361–62
pimozide 197
pindolol 510
Pini, A. 268, 349
Pioneer on Death in America 611, 612
Pippenger, C. E. 328, 343
Pirayavaraporn, S. 312, 359
piroxicam 486
plantar fasciitis 241–44
  causes of 241–43
  treatment for 243
Ponstel 258

Portenoy, R. K. 324, 341, 348, 355
Porter, J. 281, 323, 355
post-anesthesia care unit (PACU) 279
postoperative pain management 263–381
  assessment and reassessment 270–78
  concurrent medical conditions 326–29
  elderly 320–23
  executive summary 264–66
  infants, children, and adolescents 300–320
  introduced 266–70
  outpatient 331–34
  prevention and control 278–91
  shock, trauma, and burns 329–31
  site-specific control 291–300
  substance abuse 323–26
posture 85
Powell, S. 289, 352
prednisone 424
prescription drugs
  brand names
    endorsement disclaimers of 410
prescription medications
  for cancer pain 407, 415–24
  for cluster headaches 85
  for headaches 121–22
  for leg cramps 230
  for low back pain 162
  for migraine headaches 83
  migraine headaches and 105
  narcotics as 10
  for sciatic pain 145
  see also narcotics; over-the-counter drugs
Preshaw, R. 296, 353
preventive measures
  for backaches 146–47
  for headaches 125–27
  for hemorrhoids 249
  for low back problems 181
  for neck problems 190
Price, D. D. 321, 348
Principles of Analgesic Use in the Treatment of Acute Pain and Cancer Pain 619

Proceedings of First International Symposium on Pediatric Pain 350
Proceedings of Fourth World Conference on Pain 353
Proceedings of Sixth World Congress on Pain 340
Progestasert 515
progesterone 253, 515
progressive muscle relaxation 529
Project on Death in America 609, 611
promethazine 309
propoxyphene 43
  see also Darvon
propranolol 508, 510
propranolol hydrochloride (Inderal) 83, 87
prostaglandins 465–66, 484
  arthritis and 219, 484
  aspirin and 42, 489–90, 544
  menstrual pain and 253, 2570258
  released by injured tissues 77
proteins
  enkephalins
    described 37
  speed-up of pain messages and 5
Prozac see fluoxetine (Prozac)
Pruitt, S. 311, 350
Przewlocki, R. 268, 355
Psychiatric Association of Spine, Sports and Occupational Rehabilitation (PASSOR) 170, 620
psychogenic headache see tension-type headaches
psychogenic pain treatment 51–52
psychological cravings see addictions
psychological treatments for pain 44–46
psychosocial factors
  low back pain and 161
  pain assessment and 450
Psychosomatics 343
psychotherapy, meaning of pain and 44
Public Health Service (PHS) 218, 264
  studies 496
Purcell-Jones, G. 301, 317, 355
Pursell, C. H. 287, 288, 349
Pybus, D. A. 295, 298, 356
pyrilamin maleate 258

Index

Q

quadriceps, knee pain and 239–40
quasi-experimental study, described 362
Quay, N. B. 313, 356
Questions and Answers About Manipulation 185
Quinamm 230
quinine 230

R

radiculopathy 156, 188
  acute low back pain and 168
  corticosteroids and 162
Radnay, P. 281, 354
RAND Corporation 184
Rane, A. 327, 348
Rarick, Lisa, MD 257, 258
Rawal, N. 283, 356
Reading, A. E. 271, 356
Ready, L. B. 268, 356
Reay, B. A. 298, 356
recurrent pain
  back problems and 182
  trigeminal neuralgia and 201–3
referred pain 142–43
reflexes
  low back pain diagnosis and 156
  pain signals and 76
regional anesthesia 387
Reidenberg, M. M. 282, 350, 359
Reinscheid, R. K. 72
relaxation therapy 454, 473
  for cancer pain 425–28, 438–40
  for chronic pain 527–40
  described 362
  exercises 380–81
  for fibromyalgia 210
  for insomnia 527–40
  for jaws 288
  for pain relief 12, 16, 44–45
  for postoperative pain 278, 287–88
  tension-type headaches and 91, 92
Relief from Migraine 622
Rem, J. 267, 351

repetitive strain injuries (RSI) 217–22
  information sources for 623–24
Report of the Working Party on Pain After Surgery 356
Research in Nursing and Health 66, 67, 350, 359
Restoril 112
Reviews of Infectious Diseases 344
Reye, Douglas, MD 493, 494, 495
Reye syndrome 493–98, 548
Reynolds, G. J. 301, 342
Rezvani, A. 304, 347
Rheumatic Diseases Clinics of North America 356
rheumatoid arthritis 50, 219
  see also arthritis pain
Rice, V. 287, 350
Rideout, E. 320, 343
Riopan 505
Ripamonti, C. 329, 360
Ritchie, J. 311, 345
Rivotril 197
Robertson, E. 288, 354
Robert Wood Johnson Foundation 606, 611
Rodary, C. 304, 347
Rodman, J. 317, 318, 352
Rogers, A. G. 282, 322, 350, 351
Rolaids 505
Rooke, G. A. 268, 356
Rooney, S. M. 289, 356
Rosales, J. K. 313, 347
Rosen, H. 280, 356
Ross, D. M. 311, 356
Roth, S. H. 322, 356
Rothman, David 605
Rotman, H. 280, 349
Routh, D. 307, 357
Rowe, Peter C., MD 496
Rowlingson, J. C. 290, 359
Roy, W. L. 313, 317, 343
Royal Alexandra Hospital for Children, New South Wales, Australia 493
Royal College of Surgeons of England 268, 356
rubber band ligation 248

Rufen 258
Ruit, P. 355
Rush-Presbyterian-St. Luke's Medical Center, Chicago 21, 23
Russell, G. A. 301, 342
Russell, R. I. 280, 343
Russo, D. 315, 342
Ryan, E. 311, 356

S

Saal, S. 282, 359
Sabanathan, S. 280, 295, 356–57
Sachar, E. J. 267, 282, 353
sacroiliac joint 137, 142
sacrum, described 137
Sadar, E. 289, 343
saddle anesthesia 153
Safety and Health Assessment and Research for Prevention 624
safety issues
  anesthesia and 385–87
  lifting and carrying *181*
Sahlstedt, B. 300, 354
Saksena, R. 298, 343
Saldeen, T. 300, 354
salsalate 280
Samuels, Todd, L., MD 137
Sanborn, Timothy, MD 232–33
Sanders, A. J. 214
Sandler, A. N. 295, 358
Saniabadi, A. R. 280, 343
Sankaran, Neeraja 70
Sansert 83, 85, 86
Saper, Joel, MD 96
Savedra, M. 301, 360
Savedra, M. C. 63, 67, 303, 304, 305, 357, 359
Sawa, J. 327, 348
Schechter, N. L. 301, 302, 306, 307, 309, 311, 357, 361
Schenker, J. G. 290, 345
Schillinger, J. 304, 353
Schmidt, C. D. 267, 352
Schmitt, F. 271, 286, 357
Schneidman, D. S. 267, 355
Schnurrer, J. A. 301, 357
Schofield, N. 313, 357

Schonberger, Lawrence B. MD 496, 498
Schwartzman, R. J. 214
sciatica 137, 173, *236*
  surgical treatment for 164
sciatic pain 145
Science 72
Science and Immortality 605
Scientific American 605n
scientific review 362
sclerotherapy 248
scoliosis 143
scopalamine 513
Scott, J. 275, 357
Scott, N. B. 296, 357
Scott, Suzanne 131n
Scottish Medical Journal 343
Scripps Clinic and Research Foundation, La Jolla 197
Sear, J. W. 327, 357
Seattle Veterans Affairs Medical Center 169
sedatives 112, 124–25
Segal, Marian 516
Selby, D. 287, 352
self-controlled medication
  as delivery system 15
  results of 28
  see also patient-controlled analgesia (PCA)
self-reports, pain assessments and 62
self-treatment, for headaches 127
Semple, A. J. 298, 356
sensory innervation 97
sensory overload, pain relief and 11
serotonin 43, 544
  decrease of pain with 5
  migraine headaches and 75, 82
  pain awareness and 77
Sethna, N. F. 315, 342
sexuality issues 576–78, 597–98
Shankar, B. S. 330, 358
Shaw, A. 301, 346
Shaw, E. 307, 357
Sheftell, Fred 101
Sheltering Arms Day Rehabilitation Program 219
Shepard, K. V. 328, 343

Index

Sherzer, L. 307, 357
shingles 7, 11, 51, 544
  see also herpes simplex
Shnider, S. M. 304, 341
shock, pain management and 329–31
shoes, plantar fasciitis and 242
Short, L. M. 269, 322, 344
shoulder pain 213
Shulman, M. 295, 358
sick headaches 79
side effects
  of anticonvulsant medications 10
  of antidepressants 10
  of aspirin 412
  of beta blockers 509
  of chemotherapy 50
  of headache medications *123*
  of narcotics 10, 420–22
  of nonsteroidal anti-inflammatory drugs 485
  of nonsteroidal anti-inflammatory drugs (NSAID) 280
  of opioids 544
  of over-the-counter drugs 125
  of preventive medications *126*
  of synthetic analgesics 11
Siegel, L. 311, 358
Siegel, S. E. 305, 351
Silberstein, Marsha, MD 85
Silberstein, Stephen, MD 85
Silverberg, Stanley, MD 228, 230, 231
Simethicone 505
Simon, B. 290, 359
Sinequan 424
Singer, G. 287, 288, 352
Sippell, W. G. 269, 301, 340
sitz baths 247, 249
Sjogren, P. 294, 358
Sjostrand, U. H. 283, 356
Skacel, P. O. 331, 358
Skelton, J. 290, 359
skin 4
  nerve fibers in 33–34, *35*
  see also nociceptors
skin patches 15, 390, 513–14
skin stimulation, for cancer pain 431–34
Slattery, J. T. 317, 352

Slavin, R. E. 365, 367
Slawson, K. B. 280, 344
sleep
  headaches and 118
  low back problems and 180
  relationship with headaches 111–13
  see also insomnia
sleep diaries 112–13
slipped discs
  low back pain and 136–37
  surgical treatment for 145
  see also spinal discs; vertebrae
Smith, C. M. 289, 358
Smith, Frederick, MD 230, 233
Smith, Lee E., MD 245, 246, 247, 248–49
Smith, M. J. 289, 358
snack food, headaches and 116
Snow, B. R. 288, 358
social isolation 574–75, 596–97
Socio-Economic Factbook for Surgery, 1991-1992 355
Soderstrom, C. A. 330, 358
sodium valproate 197
Soldin, S. 317, 352
Soloman, R. 289, 358
Solomon, Seymour, MD 94, 101
Soros, George 609
Souron, R. 316, 354
sour stomach 503
SPA *see* stimulation-produced analgesia (SPA)
specialists
  low back pain treatment and 168–69
  in pain management 8, 404, 462–63
Spellman, M. 317, 348
Spence, A. A. 283, 339
spinal canal *236*
  narrowing of 235–36
spinal cord *140*
  cancer pain treatment and 423
  described 78
  endorphin production and 5
  low back problems and 175
  lower back pain and 141
  pain pathways of
    early treatment and 9

spinal cord, continued
  pain signals in 4
  reflex inhibition of 70
  surgical severing of nerve fibers 47, 48
  see also brain; central nervous system
spinal cord stimulation (SCS) 517–21, 518, 519
  described 519–20, 520
spinal discs 141
spinal fusion 145, 169
  cervical spine disorders and 189
spinal infusion, for pain relief medications 15
spinal manipulation
  for low back problems 177–78
  see also chiropractic manipulation; manipulative therapy
spinal stenosis 235–38
  causes of 235–36
  diagnosis of 157
  surgical treatment for 145
  treatment for 146, 237–38
spine 138
  lower back pain and 137–41
  neck pain and disorders of 187–90
Spine 352
splints
  for plantar fasciitis 243
  for repetitive strain injuries 223
spondylolisthesis 236
spondylolysis 158
spondylosis 188
sports injuries
  back pain and 158–59
  knee pain and 239
spreading depression, described 94
Sriwatanakul, K. 267, 275, 358, 359
St. Joseph Mercy - Oakland *SmartHealth* 239n
Stadol 281
standards of care, for pain assessments 56–57
Stark, Stuart, MD 80, 81, 82, 85
Stehlin, Dori 249, 475, 486
Stein, J. 289, 360
Stephenson, Marilyn, RD 246

steroids, long-term use of 50
Stevens, B. 303, 359
Stewart, Walter 101
Stimmel, Barry, MD 468–69
stimulation-produced analgesia (SPA) 39
stool softeners 246–48, 249
straight-leg raising test 151, 156
stress 575–76
  effect on pain of 12
  family response to pain and 594–95
  low back problems and 180
  migraine headaches and 83
  placebo effect and 41
  relaxation therapy and 528
  reports of little pain and 77
  tension-type headaches and 80, 85, 89
stress headache see tension-type headaches
stretch exercises
  for plantar fasciitis 243–44
  for repetitive strain injuries 224
Study to Understand Prognoses and Preferences for Outcomes and Risks of Treatments (SUPPORT) 606, 607
substance abuse, pain management and 323–26, 580–83
substance P
  migraine headaches and 82
  released by injured tissues 77
suicide headache see cluster headaches
sulindac 486
Sullivan, J. J. 315, 316, 348
sumatriptan
  serotonin and 75
sumatriptan succinate (Imitrex) 11, 87
Sumerian Healers 5
Sumner, E. 301, 317, 355
super sleep, described 112
SUPPORT see Study to Understand Prognoses and Preferences for Outcomes and Risks of Treatments (SUPPORT)
suppositories, pain medication and 416

Index

Surgeon General 496, 498
surgery
  abdominal and perineal surgery
    postoperative pain management and 297–98
  acute pain from 467
  anesthesia and 385–87
  cancer pain and 398
  cardiac surgery
    pain management and 296–97
  chest and chest wall surgery
    postoperative pain management and 294–97
  chronic pain and 7, 554–55
  control of acute pain after 9, 263–381
  head and neck surgery
    postoperative pain management and 291–94
  for leg cramps 232
  musculoskeletal surgery
    postoperative pain management and 298–300
  soft tissue surgery
    postoperative pain management and 300
  thoracic surgery
    pain management and 294–96
  as treatment for pain 12, 46–49
Surgery 344, 358
Surgery, Gynecology and Obstetrics 214, 355
surgical implants, for pain relief medications 15
surgical pain
  Demerol and 28
  information sources for 626–27
  treatment for 21–22
  see also postoperative pain
surgical treatment
  for back pain 144–45, 150
  for Bell's palsy 207
  for cervical spine disorders 189
  for hemorrhoids 248
  for herniated disks 169
  for low back pain 164
  for low back problems 181
  for plantar fasciitis 243

surgical treatment, continued
  for repetitive strain injuries 224
  for spinal stenosis 238
  tic douloureux and 197
Svensson, J. O. 327, 348
Swezey, Annette M. 170
Swezey, Robert L., MD 170
Swinford, P. 288, 359
Sydow, F. W. 267, 359
symptoms
  of Bell's palsy 207
  cancer pain and 399–400
  of cervical spine disorders 188
  of cluster headaches 80, 84
  discussing with health care providers 175–76
  eye pain as 98
  headaches as 95
  of migraine headaches 81, 93–94, 105
synthetic analgesics 11
synthetic morphine 16
synthetic narcotics (opioids) 10
  see also narcotics
Syrjala, K. L. 274, 343, 359
Szeto, H. 282, 359
Szyfelbein, S. K. 330, 331, 341

T

tactile strategies, described 363
Tagariello, V. 295, 298, 342
tailbone (coccyx) 137
Tambuscio, B. 290, 345
"Taming Menstrual Cramps" 466
Tampa General Hospital Rehabilitation Center 549, 549n
Taylor, A. G. 290, 359
team approach to pain management 8, 447–59, 543
Tegretol 194, 196, 202, 424
  see also carbamazepine
temporary pain 7
  see also acute pain
temporomandibular joint 85, 90
tendinitis 223, 483
tennis elbow 222
TENS *see* transcutaneous electrical nerve stimulation (TENS)

tension-type headaches 85, 89–92
  described 80
  types of 91
terminal illnesses 5, 9, 10, 605–13
Teske, K. 61, 67
Tesler, M. 305, 357
Tesler, M. D. 63, 67, 303, 304, 357, 359
tests
  for carpal tunnel syndrome 218
  for chronic pain 555–56
  evaluation of pain and 8
  for low back pain 151
  for low back problems 180–81
  for spinal stenosis 237
  see also evaluations
thalamus 544, 546–47
  described 78
  pain signals in 4
Theodor, Emanuel 231
thermal angioplasy 232–33
thermocoagulation treatment, for neurogenic pain 51
thermography, as treatment for psychogenic pain 52
thoracic outlet syndrome 213–15
Thorazine 309
thromboembolism 299
Thurston, N. 296, 353
tic douloureux (trigeminal neuralgia) 43, 194–203
  described 33
  treatment for 51
timolol 507, 510
tired eyes (asthenopia) 98
Titralac 505
Tjellden, N. U. 269, 299, 341
TN see *tic douloureax;* trigeminal neuralgia (TN)
TN Alert 203
Todd, Dennis, PhD 549
Tofranil 424
  see also imipramine (Tofranil)
Toledo-Pereyra, L. H. 280, 285, 359
Toll, L. 72
tolmetin 486
Tompkins, J. M. 303, 341
Tomsak, Robert L., MD, PhD 99

Topics in Clinical Nursing 360
Torda, T. A. 295, 298, 356
Tornquist, E. M. 344, 346, 348, 356
Tousignant, G. 313, 350
traction, low back pain problems and 178
tramadol (Ultram) 11
transcendental meditation 529
  see also meditation therapy
transcutaneous electrical nerve stimulation (TENS) 454–55, 547
  for arthritis pain 51
  for cancer pain 435
  defined 363
  low back pain problems and 178
  for pain relief 11, 23, 38–39, 472–73
  for postoperative pain 279, 289–90
trauma
  chronic pain and 7
  low back pain and 153
  pain management and 329–31
trazodone (Desyrel) 10
Tree-Trakarn, T. 312, 359
Trends in Neurosciences 346
Trental 232
Trifillis, A. L. 330, 358
trigeminal nerve
  disorder of 194
  migraine headaches and 83
  parts of 98
  surgery and 198
Trigeminal Neuralgia Association 194n, 195n, 198n, 201n, 623
  Medical Advisory Board 197, 201
trigeminal neuralgia (TN) 194–203
  treatment for 195–97, 198
  see also *tic douloureux*
trigeminal neurons, nociceptin and 70
trigger finger 218, 223
triggers
  for headaches 116, 128
  for migraine headaches 83
Trileptal 197
Trilisate 416
Triplett, J. L. 311, 359
Troletti, G. 290, 345
Tums 505

664

Index

Tylenol 83, 257, 258, 410, 465
 see also acetaminophen
Tyler, D. 346, 350
Tyler, D. C. 315, 349, 352

U

U. S. Preventive Services Task Force 491–92
U. S. Supreme Court 606, 610
Ultram 11
ultrasound
 evaluation of pain and 8
 low back pain problems and 178
 for plantar fasciitis 243
Understanding Acute Low Back Problems 182, 185
United Hospital Fund 609
University of Alabama, Birmingham 211
University of California, Los Angeles Pain Control Unit 429
University of California, San Diego 201
University of California, San Francisco 40, 546
 School of Nursing 357
University of Colorado 113
University of Colorado, Denver 365
University of Florida College of Medicine 19
University of Maryland, Baltimore 365
University of Michigan Medical Center, Ann Arbor 210
University of Michigan Medical School, Ann Arbor 516
University of North Carolina, Greensboro, School of Nursing 67
University of Pittsburgh 198, 200
University of Washington, Seattle 52
University of Washington School of Pharmacy, Seattle 512
University of Washington Schools of Medicine and Public Health 169
University of Wisconsin, Madison Pain Research Group 22
University of Wisconsin Pain and Policy Studies Group 610

Unruh, A. M. 303, 354
upset stomach 503
Utah Workers' Compensation Board 184
uveitis (intraocular inflammation) 97, 99

V

Valium 112, 230
Van Aernam, B. 270, 359
Vandam, L. D. 331, 344
VanderArk, G. 289, 359
Vanderbilt University, Nashville, TN 211
Vanderveen, John, PhD 219
Vane, John, PhD 489
van Egmond, J. 295, 348
varicose veins
 leg cramps and 231
Ventafridda, V 329, 360
verbal descriptor scales (VDS) 63–64
Versed 392
vertebrae *139*
 low back problems and 173
 lower back pain and 139–41
veterans
 pain relief for 6
videotapes
 No More Back Pain 170
Viernstein, M. 289, 358
Vincenti, E. 290, 345
Vinci, R. 307, 341
Visintainer, M. 313, 360
Visiting Nurses Association 402
Vistaril 424
visual analog scales (VAS) 63–64
visualization exercises
 as pain relief method 28
 for postoperative pain 278
visualization therapy
 for cancer pain 429–30
 for postoperative pain 288
vitamin supplements
 potassium 229
volunteers
 pain treatment and 53–54
 terminal illnesses and 612

Von Korff, M. 171
Voshall, B. 270, 286, 360

W

Wall, P. D. 269, 360
Wall, Patrick D. 546
Wallenstein, S. L. 322, 351
Wang, X. -M. 71
Wang, Y. S. 171
Ward, J. A. 303, 304, 305, 357, 359
Warfield, C. 289, 360
Warfield, Carol, MD 23
Waring, C. 307, 341
Warren Grant Magnuson Clinical Center 449
Wasylak, T. J. 296
Watt-Watson, J. H. 56, 57, 67
Wattwil, M. 267, 360
Way, E. L. 317, 360
Way, W. L. 317, 360
Wayslak, T. J. 269, 283, 360
Webster, J. A. 280, 356
Weck, Egon 548
Wedel, D. J. 300, 354
Weekes, D. 301, 360
Weeks, J. L. 300, 354
Wegner, C. 305, 357
Weigel, George 203
Weinstock, Cheryl Platzman 221
Weintraub, M. 267, 359
Weintraub, Michael, MD 478, 479, 481
Weis, O. F. 267, 275, 358, 359
Weissman, D. E. 326, 360
Welch, C. E. 270, 286, 344
Wells, N. 63, 67, 287, 288, 354, 360
West, B. A. 290, 359
West, C. M. 61, 66
Western Journal of Nursing Research 66
Wetzel, R. 312, 353
Wewers, M. E. 63, 67
whirlpool treatment
  pain relief and 12
White, J. 313, 357
WHO *see* World Health Organization (WHO)

Wiese, R. A. 344, 346, 348, 356
Wigraine 83, 86
Wigram, J. R. 290, 360
Wild, L. M. 268, 356
Wilkie, D. J. 304, 359
Wilkie, D. S. 63, 67
Williams, J. S. 255, 280
Williams, Rebecca D. 394
Willis, Hayes 221
Wolfer, J. 313, 360
Wolff, Harold 90
Wolskee, P. J. 275, 347
Wood, M. M. 282, 323, 360
Wood, R. 171
Woolf, C. J. 269, 360
Woolridge, P. J. 271, 286, 357
work issues
  low back problems and 179
World Health Organization (WHO) 610
Wright, Curtis, MD 392, 393, 468, 469, 470
Wright, D. 296, 353
Wyche, M. Q., Jr. 267, 353

X

Xanax 112, 424
X-rays
  for back pain 144
  cervical spine disorders and 188
  evaluation of pain and 8
  low back pain and 160
  low back problems and 180
  myelogram, described 49

Y

Yadav, S. N. 290, 343
Yang, G. W. 289, 352
Yaster, M. 312, 313, 353, 360
Yee, J. D. 315, 342
yoga 12, 529
You Don't Have to Suffer 29, 626
Young, P. S. 295, 358

Index

Z

Zamula, Evelyn 147, 498
Zeltzer, L. 305, 352
Zeltzer, L. K. 306, 309, 311, 361
Zhang, K. M. 71
Ziebarth, D. 314, 347
Zostrix 11
   see also capsaicin

Environmentally Induced Disorders Sourcebook

Basic Information about Diseases and Syndromes Linked to Exposure to Pollutants and Other Substances in Outdoor and Indoor Environments Such As Lead, Asbestos, Formaldehyde, Mercury, Emissions, Noise, and More

Edited by Allan R. Cook. 620 pages. 1997. 0-7808-0083-4. $75.

Fitness & Exercise Sourcebook

Basic Information on Fitness and Exercise, Including Fitness Activities for Specific Age Groups, Exercise for People with Specific Medical Conditions, How to Begin a Fitness Program in Running, Walking, Swimming, Cycling, and Other Athletic Activities, and Recent Research in Fitness and Exercise

Edited by Dan R. Harris. 663 pages. 1996. 0-7808-0186-5. $75.

Food & Animal Borne Diseases Sourcebook

Basic Information about Diseases That Can Be Spread to Humans through the Ingestion of Contaminated Food or Water or by Contact with Infected Animals and Insects, Such As Botulism, E. Coli, Hepatitis A, Trichinosis, Lyme Disease, and Rabies, along with Information Regarding Prevention and Treatment Methods, and a Special Section for International Travelers Describing Diseases Such as Cholera, Malaria, Travelers' Diarrhea, and Yellow Fever, and Offering Recommendations for Avoiding Illness

Edited by Karen Bellenir and Peter D. Dresser. 535 pages. 1995. 0-7808-0033-8. $75.

"A comprehensive collection of authoritative information." — *Emergency Medical Services, Oct '95*

"Targeting general readers and providing them with a single, comprehensive source of information on selected topics, this book continues, with the excellent caliber of its predecessors, to catalog topical information on health matters of general interest. Readable and thorough, this valuable resource is highly recommended for all libraries." — *Academic Library Book Review, Summer '96*

Gastrointestinal Diseases & Disorders Sourcebook

Basic Information about Gastroesophageal Reflux Disease (Heartburn), Ulcers, Diverticulosis, Irritable Bowel Syndrome, Crohn's Disease, Ulcerative Colitis, Diarrhea, Constipation, Lactose Intolerance, Hemorrhoids, Hepatitis, Cirrhosis and Other Digestive Problems, Featuring Statistics, Descriptions of Symptoms, and Current Treatment Methods of Interest for Persons Living with Upper and Lower Gastrointestinal Maladies

Edited by Linda M. Ross. 413 pages. 1996. 0-7808-0078-8. $75.

"... very readable form. The successful editorial work that brought this material together into a useful and understandable reference makes accessible to all readers information that can help them more effectively understand and obtain help for digestive tract problems." — *Choice, Feb '97*

Genetic Disorders Sourcebook

Basic Information about Heritable Diseases and Disorders Such As Down Syndrome, PKU, Hemophilia, Von Willebrand Disease, Gaucher Disease, Tay-Sachs Disease, and Sickle-Cell Disease, along with Information about Genetic Screening, Gene Therapy, Home Care, and Including Source Listings for Further Help and Information on More Than 300 Disorders

Edited by Karen Bellenir. 642 pages. 1996. 0-7808-0034-6. $75.

"... geared toward the lay public. It would be well placed in all public libraries and in those hospital and medical libraries in which access to genetic references is limited." — *Doody's Health Sciences Book Review, Oct '96*

"Provides essential medical information to both the general public and those diagnosed with a serious or fatal genetic disease or disorder." — *Choice, Jan '97*

Head Trauma Sourcebook

Basic Information for the Layperson about Open-Head and Closed-Head Injuries, Treatment Advances, Recovery, and Rehabilitation, along with Reports on Current Research Initiatives

Edited by Karen Bellenir. 414 pages. 1997. 0-7808-0208-X. $75.

Health Insurance Sourcebook

Basic Information about Managed Care Organizations, Traditional Fee-for-Service Insurance, Insurance Portability and Pre-Existing Conditions Clauses, Medicare, Medicaid, Social Security, and Military Health Care, along with Information about Insurance Fraud

Edited by Wendy Wilcox. 530 pages. 1997. 0-7808-0222-5. $75.

Continues next page

REFERENCE

DO NOT REMOVE FROM LIBRARY

Immune System Disorders Sourcebook

Basic Information about Lupus, Multiple Sclerosis, Guillain-Barré Syndrome, Chronic Granulomatous Disease, and More, along with Statistical and Demographic Data and Reports on Current Research Initiatives

Edited by Allan P. ...
0209-8. $75.

"The great strengths of the book are its readability and its inclusion of places to find more information. Especially recommended." — *RQ, Winter '96*

"Recommended for public and academic libraries." — *Reference Book Review, '96*

"... useful for public and academic libraries and consumer health collections."
— *Medical Reference Services Quarterly, Spring '97*

Kidney & ... &Disorders ...

*Basic Information ...
Incontinence, ...
Disease, Dialysis ...
and Demographic ...
Research Initiatives*

Edited by Linda ...
0079-6. $75.

..., Cataracts, Macular ... efractive Disorders, ... and Demographic ... earch Initiatives

... ages. 1996. 0-7808-

Learning D...

*Basic Information ...
Dyslexia, Hyper...
Disorder, along ...
Data and Report...*

Edited by Linda ...
0210-1. $75.

...ok

...es and Conditions
...g Cavities, Gum
...ers, Fever Blisters,
... Breath, Temporo-
...Craniofacial Syn-
...Data on the Oral
..., Emergency First
... Procedures and

...ages. 1997. 0-7808-

Men's Health Sourcebook

*Basic Information ...
Men, Including ...
Other Sexual D...
Snoring, Sleep A...*

Edited by Allan ...
0212-8. $75.

...ns of Acute and
...es, Back Pain,
...in, and Cancer
...tions Such As
...Transcutaneous
...Forms of Pain
...ging, Behavior
...ues

... 1997. 0-7808-

Mental Health Disorders ...

*Basic Information ...
Bipolar Disorde...
pulsive Disorde...
orders, Paranoia ...
Eating Disorders ...
Information abou...*

Edited by Karen ...
0040-0. $75.

"... provides inf... ...range of mental disorders, presented in nontechnical language."
— *Exceptional Child Education Resources, Spring '96*

"The text is well organized and adequately written for its target audience." — *Choice, Jun '96*

...cebook

...regnancy, Fetal
...and Delivery,
...ncy in Mothers
...of Pregnancy,
...tion and Exer-
...omfort, Multi-
ple Births, Cesarean Sections, Medical Testing of Newborns, Breastfeeding, Gestational Diabetes, and Ectopic Pregnancy

Edited by Heather Aldred. 752 pages. 1997. 0-7808-0216-0. $75.

Ref. $75.00
RB
127   Paine Sourcebook.
P346

24694

REFERENCE

DO NOT REMOVE FROM LIBRARY

REFERENCE

DO NOT REMOVE FROM LIBRARY

SOUTH COLLEGE
709 Mall Blvd.
Savannah, GA 31406